Clinical Guide to
Nutrition Care in Kidney Disease

THIRD EDITION

Renal Dietitians Dietetic Practice Group
National Kidney Foundation Council on Renal Nutrition
Editors: Janelle E. Gonyea, RDN, LD, FNKF
    Stacey C. Phillips, MS, RD

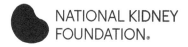
NATIONAL KIDNEY FOUNDATION.

eat right. Academy of Nutrition and Dietetics

eat right. Academy of Nutrition and Dietetics

Academy of Nutrition and Dietetics
120 S. Riverside Plaza, Suite 2190
Chicago, IL 60606

Clinical Guide to Nutrition Care in Kidney Disease, Third Edition

ISBN 978-0-88091-201-3 (print)
ISBN 978-0-88091-073-6 (eBook)

Catalog Number 344423 (print)
Catalog Number 344423e (eBook)

10   9   8   7   6   5   4   3   2   1

For more information on the Academy of Nutrition and Dietetics, visit www.eatright.org.

Library of Congress Cataloging-in-Publication Data
Names: Phillips, Stacey, editor. | National Kidney Foundation. Council on
  Renal Nutrition, editor.
Title: Clinical guide to nutrition care in kidney disease / Renal Practice
  Group, National Kidney Foundation Council on Renal Nutrition ; editors,
  Stacey Phillips, MS, RD, and Janelle Gonyea, RDN, LD.
Description: Third edition. | Chicago, IL : Academy of Nutrition and
  Dietetics, [2022] | Includes bibliographical references and index.
Identifiers: LCCN 2022020485 (print) | LCCN 2022020486 (ebook) | ISBN
  9780880910736 (paperback) | ISBN 9780880912013 (ebook)
Subjects: LCSH: Kidneys--Diseases--Nutritional aspects. |
  Kidneys--Diseases--Diet therapy.
Classification: LCC RC903 .C5585 2022 (print) | LCC RC903 (ebook) | DDC
  616.6/10654--dc23/eng/20220713
LC record available at https://lccn.loc.gov/2022020485
LC ebook record available at https://lccn.loc.gov/2022020486

Contents

Frequently Used Terms and Abbreviations

AACE	American Association of Clinical Endocrinologists	**DKD**	diabetic kidney disease
AADE	American Association of Diabetes Educators	**DM**	diabetes mellitus
ACC	American College of Cardiology	**DN**	diabetic neuropathy
ACE	angiotensin-converting enzyme	**DPI**	dietary protein intake
ADA	American Diabetes Association	**DR**	diabetic retinopathy
ADCES	Association of Diabetes Care & Education Specialists	**DRI**	Dietary Reference Intake
AF	atrial fibrillation	**DXA**	dual-energy x-ray absorptiometry
AGE	advanced glycation end	**EASD**	European Association for the Study of Diabetes
AHA	American Heart Association	**EH**	enteric hyperoxaluria
AKI	acute kidney injury	**EN**	enteral nutrition
AMDR	acceptable macronutrient distribution ranges	**ESA**	erythropoietin-stimulating agents
AN	autonomic neuropathy	**ESKD**	end-stage kidney disease
APD	automated peritoneal dialysis	**FDA**	US Food and Drug Administration
ARB	angiotensin II receptor blockers	**FSGS**	focal segmental glomerulosclerosis
ASPEN	American Society for Parenteral and Enteral Nutrition	**GA**	glycated albumin
AUA	American Urological Association	**GAN**	gastrointestinal autonomic neuropathy
BG	blood glucose	**GDM**	gestational diabetes mellitus
BIA	bioelectrical impedance analysis	**GDP**	glucose degradation products
BMD	bone mineral density	**GFR**	glomerular filtration rate
BMI	body mass index	**GRV**	gastric residual volume
BP	blood pressure	**GV**	glycemic variability
BUN	blood urea nitrogen	**HCFC**	high concentrated fructose corn
CAC	coronary artery calcification	**HDL**	high-density lipoprotein
CAD	coronary artery disease	**HF**	heart failure
CAN	cardiovascular autonomic neuropathy	**HHD**	home hemodialysis
CAPD	continuous ambulatory peritoneal dialysis	**IBD**	inflammatory bowel disease
CaSR	calcium-sensing receptors	**IBW**	ideal body weight
CCPD	continuous cyclic peritoneal dialysis	**ICHD**	in-center hemodialysis
CGM	continuous glucose monitoring	**ICU**	intensive care unit
CHD	coronary heart disease	**IDWG**	intradialytic weight gain
CHF	congestive heart failure	**IFG**	impaired fasting glucose
CKD	chronic kidney disease	**IH**	idiopathic hypercalcuria
CRP	C-reactive protein	**ILE**	intravenous lipid emulsion
CRRT	continuous renal replacement therapy	**INR**	international normalized ratio
CT	computed tomography	**IR**	insulin resistance
CVD	cardiovascular disease	**IRS**	insulin resistance syndrome
DASH	Dietary Approaches to Stop Hypertension	**ISRNM**	International Society of Renal Nutrition and Metabolism
		KDIGO	Kidney Disease Improving Global Outcomes

KDOQI	Kidney Disease Outcomes Quality Initiative
KRT	kidney replacement therapy
LDL	low-density lipoprotein
LEA	lower-extremity amputation
LVH	left ventricular hypertrophy
MBD	mineral bone disease
MD	maintenance dialysis
MI	myocardial infarction
MNT	medical nutrition therapy
MS	metabolic syndrome
MUAC	mid-upper arm circumference
NFPE	nutrition focused physical exam
NHANES	National Health and Nutrition Examination Survey
NIPD	nocturnal intermittent peritoneal dialysis
NODAT	new-onset diabetes after transplantation
NPH	neutral protamine Hagedorn
OGTT	oral glucose tolerance test
ONS	oral nutrition supplements
PA	physical activity
PAD	peripheral artery disease
PAL	physical activity level
PCR	protein catabolic rate
PD	peritoneal dialysis
PEG	percutaneous endoscopic gastrostomy
PET	peritoneal equilibration test
PH	primary hyperoxaluria
PN	parenteral nutrition
PNA	protein equivalent of nitrogen appearance
PPN	peripheral parenteral nutrition
PRAL	potential renal acid load

PTH	parathyroid hormone
PVD	peripheral vascular disease
RBC	red blood cell
RDN	registered dietitian nutritionist
RFS	refeeding syndrome
RKF	residual kidney function
RR	risk ratio
RTA	renal tubular acidosis
SCCM	Society of Critical Care Medicine
SD	standard deviation
SDI	standard dietary intake
SDS	standard deviation scores
SGA	subjective global assessment
SIADH	syndrome of inappropriate antidiuretic hormone
SMBG	self-monitoring of blood glucose
SO	soybean oil
SPS	sodium polystyrene sulfonate
TLC	therapeutic lifestyle change
TNA	total nitrogen appearance
TPD	tidal peritoneal dialysis
TW	target weight
UL	Tolerable Upper Intake Level
USRDS	United States Renal Data System
UTI	urinary tract infection
VC	vascular calcification
VDR	vitamin D receptor
VLDL	very low-density lipoprotein
WHI	Women's Health Initiative
WHO	World Health Organization
WHR	waist-to-hip ratio

About the Editors

Janelle E. Gonyea, RDN, LD, FNKF, received her dietetics degree from Michigan State University in East Lansing, MI, and completed her dietetic internship at Mayo Clinic Hospital, Saint Marys Campus in Rochester, MN. She has 30 years of experience as a renal dietitian at the Mayo Clinic in Rochester, MN, working with chronic kidney disease patients in all stages of their disease process and across all treatment options. In addition to patient care, she authored medical nutrition therapy (MNT) protocols, chaired committees in charge of developing patient education materials and programming for the Division of Nephrology and Hypertension receiving the Mayo Clinic Department of Medicine Outstanding Education Award and educated countless nephrology colleagues, medical students, nephrology fellows and dietetic interns, holding the rank of Assistant Professor of Nutrition for the Mayo Clinic College of Medicine.

In addition to her clinical dietitian role, Janelle has served on the executive committee of the Council on Renal Nutrition for the National Kidney Foundation as editor of the *RenaLink* professional council newsletter, planning committee chair for the annual Spring Clinical Meeting as well as coordinator for the preconference workshop. Janelle was recognized for her work with the Council on Renal Nutrition by receiving the Susan C. Knapp Excellence in Education Award and Outstanding Service Award. She has also authored numerous articles for patient and professional publications and often speaks at regional and national meetings on various topics related to renal nutrition. Janelle has volunteered as program content creator and reviewer for various patient and professional organizations and received the American Association of Kidney Patients Dietitian Medal of Excellence. Currently she serves as a committee member for the update of the Academy of Nutrition and Dietetics National Kidney Diet, on the Medical Review Committee for the Midwest Kidney Network, as a charter member of the American Kidney Fund's Dietitian Advisory Group and as coeditor for the American Association of Kidney Patients' *AAKP Delicious!* recipe series. Janelle has had a lifelong passion for all things related to nephrology and enjoys the opportunities she has been given to collaborate with others to promote patient advocacy and advancement of care for kidney disease.

Stacey C. Phillips, MS, RDN, has been a registered dietitian nutritionist for over 16 years working for Mercy Health Saint Mary's in Grand Rapids, MI. She received her undergraduate degree from the University of Illinois at Urbana-Champaign, completed her dietetic internship at the Mayo Clinic School of Health Sciences in Rochester, MN, and earned her master's degree in dietetics through Central Michigan University. In her role as a clinical dietitian, Stacey has worked with patients in all stages of chronic kidney disease including kidney transplant recipients and living kidney donors as well as in the areas of general medicine, older adult, oncology, and long-term acute care. Her interest in renal nutrition developed from enjoying this rotation during her own internship due to some dedicated preceptors and through her current work Stacey has mentored over 70 dietetic interns as they rotate through their older adult and renal nutrition rotations.

Outside of her clinical work, Stacey has been involved with the Renal Dietitians Dietetics Practice Group through the Academy of Nutrition and Dietetics in several different roles including the Renal Nutrition Forum Editorial Board, Treasurer, Awards Chair, and Marketing and Communications Chair and was recognized with the 2021 Renal Dietitians Dietetics Practice Group Outstanding Service Award. She has served as coeditor of the American Association of Kidney Patients' *AAKP Delicious!* recipe series and was awarded the 2019 American Association of Kidney Patients Dietitian Medal of Excellence. In addition, Stacey has been a member of the National Kidney Foundation and served as the Patient Education Editor for the *Journal of Renal Nutrition*. Currently, she enjoys a number of consultant roles including as a subject matter expert for Dietitians on Demand, a Health Coach for the University of Michigan Controlling Hypertension Through Education and Coaching in Kidney Disease (CHECK-D) Study and as a nutrition reviewer for several different professional organizations. She is also a contributor to online medical information, peer-reviewed journals, and Academy of Nutrition and Dietetic publications. With each of these roles, Stacey has enjoyed working with a dynamic group of registered dietitians all with the same mindset of improving the available resources for professionals and patients.

Contributors

Sarita Bajpai, PhD, RDN, CD, CNSC
Clinical Dietitian Specialist, IU Health
Indianapolis, IN

Christine Benedetti, MS, RDN, CSR, LD, FNKF
Clinical Dietitian, Children's Healthcare of Atlanta
Atlanta, GA

Judith Beto, PhD, RDN, FAND
Research Associate, Loyola University Healthcare
Maywood, IL

Deborah Brommage, MS, RDN, LDN
Senior Scientific Director, National Kidney Foundation
Boynton Beach, FL

Joan Brookhyser Hogan, RD, CD
Registered Dietitian, Food 4 Life Nutrition Counseling
Tacoma, WA

Michelle Bump, MS, RD, LD
Director, Didactic Program in Dietetics;
Clinical Coordinator, Dietetic Internship,
Oregon State University
Corvallis, OR

Jenni Carvalho-Salemi, MPH, RDN, LD, CSP
Director, SAGE Research Group
Lutz, FL

Carolyn C. Cochran, RDN, LD, MS, CDCES, FNKF
Senior Clinical Dietitian, Dallas Nephrology
Associates, Dallas Transplant Institute
Dallas, TX

Sara Colman Carlson, RDN, CDCES
Manager, DaVita, Inc
Huntington Beach, CA

Rebecca Chrasta, MCN, RDN, LD
Registered Dietitian, Parkland Health
Dallas, TX

Joanne Cooke, MS, RD, CSR, FAND
Advanced Practice Renal Dietitian,
Kansas City VA Medical Center
Kansas City, MI

Ann Beemer Cotton, MS, RD, CNSC
Clinical Dietitian Specialist in Critical Care,
IU Health, Methodist Hospital
Indianapolis, IN

Desiree de Waal, MS, RD, CD, FAND
Renal Dietitian, University of Vermont Medical Center
Burlington, VT

Marian Glick-Bauer, MS, RD, CDN, CSR, CNSC
Clinical Dietitian, North Shore University Hospital,
Northwell Health
Manhasset, NY

Donna E. Gjesvold, RDN, LD, CCTD
Clinical Dietitian, Hennepin Healthcare, Kidney Center
Minneapolis, MN

D. Jodi Goldstein-Fuchs, DSc, CNN-NP, NP-C, RD
Nephrology Nurse Practitioner, Lucille Packard
Children's Hospital, Stanford, Pediatric Nephrology
Palo Alto, CA

Janelle E. Gonyea, RDN, LD, FNKF
Clinical Dietitian
Rochester, MN

Haewook Han, PhD, RD, LDN, FNKF
Department of Nephrology, Atrius Health;
Director of Combined MS in Nutrition & Dietetic
Internship, Friedman School of Nutrition
Science and Policy, Tufts University
Boston, MA

Peggy Hipskind, MA, RD, LD
Advanced Practice II Clinical Dietitian, Cleveland Clinic
Cleveland, OH

Wai Yin Ho, MSEd, MS, RDN, LD
Learning Experience Designer
Charleston, SC

Kathleen Hunt, RD, CSR
Renal Dietitian, Kaiser Permanente
Hayward, CA

Pamela S. Kent, MS, RD, CDCES, LD
Director of Population Health-Ohio Somatus
Vermilion, OH

Judith Kirk, MS, RDN, CDN, CSR, FNKF
Clinical Nutrition Specialist, Solid Organ Transplant
Dietitian, University of Rochester Medical Center
Rochester, NY

Meredith Larsen, MS, RDN, LD, FNKF
Program Manager, Nutritional Services, DaVita Inc
Cedar Park, TX

Kristin Leonberg, MS, RD, CSR, CDCES
Global Scientific Communications, Rare Disease
Cambridge, MA

Rachael R. Majorowicz, RDN, CSR, LDN, FNKF
Renal Dietitian, Mayo Clinic
Rochester, MN

Heidi Mathes, RD, LD, CNSC
Clinical Dietitian Specialist, Mercy One West
Des Moines Medical Center
West Des Moines, IA

Lesley McPhatter, MS, RDN, CSR
Assistant Clinical Nutrition Manager, Renal Nutrition,
University of Virginia/Morrison Healthcare
Lynchburg, VA

Eileen Moore, RD, LD
Clinical Liaison Director, Renal Products,
Pentec Health Inc
Glen Mills, PA

Aida L. Moreno-Brown, MS, RD, LD
Nutrition Manager, Fresenius Medical Care, University
of Texas at El Paso; El Paso Community College
El Paso, TX

Walter P. Mutter, MD
Chief of Nephrology, Newton-Wellesley Hospital
Newton, MA

Samer Nasser, MD, FASN
Nephrologist, Harvard Vanguard Medical Associates,
Beth Israel Deaconess Medical Center
Boston, MA

Hannah Norris, RDN, CSR
Transplant Dietitian, Banner University Medical Center,
Phoenix, Transplant Institute
Phoenix, AZ

Jessie M. Pavlinac, MS, RDN-AP, CSR, LD, FNKF, FAND
Adjunct Instructor, Oregon Health & Science University;
Adjunct Instructor, Rutgers University;
Adjunct Instructor, Oregon State University
Corvallis, OR

Stacey C. Phillips, MS, RDN
Clinical Dietitian, Mercy Health Saint Mary's
Grand Rapids, MI

Sara Prato, MS, RDN
Dietitian, Puget Sound Kidney Centers
Mountlake Terrace, WA

Melissa Prest, DCN, MS, RDN, CSR, LDN
Foundation Dietitian,
National Kidney Foundation of Illinois
Chicago, IL

Mary Rath, MEd, RD, LD, CNSC
Nutrition Support Dietitian, Cleveland Clinic
Cleveland, OH

Sharon R. Schatz, MS, RD, CSR, CDCES
Retired Renal Dietitian III,
DaVita Kidney Care Home Program
Cherry Hill, NJ

Kathy Schiro Harvey, MS, RDN, CSR
Director of Nutrition Services,
Puget Sound Kidney Centers
Mountlake Terrace, WA

Elizabeth C. Shanaman, RDN, CD, FNKF
Manager of Nutrition and Fitness Services,
Northwest Kidney Centers
Seattle, WA

Brittany Sparks, RDN, CSR
Private Practice Renal Dietitian, Nutrition by
Brittany, LLC
Denver, CO

Jean Stover, RD, LDN
Renal Dietitian, DaVita Kidney Care
Philadelphia, PA

Gail Torres, MS, RD, RN
Senior Clinical Communications Director,
National Kidney Foundation
New York, NY

Karen Wiesen, MS, RDN, LDN, FNKF
Renal Dietitian/Inpatient Dietitian Supervisor,
Geisinger Medical Center
Danville, PA

Victor Yu, PhD, RD, BC-ADM
Renal Dietitian and Professor of Nutrition,
Fresenius Kidney Care and Georgia Military College
North Augusta, SC

Lindsey Zirker, MS, RD, CSR
Renal Dietitian and Consultant,
The Kidney RD, RenAlign
Ammon, ID

Reviewers

Dominique Adair, MS, RD
Clinical Director, Cricket Health
New York, NY

Lubna Akbany, RD, CSR
Consulting Renal Dietitian
Newport Beach, CA

Vishal Bagchi, MBA, RD, LD
Dialysis Consultant, Nutricia/Danone North America
Dallas, TX

Deborah Benner, MA, RD, CSR
Vice President, Clinical Support, DaVita Inc
Yorba Linda, CA

Melanie Betz, MS, RD, CSR, CSG, LDN
Chronic Kidney Disease Nutrition and Education
Specialist, University of Chicago Medicine
Chicago, IL

Gloria M. Bissler, RD, LD
Renal Dietitian, Dialysis Clinic, Inc
Cincinnati, OH

Krista Blackwell, MD, RD, LDN, CNSC
Dietitian II, Sodexo
Silver Spring, MD

Amy Clatanoff Brown, RD, CSR, LDN
Renal Dietitian, Fresenius Kidney Care
Yarmouthport, MA

Cathleen Burns, DCN, RDN, LDN
Nutrition Consultant
Acushnet, MA

Laura D. Byham-Gray, PhD, RDN, FNKF
Professor and Vice Chair of Research,
Rutgers University
Newark, NJ

Greg Cannon, MS, RD, LD/N
Renal Dietitian, Fresenius Kidney Care
Melbourne, FL

Winnie Chan, PhD, RD, FNKF
Postdoctoral Research Fellow,
University of Birmingham
Birmingham, United Kingdom

Jan C. Beyer, MS, RD, LDN, CNSC
Clinical Dietitian, Centennial Medical Center—
Tristar Division
Nashville, TN

Claudia D'Alessandro, BSc, RDN
Renal Dietitian Nutritionist, University of Pisa
Pisa, Italy

Desiree de Waal, MS, RD, CD, FAND
Renal Dietitian, University of Vermont Medical Center
Burlington, VT

Doris Delgado, RDN
Nutrition Therapy Consultant, Patient Care American
Los Angeles, CA

Toni DeVane, MS, RDN, CSR, LDN, CNSC
Lead Renal Clinical Case Manager, Pentec Health
Glen Mills, PA

April Diederich, RDN, CSR
Assistant Director, Marilyn Magaram Center,
California State University, Northridge
Northridge, CA

Andrea Dombrowski, MS, RD, LD
Renal Dietitian, Satellite Healthcare
Austin, TX

Tiffany Donahue, RD, CSR, LDN
Clinical Dietitian Specialist,
Hospital of the University of Pennsylvania
Philadelphia, PA

Julie Driscoll, RDN, CSG, CSR
Assistant Health Services Administrator,
Federal Bureau of Prisons
Ayer, MA

Sara Erickson, RD, CSR, LDN
Clinical Nutrition Supervisor,
Atrium Health Levine Children's Hospital
Charlotte, NC

Bonnie K. Everett, MS, RD, CSR, LD
Renal Dietitian, Fresenius Kidney Care
Canton, MI

Kathleen M. Hill Gallant, PhD, RD
Associate Professor, University of Minnesota
St Paul, MN

Patricia Mae Garcia, MS, RD
Registered Dietitian, San Ysidro Health PACE,
Fresenius Kidney Care
Chula Vista, CA

Sarvnaz Medarresi Gharami, MS, RD, LDN
Nutrition Manager, Fresenius Medical Care
Roxbury, MA

Marian Glick-Bauer, MS, BD, CDN, CSR, CNSC
Clinical Dietitian, North Shore University Hospital,
Northwell Health
Manhasset, NY

Vida Goudarzi, MS, RDN, CSR
Satellite Healthcare
San Jose, CA

Lisa Gutekunst, MSEd, RD, CSR, CDN, FNKF
Dietitian, US Renalcare Research
Buffalo, NY

Heidi J. Haas, MS, RD, LD
Renal Dietitian, Grand River Medical Group—
Tri-State Dialysis
Dubuque, IA

Ana Maria Hernandez-Rosa, MS, RDN, LDN
Renal Dietitian, Fresenius Kidney
Care/American Renal Associates
Tampa, FL

Lois Hill, MS, RDN, LD, LDE, FAND
Owner, Nutrition Solutions
Lexington, KY

Dorothy C. Humm, MBA, RDN, CDN
Founder, The Preferred Nutritionist Organization
Brockport, NY

Ruth Kander, BSc (Hons), RD, MBDA, AFHEA
Renal Specialist Dietitian, Imperial College
Healthcare NHS Trust
London, United Kingdom

Jennifer Kernc, RD, CSR, LD, FAND
Vice President Market Development, InterWell Health
Waltham, MA

Jillian Klein, MS, RD
Clinical Dietitian, Trinity Health Muskegon
Muskegon, MI

Laura Koch, MS, RD, LMNT
Renal Dietitian, Dialysis Center of Lincoln, Inc
Lincoln, NE

Constance A. Laux, MEd, RDN, LD
Renal Dietitian, Davita Fort Wayne South
Fort Wayne, IN

Helen Lui, MS, RD
Renal Dietitian, Fresenius Kidney Care
Methuen, MA

Christiane L. Meireles, PhD, RD
Clinical Assistant Professor, University of Texas Health
Science Center, School of Nursing
San Antonio, TX

Diane L. Mettler, RD, CSR
Clinical Dietitian, The University of Colorado Hospital
Aurora, CO

Lynn Munson, MS, RD, LD
Renal Dietitian, Kidney Specialists of Minnesota
Brooklyn Center, MN

Margaret Murphy, PhD, RD, LD, FAND
Assistant Professor/Pediatric Renal Dietitian,
University of Kentucky Healthcare
Lexington, KY

Marjorie A. Naples, RD, CDN
Renal Dietitian, American Renal Associates,
Dialysis Center of Oneida
Oneida, NY

Christina L. Nelms, MS, RDN, LMNT
Pediatric Renal Nutrition Educator and Consultant,
PedsFeeds, LLC and University of Nebraska
Kearney, NE

Amy Myrtue Nelson, MPH, RD, CSR, CD
Renal Dietitian, Fresenius Kidney Care
Olympia, WA

Helen M. O'Connor, MS, RDN
Research Dietitian, Mayo Clinic
Rochester, MN

Laura Olejnik, MS, RD, LDN, CNSC
Renal Specialist, Akebia Therapeutics
Cambridge, MA

Joni Pagenkemper, MS, RD/LMNT, CDCES
Certified Diabetes Care and Education Specialist
Lincoln, NE

Chhaya Patel, MA, RDN
Sr, Program Manager Clinical Services,
ORCA Divisional Lead RD, Davita
Walnut Creek, CA

Jessica Prohn, MS, RD, CSR, LDN
Renal Dietitian, Cricket Health
Camrbidge, MA

Megan Reynolds, MS, RD, CSR, LD
HEALTHY HELPings Nutrition Services
Westlake, OH

Cate Rhodes, MS, RDN, LDN, CNSC
Clinical Dietitian III, Cone Health
Greensboro, NC

AnnaMarie Rodriguez, RDN, LD, FAND
Dietitian/Nutrition Consultant, Nutrition Directions LLC
Sturtevant, WI

Rebecca Schaffer, MS, RDN, LD
Clinical Dietitian, Mayo Clinic
Rochester, MN

Noelle Schleder, MS, RDN
Nutrition Coach, Stronger U Nutrition
Traverse City, MI

Natalie Sexton, MS, RDN, CSR, LD
Registered Dietitian, DaVita
Gilmer, TX

Susanna Slukhinsky, RD, CSR, CDN
Clinical Dietitian, Susanna Slukhinsky Nutrition
Brooklyn, NY

Sue Steiner, RD, LMNT, CSR, CDCES
Renal Dietitian, Dialysis Clinics Inc
Bellevue, NE

Cynthia J. Terrill, RDN, CSR, CD
Pediatric Renal Dietitian,
University of Utah School of Medicine
Salt Lake City, UT

Maria Tointon, RDN, CSR
Renal Dietitian, U.S. Renal Care
Honolulu, HI

Jessica D. Tower, MS, RD, CSR, LD, CCTD
Clinical Nutrition Specialist III, Children's Mercy Hospital
Kansas City, MO

Dana Trotta, MS, RD, CSR, LDN, FNKF
Renal Dietitian, American Renal Associates
Narragansett, RI

Girija Vijaykumar, RD
Renal Dietitian, Pure Life Renal
Lansdowne, VA

Jennifer Vyduna, MS, RDN, CNSC
Lead Renal Clinical Case Manager, Pentec Health
Glen Mills, PA

Joanne L. White, RDN, LDN, CSR
Registered Dietitian Nutritionist Consultant
Wilmington, NC

Gretchen Wiese, MS, RDN
Associate Dietitian, Fresenius Kidney Care
Indianapolis, IN

Karen Wiesen, MS, RDN, LDN, FNKF
Inpatient Dietitian Supervisor and Renal Dietitian,
Geisinger Medical Center
Danville, PA

Melissa Young, MS, RDN, CSR, LDN
VA Dietitian
Asheville, NC

Lindsay Zirker, MS, RD, CSR
Renal Dietitian and Consultant, The Kidney RD, RenAlign
Ammon, ID

Preface

Nearly four decades ago, the Renal Dietitians Dietetic Practice Group of the Academy of Nutrition and Dietetics and the Council on Renal Nutrition of the National Kidney Foundation began development of a clinical guide to assist dietetic professionals managing the nutrition care of persons with kidney disease. At that time, renal dietitians were surveyed and they identified three key objectives for the publication. The *Clinical Guide to Nutrition Care in Kidney Disease* should address the following objectives:

1. Contain practical information that is useful in day-to-day clinical practice.
2. Represent a consensus formed by clinical practitioners based on current scientific literature and experience.
3. Focus on characteristics unique to the kidney disease population.

This edition, as well as previous editions, was written with these key objectives in mind.

The *Clinical Guide to Nutrition Care in Kidney Disease* also recognizes that registered dietitian nutritionists (RDNs) who practice in the realm of nephrology nutrition provide both preventive and therapeutic nutrition care for individuals of all ages who present with a variety of kidney disorders, requiring a continuum of treatment options to successfully manage established kidney disease. Consequently, this third edition of *Clinical Guide to Nutrition Care in Kidney Disease* continues to expand content to keep pace with the rapidly evolving field of nephrology. Enduring content areas have been updated to reflect the newly published Kidney Disease Outcomes Quality Initiative (KDOQI) Clinical Practice Guideline for Nutrition in CKD: 2020 Update. Updates also support the efforts of practitioners to achieve goals set forth by the July 2019 Executive Order on Advancing American Kidney Health which focuses on the prevention of progressive chronic kidney disease (CKD) and the promotion of home dialysis modalities as well as kidney transplantation in the event that CKD progresses to the point where kidney replacement therapy is required, ultimately improving medical care and quality of life for individuals with kidney disease.

The number of topics have been expanded to reflect the ever-broadening scope of practice for RDNs employed in outpatient clinics, transplant centers, dialysis facilities, long-term care facilities, and hospitals. New topics found in the third edition include nutritional management of kidney stones, guidelines for patients following plant-based diets to support recommended dietary patterns in the 2020 KDOQI update, CKD and gut health, information regarding herbal and botanical use in patients with transplant as well as malnutrition criteria, nutrition focused physical examination, and an overview of oral nutrition supplements for use in patients with kidney disease to help prevent or treat malnutrition that is commonly identified in this patient population.

This third edition of the *Clinical Guide to Nutrition Care in Kidney Disease* will provide continuing education credits for those who desire to pursue this option and assist RDNs who are preparing to take the credentialing examination to become a Certified Board Specialist in Renal Nutrition. With the aforementioned enhancements, we hope that you will find this third edition of the *Clinical Guide to Nutrition Care in Kidney Disease* to be an invaluable resource as you care for individuals with kidney disease.

A special thank you to previous clinical guide coeditors Karen Wiesen, MS, RDN, LDN, FNKF, Jean Stover, RD, LDN, and Laura Byham-Gray, PhD, RDN, FNKF, for their guidance and support with the third edition.

Acknowledgements

We would like to acknowledge a number of individuals, as without their support, publication of the third edition of this clinical guide would not have been possible. First, we would like to thank the previous coeditors of the clinical guide, Laura Byham-Gray, PhD, RDN, FNKF; Jean Stover, RD, LDN; and Karen Wiesen, MS, RDN, LDN, FNKF. Not only have they provided us with the first and second edition of this publication, but each was more than happy to help answer questions as we navigated through the publication process. Next, we would also like to thank the Academy of Nutrition and Dietetics Product Strategy and Development team including Betsy Hornick, MS, RDN, Emily Motycka, Erin Fagan Faley, and Stacey Zettle, MS, RDN, LDN. Each provided invaluable support and encouragement from the beginning to the end of this project. Lastly, thank you to all of our authors and reviewers for volunteering your time and expertise to write and provide feedback on this next edition. The field of nephrology nutrition continues to evolve, and with your support the *Clinical Guide to Nutrition Care in Kidney Disease* remains a great resource for registered dietitian nutritionists.

Overview of Kidney Disease and Nutrition Assessment

CHAPTER 1

Overview: Pathophysiology of the Kidney

Janelle E. Gonyea, RDN, LD, FNKF, and Brittany Sparks, RDN, CSR

Basic Kidney Anatomy

The kidneys are located symmetrically on either side of the vertebrae, starting at the 12th thoracic vertebra and extending down to the third lumbar vertebra. Each adult kidney measures approximately 11 cm to 12 cm long, 5 cm to 7.5 cm wide, 2.5 cm to 3 cm thick, and weighs approximately 115 g to 170 g. Each kidney has two general regions: the cortex, and the medulla (see Figure 1.1). The medulla is divided into cone-shaped regions called renal pyramids.[1] Blood is supplied to healthy kidneys through the renal artery, which enters the kidney at the hilus. Approximately 20% of cardiac output circulates to the kidneys. This is far more blood flow than necessary to supply needed oxygen to the kidneys, but it is required for excretory function.[2] Urine that has been formed collects in the lower portion of the renal pelvis, which is the expanded upper region of the ureter. It then exits the kidney via the ureter that extends for a length of 22 cm to 30 cm, providing a connection to the bladder.[3]

The basic functional unit of the kidney is the nephron (see Figure 1.2 on page 2). On average, each human kidney contains 900,000 to 1 million nephrons, which are located in both the cortex and the medulla.[4] Within each nephron, there are several well-known microscopic components (see Box 1.1 on page 2).

FIGURE 1.1 | Anatomy of a kidney

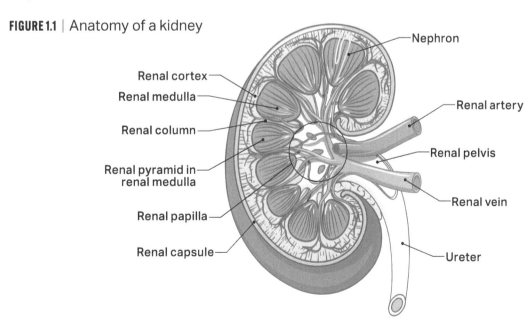

- Nephron
- Renal cortex
- Renal medulla
- Renal column
- Renal pyramid in renal medulla
- Renal papilla
- Renal capsule
- Renal artery
- Renal pelvis
- Renal vein
- Ureter

FIGURE 1.2 | Nephron

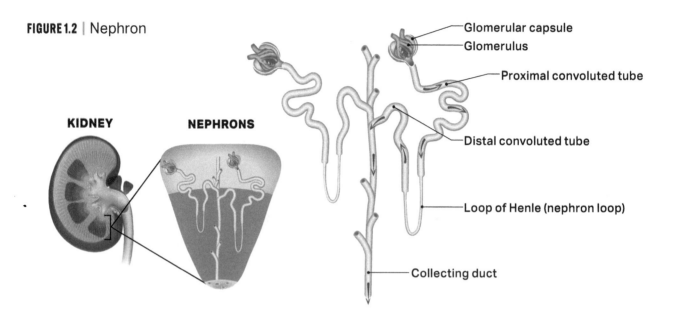

BOX 1.1 | Functional Units of the Nephron[4]

NEPHRON COMPONENT	FUNCTION
Glomerulus/ Bowman's capsule/ renal corpuscle	Serves as the kidney's filtering unit
	Made of a network of capillaries surrounded by a narrow wall of epithelial cells
	Forms approximately 125 mL/min of filtrate within the glomerulus
	Bowman's capsule, with its basement membrane, encompasses the glomerulus (Together they are known as the renal corpuscle)
Proximal convoluted tubule	Is a direct continuation of the epithelium of the Bowman's capsule
	Controls reabsorption of filtered glucose, amino acids, sodium, bicarbonate, potassium, chloride, calcium, phosphate, water, and other solutes
	Manages secretion of renally excreted drug metabolites
	Produces ammonium
Loop of Henle	Concentrates urine which may be diluted later in the excretory system
	Unable to permeate water—but sodium can be pumped out
	Influences movement of water in or out of the water–permeable collecting duct
Distal tubule	Comprised of three parts: 1. the thick ascending limb of the loop of Henle 2. the macula densa 3. the distal convoluted tubule
	Has ability for active transport of sodium chloride in the thick ascending limb of the loop of Henle
	Concentrates urine by absorbing approximately 99% of the water that is filtered by the kidneys back into the body
	Thick ascending limb of loop of Henle functions are governed by hormones, including vasopressin, parathyroid hormone, and calcitonin
Collecting duct	Contains two types of cells: principal cells and intercalated cells
	Controls reabsorption of sodium chloride and the secretion of potassium via principal cells
	Regulates acid-base balance via secretion of hydrogen and bicarbonate in intercalated cells

Kidney Functions

The major functions of the kidneys can be described as excretory, acid-base balance, endocrine, and fluid and electrolyte balance.

Excretory functions of the kidneys include removing excess fluid and waste products. While approximately 180 L of filtrate pass daily through the kidneys, only 1 to 2 L are removed in the urine each day.[5] The remaining fluid is retained in the body to support tissues. Substances removed with the urine include urea, vitamins and minerals consumed in excess of the body's requirements, and metabolites of some drugs and poisons. If the blood levels of any needed substances are low, the kidneys promote homeostasis by conserving them to maintain levels within narrowly defined limits.

Acid-base balance is maintained through a buffer system, which keeps the blood's pH level at approximately 7.4. Bicarbonate carries hydrogen ions to the kidney, where they are removed from extracellular fluid in the tubules, then reabsorbed in the proximal tubule, and then returned as needed to the bloodstream. In addition, phosphate buffers intracellular fluid, which is concentrated in the tubules as water is removed. Other organic compounds, such as citrate, also support acid-base balance. Finally, metabolites of amino acids may be used to moderate acid or base reactions.[6]

Several hormones are included in the endocrine function of the kidneys. Calcitriol, or 1,25-dihydroxy-vitamin D3, is produced in the kidney and subsequently enhances calcium absorption. In healthy kidneys, the activation of vitamin D and the excretion of excess phosphorus set the stage for maintaining healthy bones (see Chapter 10 for more details).

Anemia of patients with chronic kidney disease (CKD) is related to altered production of erythropoietin (EPO) in the diseased kidney. Normally, EPO acts on bone marrow to increase the production of red blood cells, thus enhancing the transportation of oxygen throughout the body's tissues. In patients with CKD, decreased production of EPO can lead to anemia (see Chapter 2 for more details).

The kidneys play an important role in maintaining fluid and electrolyte balance. Antidiuretic hormone (ADH), also known as arginine vasopressin, is released from the posterior pituitary gland and helps regulate water that is reabsorbed into the body. When fluid volume (blood or other fluids) is low, ADH is secreted and reduces urine flow, increasing the reabsorption of water in the collecting duct. This mechanism maintains the body's osmolality within a very tight range.

When extracellular volume decreases, the perfusion of all body tissues—including the kidney—is reduced. Consequently, the glomerular filtration rate (GFR) is lower, resulting in decreased removal of sodium chloride. This activates the trio of hormones of the renin-angiotensin-aldosterone system to increase blood pressure to maintain adequate tissue perfusion.[7]

A person with advanced kidney function impairment may experience edema, uremia (accumulation of waste products in the blood), metabolic acidosis, hypertension, anemia, bone disease, and increased sensitivity to certain medications, vitamins, minerals, and dietary supplements, which can reach toxic levels in the body.

[handwritten margin note: Passage of fluid through circulatory system or lymph to organs or tissues.]

Types of Kidney Failure

The onset of kidney failure can be sudden, as in acute kidney injury (AKI), or progressive, leading to CKD. Patients with AKI will potentially regain their kidney function with medical treatment of the underlying cause of insult. However, if a decrease in GFR or an increase in serum creatinine persists for more than 3 months after the diagnosis of AKI, the kidneys are not expected to recover, resulting in CKD. Typically, CKD cannot be reversed but may be stabilized with certain etiologies. Additional challenges for patients with significant proteinuria should also be addressed. Medical nutrition therapy (MNT) is important in both the management of AKI and CKD and will be discussed in detail in Chapters 3 and 4.

ACUTE KIDNEY INJURY

AKI generally has a rapid onset of symptoms occurring over a period of hours to days. AKI may start with a small increase in serum creatinine and progress to reduced urine volume (oliguria) and ultimately to a complete absence of urine output (anuria).[8] AKI can occur in previously healthy kidneys. With proper nutrition management and appropriate dialytic support, ranging from intermittent hemodialysis to continuous venovenous hemodiafiltration, the kidneys can often repair themselves (see Chapter 4).[9] However, AKI can often be superimposed on underlying CKD secondary to diabetes, hypertension, and other comorbidities. In this scenario, the goal is to return kidney function to baseline by removing the offending agent and avoiding chronic dialysis. AKI is associated with a high degree (40%–70%) of morbidity and mortality, despite advancing technology in kidney replacement therapy (KRT).[10,11] AKI is also associated with increased risk for development of CKD, even when there is complete recovery of kidney function.[10-13]

In the United States, AKI most commonly occurs in hospitalized and critically ill patients and is often secondary to ischemic events and consequent injury to the kidney. However, AKI can arise from many different etiologies. AKI can be characterized by the type of underlying insult to the kidney and is categorized as either prerenal, intrinsic or tubulointerstitial, or postrenal.[14-16] Prerenal AKI results from decreased kidney perfusion in an otherwise normal kidney, perhaps due to altered cardiac function and altered glomerular blood flow; with treatment, it can be quickly reversed. AKI may have a kidney origin due to underlying structural or functional changes in the kidney, and postrenal etiologies of AKI may include urethral strictures, tumors, clots, or stones restricting flow to or from the urinary tract.[14,16] Identifying where the damage may be occurring within the kidney is key to treatment (see Chapter 4 for a more detailed discussion on AKI).

CHRONIC KIDNEY DISEASE

In 1997, the National Kidney Foundation Kidney Disease Outcomes Quality Initiative (NKF-KDOQI) began publishing evidence-based clinical practice guidelines. These guidelines were developed and implemented by physicians and health care providers within the nephrology community. In 2002, NKF-KDOQI outlined a standard for classifying stages of CKD.[17] A decade later, the Kidney Disease: Improving Global Outcomes (KDIGO) organization offered an update to the initial guidelines. The classification for CKD appears in Table 1.1.[18]

TABLE 1.1 | Stages of Chronic Kidney Disease[18]

Stage	Glomerular filtration rate (mL/min/1.73 m²)	Description
G1	≥90	Kidney damage with normal or increased glomerular filtration rate (GFR)
G2	60-89	Mild decrease in GFR
G3a	45-59	Mild-to-moderate decrease in GFR
G3b	30-44	Moderate-to-severe decrease in GFR
G4	15-29	Severe decrease in GFR
G5	<15	Kidney failure

It is important to note that some decrease in kidney function is a normal part of aging. CKD stage 1 and even CKD stage 2 may be observed in otherwise healthy individuals aged 60 years and older. However, even in older adults, reduced kidney function should be monitored to allow appropriate intervention if the decrease in GFR continues into later stages of CKD.[19]

Patients with CKD continually lose GFR over a period of months to years. In many of the underlying conditions, progression of the disease continues even if the kidney is no longer exposed to the initial insult. Eventually, CKD may progress to stage 5, requiring KRT, such as dialysis or transplantation, to sustain life (see Chapters 5, 6, 7 and 8 for more details).

Nephrotic Syndrome

Nephrotic syndrome (NS) is one of the most serious challenges in clinical nephrology.[20] NS is not a disease but rather a collection of symptoms that may be recognized in patients with CKD of several different etiologies. Box 1.2 shows the clinical characteristics of NS.[21] Nephrotic range proteinuria is a common characteristic of NS, which is classified as greater than 3 g urinary protein loss in a 24-hour time frame. With NS, fundamental alterations of the kidney's glomerular basement membrane allow persistent loss of large amounts of protein and other large molecules to pass into the urine. Normal urinary protein losses are approximately 150 mg/d.[22] Conditions often associated with NS include diabetes mellitus, glomerular diseases, amyloidosis, minimal change disease, and focal segmental glomerulosclerosis (FSGS).[22]

BOX 1.2 | Clinical Characteristics of Nephrotic Syndrome

Proteinuria (>3 g/d of urinary protein losses, with proportionally lesser amounts for children)

Hypoalbuminemia

Hypertension

Hyperlipidemia

Edema

A urinalysis is typically performed to determine the type and the amount of protein in the urine. This test helps to specify the kind of kidney damage that may be occurring and the necessary treatment. Low-molecular-weight protein losses are often associated with etiologies that affect the kidney tubules and often do not reach nephrotic range proteinuria.[22]

"Albuminuria" is the term used to describe when albumin, a large-molecular-weight protein, is lost in the urine at levels higher than 30 mg/d. Albuminuria is classified as either moderately increased albuminuria with urine albumin levels between 30 mg/d and 300 g/d or severely increased albuminuria, when levels are more than 300 mg/d. These terms are now being used in place of microalbuminuria and macroalbuminuria.[22] Albuminuria is considered to be problematic as it is associated with increased incidence of all-cause mortality, left ventricular hypertrophy, stroke, and vascular calcification.[22] Albuminuria typically results from damage to the filtration barrier and can often be seen in patients with diabetes mellitus and NS.[16]

Since proteinuria, including albuminuria, represents such a high risk factor for cardiovascular disease and CKD progression, the treatment of NS must include reduction of urinary protein losses. Medical intervention may involve corticosteroids and immunosuppressive agents in several specific etiologies. Angiotensin-converting enzyme inhibitors and angiotensin receptor blockers may also be used to reduce urinary protein losses and control blood pressure and fluid balance. The latter agents may be prescribed to reduce proteinuria even when blood pressure is normal.[21]

The etiology of hyperlipidemia in NS is related to excess production and reduced catabolism of apolipoprotein B–containing lipoproteins (including chylomicrons and very low-density lipoproteins). Some patients present with elevated levels of cholesterol and triglycerides.[23] Hyperlipidemia is associated with an increased risk for vascular disease and, therefore, hydroxymethylglutaryl coenzyme A reductase inhibitors are often used for lipid control. With some disorders, particularly FSGS, there may be a proteinuric factor, and the removal of this factor may help manage proteinuria and subsequent hyperlipidemia.[24]

MNT for NS includes avoiding excessive protein intake, as large protein loads can exacerbate proteinuria. For those with CKD stage 1 and stage 2 with NS, a protein intake of 0.8 g/kg/d of body weight is recommended.[25,26] Refer to Chapter 3 for more information on recommended protein needs for treating patients with CKD stages 3 through 5. Sodium restriction can be beneficial. One study recommends limiting sodium to 100 mmol/d or less than 2,300 mg/d in those with proteinuria; however, the overall goals should be based on fluid status and the need to control edema.[27] Potassium, other electrolytes, and minerals need to be monitored, and the patient's diet should be individualized. Monitoring for vitamin D insufficiency and deficiency in patients with NS is important, as studies have shown increased risk due to increased loss of vitamin D–binding proteins in the urine.[27-30] In patients with nephrotic range proteinuria, vitamin D supplementation with either cholecalciferol, ergocalciferol, or other safe and effective 25-hydroxyvitamin D precursors may be necessary to maintain adequate serum levels.[27] Nutrition therapy for the associated hyperlipidemia may not normalize serum cholesterol levels, and pharmacological therapy, as previously described, is generally required.[25,26,30,31] More research and clinical trials are needed to identify optimal treatment for NS, especially for vitamin and mineral supplementation.

Summary

This chapter has provided an overview of normal kidney function and various consequences of kidney disease, along with many potential etiologies for compromise in kidney function including AKI, CKD, and NS. More detailed information regarding medical treatment and MNT required at these various stages will be found throughout this publication.

References

1. Fenton RA, Praetorius J. Anatomy of the kidney. In: Skorecki K, Chertow GM, Marsden PA, Taal MW, Yu ASL, eds. *Brenner and Rector's The Kidney.* 10th ed. Elsevier; 2016:42.
2. Munger KA, Maddox DA, Brenner BM, Kost CK Jr. The renal circulations and glomerular ultrafiltration. In: Skorecki K, Chertow GM, Marsden PA, Taal MW, Yu ASL, eds. *Brenner and Rector's The Kidney.* 10th ed. Elsevier; 2016:83.
3. Elkoushy MA, Andonian S. Surgical, radiologic, and endoscopic anatomy of the kidney and ureter. In: Wein AJ, Kavoussi LR, Partin AW, Peters CA, eds. *Campbell-Walsh Urology.* 11th ed. Elsevier; 2016:974.
4. Fenton RA, Praetorius J. Anatomy of the kidney. In: Skorecki K, Chertow GM, Marsden PA, Taal MW, Yu ASK, eds. *Brenner and Rector's The Kidney.* 10th ed. Elsevier; 2016:45-75.
5. Koeppen BM, Stanton BA. Renal transport mechanisms: NaCl and water reabsorption along the *nephron.* In: *Renal Physiology.* 5th ed. Elsevier Mosby; 2013:45-46.
6. Koeppen BM, Stanton BA. Regulation of acid–base balance. In: *Renal Physiology.* 5th ed. Elsevier Mosby; 2013:131-152.
7. Koeppen BM, Stanton BA. Regulation of body fluid osmolality: regulation of water balance. In: *Renal Physiology.* 5th ed. Elsevier Mosby; 2013:75-82.
8. Levin A, Warnock DG, Mehta RL, et al. Acute Kidney Injury Network Working Group: improving outcomes from acute kidney injury: report of an initiative. *Am J Kidney Dis.* 2007;50(1):1-4. doi:10.1053/j.ajkd.2007.05.008
9. The VA/NIH Acute Renal Failure Trial Network. Intensity of renal support in critically ill patients with acute kidney injury. *N Engl J Med.* 2008;359(1):7-20. doi:10.1056/NEJMoa0802639
10. Palevsky PM, Liu KD, Brophy PD, et al. KDOQI US commentary on the 2012 KDIGO clinical practice guideline for acute kidney injury. *Am J Kidney Dis.* 2013;61(5):649-672. doi:10.1053/j.ajkd.2013.02.349
11. Uchino S, Kellum JA, Bellomo R, et al. Acute renal failure in critically ill patients: a multinational, multicenter study. *JAMA.* 2005;294(7):813-818. doi:10.1001/jama.294.7.813
12. Heung M, Steffick DE, Zivin K, et al. Acute kidney injury recovery pattern and subsequent risk of CKD: an analysis of veterans health administration data. *Am J Kidney Dis.* 2016;67(5):742-752. doi:10.1053/j.ajkd.2015.10.019
13. Mehta S, Chauhan K, Patel A, et al. The prognostic importance of duration of AKI: a systematic review and meta-analysis. *BMC Nephrol.* 2018;19(1):91. doi:10.1186/s12882-018-0876-7
14. Himmelfarb J, Joannidis M, Molitoris B, et al. Evaluation and initial management of acute kidney injury. *Clin J Am Soc Nephrol.* 2008;3(4):962-967. doi:10.2215/CJN.04971107
15. Basile DP, Anderson MD, Sutton TA. Pathophysiology of acute kidney injury. *Compr Physiol.* 2012;2(2):1303-1353. doi:10.1002/cphy.c110041
16. Kidney Disease: Improving Global Outcomes (KDIGO) Acute Kidney Injury Work Group. KDIGO Clinical Practice Guideline for Acute Kidney Injury. *Kidney Int Suppl.* 2012;2(suppl 1):78-80. doi:10.1038/kisup.2012.1

17. National Kidney Foundation. K/DOQI clinical practice guidelines for chronic kidney disease: evaluation, classification, and stratification. *Am J Kidney Dis.* 2002;39(2 suppl 1):S1-S266.

18. KDIGO 2012 clinical practice guideline for the evaluation and management of chronic kidney disease. *Kidney Int.* 2013;3(1):5. doi:10.1038/kisup.2012.74

19. Glassock RJ, Winearls C. Aging and the glomerular filtration rate: truths and consequences. *Trans Am Clin Climatol Assoc.* 2009;120:419-428.

20. Schwarz A. New aspects of the treatment of nephrotic syndrome. *J Am Soc Nephrol.* 2001;12(suppl 17):S44-S47.

21. Orth SR, Ritz E. Medical progress: the nephrotic syndrome. *N Engl J Med.* 1998;338:1202-1211. doi:10.1056/NEJM199804233381707

22. Gilbert SJ, Weiner DE, Bomback AS, Perazella MA, Tonelli M. *National Kidney Foundation's Primer on Kidney Diseases.* 7th ed. Elsevier; 2018:46-49.

23. Crew RJ, Radhakrishnan J, Appel G. Complications of the nephrotic syndrome and their treatment. *Clin Nephrol.* 2004;62(4):245-259. doi:10.3345/kjp.2011.54.8.322

24. Keane WF. Proteinuria: its clinical importance and role in progressive renal disease. *Am J Kidney Dis.* 2000;35(4 suppl 1):S97-S105. doi:10.1016/S0272-6386(00)70237-X

25. Kidney Disease: Improving Global Outcomes (KDIGO) Glomerulonephritis Work Group. KDIGO clinical practice guideline for glomerulonephritis. *Kidney Int Suppl.* 2021;2(suppl 2):S139-274. doi:10.1038/kisup.2012.9

26. Fouque D. Nephrotic syndrome and protein metabolism. *Nephrologie.* 1996;17(5):279-282.

27. National Kidney Foundation. K/DOQI Clinical Practice Guideline for Nutrition in Chronic Kidney Disease: 2020 Update. *Am J Kidney Dis.* 2020;76(3 suppl 1):S1-S107. doi:10.1053/j.ajkd.2020.05.006

28. Selewski DT, Chen A, Shatat IF, et al. Vitamin D in incident nephrotic syndrome: a Midwest Pediatric Nephrology Consortium study. *Pediatr Nephrol.* 2016;31(3):465-472. doi:10.1007/s00467-015-3236-x

29. Barragry JM, France MW, Carter ND, et al. Vitamin D metabolism in nephrotic syndrome. *Lancet.* 1977;2:629-32. doi:10.1016/s0140-6736(77)92498-9

30. Molfino A, Don BR, Kaysen GA. Nutritional and non-nutritional management of the nephrotic syndrome. In: Kopple JD, Massry SG, Kalantar-Zadeh K, eds. *Nutritional Management of Renal Disease.* 3rd ed. Elsevier; 2012:26.

31. Kaysen GA. Nutritional management of nephrotic syndrome. *J Ren Nutr.* 1992;2(2):50-58. doi:10.1016/S1051-2276(12)80212-3

CHAPTER 2

Nutrition Assessment in Chronic Kidney Disease

Deborah Brommage, MS, RDN, LDN, Heidi Mathes, RD, LD, CNSC, and Gail Torres, MS, RD, RN

Introduction

Nutrition assessment is the first step in the Nutrition Care Process.[1] Therefore, it is recommended that all nutrition professionals follow the steps necessary to achieve a complete and valid assessment to create a lasting record that allows for ongoing monitoring of patient outcomes.

Assessment criteria will vary, depending on the stage of kidney dysfunction. For example, in chronic kidney disease (CKD) stage 1, acceptable serum calcium and phosphorus levels will be different than in CKD stage 4 or stage 5.[2] The 2008 Centers for Medicare & Medicaid Services Conditions for Coverage for patients with CKD stage 5 receiving dialysis provide detailed guidelines that elucidate the time frame, frequency, and comprehensiveness of interdisciplinary assessments. These guidelines include specific criteria for registered dietitian nutritionists (RDNs) to use in assessing, monitoring, and reassessing nutritional status and developing a nutrition care plan based on a patient's dialysis initiation date, medical stability, and changes in health status.[3] The 2020 Kidney Disease Outcomes Quality Initiative (KDOQI) Guideline for Nutrition in CKD recommends a comprehensive nutrition assessment at least within the first 90 days of starting dialysis, annually, or when indicated by nutrition screening or provider referral for adults with CKD stages 3 through 5D or posttransplant.[4]

Standardization of the diagnosis of adult nutritional status starts with recognizing that the inflammatory response plays a role in modulating acute-phase proteins commonly used as markers of nutritional status (see section on Serum Proteins). Therefore, an etiology-based approach to diagnose the nutritional status in adults is based on whether inflammation is present. For example, a diagnosis of malnutrition can be defined in the context of starvation-related malnutrition (no inflammation), chronic diseases or conditions (mild to moderate degree of inflammation), and acute illness or injury (marked inflammatory response).[5]

Expert consensus has identified the following six characteristics that reflect nutritional status vs the inflammatory response: insufficient energy intake, weight loss, loss of muscle mass, loss of subcutaneous fat, localized or generalized fluid accumulation that may sometimes mask weight loss, and diminished functional status as measured by handgrip strength.[5] Therefore, nutrition assessment involves the evaluation of multiple parameters, including an extensive patient history, nutrition focused physical exam (NFPE), and biochemical and hematologic values. Other areas that will affect the provision of medical nutrition therapy (MNT) for the patient with CKD include socioeconomic factors, education level, health literacy, and learning ability. A comprehensive nutrition assessment leads to a plan of achievable goals that are workable and acceptable to the patient.

This chapter is designed to help the reader understand the basics of nutrition assessment for the adult with kidney disease (see Chapter 13 for parameters applicable to children). Included within this chapter are the basic areas of patient history, NFPE, biochemical parameters, and nutrition assessment tools.

Patient History

The patient's history gives a perspective about past and present nutritional status, current changes, and areas that need to be addressed in order to develop a nutrition plan of care. Histories provide information concerning comorbid conditions, medications, hospitalizations, adequacy of current dietary intake and any changes in oral intake, gastrointestinal (GI) conditions that interfere with intake, changes in height and weight, economic status, socialization, functional status, and information from the NFPE.

MEDICAL AND PSYCHOSOCIAL HISTORY

Much of the patient's history is obtained by reviewing the medical record and interviewing the patient and, as appropriate, the family, or caregiver. The interview is the first opportunity for the patient and the RDN to establish rapport and build trust. Once the relationship has been developed, the patient will be more at ease with sharing information regarding medical and diet history.

The medical history provides information on disease states that may impact diet and nutrition. Since diabetes and hypertension are the leading causes of CKD, these comorbidities are commonly seen in this patient population and can have a profound impact on nutritional status and dietary intervention. Concurrent diseases and their corresponding medications may also contribute to drug–nutrient and drug–drug interactions that can alter nutrient absorption and utilization, as well as cause GI side effects. GI conditions may interfere with food ingestion, nutrient absorption, and elimination patterns.

The RDN should use the psychosocial history to assess the patient's ability to obtain, prepare, ingest, and enjoy food and evaluate the patient's mental health, educational level, and functional status. It is important to know who shops for the food and prepares the meals as well as other pertinent socioeconomic and cultural factors that may affect food choices. The social aspects of a person's life need to be assessed in order to understand what and who helps the patient and how to achieve optimal care for the patient. Finally, knowing a person's abilities and psychosocial situation can enhance the understanding of who they are and how they eat, and the evaluation of their dietary intake.

For example, because the social aspects of a meal may influence a patient's intake, it is important that the RDN assess whether the patient is eating alone or with others. Functional status can be assessed using tools such as the Katz Activities of Daily Living.[6] Religious and cultural beliefs can also affect food preferences and dietary intake and, therefore, need to be evaluated.[7,8] It is important to discuss any firsthand experiences that other care team members may be having with the patient (eg, observed food intolerances or problems with feeding) so that timely solutions can be implemented.

APPETITE ASSESSMENT

Appetite assessment tools may help clinicians assess and monitor appetite in patients with CKD because change in appetite impacts dietary intake. Two appetite assessment tools that perform well in patients treated with hemodialysis (HD) include the Functional Assessment of Anorexia/Cachexia Therapy (FAACT) score and the Visual Analog Scale (VAS).[9,10] The FAACT utilizes 12 questions related to appetite and food intake, which provide a qualitative and quantitative diagnosis of anorexia. A total score of 30 or less indicates the presence of anorexia. The VAS uses a rating scale of 0 mm (no hunger) to 100 mm (hunger). While this tool provides a quantitative "measure" of appetite, there is no defined cutoff value for diagnosing anorexia. Zabel et al[10] showed that the mean VAS score reported by patients receiving dialysis with poor appetite was 50 mm or less. The VAS may be more useful in daily practice because it takes only a few seconds to perform and does not require specific competencies.[10,11]

The Dialysis Practice Patterns Outcomes Study (DOPPS) data show that there is a twofold higher risk of hospitalization among patients who struggle with an extreme lack of appetite compared with those who do not.[12]

DIET HISTORY

Diet histories help determine adequacy of intake and nutrient content. They provide a review of usual food intake, food intake patterns, and factors that affect intake. Diet histories should assess the patient's "normal" eating habits and any changes in those patterns. The RDN should assess the patient's ability to chew, swallow, taste, and smell food, any changes in appetite (see the section on Appetite Assessment) and eating patterns, use of dietary supplements, and alternative or complementary therapies (see Chapter 19), previous dietary restrictions or diet instructions, and comprehension of previous counseling sessions. Knowledge of food preferences, allergies and intolerances, alcohol use, and pica are also important because all can affect food intake.

The reliability and the validity of the data depend on the patient's ability to provide accurate and relevant data and the interviewer's skills to elicit information from the patient.[12-14] According to the National Kidney Foundation KDOQI guidelines, dietary interviews and food diaries are "the most reliable and valid measure of dietary intake" among patients with CKD.[4] The data gathered on dietary intake should be incorporated into the plan of care, inclusive of educational needs and goals. Following are five methods for assessing dietary intake typically used in patients with CKD.

3-day food records/diary This prospective dietary intake method entails having the patient document dietary intake as it occurs for a period of 3 days. This approach relies on accurate reporting that includes portion sizes. The days should include one weekday and one weekend day, and for patients on maintenance HD (MHD), one

dialysis day and one nondialysis day. The clinician will review the food records with the patient and then assess the nutrient intake from the record.[10-12] The KDOQI guidelines recommend periodic 3-day food records as the preferred method for measuring protein and energy intake for patients receiving dialysis.[4]

24-hour food recall For this retrospective method, the patient is asked to list specific foods eaten in the previous 24 hours or, possibly, on specific days, such as dialysis days vs nondialysis days. The responses are evaluated for nutrient intake.[4,14] The KDOQI guidelines state that 24-hour recall may be considered as an alternative method for assessing dietary energy and protein intake.[4]

Food frequency questionnaire This retrospective questionnaire is used to establish how frequently a patient eats certain foods—ie, daily, weekly, or monthly. The food frequency questionnaire is helpful as a complement to food records/diary.[4]

Normalized protein catabolic rate This may be used as an alternative method for assessing protein intake in patients with CKD.[4]

24-hour urine collection This method is reliable for measuring urine urea nitrogen (UUN), sodium, and potassium in order to confirm accuracy of dietary intake estimates in nondialyzed patients with CKD.[4]

ANTHROPOMETRICS AND PHYSICAL EXAM

The NFPE provides information about the adequacy of a patient's weight status, nutritional status, and the distribution of body fat and lean muscle mass. The NFPE can be used to identify nutritional excesses or deficiencies in energy or somatic protein reserves. This is especially critical in patients with a chronic illness, such as CKD. These measurements can also be used to compare individuals to other population groups or to record changes in one person over time. These measurements include anthropometric measurements and physical exam.

ANTHROPOMETRIC AND OTHER MEASUREMENTS

Anthropometric and other measurements to assess body composition include weight, height, skeletal frame size, body mass index (BMI), skinfolds, circumferences, and creatinine kinetics.[4] These parameters should be routinely measured. Some advanced methods for measuring body composition may require special equipment and trained personnel, can be costly, and are seldom used outside of research facilities. These methods include bioelectrical impedance analysis (BIA) and dual-energy x-ray absorptiometry (DXA).[4,13-16]

Body Weight

Body weight (BW) can be difficult to determine in patients with CKD because as kidney function declines, the ability to eliminate excess fluid is lost. For patients being treated with kidney replacement therapies, the BW recorded and monitored over time should be obtained when body fluid compartment levels are balanced.[4] For patients who receive HD, this weight should be obtained after dialysis; for patients who receive peritoneal dialysis (PD), the weight is obtained after drainage of dialysate with the peritoneum empty. The KDOQI guidelines suggest that in adults with CKD stages 1 through 5D and in patients post transplant who are clinically stable, it is advisable to measure BW and BMI and monitor for changes in BW/BMI and body composition as needed[4]:

- At least monthly in patients requiring MHD and PD
- At least every 3 months in patients with CKD stages 4 and 5 and post transplant
- At least every 6 months in patients with CKD stages 1 through 3

Weight loss should be assessed and provided in terms of percent weight loss as follows[17]:

$$\% \text{ Weight Loss} = \left[\frac{(\text{Previous body weight} - \text{Current body weight})}{\text{Previous body weight}}\right] \times 100$$

If the patient is just starting dialysis, percentage of weight loss due to fluid removal needs to be established. Attempts should be made to determine the patient's usual body weight (UBW) prior to developing symptoms of uremia and CKD-associated edema. Once UBW has been established, the percent UBW should be calculated as follows:

$$\% \text{ Usual body weight} = \left(\frac{\text{Current body weight}}{\text{Usual body weight}}\right) \times 100$$

The percent UBW will indicate if there has been any weight loss that may indicate a decline in nutritional status.[4] Standard body weight (SBW) can be obtained using the Second National Health and Nutrition Examination Survey (NHANES II) (see Tables 2.1 through 2.4). The data are validated and standardized and use a large database of ethnically diverse groups. However, the data are given only on what individuals weigh, not on what they should weigh in order to reduce morbidity and mortality.[4] The desirable BW can be obtained using BMI (see section on Body Mass Index).

TABLE 2.1 | Standard Body Weights (kg) for Men Aged 25 Through 54 Years: Second National Health and Nutrition Examination Survey Data

Height (cm)	Frame size (kg)		
	Small	Medium	Large
157	64	68	82
160	61	71	83
163	66	71	84
165	66	74	79
168	67	75	84
170	71	77	84
173	71	78	86
175	74	78	89
178	75	81	87
180	76	81	91
183	74	84	91
185	79[a]	85	93
188	80[a]	88	92

[a] Estimated using linear regression formula.

Adapted with permission from Frisancho AR. New standards of weight and body composition by frame size and height for assessment of nutritional status of adults and the elderly. *Am J Clin Nutr.* 1984;40:808-819.

TABLE 2.2 | Standard Body Weights for Men Aged 55 Through 74 Years: Second National Health and Nutrition Examination Survey Data

Height (cm)	Frame size (kg)		
	Small	Medium	Large
157	61	68	77
160	62	70	80
163	63	71	77
165	70	72	79
168	68	74	80
170	69	78	85
173	70	78	83
175	75	77	84
178	76	80	87
180	69	84	84
183	76[a]	81	90
185	78[a]	88	88
188	77[a]	95	89

[a] Estimated using linear regression formula.

Adapted with permission from Frisancho AR. New standards of weight and body composition by frame size and height for assessment of nutritional status of adults and the elderly. *Am J Clin Nutr.* 1984;40:808-819.

TABLE 2.3 | Standard Body Weights for Women Aged 25 Through 54 Years: Second National Health and Nutrition Examination Survey Data

Height (cm)	Frame size (kg)		
	Small	Medium	Large
147	52	63	86
150	53	66	78
152	53	60	87
155	54	61	81
157	55	61	81
160	55	62	83
163	57	62	79
165	60	63	81
168	58	63	75
170	59	65	80
173	62	67	76
175	63[a]	68	79
178	64[a]	70	76

[a] Estimated using linear regression formula.

Adapted with permission from Frisancho AR. New standards of weight and body composition by frame size and height for assessment of nutritional status of adults and the elderly. *Am J Clin Nutr.* 1984;40:808-819.

TABLE 2.4 | Standard Body Weights for Women Aged 55 Through 74 Years: Second National Health and Nutrition Examination Survey Data

Height (cm)	Frame size (kg)		
	Small	Medium	Large
147	54	57	92
150	55	62	78
152	54	65	78
155	56	64	79
157	58	64	82
160	58	65	80
163	60	66	77
165	60	67	80
168	68	66	82
170	61[a]	72	80
173	61[a]	70	79
175	62[a]	72[a]	85[a]
178	63[a]	73[a]	85[a]

[a] Estimated using linear regression formula.

Adapted with permission from Frisancho AR. New standards of weight and body composition by frame size and height for assessment of nutritional status of adults and the elderly. *Am J Clin Nutr.* 1984;40:808-819.

There is much controversy about what is the "correct" weight to use when estimating a patient's energy and protein needs in the various stages of CKD. The Academy of Nutrition and Dietetics Evidence Analysis Library has outlined some of the key concerns and suggestions for clinical use. Certain ethnic groups living in the United States, for example, cannot be accurately assessed using some of the most common predictive formulas available.[13] Good clinical judgment may be the best guide for determining these values on an individual basis.[18,19] In individuals who are very obese or underweight, the use of current, unadjusted BW when determining actual nutrient intake or prescribing energy and protein needs may be inappropriate. The metabolic rate is lower for fat mass (FM) than for fat-free mass (FFM), and the task of achieving appropriate nutrient requirements is compounded in hospitalized and chronically ill patients.

Experts have suggested that 25% of excess BW above ideal/SBW is metabolically active tissue. However, no research evidence supports this adjustment in weight for use in CKD, and it may either overestimate or underestimate energy and protein requirements.[4] Adjusted body weight (ABW) equations are stated as references in the KDOQI Clinical Practice Guideline for Nutrition in CKD, and there is a lack of clinical evidence that supports one method over the other. The adjustment of BW is based on a theory; therefore, it is important that clinicians understand the debate and that these are potential methods in the literature that have been used. The use of these equations requires careful clinical interpretation and, if incorporated into the nutrition care plan, depends on clinical decisions, patient goals, and overall health status. ABW equations that have been used are listed below.[19]

Using IBW based on the Hamwi method

Adjusted body weight = Ideal body weight + [(Actual body weight – Ideal body weight) × 0.25]

Using SBW based on NHANES II data See Tables 2.1 through 2.4.

Adjusted body weight = Edema-free body weight + [(Standard body weight – Edema-free body weight) × 0.25]

Regardless of what source is used to determine the weight on which to assess the patient and make nutrition recommendations, amputations must be considered, and adjustments must be made as part of that assessment (see Table 2.5).[16] To estimate BW after amputation, consider the following:

Example: Preamputation body weight is 75.5 kg with one below-the-knee amputation:
75.5 kg × 5.9% = 4.5 kg
75.5 kg – 4.5 kg = 71 kg

TABLE 2.5 | Amputation Adjustments

Body segment	Average percentage (%) of total body weight
Entire arm	5.0
Forearm + hand	2.3
Entire leg	16.0
Thigh	10.1
Lower leg, below knee	5.9
Foot	1.5

Interdialytic Weight Gains

As kidney function diminishes, the body loses its ability to eliminate excess fluid. Patients who receive HD may gain several kilograms of fluid between treatments. This fluid gain is referred to as interdialytic weight gain (IDWG). When assessing the nutritional status of a patient on HD, it is important to assess IDWG. Excessive IDWG, a fluid gain of more than 4% to 4.5% of BW, reflects excessive fluid intake that can potentially cause false laboratory values and lead to hypertension, peripheral edema, worsening ascites, congestive heart failure, and pleural effusion.[20,21] Low IDWG reflects minimal fluid and food intake.[22] Low IDWG can also cause laboratory values to be falsely high due to dehydration. Adjustments in the estimated edema-free BW may be needed after careful inspection of both pre- and post-HD weights, IDWGs, and the treatment course. For example, a patient who gains minimal weight between treatments and consistently leaves the unit weighing less than his or her dry weight may be losing lean body mass (LBM) due to a suboptimal dietary intake, which will require a downward adjustment of edema-free BW.

Height

Initial measurement of height is essential. For patients who are unable to stand, recumbent bed height, arm span, demi–arm span (demi-span), height estimation from forearm, or knee height measurements may provide an estimate of stature.[23] Knee height correlates with stature and may be used to estimate height. A knee height caliper should be used to measure knee height. Measure the distance from the heel to the top of the knee on the outside of the left leg, and then use the following formulas[23]:

Male height = 64.19 – (0.04 × Age) + (2.02 × Knee height)
Female height = 84.88 – (0.24 × Age) + (1.83 × Knee height)

where height is measured in centimeters and age is measured in years.

Arm span is approximately equal to height in men and women, with an approximate variation in the results of up to 6%.[24] Fully extend the arms to the side so that they are parallel to the ground. Measure the distance from the tip of the middle finger on one hand to the tip of the middle finger on the other hand.[24] Demi-span is the distance from the middle of the sternal notch to the tip of the middle finger in the arm that does not have a dialysis access site. When measuring, the arm must be horizontal and level with the shoulders.[23] The following formulas are then used to calculate height[23]:

$$\text{Male height} = (1.40 \times \text{Demi-span}) + 57.8$$
$$\text{Female height} = (1.35 \times \text{Demi-span}) + 60.1$$

where height and demi-span are measured in centimeters.

Height can also be estimated from the forearm by measuring between the point of the elbow and the midpoint of the prominent bone of the wrist. These values are then used with a reference table to determine height.[23] Yearly measurement of height for those who can stand is important because decreasing stature may reflect bone disease.

Estimation of Frame Size

Frame size is determined using height and weight tables and may be estimated using either wrist circumference or elbow breadth.[16] A useful and quick procedure for estimating frame size is having the patients gauge themselves by encircling the nondominant wrist with the thumb and index finger of the dominant hand at the level of the radius and ulnar styloid process.[16]

- Small frame: Thumb and index finger overlap
- Medium frame: Thumb and index finger touch
- Large frame: Thumb and index finger do not touch

Body Mass Index

BMI is affected by muscle mass, FM, and bone. Deviations from expected levels for muscle mass can obfuscate the relationship between BMI and outcomes.[25] BMI can be calculated as follows[16]:

$$\text{Body mass index} = \frac{\text{Weight in kg}}{\text{Height in meters}^2}$$

or

$$\text{Body mass index} = \left(\frac{\text{Weight in lb}}{\text{Height in inches}^2} \right) \times 703$$

The World Health Organization defines standard weight status according to BMI ranges for adults. According to the KDOQI guidelines, the same standard should be used for patients with CKD as follows: <18.5 for underweight; 18.5 through 24.9 for normal (desirable) weight; 25.0 through 29.9 for overweight; and ≥30 for obese. However, these values may be lower for Asian populations.[4] In the general population, BMI of 30 or more is associated with increased morbidity and mortality, especially from cardiovascular disease (CVD).[26] In contrast, in patients with CKD stage 5D who receive HD, higher BMI is associated with lower mortality.[4,27,28] However, this obesity paradox has not been studied across all racial–ethnic subgroups and requires further examination to understand its pathophysiologic mechanisms and determine therapeutic targets for improved patient outcomes.[29]

Per KDOQI, underweight status (based on BMI) can be used to predict higher mortality for patients with CKD stage 5D who receive HD or PD. In patients with CKD post transplant, underweight and overweight/obesity status may be used to predict higher mortality. In patients with CKD stages 1 through 5D and post transplant, BMI alone is not sufficient to determine protein energy wasting (PEW) unless the BMI is very low (<18). In certain patients (eg, those with polycystic kidney disease), BMI measurement is not suitable.[4]

Waist Circumference

Abdominal fat deposition is associated with increased inflammation, PEW, and poorer outcomes in patients undergoing MHD.[30] Waist circumference, established by the Centers for Disease Control and Prevention, is another way to determine abdominal fat content and is an independent risk factor for CVD when disproportional to total body fat.[31] Waist circumference is determined by measuring the distance around the smallest area below the rib cage and above the umbilicus with a nonstretchable tape measure. High CVD risk is reported when the waist circumference is greater than 40 in (>101.6 cm) in males and 35 in (88.9 cm) in females.[32] In patients with CKD stage 5D, waist circumference may be used to assess abdominal obesity, but its reliability in assessing changes over time is low. Waist circumference is not suitable in certain patients such as those with polycystic kidney disease.[4]

Skinfold Thickness

Skinfold thickness is a well-established clinical method for measuring subcutaneous fat when edema is not present. Measurements, using good quality calipers, include the triceps, biceps, subscapular skinfolds, and iliac crest.[4] Measuring body fat stores helps to evaluate the patient's energy status, and tracking measurements over time can aid in early detection of malnutrition.

Excess fluid and the location of the vascular access may affect anthropometric measurements. For patients with CKD stage 5D, experts recommended that measurements be obtained after dialysis in the nonaccess arm. Triceps skinfold is often used in the CKD setting because it is a quick, convenient, and reliable general indicator of somatic reserves.

Conicity Index

Conicity index (CI) is a measure of abdominal obesity. According to the KDOQI standards, this measurement may be used in patients with CKD stage 5D on HD to assess nutritional status and as a predictor of mortality. CI is based on the following formula[4]:

$$\text{Conicity index} = \frac{\text{Waist circumference in meters}}{0.190 \times \sqrt{\text{Weight in kg/Height in meters}}}$$

Creatinine Kinetics

Creatinine kinetics may be used to estimate muscle mass in patients with CKD stage 5D. It is based on the principle that creatine production is in proportion to LBM and that, in steady state, creatinine production = creatine excretion (urinary and dialytic) + metabolic degradation.[33] However, this measurement is influenced by very high or very low dietary intake of meat and creatine supplements. In patients who receive HD, creatinine kinetics based on pre- and post-HD serum creatinine measurements is more reliable for patients who are anuric.[4] Other tools may assist with the evaluation of body composition in patients with CKD.[13] BIA is used to assess LBM, fat reserves, and total body water. DXA is used to measure bone, bone mineral content, FM, and LBM.[16,34] As mentioned previously, these methods are most often restricted to controlled studies and are not generally available in the routine clinical setting.

NUTRITION FOCUSED PHYSICAL EXAM

Physical signs of nutritional status can be assessed using a systematic head to toe examination of a patient's physical appearance. This includes a careful evaluation of hair, skin, nails, eyes, and mouth to uncover signs of malnutrition, nutrient deficiencies, or nutrient toxicities. Key nutrients of concern include the following[16]:

- protein (hair, skin, nails)
- vitamin A (eyes, gums, skin)
- iron (tongue, nails, inner eyelids)
- vitamin C (skin, gums, hair)
- zinc (hair, nails, skin)
- essential fatty acids (hair, skin, nails)
- vitamin B complex (lips, tongue)

Other components of the physical exam include assessment of muscle and fat stores. The main exam areas are as follows[16]:

- Subcutaneous fat loss: below the eyes, triceps/biceps
- Muscle loss: temple, clavicle, shoulder, scapula, interosseous muscle, knee, quadriceps, calf

Finally, assessing the presence of edema involves examination and palpitation of the extremities. Evaluation for peripheral edema is important, especially in the dialysis setting for quantifying weight loss in view of fluctuating fluid balance.[16]

For additional instruction on the NFPE, see the video *How to Perform a Nutrition Focused Physical Exam* by Iowa State University Dietetic Internship (available at https://.vimeo.com/174861683).

Energy and Nutrient Requirements

Nutrient requirements must be individually assessed based on the patient's stage of CKD, comorbid conditions, age, activity level, and body size. To determine daily energy expenditure, indirect calorimetry is the gold standard for clinical practice. However, indirect calorimetry requires a steady-state protocol to measure resting energy expenditure (REE). Because achieving strict criteria for a steady-state interval may be difficult for patients who receive MHD, due to discomfort either from the test itself or their health status, the determination of steady state may be abbreviated from 10 minutes to 5 minutes.[35]

When indirect calorimetry cannot be performed in a clinical setting, a valid predictive energy formula is of utmost importance. The following two predictive energy equations are specific to patients who receive HD:

Byham-Gray et al[36]

$$\text{Resting energy expenditure} = \\ 404.58 + 15.44 \text{ (Fat free mass)} - 6.62 \text{ (Age)} + \\ 194.45 \text{ (Albumin)} + 4.58 \text{ (C-reactive protein)}$$

For this equation, note that FFM was measured in kg, age in years, albumin in g/dL, and C-reactive protein in mg/dL.

Vilar et al[37]

$$\text{Resting energy expenditure} = \\ -2.497 \times \text{Age} \times \text{Factor}_{age} + 0.011 \times \text{Height}^{2.023} + \\ 83.573 \times \text{Weight}^{0.6291} + 68.171 \times \text{Factor}_{sex}$$

For this equation, note that Factor_{age} is 0 if age is <65 years or 1 if ≥65 years; height is measured in centimeters, weight in kg; Factor_{sex} is 0 if female or 1 if male.

While it is reasonable to use these disease-specific predictive energy equations to assess REE in the absence of indirect calorimetry for CKD stage 5D, evidence-based guidelines recommend estimating energy needs in CKD stages 1 through 5D or post transplant in patients who are metabolically stable using a kilocalorie per kilogram formula (see Table 2.6).[4]

TABLE 2.6 | Energy Needs for Individuals With Kidney Disease[16,38]

Type of kidney disease	Energy needs (kcal/kg)	Notes
Acute[a]	20-30	Depends on stress/nutritional status
Chronic kidney disease	25-35	
Hemodialysis	25-35	
Peritoneal dialysis	25-35	Includes dialysate kilocalories
Transplant[b]	23-35	Maintain desirable body weight, limit fat to 30% of kilocalories

[a] See reference 38.
[b] See reference 16.

Biochemical Parameters

Clinicians need to monitor several biochemical parameters on an ongoing basis to assess the nutritional status of patients with CKD (see Table 2.7).[16] Laboratory results guide the nutrition professional in managing the patient. To ensure accuracy, protocols must be followed when blood samples are obtained and handled. For example, when drawing blood for evaluating serum potassium levels, it is important that the blood does not hemolyze or the value will be falsely elevated. Reference ranges are established to indicate when a value for a laboratory test is within the range for good health. Values above or below these ranges require further inspection. The clinical staff must determine the cause and take steps to manage the abnormality. The reference ranges for CKD in this book are set by the KDOQI and Kidney Disease Improving Global Outcomes (KDIGO) guidelines (see Table 2.7). Individual laboratories have their own "normal" reference laboratory values based on their particular procedures and laboratory equipment. These reference ranges typically do not correlate with CKD ranges as they are set for "healthy" individuals. The RDN evaluates the results of the following laboratory tests to determine the nutritional status in the patient with CKD.

TABLE 2.7 | Summary of Biochemical Parameters for Chronic Kidney Disease[16]

Test	Normal range	Chronic kidney disease range
Creatinine	Male: 0.6-1.2 mg/dL Female: 0.5-1.01 mg/dL	2-15 mg/dL (based on muscle mass, glomerular filtration rate/dialysis)
Albumin	3.5-5.5 g/dL	Within normal limits for laboratory, goal >4 g/dL
Transthyretin (prealbumin)	15-36 mg/dL	≥30 mg/dL
C-reactive protein (CRP)	<0.5 mg/dL	Same
Transferrin saturation	Male: 20%-50% Female: 15%-50%	Consider iron supplementation when <30%
Glucose	74-106 mg/dL fasting	Within normal limits; ≤200 nonfasting
Parathyroid hormone (PTH), intact	10-65 pg/mL	2-9 times upper normal limit; avoid extremes
Calcium	9-10.5 mg/dL	Within normal limits (Avoid sustained levels above lab normal)
Phosphorus	3.0-4.5 mg/dL	Lower toward normal range chronic kidney disease stage 3-5D
Alkaline phosphatase	36-92 U/L	Within normal limits
Vitamin D 25-hydroxy-cholecalciferol	15-80 ng/mL	Unknown, but ≥20 ng/mL
Potassium	3.5-5.0 mEq/L	Within normal limits (<6.0 mEq/L predialysis)
Sodium	136-145 mEq/L	Within normal limits
Cholesterol	<150-199 mg/dL	No specific therapeutic range recommended
Triglycerides (dialysis: usually nonfasting)	Male: 40-160 mg/dL Female: 35-135 mg/dL	<500 mg/dL
Hemoglobin	Male: 14-17 g/dL Female: 12-16 g/dL	~9-11 g/dL Variable based on patient's needs, symptoms, risks Food and Drug Administration <11 g/dL
Iron	Male: 80-180 mcg/dL Female: 60-160 mcg/dL	Within normal limits
Ferritin	Male: 12-300 ng/mL Female: 10-150 ng/mL	Peritoneal dialysis/chronic kidney disease ≥100 ng/mL Hemodialysis 200-500 ng/mL Kidney Disease Improving Global Outcomes (KDIGO): consider iron supplement if serum levels drop below stated range
Blood urea nitrogen (BUN)	10-20 mg/dL	Variable; typically above normal range
Adequacy • hemodialysis • peritoneal dialysis		Kt/V ≥1.2 (minimally adequate) Kt/V ≥1.7

KIDNEY FUNCTION

Serum Creatinine

Creatinine, which has large daily intravariation, is the nitrogenous waste product from the metabolism of creatine in muscle and from dietary meat intake. It is a sensitive marker of kidney function (ie, serum creatinine level increases as kidney function declines). The body produces creatinine at a constant rate proportional to body muscle mass.[39]

In kidney failure, once the dialysis regimen has been established, creatinine values plateau to a steady state. A sudden increase of creatinine along with a change in blood urea nitrogen (BUN), blood pressure, or serum potassium levels may reflect a need to assess dialysis access status or consider a change in the dialysis treatment plan. A decrease in serum creatinine over time may reflect a loss of LBM. When changes in serum creatinine occur, clinicians should investigate weight loss, amputations, residual kidney function, patient adherence to the dialysis prescription, and changes in treatment plans.

Glomerular Filtration Rate

The glomerular filtration rate (GFR) is the amount of glomerular filtrate formed per minute based on the total kidney surface area available for filtration (number of functioning glomeruli). The approximate normal value for GFR is 130 mL/min/1.73 m^2 for men and 120 mL/min/1.73 m^2 for women, but the value differs even among normal individuals. Estimated GFR (eGFR) reflects kidney function and predicts the onset of CKD.[39] The use of race has been omitted as a variable in the new eGFR calculations. The National Kidney Foundation (NKF) and American Society of Nephrology (ASN) taskforce concluded that the new equation that includes creatinine and cystatin C is a better predictor of eGFR across Black and non-Black individuals than either creatinine or cystatin C alone. The NKF website (www.kidney.org/professionals/KDOQI/gfr_calculator) and app (www.kidney.org/apps/professionals/egfr-calculator) include the following eGFR calculators:

- CKD-EPI creatinine equation (2021)–preferred method

- CKD-EPI creatinine-cystatin equation (2012)
- CKD-EPI cystatin C equation (2012)

GFR decreases 10% for each decade after the age of 30 years, and the human body can sustain a significant decrease in this function before there are any discernible symptoms. As GFR decreases to less than 40 mL/min/1.73 m^2 to 50 mL/min/1.73 m^2, the amount of toxins in the blood and body tissues accumulates. These toxins are responsible for the following symptoms:

- nausea
- vomiting
- itching
- malaise
- anorexia
- bone and heart disease
- increased blood pressure
- edema
- acidosis
- cardiac arrhythmias
- sleep disturbances

A decrease in GFR to less than 15 mL/min/1.73 m^2 indicates CKD stage 5 or kidney failure. Clinicians should base the decision to start dialysis on the signs and symptoms of uremia, evidence of PEW, and the ability to safely manage metabolic abnormalities and volume overload with medical therapy, rather than on a specific level of kidney function in the absence of such signs and symptoms.[20]

SERUM PROTEINS

Proteins in plasma and extravascular fluids approximate 3% of total body protein; however, visceral organ protein constitutes approximately 10%. Since albumin and other plasma proteins are synthesized in the liver, plasma proteins can be thought of as functional indexes of hepatic protein status. Although serum hepatic proteins have been associated with nutritional status, evidence demonstrates that inflammation affects hepatic protein metabolism. Therefore, in the presence of inflammation, serum hepatic protein levels do not necessarily reflect nutritional status and protein intake, nor do they accurately measure nutritional repletion.[41]

Serum Albumin

Albumin is a measure of total body protein, both muscle and visceral. It is a good prognostic indicator and may be considered as a complimentary tool for assessing nutritional status.[4] With a long half-life (averaging 14–21 days) and a large body pool (4–5 mg/kg), serum albumin may not give an accurate measure of the patient's actual protein status. Serum albumin is a negative acute-phase reactant, meaning that its production is negatively influenced by situations that may cause inflammation and by stress, including dialysis.[41] Therefore, low serum albumin in isolation is not sufficient to assess nutritional status but may be used as a predictor of higher risk for hospitalization and mortality.[4] Interpretation of serum levels is greatly impacted by fluid status. Low levels of serum albumin may be found in the following situations[16]:

- decreased protein production: malnutrition, malabsorption, chronic liver disease (eg, cirrhosis), or when an acute-phase response occurs
- increased protein loss: protein-losing states (eg, nephrotic syndrome, protein-losing enteropathy), severe burns, malabsorption and during operative procedures
- redistribution: during sepsis, albumin may be lost to the extravascular compartment due to increased vascular permeability, and in ascites, albumin is lost to the abdominal cavity (this may require paracentesis)
- increased peritoneal permeability: a greater loss of albumin occurs across the peritoneal membrane; thus, protein needs are higher in PD than in HD (Note: in the event of peritonitis, losses may be increased as much as tenfold due to inflammation, and this condition can continue for a few months after the infection resolves.)

Oncotic pressure, which is maintained by albumin, is responsible for the transport of drugs, hormones, enzymes, minerals, and trace elements. When the protein content of plasma is exceptionally low (low oncotic pressure), water can shift into the interstitial spaces, causing edema.[42] Elevated serum albumin levels may reflect dehydration. Therefore, it is important to include the patient's hydration status in the overall nutrition assessment.

Serum Prealbumin (Transthyretin)

Serum prealbumin is another plasma protein that may be used to assess protein status. It is a transport protein for thyroid hormones and is bound to retinol. Compared with serum albumin, serum prealbumin has a much shorter half-life (2–3 days) and a smaller body pool. However, similar to albumin, it should not be interpreted in isolation to assess nutritional status since it is influenced by nonnutritional factors.[4] It is less affected by liver disease or hydration status, but in patients with CKD, the transthyretin level may be falsely high due to decreased kidney catabolism.

SERUM GLUCOSE

Glucose is the principal energy source in the body. The blood level fluctuates with food intake and insulin action. The criteria for the diagnosis of diabetes mellitus include a fasting plasma glucose (FPG) level of 126 mg/dL or greater, glycated hemoglobin (HbA1c) of greater than or equal to 6.5%, 2-hour plasma glucose of greater than or equal to 200 mg/dL during an oral glucose tolerance test, or a random plasma glucose of greater than or equal to 200 mg/dL in a patient with classic symptoms of hyperglycemia or hyperglycemic crisis.[43] Other factors that may influence glucose include chronic hepatic problems, hyperthyroidism, malignancy, acute stress, emotional distress, burns, diabetic acidosis, pancreatic insufficiency, and PD. Low glucose levels may indicate hyperinsulinemia, alcohol abuse, pancreatic tumors, liver failure, pituitary dysfunction, malnutrition, and extreme exercise.[16] There is also an increased risk of hypoglycemia in CKD stages 3 through 5 due to decreased kidney clearance of insulin and some of the oral agents used to treat diabetes mellitus and impaired kidney gluconeogenesis.[44] Refer to Chapter 9 for more information on diabetes mellitus.

HbA1c (hemoglobin to which glucose is bound) cannot be reversed. There is a strong correlation between elevations in plasma glucose and HbA1c.[45] The formula for estimated average glucose based on HbA1c is as follows[46]:

$$\text{Estimated average glucose mg/dL} = 28.7 \times \text{Hemoglobin A1c} - 46.7$$

Since HbA1c is indicative of the long-term regulation of plasma glucose, it is used to measure the effectiveness of diabetes therapy. However, any factor that shortens the life span of the erythrocyte, such as CKD, also reduces HbA1c. In patients with CKD, HbA1c should be interpreted considering the potentially shortened erythrocyte survival time, blood loss, and hemolysis.[16] KDOQI recommends a therapeutic target HbA1c of ~7.0% for patients with CKD to prevent or delay the progression of diabetic kidney disease and other complications associated with diabetes mellitus.[44] However, the use of HbA1c is not currently recommended to diagnose diabetes mellitus in patients with CKD because the association between FPG and HbA1c in individuals with mild glucose intolerance or normal glucose tolerance is less clear.[47]

CHRONIC KIDNEY DISEASE MINERAL AND BONE DISORDER

Chronic kidney disease mineral and bone disorder (CKD–MBD) is a systemic disorder manifested by either one or a combination of the following[48]:

- abnormalities of calcium, phosphorus, parathyroid hormone (PTH), or vitamin D metabolism
- abnormalities in bone turnover, mineralization, volume, linear growth, or strength
- vascular or other soft tissue calcification

CKD–MBD is a complex disorder integrating calcium, phosphorus, PTH, and vitamin D and requires close monitoring of these parameters for proper management. KDIGO guidelines recommend that clinicians base therapeutic decisions on trends, rather than on a single laboratory value.[2] Refer to Chapter 10 for more details about bone and mineral metabolism.

Parathyroid Hormone

PTH is secreted by the parathyroid gland and regulates bone physiology. PTH acts directly on kidney and bone and indirectly on the GI tract through its effects on synthesis of 1,25-dihydroxycholecalciferol to regulate calcium. An optimal level of PTH in CKD stages 3 through 5D is not known; however, patients with PTH levels progressively rising or persistently above the upper normal limit for the assay are at risk for secondary hyperparathyroidism.[49]

Vitamin D

Vitamin D helps maintain calcium homeostasis by increasing absorption in the GI tract and must be in the active form to make this reaction occur. Vitamin D (cholecalciferol) needs two hydroxyl groups added to create the active form 1,25-dihydroxycholecalciferol (or calcitriol), with hydroxylation taking place in the liver and the kidney. As CKD progresses, the prevalence of both 25-hydroxyvitamin D3 and 1,25-dihydroxyvitamin D3 deficiency increases. The prevalence of 25-hydroxyvitamin D3 deficiency remains relatively stable until the eGFR falls below 30 mL/min/1.73 m^2, while 1,25-dihydroxyvitamin D3 deficiency is evident at all reduced eGFR levels.[50] A decrease in vitamin D levels, in turn, diminishes the absorption of calcium in the GI tract. When the parathyroid gland recognizes a low serum calcium level, it triggers the parathyroid to secrete its hormone, causing the release of calcium from the bone.[51]

Calcium

Calcium is the most abundant mineral in the human body. It comprises approximately 1.5% to 2% of BW and 39% of all body minerals. Ninety-nine percent of calcium exists in the bones and teeth. The remaining 1% acts as a cation in the extracellular fluids. Total plasma calcium has three components: protein-bound 47%, ionized (free) 43%, and complexed 10%. The extent of protein binding varies with protein concentrations and pH. The calcium in the fluid surrounding muscle fibers regulates muscle contraction. Calcium ions enable nerve conduction and are a factor in the blood-clotting cascade. Calcium is also a cofactor for many enzyme reactions; it is a hormone trigger, and it acts in energy coupling cycles.[51] The majority of protein-bound calcium is attached to albumin. A low serum albumin results in low serum calcium, without a change in ionized calcium. Corrected calcium offers no superiority over total calcium alone and is less specific than ionized calcium measurements. Since ionized calcium is not available routinely and is not considered to be practical or cost effective, total calcium is adequate for routine monitoring.[2]

Phosphorus

Phosphorus is a critical mineral. In the body, 85% of phosphate is combined with calcium to form bone tissue. Less than 1% is found in the extracellular fluid. The remainder is found in the intracellular soft tissue, particularly in muscle. This mineral is vital to energy production and storage and is a component of fats, proteins, and cell membranes. Phosphorus control is maintained in the body by PTH, calcitriol, and fibroblast growth factor-23 (FGF23).[50]

A high serum phosphorus poses substantial health risks, making it a major issue in the overall nutrition assessment of patients with CKD. In a study of patients with CKD stages 3 through 5 who were not on dialysis, elevated serum phosphorus was a predictive factor for coronary artery calcification.[49,52] As kidney function decreases, the body loses its ability to adequately filter excess phosphorus into the urine, and it begins to accumulate in the blood. As the level increases, PTH is released, which then stimulates calcium to be released from bone.

It is important to diminish GI absorption of phosphorus by applying a dietary phosphorus restriction and by dosing phosphate binders at the time of food ingestion. Phosphate binders will form an insoluble complex, and the phosphorus will be excreted in the stool.[50] An estimate of phosphorus that must be controlled by binders is equal to the amount of phosphorus absorbed (50%–60% of intake) minus the amount of phosphorus removed during dialysis. The amount of phosphorus removed with dialysis depends on dialyzer clearance and dialysis frequency, duration, and modality. It is imperative that patients on dialysis be diligent with their phosphate binder regimen and dietary phosphorus restriction to manage phosphorus retention.

It is also important to consider that when patients are eating poorly, their phosphorus levels may fall below normal. In this case, phosphate binders should be discontinued, and phosphorus repletion may be required if the depletion is severe.

ELECTROLYTES

Potassium

Potassium is the primary intracellular cation. Extracellular potassium influences muscle activity, especially the cardiac muscle.[53] Hypokalemia (<3.5 mEq/L) or hyperkalemia (>5.5 mEq/L) may induce muscle weakness and cardiac arrhythmia. Hyperkalemia may cause cardiac arrest. The kidneys are the major route of elimination for this ion. When this ability decreases, there is an obvious increase in the serum levels. Possible nondietary causes of hyperkalemia include the following[16]:

- metabolic acidosis (low serum CO_2 level)
- high serum glucose: shift between cell and serum
- insulin deficiency or resistance (in persons with diabetes mellitus)
- inadequate dialysis
- dialysate potassium concentration (ie, too high)
- drug content or interactions (eg, effects of β-blocking drugs or drugs inhibiting aldosterone, angiotensin-converting enzyme (ACE), or distal nephron sodium reabsorption, such as ACE inhibitors or potassium-sparing diuretics, cyclosporine, tacrolimus, or severe digitalis toxicity)
- tissue destruction (eg, rhabdomyolysis, burns, and tumor lysis syndrome)
- catabolism/starvation (ie, cell breakdown and release of potassium into serum)

- concomitant disease (eg, Addison disease and sickle cell anemia)
- chronic constipation
- infection
- GI bleeding
- blood transfusion

The validity of laboratory values should also be checked, especially if the blood sample is hemolyzed. If the blood sample was hemolyzed, there would be lysis of the red blood cells (RBCs) and all the potassium inside the cells would be mixed with the serum, giving a falsely elevated result.

Sodium

Sodium is the principal extracellular cation responsible for fluid homeostasis. Functions of sodium include preservation of normal muscle function and maintenance of acid-base balance, osmotic pressure of body fluids, and permeability of cells. With advancing nephron loss in patients with CKD, the atrial natriuretic peptides lose their effectiveness, and sodium retention results in intravascular volume expansion, edema, and worsening hypertension.[53]

The serum sodium level is not a reliable indicator of sodium intake or sodium status in patients with CKD. Fluid retention (edema) due to decreased urine production can mask an elevated total body sodium level, thereby causing the serum level to appear normal. Serum levels must be interpreted in conjunction with the patient's current fluid status.

LIPIDS

Lipid abnormalities are common in patients with CKD and depend on several risk factors, including GFR level, diabetes mellitus, severity of proteinuria, immunosuppressive agents, dialysis modality, other comorbidities, and nutritional status.[16] A lipid profile is recommended for patients newly diagnosed with CKD, but follow-up measurement of lipids is not required for the majority of patients.[54] Refer to Chapter 11 for more details concerning dyslipidemias in kidney disease.

Cholesterol

Cholesterol is essential for the development of cell membranes and hormones. Low-density lipoprotein (LDL) is often called "bad" cholesterol because high serum levels are thought to contribute to heart disease. High-density lipoprotein (HDL) is often called "good" cholesterol because it removes LDL. Low or declining serum total cholesterol to less than 100 mg/dL in patients with CKD is associated with protein–energy malnutrition, increased mortality risk, acute infection, and inflammation.[55] Medical treatment goals and the influence of lipid-lowering medications and sevelamer (a phosphate binder that has been shown to lower serum cholesterol levels) should also be considered when evaluating low total cholesterol levels.[56] High cholesterol is associated with nephrotic syndrome, glucocorticoid use, excessive saturated fat intake, and disorders of lipid metabolism.[16]

Triglycerides

A triglyceride is composed of three fatty acids joined to a glycerol side chain. Triglycerides are neutral and insoluble (hydrophobic). These neutral fats can be transported safely in the blood and stored in the fat cell (adipocyte) as an energy reserve. Excess levels of these fats in the serum may indicate a metabolic abnormality that can contribute to CVD.[57] Risk factors for high triglyceride levels include liver disease, gout, pancreatitis, nephrotic syndrome, diabetes mellitus, steroid use, PD, and excessive alcohol use. Low values of these fats in the serum are seen in malnutrition and malabsorption.[16]

ANEMIA MANAGEMENT

Pathophysiology

Anemia is one of the major clinical pathologic conditions associated with CKD. It is a common complication and contributes to increased morbidity and mortality in patients with CKD. Renal anemia is typically an isolated hypoproliferative anemia with no leukopenia or thrombocytopenia.[58] The RBCs are normocytic (ie,

RBC volume is normal) and also normochromic (ie, normal concentration and quantity of hemoglobin), although the span and the rate of RBC production is reduced.[58] Inflammation and iron treatment can stimulate hepcidin, decreasing GFR and the opposing suppressive effects of erythropoietin and erythroferrone on hepcidin production. When plasma hepcidin concentrations are high, this causes decreased ferroportin on cell membranes, thus inhibiting duodenal iron absorption and diminishing iron availability for erythropoiesis.

Anemia is more frequent in patients with lower GFR, especially those with advanced kidney disease requiring long-term dialysis.[59] In patients who have CKD-associated anemia (regardless of age and CKD stage), the following tests are recommended during initial evaluation of the anemia[60]:

- complete blood count
- absolute reticulocyte count
- serum ferritin level
- serum transferrin saturation (TSAT)
- serum vitamin B12 and folate levels

Anemia typically develops independently of the cause of kidney disease; however, there are some exceptions. Patients with diabetes mellitus develop anemia more frequently in the earlier stages of CKD and are more severely dependent on the level of kidney impairment. Conversely, in patients with polycystic kidney disease, hemoglobin (Hgb) is on average higher than in other patients with similar degrees of kidney failure, and polycythemia may occasionally develop.[58]

Hematological Parameters and Therapy

Hemoglobin (Hgb), a conjugated protein-containing four heme groups and globin, is the oxygen-carrying pigment of the erythrocytes. In normal circumstances, erythrocytes are produced by the bone marrow and released into circulation, where they survive for approximately 120 days. The hormone erythropoietin (EPO), produced by the kidney and the liver, is one of the main triggers for production of erythrocytes. In anemia associated with CKD, there can be insufficient production and release of the glycoprotein hormone EPO by kidney glomerular epithelial cells. A failure of EPO production can occur in response to chronically reduced Hgb concentrations and decreased oxygen sensing in kidney EPO producing cells.[58,59] EPO induces erythroid precursor cells to differentiate, causing an increase in new RBC production. An undersecretion of EPO contributes to a suppression of an essential signal that triggers RBC production.[61,62] When this hormone is lacking, production of erythrocytes is diminished. Erythrocytes carry oxygen to all of the other cells in the body; so when their number decreases, the resulting anemia increases, and the signs and symptoms are exacerbated. For adult patients with CKD, the KDIGO guidelines suggest that erythropoiesis-stimulating agent (ESA) therapy be initiated when Hgb is less than 10 g/dL. ESA therapy should not be used to maintain Hgb levels greater than 11.5 g/dL and/or be used to intentionally increase the Hgb concentration over 13 g/dL.[63]

An ESA is a synthetic exogenous agent that enhances the process of erythropoiesis in the absence of sufficient EPO and has greatly reduced the anemia of dialysis. Before ESA therapy is considered in patients with CKD, it is essential to exclude and correct any other cause of anemia other than EPO deficiency, such as hematinic deficiencies, which commonly include inadequate levels of iron, folate, and vitamin B12.[58]

Despite adequate vitamin and mineral intake, some patients may not respond appropriately to EPO therapy. The causes of inadequate response may include the following[64]:

- iron deficiency, including chronic blood loss or iron malabsorption
- infection or inflammation
- malnutrition, including folate or vitamin B12 deficiency
- aluminum toxicity
- severe secondary hyperparathyroidism
- hemoglobinopathies (ie, sickle cell anemia, α- and β-thalassemia)
- malignancies
- hemolysis
- pure RBC aplasia

Following strict protocols, patients receive varying doses of ESA based on serum values of Hgb and iron.[63]

Emerging strategies for managing anemia include hypoxia-inducible factor prolyl hydroxylase (HIF-PH) enzyme inhibitors, a new class of agents which stimulates endogenous EPO production by the liver.[65] A common complication of EPO is an elevation of blood pressure due to the increased blood viscosity from increased RBC mass. This existence or exacerbation of hypertension is not a contraindication to ESA therapy, but it should be treated with more aggressive pharmacologic therapy, increased ultrafiltration on dialysis, or a decrease in the ESA dose (sometimes all three simultaneously) to allow for physiologic vasomotor adaptation.[66]

Iron The most commonly encountered reversible cause of chronic anemia in patients with CKD, other than anemia related directly to CKD, is iron deficiency anemia.[58] Iron is an essential ingredient for heme synthesis, and adequate amounts of this mineral are required for the manufacture of new RBCs. Iron in the adult human body is found in two major pools: (a) functional iron in Hgb, myoglobin, and enzymes, and (b) storage iron in ferritin, hemosiderin, and transferrin.[67] Under enhanced erythropoietic stimulation, greater amounts of iron are used, and many patients with CKD have inadequate stores of available iron to satisfy the increased demands of the bone marrow. Iron absorption capacity in patients with CKD is considerably lower than in nonuremic individuals, particularly in the presence of systemic inflammation.[63] Additional contributing factors include the following[68]:

- folic acid deficiency
- aluminum toxicity
- vitamin B12 deficiency
- menstrual bleeding
- GI bleeding
- inadequate nutrient intake
- inadequate absorption of iron
- secondary and tertiary hyperparathyroidism
- use of certain medications (ie, renin-angiotensin-aldosterone system [RAAS] inhibitors)

Due to the anemia associated with CKD and the use of ESA, there is an increased need for supplemental iron. Per KDIGO guidelines, iron supplementation should be selected based on the potential benefits (ie, reducing the number of blood transfusions or avoiding blood transfusions, minimizing ESA therapy, or limiting symptoms from anemia) vs the risks concerning reactions to the supplementation. Intravenous (IV) iron should be administered to restore and maintain iron stores for patients who receive HD, unless there is a documented allergic reaction. The route of iron administration can be either IV or oral in patients with CKD who are not on dialysis or who are on PD or home HD.[63]

Oral iron is usually prescribed in three divided doses and is best absorbed on an empty stomach. This is especially true because iron is easily bound to phosphate binders taken with meals. Therefore, it is recommended that traditional oral iron supplements be taken 2 hours apart from meals and phosphate binders.[65] In patients with CKD who do not receive dialysis, oral iron supplementation is often ineffective due to inadequate absorption and resulting GI intolerance. The KDIGO guidelines suggest that a 1- to 3-month supplementation of oral iron therapy can be administered initially as an alternative to IV therapy.[63] The development of absorbable iron-based phosphate binders provides the opportunity to replete iron stores and bind phosphorus.[69] Iron-based phosphate binders are taken with meals and may have fewer GI side effects.[69,70]

Ferritin Serum ferritin represents iron that is stored in cells and can be extracted for release. Under steady-state conditions, the serum ferritin level correlates with total body iron stores, making serum ferritin a relevant estimate of iron stores.[63] In patients with CKD, iron tends to be held in the storage pool but is not readily available for erythropoiesis. In such cases, the transferrin saturation and serum ferritin may be normal, and serum ferritin actually underestimates iron needs.[62] Elevated ferritin levels may indicate iron overload, which sometimes occurs when patients have received blood transfusions or IV iron. However, ferritin is an acute-phase reactant, so elevated levels may also be a marker of inflammation rather than iron overload. For patients with CKD who do not receive dialysis and for patients on PD, the lower limit of normal for ferritin is 100 ng/mL. The range for ferritin for patients who receive HD is 200 to 500 ng/mL.[63]

KDIGO provides extensive guidelines for monitoring and adjusting IV iron dosing in the management of iron status and anemia based on percent transferrin saturation and serum ferritin levels.[63]

Transferrin saturation Percent transferrin saturation (%TSAT) is determined by the following formula:

$$\text{Percent transferrin saturation} = \left(\frac{\text{Serum iron}}{\text{Total iron binding capacity}} \right) \times 100$$

TSAT reflects the iron that is available for erythropoiesis and is useful in determining the need for iron agents. A TSAT of less than 30% indicates a need for iron supplementation. The KDIGO guidelines do not recommend the routine use of iron supplementation in patients with TSAT greater than 30% or serum ferritin greater than 500 ng/mL because the benefits and the risks of doing so have not been thoroughly explored. Ferritin and %TSAT are the best available measures of body iron stores.[63]

DIALYSIS ADEQUACY

Numerous studies have demonstrated a correlation between morbidity and mortality and the delivered dose of dialysis. The preferred method for measuring on a monthly basis the delivered dose of HD is formal urea kinetic modeling (UKM). Other methods may be used if they produce similar results and do not significantly overestimate the modeled dose.[20] Clinical practice guidelines recommend that PD UKM be measured within 1 month of treatment and at least once every 4 months thereafter.[71]

Blood Urea Nitrogen

Urea is a product of protein catabolism. Since urea nitrogen is readily measurable in serum, BUN (sometimes referred to as serum urea nitrogen) is the most frequently assessed parameter for calculating dialysis dose and adequacy in patients who receive dialysis.[20]

Elevation of this value may indicate the following[16]:
- high dietary protein intake
- GI bleeding
- decreased clearance of dialysis
- dehydration
- increased catabolism

Decreased BUN may indicate the following:
- low dietary protein intake
- loss of protein due to emesis or diarrhea
- protein anabolism
- overhydration
- hepatic failure
- residual kidney function

Due to these multiple factors affecting serum levels, BUN cannot be used in isolation to assess adequacy of nutritional status or adequacy of HD.

Kt/V

Kt/V is best described by KDOQI as "the fractional clearance of urea as a function of its distribution volume."[20] K represents the delivered dialyzer urea clearance measured in L/min plus residual kidney clearance unless the patient is anuric, t is the treatment time (in minutes), and V is the patient's volume (in mL) of the distribution of urea.

UKM calculations are performed by the laboratory or by software applications. Practitioners should measure the delivered dose of dialysis to ensure that patients receive the prescribed and most adequate dose of dialysis for their condition, body size, and residual kidney function. Interpretation may vary, depending on treatment modality (see Chapters 5, 6, and 7). If dialysis adequacy is not achieved, then the treatment plan must be adjusted.[20,71]

As an added benefit, Kt/V provides another important tool in the nutrition assessment of the patient receiving dialysis: normalized protein nitrogen appearance (nPNA). This mathematical representation may not be valid to assess the amount of daily protein intake in patients who receive dialysis, but it may be a useful measure of net protein degradation, and is predictive of morbidity and mortality.[72,73]

Urea Reduction Ratio

Urea reduction ratio (URR) is used to assess adequacy of HD. It is a simple measure of the change in urea concentration between pre- and post-HD blood tests. It has been shown to be a statistically significant predictor of mortality. However, it does not account for the ultrafiltration factor in the final delivered dose of dialysis or residual kidney function and it does not allow for determination of nPNA.[20] The following formula is used to calculate the URR:

$$\text{Urea reduction ratio} = \left(\frac{\text{Pre-BUN} - \text{Post-BUN}}{\text{Pre-BUN}} \right) \times 100$$

Nutrition Assessment Tools

Nutrition professionals should consider several nutritional parameters when assessing the nutritional status of a patient with CKD. No parameter by itself is useful in predicting nutritional status or malnutrition; therefore, it is important to view several parameters together.

Several tools have been validated for predicting malnutrition in patients with CKD, including subjective global assessment (SGA), malnutrition–inflammation score (MIS), and handgrip strength. In addition, the PEW score is a screening tool for determining the risk of PEW. In a study of patients who receive HD, both the 7-point SGA and the PEW score could identify PEW risk. While the 7-point SGA was more specific, the PEW score was more sensitive. Therefore, some patients with PEW risk may be missed if the 7-point SGA is used as the only diagnostic tool for identifying PEW risk because of its lower sensitivity than the PEW score.[74]

SUBJECTIVE GLOBAL ASSESSMENT

SGA was originally developed to assess the nutritional status of surgical patients.[75] SGA provides a nutritional score based on two components: a medical history and a physical assessment. The medical history includes

progression of weight loss, eating habits, GI symptoms, physiological functioning, and simple analysis of metabolic stress. The physical assessment includes loss of subcutaneous fat and muscle mass (see section on Nutrition Focused Physical Exam). After evaluation, the patient is scored as either well nourished (A), mild to moderately malnourished (B), or severely malnourished (C).[15] The SGA has since been validated in a variety of patient populations, including CKD, as a predictor of malnutrition and relative risk of death.[16,76] The point rating system has been adapted to the following 7-point scale, instead of an ABC scale, for more accuracy and sensitivity to change.[4,16]

- 6 or 7 = very mild nutritional risk to well nourished
- 3, 4, or 5 = mild to moderately malnourished
- 1 or 2 = severely malnourished

The KDOQI guidelines recognize SGA as a valid and clinically useful measure of protein–energy nutritional status in the maintenance of patients who receive dialysis.[4] The KDOQI guidelines also suggest use of a four-item 7-point scale. The medical history reviews weight change during the previous 6 months, dietary intake, and GI symptoms. The physical exam includes visual assessment of subcutaneous tissue and muscle mass. SGA is beneficial because it is a cost effective, reproducible, and validated measure of nutritional status in patients with CKD stage 5D.[4,77]

MALNUTRITION–INFLAMMATION SCORE

MIS is another measure of nutritional risk that the KDOQI guidelines suggest may be used in patients with CKD, in those who receive dialysis, and in posttransplant populations.[4] This nutritional scoring tool includes components similar to SGA, such as anthropometrics and dietary intake patterns, with the addition of biochemical parameters.[78,79] A higher MIS score indicates worse nutritional status. Research using MIS shows that frailty is closely associated with PEW, muscle wasting, and cachexia; and muscle loss is more closely associated with negative outcomes than fat loss.[80]

There is a paradoxical relationship between the normal cardiovascular risk factors in the general population and persons who receive MHD.[81] For example, patients who receive MHD have not shown a significant improvement in their morbidity and mortality when their medical management has followed "conventional" pathways to control hypercholesterolemia, hyperhomocysteinemia, obesity, and hypertension.

PROTEIN ENERGY WASTING SCORE

PEW is characterized by multiple clinical, biochemical, and nutritional factors. As indicated by the International Society of Renal Nutrition and Metabolism, a diagnosis of PEW must utilize (a) biochemical measures (ie, serum albumin, prealbumin, and cholesterol); (b) measures of BMI, unintentional weight loss, and total body fat; (c) measures of muscle mass (ie, midarm circumference and creatinine appearance); and (d) measures of dietary intake. The paradox of these findings shows that low cholesterol and low BMI have been consistently associated with increased mortality risk, especially in the MHD population.[55] There is also a higher occurrence of inflammation.[82]

The PEW score is a simplified screening tool for identifying PEW risk in patients who receive HD.[83] The four components and their respective threshold values for the PEW score are as follows: serum albumin 3.8 g/dL, BMI of 23, serum creatinine normalized by body surface area (Scr/BSA 380 mmol/L/m^2), and nPNA 0.8 g/kg/d. For each component, a value greater than the threshold value receives 1 point for that component. A value that is less than the threshold value receives 0 points for that component. Therefore, the total PEW score ranges from 0 to 4 and the overall ratings are as follows[83]:

- Score 4 = normal nutritional status
- Score 3 = slight wasting
- Score 2 = moderate wasting
- Score 0–1 = severe wasting

According to the KDOQI guidelines, this score may help clinicians identify the subgroups of patients with a high mortality rate in order to recommend nutrition support.[4]

HANDGRIP STRENGTH

Handgrip strength is measured by handheld dynamometers and is reliable for measuring upper extremity strength.[84] Handgrip strength can be used to determine nutritional status since muscle functionality may precede loss of muscle or muscle wasting.[85] Evidence also supports that lower handgrip strength values are associated with higher MIS scores.[86] Handgrip strength should be assessed using the patient's dominant hand or nonfistula arm and may not be accurate in patients with arthritis.[85] KDOQI guidelines suggest that handgrip strength may be used as an indicator of protein–energy status and functional status when baseline data are available for comparison.[4]

Summary

Achieving the best possible outcomes for patients with CKD begins with a comprehensive nutrition assessment. Timely evaluation to detect suboptimal nutrition-related biochemical and physical parameters allows for early intervention and the ability to improve outcomes for comorbidities such as malnutrition and PEW, bone and mineral metabolism disorders, diabetes mellitus, and anemia. Although a single parameter may provide significant information regarding nutritional status, it is necessary to consider multiple parameters and monitor trends to assess thoroughly the nutritional status of patients with kidney disease.

References

1. The Academy of Nutrition and Dietetics. Nutrition Care Process (NCP). Accessed November 6, 2018. www.eatrightpro.org/practice/practice-resources/nutrition-care-process

2. Kidney Disease: Improving Global Outcomes (KDIGO) CKD-MBD Update Work Group. KDIGO 2017 Clinical practice guideline update for the diagnosis, evaluation, prevention, and treatment of chronic kidney disease–mineral and bone disorder (CKD-MBD). *Kidney Int Suppl.* 2017;7(1):1-59. doi:10.1016/kisu.2017.04.001

3. Department of Health and Human Services, Centers for Medicare & Medicaid Services, 42 CFR Parts 405, 410, 413, 414, 488. Medicare and Medicaid Programs; Conditions for Coverage for End-Stage Renal Disease Facilities; Final Rule. Federal Register, April 15, 2008. Accessed September 20, 2020. www.cms.gov/Regulations-and-Guidance/Legislation/CFCsAndCoPs/downloads/esrdfinalrule0415.pdf

4. Ikizler TA, Burrowes JD, Byham-Gray L, et al; KDOQI Nutrition in CKD Guideline Work Group. KDOQI clinical practice guideline for nutrition in CKD: 2020 update. *Am J Kidney Dis.* 2020;76(3)(suppl 1):S1-S107. doi:10.1053/j.ajkd.2020.05.006

5. White JV, Guenter P, Jensen G, Malone A, Schofield M, Academy Malnutrition Work Group, A.S.P.E.N. Malnutrition Task Force, A.S.P.E.N. Board of Directors. Consensus statement: Academy of Nutrition and Dietetics and American Society for Parenteral and Enteral Nutrition: characteristics recommended for the identification and documentation of adult malnutrition (undernutrition). *JPEN J Parenter Enteral Nutr.* 2012;36(3):275-283. doi:10.1177/0148607112440285

6. Katz Activities of Daily Living. National Palliative Care Research Center website. Accessed November 5, 2018. http://.npcrc.org/files/news/katz_index_of_independence_in_activities_of_daily_living.pdf

7. Nordström K, Coff C, Jönsson H, Nordenfelt L, Görman U. Food and health: individual, cultural, or scientific matters? *Genes Nutr.* 2013;8(4):357-363. doi:10.1007/s12263-013-0336-8

8. Burrowes JD. Issues Affecting dietary adherence. In: Byham-Gray LD, Burrowes JD, Chertow GM, eds. *Nutrition in Kidney Disease.* Humana Press; 2014:405-411.

9. Arezzo di Trifiletti A, Misino P, Giannantoni P, et al. Comparison of the performance of four different tools in diagnosing disease-associated anorexia and their relationship with nutritional, functional and clinical outcome measures in hospitalized patients. *Clin Nutr.* 2013;32(4):527-532. doi:10.1016/j.clnu.2012.11.011

10. Zabel R, Ash S, Bauer J, King N. Assessment of subjective appetite sensations in hemodialysis patients. Agreement and feasibility between traditional paper and pen and a novel electronic appetite rating system. *Appetite.* 2009;52(2):525-527. doi:10.1016/j.appet.2008.10.010

11. Molfino A, Kaysen GA, Chertow GM, et al. Validating appetite assessment tools among patients receiving hemodialysis. *J Ren Nutr.* 2016;26(2):103-110. doi:10.1053/j.jrn.2015.09.002

12. Lopes AA, Elder SJ, Ginsberg N, et al. Lack of appetite in haemodialysis patients: associations with patient characteristics, indicators of nutritional status and outcomes in the international DOPPS. *Nephrol Dial Transplant.* 2007;22(12):3538-3546. doi:10.1093/ndt/gfm453

13. Academy of Nutrition and Dietetics. Evidence Analysis Library. Chronic Kidney Disease. Assessment of Food/Nutrition-Related History. Accessed November 5, 2018. www.andevidencelibrary.com

14. Moore LW. Dietary assessment in chronic kidney disease. In: Byham-Gray LD, Burrowes JD, Chertow GM, eds. *Nutrition in Kidney Disease.* Humana Press; 2014:25-48.

15. Nelson EE. Anthropometry in the nutritional assessment of adults with end-stage renal disease. *J Ren Nutr.* 1991;1(4):162-172. doi:10.1016/S1051-2276(12)80178-6

16. McCann L, ed. *Pocket Guide to Nutrition Assessment of the Patient With Kidney Disease.* 6th ed. National Kidney Foundation; 2021.

17. Kopple JD, Jones MR, Keshaviah PR, et al. A proposed glossary for dialysis kinetics. *Am J Kidney Dis.* 1995;26(6):963-981. doi:10.1016/0272-6386(95)90064-0

18. Byham-Gray LD. Weighing the evidence: energy determinations across the spectrum of kidney disease. *J Ren Nutr.* 2006;16(1):17-26. doi:10.1053/j.jrn.2005.10.004

19. Karkeck J. Adjusted body weight for obesity. American Dietetic Association Renal Dietitians Practice Group Newsletter. 1984;8:6.

20. National Kidney Foundation. KDOQI clinical practice guidelines for hemodialysis adequacy: 2015 update. *Am J Kidney Dis.* 2015;66(5):884-930. doi:10.1053/j.ajkd.2015.07.015

21. Bossola M, Pepe G, Vulpio C. The frustrating attempt to limit the interdialytic weight gain in patients on chronic hemodialysis: new insights into an old problem. *J Ren Nutr.* 2018;28(5):293-301. doi:10.1053/j.jrn.2018.01.015

22. Kalantar-Zadeh K. Nutritional management of maintenance hemodialysis patients. In: Kopple JD, Massry SG, Kalantar-Zadeh, eds. *Nutritional Management of Renal Disease*. 3rd ed. Elsevier; 2013:503-538.

23. Rx Kinetics website. Estimating height in bedridden patients. November 17, 2017. Accessed November 5, 2018. www.rxkinetics.com/height_estimate.html

24. Chhabra SK. Using arm span to derive height: impact of three estimates of height on interpretation of spirometry. *Ann Thorac Med*. 2008;3(3):94-99. doi:10.4103/1817-1737.39574

25. Janssen I, Kalzmanzyk PT, Ross R. Waist circumference and not body mass index explains obesity-related health risk. *Am J Clin Nutr*. 2004;79(3):379–384. doi:10.1093/ajcn/79.3.379di

26. Ogden CL, Carroll MD, Fryar CD, Flegal KM. Prevalence of obesity among adults and youth: United States, 2011-2014. *NCHS Data Brief*. 2015;219:1-8.

27. Doshi M, Streja E, Rhee CM, et al. Examining the robustness of the obesity paradox in maintenance hemodialysis patients: a marginal structural model analysis. *Nephrol Dial Transplant*. 2016;31(8):1310-1319. doi:10.1093/ndt/gfv379

28. Naderi N, Kleine CE, Park C, et al. Obesity paradox in advanced kidney disease: from bedside to the bench. *Prog Cardiovasc Dis*. 2018;61(2):168-181. doi:10.1016/j.pcad.2018.07.001

29. Kleine CE, Moradi H, Streja E, Kalantar-Zadeh K. Racial and ethnic disparities in the obesity paradox. *Am J Kidney Dis*. 2018;72(5 suppl 1):S26-S32. doi:10.1053/j.ajkd.2018.06.024

30. Cordeiro AC, Qureshi AR, Stenvinkel P, et al. Abdominal fat deposition is associated with increased inflammation, protein energy wasting and worse outcome in patients undergoing haemodialysis. *Nephrol Dial Transplant*. 2010;25(2):562-568. doi:10.1093/ndt/gfp492

31. Centers for Disease Control and Prevention. Assessing your weight. Centers for Disease Control and Prevention website. Updated May 15, 2015. Accessed November 5, 2018. www.cdc.gov/healthyweight/assessing/index.html

32. Sanches MR, Avesani CM, Kamimura MA, et al. Waist circumference and visceral fat in CKD: a cross-sectional study. *Am J Kidney Dis*. 2008;52(1):66-73. doi:10.1053/j.ajkd.2008.02.004

33. Keshaviah PR, Nolph KD, Moore HL, et al. Lean body mass estimation by creatinine kinetics. *J Am Soc Nephrol*. 1994;4(7):1475-1485.

34. Chumlea WC. Anthropometric and body composition assessment in dialysis patients. *Semin Dial*. 2004;17(6):466-470. doi:10.1111/j.0894-0959.2004.17607.x

35. Olejnik LA, Peters EN, Parrott JS, et al. Abbreviated steady state intervals for measuring resting energy expenditure in patients on maintenance hemodialysis. *JPEN J Parenter Enteral Nutr*. 2017;41(8):1348-1355. doi:10.1177/0148607116660981

36. Byham-Gray L, Parrott JS, Ho WY, Sundell MB, Ikizler TA. Development of a predictive energy equation for maintenance hemodialysis patients: a pilot study. *J Ren Nutr*. 2014;24(1):32-41. doi:10.1053/j.jrn.2013.10.005

37. Vilar E, Machado A, Garrett A, Kozarski R, Wellsted D, Farrington K. Disease-specific predictive formulas for energy expenditure in the dialysis population. *J Ren Nutr*. 2014;24(4):243-251. doi:10.1053/j.jrn.2014.03.001

38. KIDGO AKI Workgroup. KDIGO clinical practice guidelines for acute kidney injury. *Kidney Int Suppl*. 2012;17:1-138. doi:10.1038/kisup.2012.1

39. Inker LA, Eneanya ND, Coresh J, et al; Chronic Kidney Disease Epidemiology Collaboration. New creatinine- and cystatin C-based equations to estimate GFR without race. *N Engl J Med*. 2021;385(19):1737-1749. doi:10.1056/NEJMoa2102953

40. Stevens LA, Coresh J, Greene T, Levey AS. Assessing kidney function-measured and estimated glomerular filtration rate. *N Engl J Med*. 2006;354(23):2473-2483. doi:10.1056/NEJMra054415

41. Fuhrman MP, Charney P, Mueller CM. Hepatic proteins and nutrition assessment. *J Am Diet Assoc*. 2004;104(8):1258-1264. doi:10.1016/j.jada.2004.05.213

42. Kaysen GA, Dubin JA, Müller HG, et al; HEMO Study Group NIDDK. Inflammation and reduced albumin synthesis associated with stable decline in serum albumin in hemodialysis patients. *Kidney Int*. 2004;65(4):1408-1415. doi:10.1111/j.1523-1755.2004.00520.x

43. American Diabetes Association. Classification and diagnosis of diabetes: standards of medical care in diabetes–2019. *Diabetes Care*. 2019;42(suppl 1):S13-S28. doi:10.2337/dc19-S002

44. National Kidney Foundation. KDOQI Clinical Practice Guideline for Diabetes and CKD: 2012 update. *Am J Kidney Dis*. 2012;60(5):850-886. doi:10.1053/j.ajkd.2012.07.005

45. Makris K, Spanou L. Is there a relationship between mean blood glucose and glycated hemoglobin? *J Diabetes Sci Technol.* 2011;5(6):1572-1583. doi:10.1177/193229681100500634

46. Nathan DM, Kuenen J, Borg R, et al. A1c-Derived Average Glucose Study Group. Translating the A1C assay into estimated average glucose values. *Diabetes Care.* 2008;31(8):1473-1478. doi:10.2337/dc08-0545

47. Welsh KJ, Kirkman MS, Sacks DB. Role of glycated proteins in the diagnosis and management of diabetes: research gaps and future directions. *Diabetes Care.* 2016;39(8):1299-1306. doi:10.2337/dc15-2727

48. Moe S, Drüeke T, Cunningham J, et al. Definition, evaluation, and classification of renal osteodystrophy: a position statement from Kidney Disease: Improving Global Outcomes (KDIGO). *Kidney Int.* 2006;69(11):1945-1953. doi:10.1038/sj.ki.5000414

49. Levin A, Bakris GL, Molitch M, et al. Prevalence of abnormal serum vitamin D, PTH, calcium, and phosphorus in patients with chronic kidney disease: results of the study to evaluate early kidney disease. *Kidney Int.* 2007;71(1):31-38. doi:10.1038/sj.ki.5002009

50. Olgaard K, ed. *Clinical Guide to Bone and Mineral Metabolism in CKD.* National Kidney Foundation; 2006.

51. Goltzman D. Diagnostic approach to hypocalcemia. In: Rosen CJ, Mulder JE, eds. UpToDate. July 18, 2018. Accessed November 6, 2018. www.uptodate.com/contents/diagnostic-approach-to-hypocalcemia

52. Russo D, Corrao S, Miranda I, et al. Progression of coronary artery calcification in predialysis patients. *Am J Nephrol.* 2007;27(2):152-158. doi:10.1159/000100044

53. Haddad N, Shim R, Hebert LA. Nutritional management of water, sodium, potassium, chloride, and magnesium in kidney disease and kidney failure. In: Kopple JD, Massry SG, Kalantar-Zadeh K, eds. *Nutritional Management of Renal Disease.* 3rd ed. Elsevier; 2013:323-338.

54. Kidney Disease: Improving Global Outcomes (KDIGO) Lipid Work Group. KDIGO clinical practice guideline for lipid management in chronic kidney disease. *Kidney Int Suppl.* 2013;3(3):259-305. doi:10.1038/kisup.2013.28

55. Fouque D, Kalantar-Zadeh K, Kopple J, et al. A proposed nomenclature and diagnostic criteria for protein-energy wasting in acute and chronic kidney disease. *Kidney Int.* 2008;73(4):391-398. doi:10.1038/sj.ki.5002585

56. Walter CP, Richardson PA, Virani SS, Winkelmayer WC, Navaneethan SD. Association between intensity of statin therapy and mortality in persons with chronic kidney disease. *Nephrol Dial Transplant.* 2018;35(2):312-319. doi:10.1093/ndt/gfy237

57. Harchaoui KE, Visser ME, Kastelein JJ, Stroes ES, Dallinga-Thie GM. Triglycerides and cardiovascular risk. *Curr Cardiol Rev.* 2009;5(3):216-222. doi:10.2174/157340309788970315

58. Macdougall I, Eckardt K. Anemia in chronic kidney disease. In: Johnson R, Feehally J, Floege J, eds. *Comprehensive Clinical Nephrology.* 5th ed. Elsevier; 2015:967-974.

59. Shih H, Wu C, Lin S. Physiology and pathophysiology of renal erythropoietin-producing cells. *J Formos Med Assoc.* 2018;117(11):955-963. doi:10.1016/j.jfma.2018.03.017

60. Kliger AS, Foley RN, Goldfarb DS, et al. KDOQI US commentary on the 2012 KDIGO Clinical Practice Guideline for Anemia in CKD. *Am J Kidney Dis.* 2013;62(5):849-859. doi:10.1053/j.ajkd.2013.06.008

61. Hudnall S. Iron, heme, hemoglobin. In: *Hematology: A Pathophysiologic Approach.* Mosby; 2012:17-25.

62. Kroft SH, Monaghan SA. Red blood cell/hemoglobin disorders. In: Hsi ED, ed. *Hematopathology.* 2nd ed. Saunders; 2012:3-54.

63. Clarkson M, Magee C, Brenner B. Hematologic aspects of kidney disease and erythropoietin therapy. *Pocket Companion to Brenner and Rector's The Kidney.* 8th ed. Saunders; 2010:585-600.

64. Kidney Disease: Improving Global Outcomes (KDIGO) Anemia Work Group. KDIGO clinical practice guideline for anemia in chronic kidney disease. *Kidney Int Suppl.* 2012;2(4):288-335. doi:10.1038/kisup.2012.37

65. Gupta N, Wish JB. Hypoxia-inducible factor prolyl hydroxylase inhibitors: a potential new treatment for anemia in patients with CKD. *Am J Kidney Dis.* 2017;69(6):815-826. doi:10.1053/j.ajkd.2016.12.011

66. Wish JB. Anemia and other hematologic complications of chronic kidney disease. In: Gilbert S, Weiner D, eds. *National Kidney Foundation Primer on Kidney Disease.* 6th ed. Saunders; 2013:515-525.

67. Medline Plus. Taking iron supplements. October 31, 2018. Accessed November 6, 2018. http://medlineplus.gov/ency/article/007478.htm

68. Brugnara C, Eckardt K. Hematologic aspects of kidney disease. In: Skorecki K, Chertow G, Marsden P, et al, eds. *Brenner and Rector's The Kidney.* 10th ed. Elsevier; 2016:1875-1894.

69. Locatelli F, Del Vecchio L. Iron-based phosphate binders: a paradigm shift in the treatment of hyperphosphatemic anemic CKD patients? *J Nephrol.* 2017;30(6):755-765. doi:10.1007/s40620-017-0421-y

70. Fishbane S, Block GA, Loram L, et al. Effects of ferric citrate in patients with nondialysis-dependent CKD and iron deficiency anemia. *J Am Soc Nephrol.* 2017;28(6):1851-1858. doi:10.1681/ASN.2016101053

71. National Kidney Foundation. Clinical practice guidelines for peritoneal adequacy update, 2006. *Am J Kidney Dis.* 2006;48(1)(suppl 1):S91-S97. doi:10.1053/j.ajkd.2006.05.016

72. Kalantar-Zadeh K, Supasyndh O, Lehn RS, McAllister CJ, Kopple JD. Normalized protein nitrogen appearance is correlated with hospitalization and mortality in hemodialysis patients with Kt/V greater than 1.2. *J Ren Nutr.* 2003;13(1):15-25. doi:10.1053/jren.2003.50005

73. Misra M, Nolph K. A simplified approach to understanding urea kinetics in peritoneal dialysis. *J Ren Nutr.* 2007;17(4):282-285. doi:10.1053/j.jrn.2007.02.002

74. Sum SS, Marcus AF, Blair D, et al. Comparison of subjective global assessment and protein energy wasting score to nutrition evaluations conducted by registered dietitian nutritionists in identifying protein energy wasting risk in maintenance hemodialysis patients. *J Ren Nutr.* 2017;27(5):325-332. doi:10.1053/j.jrn.2017.04.006

75. Detsky A, McLaughlin J, Baker J, et al. What is subjective global assessment of nutritional status? *JPEN J Parenter Enteral Nutr.* 1987;11(1):8-13. doi:10.1177/014860718701100108

76. McCann L. Subjective global assessment as it pertains to the nutritional status of dialysis patients. *Dial Transplant.* 1996;4:190-198.

77. Steiber A, Leon JB, Secker D, et al. Multicenter study of the validity and reliability of subjective global assessment in the hemodialysis population. *J Ren Nutr.* 2007;17(5):336-342. doi:10.1053/j.jrn.2007.05.004

78. Kalantar-Zadeh K, Kopple JD, Block G, Humphreys MH. A malnutrition-inflammation score is correlated with morbidity and mortality in maintenance dialysis patients. *Am J Kidney Dis.* 2001;38(6):1251-1263. doi:10.1053/ajkd.2001.29222

79. Kalantar-Zadeh K, Kleiner M, Dunne E, Lee GH, Luft FC. A modified quantitative subjective global assessment of nutrition for dialysis patients. *Nephrol Dial Transplant.* 1999;14(7):1732-1738. doi:10.1093/ndt/14.7.1732

80. Obi Y, Qader H, Kovesdy CP, Kalantar-Zadeh K. Latest consensus and update on protein-energy wasting in chronic kidney disease. *Curr Opin Clin Nutr Metab Care.* 2015;18(13):254-262. doi:10.1097/MCO.0000000000000171

81. Kalantar-Zadeh K, Block G, Humphreys MH, Kopple JD. Reverse epidemiology of cardiovascular risk factors in maintenance dialysis patients. *Kidney Int.* 2003;63(3):793-808. doi:10.1046/j.1523-1755.2003.00803.x

82. Coleman S, Bross R, Benner D, et al. The Nutritional and Inflammatory Evaluation in Dialysis patients (NIED) study: overview of the NIED study and the role of dietitians. *J Ren Nutr.* 2005;15(2):231-243. doi:10.1053/j.jrn.2005.01.003

83. Moreau-Gaudry X, Jean G, Genet L, et al. A simple protein-energy wasting score predicts survival in maintenance hemodialysis patients. *J Ren Nutr.* 2014;24(6):395-400. doi:10.1053/j.jrn.2014.06.008

84. Hamilton A, Balnave R, Adams R. Grip strength testing reliability. *J Hand Ther.* 1994;7(3):163-170. doi:10.1016/s0894-1130(12)80058-5

85. Carrero JJ, Johansen KL, Lindholm B, Stenvinkel P, Cuppari L, Avesani CM. Screening for muscle wasting and dysfunction in patients with chronic kidney disease. *Kidney Int.* 2016;90(1):53-66. doi:10.1016/j.kint.2016.02.025

86. Silva LF, Matos CM, Lopes GB, et al. Handgrip strength as a simple indicator of possible malnutrition and inflammation in men and women on maintenance hemodialysis. *J Ren Nutr.* 2011;21(3):235-245. doi:10.1053/j.jrn.2010.07.004

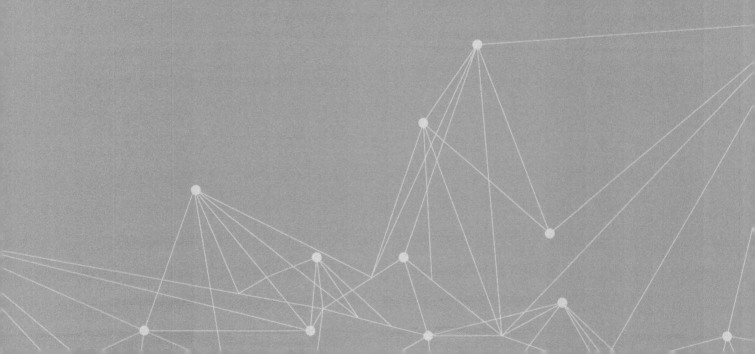

SECTION II
Nutrition Management of Kidney Disease

CHAPTER 3

Nutrition Management in Chronic Kidney Disease Stages 1 Through 5

Kathy Schiro Harvey, MS, RDN, CSR, Kristin Leonberg, MS, RD, CSR, CDCES, and Sara Prato, MS, RDN

Introduction

Chronic kidney disease (CKD) is a worldwide public health problem. The Centers for Disease Control and Prevention estimates that 15% of the US population has CKD, which is equivalent to 30 million Americans or one in seven adults.[1] Most individuals with CKD are unaware that they have the disease, as the symptoms are "hidden" until the disease has progressed to later stages and complications become apparent. The National Kidney Foundation (NKF) Kidney Disease Outcomes Quality Initiative (KDOQI) defines CKD as abnormalities of kidney structure or function lasting longer than 3 months with health implications. In addition, a greater than 3-month reduction in kidney function as estimated by the glomerular filtration rate (GFR) and the presence of proteinuria (>300 mg/d) are included in the definition. The stages of CKD are described in Chapter 1.

Approximately 680,000 people in the United States have CKD stage 5, require dialysis, or have undergone kidney transplant.[2] Most people with CKD (>29 million) are at stages 1 through 4 and are at risk of progressing to stage 5. The risk is even greater that they will develop comorbid conditions associated with CKD and die prematurely. The NKF recommends that all individuals at high risk of CKD should be screened regularly through assessment of markers of kidney damage and GFR.[3] Appropriate interventions should be initiated to prevent the development and progression of CKD and treat complications. The CKD risk factors are listed in Box 3.1.

BOX 3.1 | Risk Factors for Chronic Kidney Disease[2]

PRIMARY RISK FACTORS FOR CHRONIC KIDNEY DISEASE	SECONDARY RISK FACTORS FOR CHRONIC KIDNEY DISEASE
Diabetes mellitus	Obesity
High blood pressure	Autoimmune diseases
Family history of chronic kidney disease	Urinary tract and systemic infections
Age 60 years or older	Overuse of over-the-counter painkillers or exposure to toxic chemicals
Ethnic groups	Kidney loss, damage, injury, or infection

Certain ethnic populations that have high rates of diabetes (DM) or high blood pressure (BP) are at increased risk of CKD, such as Blacks, Hispanics, Asians, Pacific Islanders, and Indigenous Americans. The prevalence of CKD is 1.5 to 3 times higher in these groups compared to Whites.[2]

CKD involves complex, comorbid conditions, including malnutrition, DM, cardiovascular disease (CVD), hypertension (HTN), dyslipidemias, and bone and mineral metabolism disorders. Medical nutrition therapy (MNT) is the cornerstone treatment for managing CKD and its complications. People with CKD who receive MNT provided by an expert renal registered dietitian nutritionist (RDN) show less decline in

GFR compared to those who do not receive MNT. They have better markers of nutrition health, improved survival, and decreased health care costs.[4-6] Clinical guidelines recommend that all individuals with CKD receive expert dietary advice and information tailored to their specific individual situations.[3,7,8] This chapter discusses nutrition therapies appropriate for persons with CKD that can reduce comorbid complications and slow the progression to CKD stage 5. These therapies may be especially important for those with CKD who choose conservative treatment (no dialysis or transplant) to live quality and healthy lives as long as possible.

Additional information for treating those with DM and CVD is provided in Chapters 9 and 11, respectively.

Quantity vs Quality

Traditional diet therapies for persons with CKD focus on adjusting specific nutrients in the diet to help manage and balance blood chemistries and prevent buildup of toxic wastes. Diets typically include small amounts of animal protein foods along with limited amounts of fruits and vegetables and avoidance of whole grains and dairy foods to control potassium and phosphorus intake. Extra fats and sugars may be added to maintain calorie intake and satiety. Although these diets provide the appropriate mix of protein, calories, sodium, potassium, and phosphorus, they are generally not considered healthy by current nutrition standards. In recent years, research has emerged demonstrating that total diet quality may be more important and effective in treating CKD compared to limiting specific nutrient quantities. Healthy diets based on a variety of whole grains, fruits and vegetables, plant proteins (including legumes and nuts), fish, poultry, low-fat dairy foods, and plant-based oils are showing promise in preventing CKD, reducing its complications, and slowing its progression to end-stage kidney disease. Large population studies have evaluated vegetarian diets, Mediterranean diets, and the Dietary Approaches to Stop Hypertension (DASH) diet, all showing effectiveness in treating and preventing

CKD.[9-12] Studies looking at increased intake of fruits and vegetables in patients with CKD show improved acid-base balance and decreased uremic toxins.[13-15] Therefore, current CKD diet recommendations include emphasis on eating patterns consistent with overall diet quality, rather than just limiting nutrients. Within food groups, specific food choices may be required to balance sodium, potassium, and phosphorus levels, but there is little evidence that avoiding total food groups, such as whole grains, legumes, or dairy foods, is warranted. Nutrition therapies must be calculated to provide adequate calories and protein but also include a variety of whole foods consistent with overall healthy diets.

For those with CKD choosing conservative treatment rather than future dialysis or transplant, a diet balanced in quantity and quality is especially important. Patient and family priorities should be discussed and diet therapy balanced to minimize symptoms yet maximize quality of life based on individual patient wishes. Depending on the patient's overall health and kidney function, intake may need to be adjusted to limit sodium and fluid (minimize fluid retention and shortness of breath) or potassium (control hyperkalemia) or reduce protein to limit uremic symptoms. The eating pattern prescribed must be balanced and adjusted to meet the patient's clinical needs as well as quality-of-life priorities.

Malnutrition

Improving and maintaining nutrition health in people with CKD is a priority of MNT.[16-18] At the start of dialysis therapy, protein–energy malnutrition or protein energy wasting (PEW) is associated with increased mortality, as evidenced by a variety of markers of nutritional health. Early studies by Held et al[16] showed that relative risk of death more than doubled in subjects who began dialysis with serum albumin levels less than 2.5 mg/dL compared with those who began dialysis with albumin greater than 4.0 mg/dL. Kopple et al[17] reported that both average calorie intake and body mass index (BMI) in people with CKD tend to decrease as

GFR declines. Ikizler et al[18] have demonstrated that protein intake also declines with GFR. More recent studies report that low energy and/or protein intake are associated with a significant decline of nutritional parameters and an increased risk of morbidity and mortality.[19] Studies by Fried et al[20] and O'Sullivan et al[21] report that reduced lean body mass (LBM) is an important measure for protein deficit and is also predictive of increased mortality in this patient population.

Overall, as GFR drops below 60 mL/min/1.73 m^2, both calorie and protein intake spontaneously decrease. Although data are lacking regarding optimal dietary and energy patterns in order to slow the progression of CKD and maintain proper nutritional status, it is critical to assess nutrient intake and make appropriate recommendations in the earlier stages of CKD to prevent and treat PEW.

Although obesity is a major risk factor for developing CKD, once CKD is established, obesity becomes linked with greater survival. This obesity paradox is evident in the more advanced stages of CKD (stage 4 and stage 5) and has been substantiated by a large number of observational studies with large sample sizes. However, in the earlier stages of CKD (stages 1 through 3), obesity is associated with more rapid loss of kidney function and progression of CKD. Obesity is commonly associated with HTN, DM, and metabolic syndrome, which can all lead to kidney damage. Obesity also seems to contribute to proteinuria and glomerular damage. Better outcomes occur in those with BMI under 30.[22-25] Therefore, it is acceptable to promote gradual weight loss in patients with obesity and CKD, especially in stages 1 through 3. Weight loss should be achieved through a combination of increased physical activity to promote lean tissue and a high-quality diet. Rapid weight loss results in loss of lean tissue rather than fat tissue, but slow weight loss while following a healthy eating plan, in combination with resistance exercise, can help prevent muscle catabolism in patients with CKD.[26,27]

Protein Requirements

Consuming a traditional Western diet high in animal-based proteins will induce increases in GFR and ultimately lead to glomerular hyperfiltration. High protein intake increases renal blood flow and elevates intraglomerular pressure, resulting in the excretion of protein-derived nitrogenous waste products. Over a period of time, this may lead to an increase in kidney volume and weight.[28]

For more than 50 years, researchers have studied the effects of restricting protein intake on kidney function in patients with CKD. The largest study published, the Modification of Diet in Renal Disease, evaluated more than 800 participants with CKD.[29] After many years of follow-up, data evaluation, and reevaluation, the results remain inconclusive with respect to the benefits of a low-protein diet on the progression of CKD. However, several prior and subsequent studies and meta-analyses appear to support the role of limiting protein intake on the progression of CKD.[28,30-37]

Protein quality may be of more importance than total protein intake, as evidenced by current research on the effect of vegetarian, Mediterranean, and DASH diets in patients with CKD. Consuming plant proteins results in less uremic toxins, improved gut microbiome leading to decreased inflammation, and reduced metabolic acidosis and hyperphosphatemia.[10] The large National Health and Nutrition Examination Survey (NHANES) III study evaluated protein intake and CKD outcomes, and found a lower mortality rate in those participants who consumed more of their protein from plant sources.[38]

Current protein recommendations for CKD range from 0.28 to 0.43 g/kg/d with additional keto acid/amino acid analogs on a very low protein diet and from 0.55 to 0.6 g/kg/d on a low protein diet. For those with DM, recommendations are 0.6 to 0.8 g/kg/d, slightly higher to help with glycemic management.[7,8] Total protein intake is more important than protein sources, and it is no longer recommended that 50% of protein come from specific types of foods. Protein from all foods should be considered as part of the total intake, which can make meal planning more flexible (see Box 3.2 on page 36).[39,40] Be-

BOX 3.2 | Approximate Grams of Protein per Portion[39,40]

PROTEIN SIZE	PROTEIN (g)
1 oz meat, fish, poultry, cheese, seitan	7-8
1 egg	6-7
1 cup milk, yogurt, soy milk	7-8
⅓ cup tofu, tempeh	7-8
2 Tbsp peanut butter, almond butter	6-7
¼ cup nuts, cottage cheese	6-7
½ cup cooked, dried beans and peas	6-8
1 slice bread, 1 tortilla, ½ bagel	3-4
1 cup rice	4
1 cup pasta	6
1 cup cooked vegetables	2-3
1 cup fruit	1

cause these recommendations are significantly less than most typical Western diets, some people may adapt more easily if protein intake is decreased gradually to achieve goal levels, depending on usual intake. It may be beneficial to begin by altering the protein quality, substituting plant protein foods, rather than drastically reducing overall intake. In addition, overall health, activities, metabolic condition, and stress must be considered when calculating protein needs. For those individuals who require more protein (because of malnutrition, wound healing, infections, trauma, strenuous activities, etc), high-quality plant protein foods should be considered as a healthy alternative to eating more animal proteins.

When protein intake is restricted, nutritional status must be maintained with adequate energy intake to prevent iatrogenic malnutrition. Increasing the intake of fruits, vegetables, whole grains, and healthy fats will provide the requisite calories and nutrients. Depending on individual needs, food choices may need to be adapted to limit intake of sodium, potassium, and phosphorus. Unfortunately, the potassium and phosphorus content of foods does not necessarily coincide with their effect on serum levels. The phosphorus in many high phosphorus plant foods is minimally absorbed and, thus, has little impact on serum levels. Evidence supporting the effect of high potassium–containing foods on serum levels is virtually nonexistent. Therefore, when treating patients with CKD, hyperphosphatemia, and hyperkalemia, the renal RDN will need to critically evaluate not only their food intake but also their medications and overall metabolic and physical health.[41,42]

Energy Requirements

Data are lacking regarding optimal energy requirements to slow the progression of CKD and maintain proper nutritional status. Resting energy expenditure (REE) may be low, normal, or elevated in patients with CKD compared to that of the general population.[21] Inflammation and prevalence of comorbid conditions, such as poorly controlled DM and CVD, may cause an increase in metabolic rate, and elevated REE is a major risk factor for the development of PEW.[19,43]

Indirect calorimetry and reference techniques, such as dual-energy x-ray absorptiometry (DXA), are the gold standards for determining energy expenditure, but these are often laborious, invasive, and cumbersome to use routinely in the clinical setting.[44,45] Furthermore, there is not a reference standard for assessing body composition in patients with CKD.[7,8] Commonly used equations (ie, Harris-Benedict, Schofield, or Mifflin-St. Jeor) have not been extensively studied in the population with CKD. Kamimura et al[46] demonstrated that the Harris-Benedict and Schofield equations overestimated REE when compared with indirect calorimetry in 124 patients with CKD not yet on dialysis. Byham-Gray et al[45] suggested the addition of laboratory data, such as albumin, C-reactive protein, and creatinine, along with anthropometric data when estimating REE in patients with CKD who receive dialysis.

Recently, Tian et al[44] developed and evaluated two new equations based on handgrip strength (HGS) and midarm muscle circumference (MAMC) in 300 patients with CKD stages 3 through 5 for estimating LBM (see Box 3.3). The results suggested that LBM values estimated using both equations were numerical-

BOX 3.3 | Equations for Estimating Lean Body Mass in Chronic Kidney Disease[44]

Lean body mass estimated from handgrip strength

(1 if male; 0 if female) × 6.82 +
Height in cm × 0.18 + Weight in kg × 0.40 +
Handgrip strength (N) × 0.01 – 18.12

Lean body mass estimated from midarm muscle circumference

(1 if male; 0 if female) × 7.36 +
Height in cm × 0.22 + Weight in kg × 0.37 +
Midarm muscle circumference in cm × 0.24 – 26.43

---

ly close to and significantly correlated with those measured using DXA ($P < .01$).

In the absence of a validated REE formula for CKD, KDOQI and the Academy of Nutrition and Dietetics suggest energy needs of 25 to 35 kcal/kg for those who are metabolically stable in order to provide adequate calories to promote the use of protein for repair rather than energy (see Box 3.4).[7,8,47,48]

Calculating Nutrient Needs in Underweight and Obese Conditions

The data from the United States Renal Data System (USRDS) indicate an increase in the prevalence of overweight and obesity in the population with CKD.[49] The dietary management of these patients needs to address issues of excess energy consumption. As mentioned previously, obesity has complex effects in those with CKD. Patients with low BMI have increased risk of all-cause and CVD mortality, while an elevated BMI results in improved survival. These conflicting data may be a result of limitations of BMI in differentiating adipose tissue from lean mass. Patients with obesity may have more energy reserves, and this may play a role in mitigating the deleterious effects of increased REE in patients with CKD.[43] The prevention and treatment of obesity are complex, and studies on intentional weight loss to slow the progression of CKD have not been performed.

BOX 3.4 | Daily Recommended Nutrient Intakes for Chronic Kidney Disease Stages 1 Through 5[7,8]

Calories	25 to 35 kcal/kg. Individualize for metabolic stress, comorbid complications, overweight or underweight, and overall health goals.
Protein	Very low protein: 0.28 to 0.43 g/kg + keto acid/amino acid analogs Low protein: 0.55 to 0.6 g/kg, With diabetes mellitus: 0.6 to 0.8 g/kg
	Individualize for metabolic stress, comorbid complications, overweight or underweight, and overall health goals.
	Promote plant proteins. Supplement keto acid/amino acid analogs with a very low protein diet.
Sodium	1.5 to 2.3 g/d. Individualize for calorie/protein needs.
Phosphorus	Individualize to maintain normal serum level. Consider absorbability of phosphorus from food sources.
Potassium	Individualize to maintain normal serum level. Increased fiber intake may reduce absorbability of potassium from foods.
Carbohydrates	Encourage complex carbohydrates and whole grains.
	For persons with diabetes mellitus, adjust intake to maintain blood glucose goals and limit refined carbohydrates and simple sugars.
Fats	Encourage unsaturated fats (olive oil, nut and seed oils, avocado oil).
	Limit saturated fats, trans fats, and animal fats.
Vitamins and minerals	Use water-soluble vitamin supplement at Dietary Reference Intake levels, as needed. Individualize other vitamin and mineral supplements.

The KDOQI and the Academy of Nutrition and Dietetics guidelines suggest a normal weight BMI of 18.5 through 24.9.[7,8] When an individual's actual BMI is near this range, current body weight is recommended for nutrient calculations. In patients with obesity and CKD, some clinicians use adjusted body weight for calculating nutrient needs, which aims to capture what is considered to be metabolically active weight, rather than excess adiposity.[49,50] However, adjusted body weight formulas have no scientific validity and evidence-based research does not support their use. Energy recommendations calculated with an adjusted body weight are very different from calculated needs based on indirect calorimetry.[51] The Evidence Analysis Library CKD Guideline does not recommend using adjusted body weight formulas and encourages using clinical judgment if clinicians choose to do so in practice.[7] The Evidence Analysis Library Adult Weight Management Guideline by the Academy of Nutrition and Dietetics recommends using actual body weight and the Mifflin-St. Jeor equation when estimating energy needs in noncritically ill patients.[52] Therefore, it is generally recommended that actual body weight be used, whenever feasible, to determine energy needs in both underweight and overweight individuals, followed by the addition or the subtraction of calories for weight gain or loss, depending on the patient's condition and nutrition needs.[51-53]

There is no evidence-based research for determining protein needs in patients with CKD who are underweight or obese. The American Society for Parenteral and Enteral Nutrition (ASPEN) recommends using actual body weight for calculating protein needs in critically ill subjects with obesity.[54] Studies on non-ill subjects who are obese and who have no CKD also recommend actual body weight for calculating protein needs.[55,56] However, in both overweight and underweight patients with CKD, calculating 0.55 to 0.6 g of protein per kilogram actual body weight could greatly overestimate or underestimate protein needs.

Some experts have suggested that protein needs could be calculated as a percentage (eg, 10% to 12%) of estimated energy requirements once those are determined, but there is no evidence to support this method. The practitioner should exercise good clinical judgment when determining protein requirements and consider encouraging more plant protein when a higher protein intake is indicated. Clinicians must monitor patient outcomes to determine whether protein recommendations are adequate and whether they meet patient needs. As always, RDNs must be flexible to adjust goals and prescriptions according to their patient's individ-

ual conditions. Well-controlled metabolic studies and randomized, controlled trials are needed to determine actual energy requirements in patients with CKD who are obese or underweight.

Comorbidities of Chronic Kidney Disease

Individuals with CKD often have multiple comorbidities, such as DM, CVD, HTN, dyslipidemia, and bone mineral metabolism disorders. Nutrition plays an important role in the management of these comorbidities and kidney function. As previously mentioned, CKD diet recommendations should emphasize overall diet quality, rather than focusing on individual nutrients. Emerging research recommends comprehensive eating patterns (eg, the Mediterranean diet and DASH diet) for the management of chronic diseases such as CKD, DM, and CVD. These diets emphasize a variety of whole grains, vegetables, fruits, and plant proteins. Evidence suggests that these diets may be helpful in managing comorbidities of CKD, delaying progression, and preventing complications in patients with CKD.[9,11,12]

DIABETES MELLITUS

DM is the most common etiology for patients with CKD. Roughly, 40% of all individuals with CKD have DM.[49] Nutrition management must include intensive treatment of hyperglycemia to help prevent elevated albuminuria and delay kidney disease progression. Treatment of hyperglycemia includes medications, balanced nutrition, and physical activity. Depending on the stage of CKD, each of these approaches should be individualized to the patient's needs.[57,58]

A recent review of the benefits of the Mediterranean diet shows that this eating pattern can have a protective effect against the development of DM but that it also may improve glycemic control and reduce CVD risk factors in patients with DM.[59] The DASH diet, which is most well-known for reducing HTN, is now showing benefits of improved glycemic control, weight loss, and improved insulin sensitivity in patients with DM.[60]

In order to address hyperglycemia in the population with DM and CKD, the American Diabetes Association recommends adjusting the amount and the type of carbohydrates in the diet. Emphasis should be placed on reducing refined carbohydrates and added sugars and focusing on quality carbohydrates from vegetables, legumes, fruits, dairy, and whole grains.[61]

Low carbohydrate diets that include higher protein levels should be avoided due to the relationship of high-protein diets and the progression of kidney disease.[62] Current protein recommendations for people with DM and CKD are 0.6 to 0.8 g/kg/d.[3,7,8] Focusing on the quality of protein (plant vs animal) may also be beneficial, as studies have shown that plant protein diets may help preserve kidney function in patients with CKD.

CARDIOVASCULAR DISEASE

Sixty-five percent of people with CKD have CVD, which is the leading cause of death; most individuals will die prematurely of CVD, not surviving to CKD stage 5 dialysis. Nutrition interventions to treat or stabilize CVD conditions include treating traditional risk factors, such as HTN and dyslipidemias, plus the nontraditional risk factors more specific to CKD, including abnormal bone mineral metabolism (see Chapter 10).[49]

Hypertension

HTN is both a cause and a complication of CKD and CVD associated with it, with 50% to 75% of patients having BP values greater than 140/90 mm Hg. Experts generally recommend that people with kidney disease should maintain BP levels less than or equal to 130/80 mm Hg, adjusting for the level of albuminuria and age.[63] The DASH trial showed that a comprehensive eating pattern successfully reduced BP levels in adults.[64] In 2001, the DASH research group showed that adding a sodium restriction of 1.5 to 2.3 g/d to the DASH dietary plan further reduced BP levels.[65]

In 2016, the first controlled feeding study of the DASH diet in patients with moderate CKD was completed and showed that a reduced-sodium DASH diet was beneficial for BP control in patients with moderate CKD.[66] The reduced sodium content used in the study was 2.3 g/d. Additional restriction to 1.5 g/d may further lower BP; however, this may be difficult to achieve in most Western-type diets because of the prevalence of sodium additives in food production.

Compared to the typical American diet, the DASH plan is lower in fat and sodium and higher in potassium, magnesium, calcium, fiber, and antioxidants. The results from the DASH diet indicate that a whole foods approach, which may include interactions between nutrients, can be more effective in treating HTN than simply limiting or increasing a single nutrient.

The lower sodium DASH diet can be a safe and effective treatment for controlling HTN and preventing the progression of CVD. Protein- and phosphorus-containing foods may need adjustment to avoid higher than recommended intakes. As CKD progresses, adjusting potassium intake to help manage serum levels may also become necessary. Potassium excretion is usually sufficient to control serum levels in the early stages of CKD, but common BP medications (angiotensin-converting enzyme inhibitors and angiotensin II receptor blockers) can interfere with potassium excretion even when urine output is normal. These agents are recommended in patients with CKD as they not only control HTN but also reduce proteinuria, protect the kidneys, and can slow CKD progression. The side effect of increasing serum potassium often occurs in CKD stage 4 and stage 5, when diet restriction may become necessary. Although there are many common lists of high potassium-containing foods, including those with potassium additives, the evidence to support food restriction's effect on serum levels is poor. Initial studies on potassium intake and serum levels used potassium solutions, rather than whole foods. Potassium absorption and its effect on intracellular and serum levels from foods is impacted by a person's acid-base balance, glucose and insulin levels, bowel excretion, and medications. One study showed that reported potassium intake only accounted for 2% of the variance in serum potassium levels.[67] Therefore, the renal RDN will need to consider all potential causes of hyperkalemia rather than focusing only on limiting high potassium foods.

Additional lifestyle changes that can impact HTN include smoking cessation and moderation of alcohol intake. Both approaches are appropriate recommendations for people with CKD. The beneficial effects of weight loss and exercise on HTN and the progression of CKD are unknown.[63] Weight loss to obtain and maintain appropriate body weight for height (BMI of <25) is most likely beneficial along with fitness programs to improve muscle mass, flexibility, and strength. But considering the high risk of malnutrition as kidney function declines, weight loss programs should be approached with caution when CKD progresses. Maintaining adequate energy and protein intake is the first priority. In subjects with obesity, controlled, gradual weight loss might be appropriate if patients are monitored closely to ensure that they are able to consume adequate protein and that they are not losing muscle mass. This careful monitoring becomes especially critical as appetite and food intake spontaneously decline with decreasing kidney function.[17,18] Exercise programs that include resistance training can help reduce catabolism and help maintain muscle mass in individuals with CKD stage 4.[26,27]

Dyslipidemias

Abnormal lipid levels are common in people with CKD and can contribute to the progression of CKD and CVD. Research indicates that all people with CKD be evaluated for lipid disorders. Hyperlipidemia treatment recommendations include use of statin medications plus lifestyle interventions.[68,69]

Therapeutic lifestyle changes for treating dyslipidemia are similar to those for treating HTN, including diet modifications, exercise, moderate alcohol intake, and smoking cessation. As with HTN, few studies have evaluated the effect of exercise and weight loss on abnormal lipid profiles in persons with CKD, and the effect of weight reduction on dyslipidemia in subjects with obesity and CKD is unknown. Regarding diet modifications, current research suggests that eating patterns similar to the DASH and Mediterranean diets are most beneficial in treating lipid disorders.[70]

Mineral and Bone Disorders

Bone disorders and abnormalities in calcium, phosphorus, vitamin D, parathyroid hormone (PTH) metabolism, and fibroblast growth factor-23 (FGF23) begin in the early stages of CKD. Reduction in kidney function even at CKD stages 2 and 3 will result in phosphate retention, hyperphosphatemia, elevated PTH, decreased 1,25 vitamin D, and increased levels of FGF23.[71-73] Conversion of 25-hydroxyvitamin D to 1,25-dihydroxyvitamin D is reduced, lowering intestinal calcium absorption and increasing PTH. FGF23 and PTH normally enhance phosphate excretion through the kidneys, but as CKD advances, the kidneys no longer respond efficiently to either. Downregulation of vitamin D and PTH resistance at the tissue level is also evident. As GFR falls below 60 mL/min/1.73 m², serum levels of phosphorus, calcium, PTH, and vitamin D will begin to show abnormalities.[71,72]

The pathogenesis and the progression of abnormal bone metabolism in CKD are complex and convoluted, involving a combination of minerals and hormones that act on multiple organ systems throughout the body. The consequences of PTH, vitamin D, and FGF23 abnormalities include high turnover bone disease, bone resorption, osteomalacia, adynamic bone disease, overt fractures, microfractures, and bone pain.[70] More importantly, the high mortality rate of patients with CKD may be directly related to soft tissue calcification resulting from hyperphosphatemia, hypercalcemia, or high PTH. Vascular calcification has been implicated in the high rate of atherosclerosis and cardiac dysfunction seen in the population with CKD.[71-75]

Biochemical monitoring of bone health should begin in CKD stage 3, with baseline measurements of serum PTH, calcium, phosphorus, and alkaline phosphatase. Frequency of testing should be determined by baseline levels and progression of kidney disease, generally every 6 to 12 months. As CKD progresses to stage 4, frequency of testing could increase up to every 3 to 6 months, and up to monthly by stage 5, depending on serum levels and presence of biochemical abnormalities.[71,72]

25-hydroxyvitamin D should be assessed beginning at CKD stage 3. Repeat testing is dependent on baseline values and therapeutic interventions. Vitamin D deficiency should be treated, as in the general population.

For all biochemical measurements of mineral and bone disorders, therapeutic treatments should be based on serial measurements and trends, rather than single values. Progressive or persistent high serum phosphorus should be treated to lower levels toward the normal range, beginning with a low phosphorus diet. Secondary treatment for hyperphosphatemia includes phosphate binders, but calcium-based binders should be avoided, when possible, to prevent hypercalcemia.

Specific goal levels for PTH are not known. Experts recommended that when PTH is progressively increasing or persistently above the upper normal limit, patients should initially be evaluated and treated for hyperphosphatemia, high phosphorus intake, hypocalcemia, and vitamin D deficiency. Treatment with calcitriol and vitamin D analogs is not routinely recommended for patients with high PTH levels except in those with severe and progressive hyperparathyroidism at CKD stages 4 and 5.[71,72]

The restriction of dietary phosphorus in conjunction with a low-protein diet can have a direct effect on lowering serum phosphorus and PTH and is associated with a significant increase in blood levels of 1,25-dihydroxyvitamin D3.[73,76] The average phosphorus intake in the typical American diet varies from 1,000 to 1,600 mg/d based on naturally occurring phosphorus in foods, which tends to be concentrated in high protein foods such as meats, dairy products, and eggs. Although legumes, whole grains, and nuts contain significant amounts of phosphorus, it is poorly absorbed due to their high phytate and fiber content which interferes with phosphorus absorption.[41] So these foods contribute much less phosphorus to the total dietary load.[42] Phosphorus-containing food additives used in processed, convenience, and fast foods make a significant contribution to phosphorus consumption. Any diet that includes the regular use of processed foods can add an additional 500 to 1,000 mg phosphorus, thereby increasing daily consumption to nearly 1,500 to 2,600 mg/d. Phosphorus consumed in the form of food additives is readily absorbed compared to natu-

rally occurring phosphorus, thus representing a larger phosphorus burden.[77-79]

Current recommendations include limiting phosphorus intake based on laboratory values, rather than restricting to a specific daily amount.[7,8] Tracking the amount of phosphorus in foods is difficult, as this information is not included on food labels and is frequently missing from nutrient database tables. Because naturally occurring phosphorus is found in high protein foods, a protein-controlled diet that is recommended for patients with CKD tends to be lower in phosphorus compared to the typical American diet. Patients with CKD following a vegetarian low-protein diet have lower serum phosphorus levels compared to those who adhere to an animal-based low-protein diet.[42] The phosphorus content of convenience, processed, and fast foods must also be considered in planning a low phosphorus intake. Since ingredients in processed foods change often, frequent consultation with food manufacturers is needed in order to obtain accurate nutrient amounts.

Even with a dietary phosphorus restriction, phosphate binders may be required in CKD stage 3 or stage 4 to help control serum phosphorus. When taken with meals and snacks, these compounds bind phosphate in the intestine before it can be absorbed. (See Chapter 17 for additional information on phosphate binders.)

Micronutrients and Supplements

Vitamin supplementation needs in patients with CKD can vary, depending on kidney disorders, comorbid conditions, appetite, and intake. Due to compromised kidney function, some vitamin levels can be higher or lower, depending on excretion and metabolism.[80] Traditional CKD diet recommendations that restrict foods and food groups due to protein, phosphorus, and potassium content may result in suboptimal intakes of several vitamins.[81] When diet focuses on quality over quantity, it is possible to achieve healthier nutrient intakes. Thus, routine vitamin supplements may not be needed. The RDN will need to assess patients individually to determine needs, considering disease and metabolic states, stage of CKD, appetite, and overall intake. Multivitamin-mineral supplements should be avoided as they often contain extra minerals (eg, phosphorus, potassium, magnesium). Vitamin A supplements are contraindicated as they can lead to high serum and liver levels. Vitamins D and E should be individualized to specific conditions. For those patients with suboptimal intakes, it is generally safe to recommend a water-soluble vitamin supplement at Dietary Reference Intake (DRI) levels (see Table 3.1).[7,40] Biotin needs may be higher due to decreased biotin consumption when protein intake is low. Higher levels of vitamin C should be avoided due to risk of oxalosis.[82] Some clinicians prefer extra folate, pyridoxine (B6), and cobalamin (B12) to help prevent hyperhomocysteinemia, although several studies show that treating this condition with high levels of B vitamins is unwarranted and possibly harmful.[83]

Use of alternative, complementary, and herbal supplement products is common in populations with CKD. Many products are advertised as kidney protective or beneficial for kidney dysfunction. However, few of these products have been adequately studied in human beings, and even fewer have been evaluated in patients with CKD.[85,86] Because there is no regulation of the supplement industry in the United States, the purity, safety, and effectiveness of products are unknown. One study testing 44 herbal products for authenticity concluded that the majority of the products were of poor quality and contained contaminants, unlisted ingredients, and fillers.[87] Patients should be reminded that every product they consume must be filtered by their kidneys and can affect kidney health. Clinicians should routinely ask patients about their use of supplements to help identify risks. There are safe herbal products available, and the renal RDN should work with patients to find appropriate items that meet their needs. Chapter 19 provides more detailed information on dietary supplements.

Self-Management Behavior and Medical Nutrition Therapy

Nutrition management in patients with CKD involves complex diet therapies; patients must learn to balance protein, calories, sodium, phosphorus, and possibly potassium. In addition, if patients are diagnosed with DM, they must also incorporate methods to control carbohydrate intake and appropriate blood glucose levels. Practitioners should emphasize eating patterns consistent with overall diet quality rather than just limiting nutrients. The plate method has been recommended as a teaching tool to emphasize healthy eating patterns and simplify meal planning (see Figure 3.1).[88] This tool can be utilized in patients with CKD and can be adjusted, depending on individual needs. Using a healthy plate method, patients with diabetic kidney disease can plan for meals that would include the following: ½ plate nonstarchy vegetables (instead of ¼ plate vegetables and ¼ plate fruit), ¼ plate healthy protein, and ¼ plate grains, starchy vegetables, or fruit. Individuals limiting phosphorus and potassium intake can adjust the plate method to include fruits and vegetables lower in potassium, less processed foods, and a reduced amount of dairy and animal products. Patients with CKD concerned about heart issues could adjust the plate to emphasize healthy fats (eg, fish, nuts, seeds, and healthy oils). When following a vegetarian diet, patients can adjust the plate method to include vegetarian protein sources (eg, beans,

TABLE 3.1 | Vitamin Supplementation Recommendations in Chronic Kidney Disease Stages 1 Through 5[84]

Vitamin	US Dietary Reference Intakes (adults >18 yrs)[a]
Vitamin C	75-90 mg/d
Thiamin (B1)	1.1-1.2 mg/d
Riboflavin (B2)	1.1-1.3 mg/d
Niacin (B3)	14-16 mg/d
Folate (B9)	0.4 mg/d
Pyridoxine (B6)	1.3-1.7 mg/d
Cobalamin (B12)	2.4 mcg/d
Biotin (B7)	30 mcg/d
Pantothenic acid (B5)	5 mg/d

[a] Baseline needs equal to Dietary Reference Intake for adults. Higher levels may be acceptable based on specific patient's needs.

FIGURE 3.1 | Kidney healthy plate

The plate method can be used to plan high-quality, kidney healthy meals that provide adequate calories, protein, and nutrients. This plate can be adjusted for various stages and conditions of chronic kidney disease, depending on individual needs.

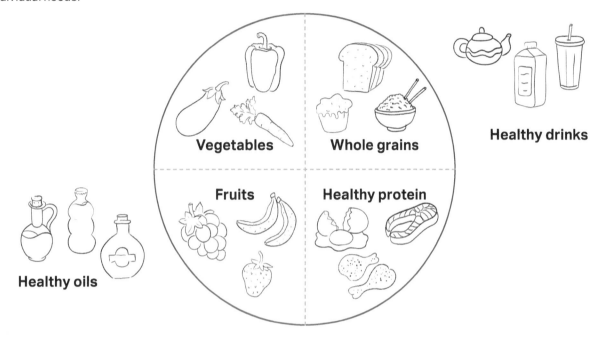

Adapted with permission from Puget Sound Kidney Centers, Everett, WA.

BOX 3.5 | Sample Kidney Healthy Meals Based on Kidney Healthy Plate

Diabetes meal	Fresh eggs scrambled with chopped onion, peppers, spinach, and zucchini
	Whole grain toast
Low potassium, low phosphorus meal	Stir-fry chicken with green beans, onions, peppers, carrots, and mushrooms
	Couscous
	Apple slices
Heart-healthy meal	Grilled salmon
	Whole grain pasta tossed with olive oil and herbs
	Sautéed bell peppers, mushrooms, spinach, onions, and garlic
Vegetarian meal	Mixed bean chili with chopped tomatoes and cilantro
	Corn bread
	Green salad with balsamic vinaigrette

lentils, tofu, nuts, and seeds). See Box 3.5 Sample Kidney Healthy Meals for examples of these meals.

Depending on the patient's overall health, clinicians may also advise lifestyle changes such as quitting smoking and increasing levels of physical activity and exercise. These are not behavioral changes that patients can learn in brief office visits with clinician: they involve intense education on new lifestyles. Partnership and collaboration between health care providers and patients are crucial in promoting self-management in patients with CKD.[89]

Studies show that MNT provided by an RDN is effective in preventing and treating malnutrition, mineral and electrolyte disorders, and minimizing the impact of other comorbid conditions (eg, HTN and DM).[4,5,7] Referrals for MNT should begin during CKD stage 3 when GFR is less than 60 mL/min/1.73 m^2. The RDN should monitor nutritional status every 1 to 3 months or more frequently, depending on risk of malnutrition or mineral and electrolyte disorders. Nutrition therapies must be adjusted to help maintain nutritional health and improve outcomes, depending on the patient's conditions. RDNs providing MNT teach self-management skills in order to promote lifestyle changes that will result in the most successful outcomes for patients with CKD.

Summary

Effective nutrition care for people with CKD stages 1 through 5 involves complex therapeutic interventions. Patients must be assessed for individual nutrition risks and needs to prevent malnutrition, electrolyte imbalances, and bone and mineral metabolism disorders. Many patients presenting with CKD are also diagnosed with comorbid conditions such as DM, CVD, HTN, and dyslipidemia. MNT must include treatment of these conditions and be coordinated with nutrition therapies relevant to CKD. The ultimate goal is to slow the progression of CKD and comorbid conditions and prevent complications of bone mineral metabolism while maintaining overall nutritional health. This can be accomplished through effective MNT provided by the RDN.

References

1. National Chronic Kidney Disease Fact Sheet, 2017. Centers for Disease Control and Prevention. National Center for Chronic Disease Prevention and Health Promotion website. Accessed October 6, 2018. www.cdc.gov/diabetes/pubs/pdf/kidney _factsheet.pdf

2. About Chronic Kidney Disease. National Kidney Foundation website. February 2017. Accessed February 6, 2021. www.kidney.org/atoz/content /about-chronic-kidney-disease

3. Inker LA, Astor BC, Fox CH, et al. KDOQI US Commentary on the 2012 KDIGO clinical practice guideline for the evaluation and management of CKD. *Am J Kidney Dis.* 2014;63(5):713-735. doi:10 .1053/j.ajkd.2014.01.416

4. de Waal D, Heaslip E, Callas P. Medical nutrition therapy for chronic kidney disease improves biomarkers and slows time to dialysis. *J Ren Nutr.* 2016;26(1):1-9. doi:10.1053/j.jrn.2015.08.002

5. Kramer H, Jimenez E, Brommage D, et al. Medical nutrition therapy for patients with non-dialysis-dependent chronic kidney disease: barriers and solutions. *J Acad Nutr Diet.* 2018;118(10):1958-1965. doi:10.1016/j.jand.2018.05.023

6. Kopple JD, Fouque D. Pro: the rationale for dietary therapy for patients with advanced chronic kidney disease. *Nephrol Dial Transplant.* 2018;33(3):373-378. doi:10.1093/ndt/gfx333

7. Academy of Nutrition and Dietetics Evidence Analysis Library. Chronic Kidney Disease. Accessed April 8, 2020. www.andeal.org/topic.cfm?menu =5303&cat=1400

8. National Kidney Foundation. K/DOQI Clinical Practice Guidelines for Nutrition in Chronic Kidney Disease: 2020 update. *Am J Kidney Dis.* 76;3(suppl 1):S1-S107. doi:10.1053/j.ajkd/2020.05.006

9. Chauveau P, Aparicio M, Bellizzi V, et al. Mediterranean diet as the diet of choice for patients with chronic kidney disease. *Nephrol Dial Transplant.* 2017;(33)5:725-735. doi:10.1093/ndt/gfx085

10. Chauveau P, Koppe L, Combe C, Lasseur C, Trolonge S, Aparicio M. Vegetarian diets and chronic kidney disease. *Nephrol Dial Transplant.* 2019;34(2):199-207. doi:10.1093/ndt/gfy164

11. Rebholz CM, Crews DC, Grams MD, et al. Dash (Dietary Approaches to Stop Hypertension) diet and risk of subsequent kidney disease. *Am J Kidney Dis.* 2016;68(6):853-861. doi:10.1053/j.ajkd.2016.05.019

12. Smyth A, Griffin M, Yusuf S, et al. Diet and major renal outcomes: a prospective cohort study. The NIH-AARP diet and health study. *J Ren Nutr.* 2016;26(5):288-298. doi:10.1053/j.jrn.2016.01.016

13. Chen W, Bushinsky DA. Addressing racial disparity in the progression of chronic kidney disease: prescribe more fruits and vegetables? *Am J Nephrol.* 2018;47(3):171-173. doi:10.1159 /000487716

14. Cupisti A, D'Alessandro CD, Gesualdo L, et al. Non-traditional aspects of renal diets: focus on fiber, alkali and vitamin K1 intake. *Nutrients.* 2017;9(5)444. doi:10.3390/nu9050444

15. Goraya N, Simoni J, Jo CH, Wesson D. A comparison of treating metabolic acidosis in CKD stage 4 hypertensive kidney disease with fruits and vegetables or sodium bicarbonate. *Clin J Am Soc Nephrol.* 2013;8(3):371-381. doi:10.2215/CJN .02430312

16. Held PJ, Port FK, Gaylin DS, et al. Evaluations of initial predictors of mortality among 4387 new ESRD patients: the USRDS Case Mix Study. *J Am Soc Nephrol.* 1991;2:328-328 abstract.

17. Kopple JD, Greene T, Chumlea WC, et al. Relationship between nutritional status and the glomerular filtration rate: results from the MDRD study. *Kidney Int.* 2000;57(4):1688-1703. doi:10.1046/j.1523-1755.2000.00014.x

18. Ikizler TA, Green JH, Wingard RL, Parker RA, Hakim RM. Spontaneous dietary protein intake during progression of chronic renal failure. *J Am Soc Nephrol.* 1995;6(5):1386-1391.

19. Carrero JJ, Stenvinkel P, Cuppari L, et al. Etiology of the protein-energy wasting syndrome in chronic kidney disease: a consensus statement from the International Society of Renal Nutrition and Metabolism (ISRNM). *J Ren Nutr.* 2013;23(2):77-90. doi:10.1053/j.jrn.2013.01.001

20. Fried LF, Boudreau R, Lee JS, et al. Kidney function as a predictor of loss of lean mass in older adults: health, aging, and body composition study. *J Am Geriatr Soc.* 2007;55(10):1578-1584. doi:10.1111/j.1532-5415.2007.01398.x

21. O'Sullivan AJ, Lawson JA, Chan M, Kelly JJ. Body composition and energy metabolism in chronic renal insufficiency. *Am J Kidney Dis.* 2002;39(2):369-375. doi:10.1053/ajkd.2002.30558

22. Rhee CM, Ahmadi SF, Kalantar-Zadeh K. The dual roles of obesity in chronic kidney disease: a review of the current literature. *Curr Opin Nephrol Hypertens.* 2016;25(3):208-216. doi:10.1097/MNH.0000000000000212

23. Stenvinkel P, Zoccali C, Ikizler TA. Obesity in CKD—what should nephrologists know? *J Am Soc Nephrol.* 2013;24(11):1727-1736. doi:10.1681/ASN.2013040330

24. Mohebi R, Simforoosh A, Tohidi M, Azizi F, Hadaegh F. Obesity paradox and risk of mortality events in chronic kidney disease patients: a decade of follow-up in Tehran lipid and glucose study. *J Ren Nutr.* 2015;25(4):345-350. doi:10.1053/j.jrn.2014.12.006

25. Kalantar-Zadeh K, Rhee CM, Chou J, et al. The obesity paradox in kidney disease: how to reconcile it with obesity management. *Kidney Int Rep.* 2017;2(2):271-281. doi:10.1016/j.ekir.2017.01.009

26. Van Huffel L, Tomson CR, Ruige J, Nistor I, Van Biesen W, Bolignano D. Dietary restriction and exercise for diabetic patients with chronic kidney disease: a systematic review. *PLoS One.* 2014;9(11):e113667. doi:10.1371/journal.pone.0113667

27. Sah SK, Siddiqui MA, Darain H. Effect of progressive resistive exercise training in improving mobility and functional ability of middle adulthood patients with chronic kidney disease. *Saudi J Kidney Dis Transpl.* 2015;26(5):912-923. doi:10.4103/1319-2442.164571

28. Ko GJ, Obi Y, Tortoricci AR, Kalantar-Zadeh K. Dietary protein intake and chronic kidney disease. *Curr Opin Clin Nutr Metab Care.* 2017;20(1):77-85. doi:10.1097/MCO.0000000000000342

29. Kovesdy CP, Kalantar-Zadeh K. Back to the future: restricted protein intake for conservative management of CKD, triple goals of renoprotection, uremia mitigation, and nutrition health. *Int Urol Nephrol.* 2016;48(5):725-729. doi:10.1007/s11255-016-1224-0

30. Ihle BU, Becker GJ, Whitworth JA, Charlwood RA, Kincaid-Smith PS. The effect of protein restriction on the progression of renal insufficiency. *N Engl J Med.* 1989;321:1773-1777. doi:10.1056/NEJM198912283212601

31. Walser M, Hill SB, Ward L, Magder L. A crossover comparison of progression of chronic renal failure: ketoacids versus amino acids. *Kidney Int.* 1993;43(4):933-939. doi:10.1038/ki.1993.131

32. Klahr S, Levey AS, Beck GJ, et al. The effects of dietary protein restriction and blood-pressure control on the progression of chronic renal disease. *N Engl J Med.* 1994;330(13):877-884. doi:10.1056/NEJM199403313301301

33. Walser M, Hill S. Can renal replacement be deferred by a supplemented very low-protein diet? *J Am Soc Nephrol.* 1999;10(1):110-116.

34. Levey AS, Green T, Beck GJ, et al. Dietary protein restriction and the progression of chronic renal disease: what have all of the results of the MDRD study shown? *J Am Soc Nephrol.* 1999;10(11):2426-2439.

35. Levey A, Greene T, Sarnak M, et al. Effect of dietary protein restriction on the progression of kidney disease: long-term follow-up of the modification of diet in renal disease (MDRD) study. *Am J Kidney Dis.* 2006;48(6):879-888. doi:10.1053/j.ajkd.2006.08.023

36. Menon V, Kopple J, Wang X, et al. Effect of a very low-protein diet on outcomes: long-term follow-up of the modification of diet in renal disease (MDRD) study. *Am J Kidney Dis.* 2009;53(2):208-217. doi:10.1053/j.ajkd.2008.08.009

37. Fouque D, Guebre-Egziabher F. Do low-protein diets work in chronic kidney disease patients? *Semin Nephrol.* 2009;29(1):30-38. doi:10.1016/j.semnephrol.2008.10.005

38. Chen X, Wei G, Jalili T, et al. The associations of plant protein intake with all-cause mortality in CKD. *Am J Kidney Dis.* 2016;67(3):423-430. doi:10.1053/j.ajkd.2015.10.018

39. Brookhyser Hogan J. *The Vegetarian Diet for Kidney Disease: Preserving Kidney Function with Plant Based Eating.* Basic Health Publications; 2010.

40. Wiggins KL. Guideline 2: Nutrition care of adult dialysis patients. In: *Guidelines for Nutrition Care of Renal Patients.* 3rd ed. American Dietetic Association; 2002.

41. St-Jules DE, Goldfarb DS, Sevick MA. Nutrient non-equivalence: does restricting high potassium plant foods help to prevent hyperkalemia in hemodialysis patients? *J Ren Nutr.* 2016;26(5):282-287. doi:10.1053/j.jrn.2016.02.005

42. Moe SM, Zidehsarai MP, Chambers MA, et al. Vegetarian compared with meat dietary protein source and phosphorus homeostasis in chronic kidney disease. *Clin J Am Soc Nephrol.* 2011;6(2):257-264. doi:10.2215/CJN.05040610

43. Naderi N, Kleine CE, Park C, et al. Obesity paradox in advanced kidney disease: from bedside to the bench. *Prog Cardiovasc Dis.* 2018;61(2):168-181. doi:10.1016/j.pcad.2018.07.001

44. Tian X, Chen Y, Yang ZK, Qu Z, Dong J. Novel equations for estimating lean body mass in patients with chronic kidney disease. *J Ren Nutr.* 2018;28(3):156-164. doi:10.1053/j.jrn.2017.09.004

45. Byham-Gray L, Parrott JS, Peters EN, et al. Modeling a predictive energy equation specific for maintenance hemodialysis. *JPEN J Parenter Enteral Nutr.* 2018;42(3):587-596. doi:10.1177/0148607117696942

46. Kamimura MA, Avesani CM, Bazanelli AP, Baria F, Draibe SA, Cuppari L. Are prediction equations reliable for estimating energy expenditure in chronic kidney disease patients? *Nephrol Dial Transplant.* 2011;26(2):544-550. doi:10.1093/ndt/gfq452

47. Byham-Gray LD. Weighing the evidence: energy determinations across the spectrum of kidney disease. *J Ren Nutr.* 2006;16(1):17-26. doi:10.1053/j.jrn.2005.10.004

48. Beto JA, Ramirez WE, Bansal VK. Medical nutrition therapy in adults with chronic kidney disease: integrating evidence and consensus into practice for the generalist registered dietitian nutritionist. *J Acad Nutr Diet.* 2014;114(7):1077-1087. doi:10.1016/j.jand.2013.12.009

49. Saran R, Robinson B, Abbott KC, et al. US Renal Data System 2017 Annual Data Report: epidemiology of kidney disease in the United States. *Am J Kidney Dis.* 2018;71(3 suppl 1):Svii,S1-S672. doi:10.1053/j.ajkd.2018.01.002

50. Ash S, Campbell KL, Bogard J, Millichamp A. Nutrition prescription to achieve positive outcomes in chronic kidney disease. *Nutrients.* 2014;6(1):416-451. doi:10.3390/nu6010416

51. Ireton-Jones C. Adjusted body weight, con: why adjust body weight in energy expenditure calculations? *Nutr Clin Pract.* 2005;20(4):474-479. doi:10.1177/0115426505020004474

52. Academy of Nutrition and Dietetics Evidence Analysis Library. "In obese adults, what is the prediction accuracy and maximum overestimation and underestimation errors compared to measured resting metabolic rate when using the Harris-Benedict formula (actual body weight)?" Accessed February 7, 2021. www.andeal.org/template.cfm?template=guide_summary&key=621&highlight=Adult%20Weight%20management&home=1

53. Schiro Harvey K. Methods for determining healthy body weight in end stage renal disease. *J Ren Nutr.* 2006;16(3):269-276. doi:10.1053/j.jrn.2006.01.008

54. McClave SA, Taylor BE, Martindale RG, et al. Guidelines for the provision and assessment of nutrition support therapy in the adult critically ill patient: Society of Critical Care Medicine (SCCM) and American Society for Parenteral and Enteral Nutrition (A.S.P.E.N.). *JPEN J Parenteral Enteral Nutr.* 2016;40(2):159-211. doi:10.1177/0148607115621863

55. Dutheil F, Lac G, Courteix D, et al. Treatment of metabolic syndrome by combination of physical activity and diet needs an optimal protein intake: a randomized controlled trial. *Nutr J.* 2012;11:72. doi:10.1186/1475-2891-11-72

56. Weijs PJM, Wolfe RR. Exploration of the protein requirement during weight loss in obese older adults. *Clin Nutr.* 2016;35(2):394-398. doi:10.1016/j.clnu.2015.02.016

57. National Kidney Foundation. KDOQI clinical practice guidelines and clinical practice recommendations for diabetes and chronic kidney disease. *Am J Kidney Dis.* 2007;49(2 suppl 2):S12-S180. doi:10.1053/j.ajkd.2006.12.005

58. National Kidney Foundation. KDOQI clinical practice guideline for diabetes and CKD: 2012 update. *Am J Kidney Dis.* 2012;60(5):850-886. doi:10.1053/j.ajkd.2012.07.005

59. Boucher JL. Mediterranean eating pattern. *Diabetes Spectr.* 2017;30(2):72-76. doi:10.2337/ds16-0074

60. Campbell AP. DASH eating plan: an eating pattern for diabetes management. *Diabetes Spectr.* 2017;30(2):76-81. doi:10.2337/ds16-0084

61. American Diabetes Association. 4. Lifestyle management: Standards of Medical Care in Diabetes-2018. *Diabetes Care.* 2018;41(suppl 1):S38-S50. doi:10.2337/dc18-S004

62. Ko GJ, Kalantar-Zadeh K, Goldstein-Fuchs J, Rhee CM. Dietary approaches in the management of diabetic patients with kidney disease. *Nutrients.* 2017;9(8):824. doi:10.3390/nu9080824

63. Taler SJ, Agarwal R, Bakris GL, et al. KDOQI US commentary on the 2012 KDIGO clinical practice guideline for management of blood pressure in CKD. *Am J Kidney Dis.* 2013;62(2):201-213. doi:10.1053/j.ajkd.2013.03.018

64. Conlin PR, Chow D, Miller ER, et al. The effect of dietary patterns on blood pressure control in hypertensive patients: results from the Dietary Approaches to Stop Hypertension (DASH) trial. *Am J Hypertens.* 2000;13(9):949-955. doi:10.1016/s0895-7061(99)00284-8

65. Sacks FM, Svetkey LP, Vollmer WM, et al. Effects on blood pressure of reduced dietary sodium and the Dietary Approaches to Stop Hypertension (DASH) diet. *N Engl J Med.* 2001;344(1):3-10. doi:10.1056/NEJM200101043440101

66. Tyson CC, Lin PH, Corsino L, et al. Short-term effects of the DASH diet in adults with moderate chronic kidney disease: a pilot feeding study. *Clin Kidney J.* 2016;9(4)592-598. doi:10.1093/ckj/sfw046

67. Noori N, Kalantar-Zadeh K, Kovesdy CP, et al. Dietary potassium intake and mortality in long-term hemodialysis patients. *Am J Kidney Dis.* 2010;56(2):338-347. doi:10.1053/j.ajkd.2010.03.022

68. Sarnak MJ, Bloom R, Mutner P, et al. KDOQI US commentary on the 2013 KDIGO clinical practice guideline for lipid management in CKD. *Am J Kidney Dis.* 2015;65(3):354-366. doi:10.1053/j.ajkd.2014.10.005

69. Marino A, Tannock LR. Role of dyslipidemia in patients with chronic kidney disease. *Postgrad Med.* 2013;125(4):28-37. doi:10.3810/pgm.2013.07.2676

70. KDIGO clinical practice guideline for lipid management in chronic kidney disease. *Kidney Int.* 2013;3(3):259-305. doi:10.1038/kisup.2013.27

71. KDIGO 2017 clinical practice guideline update for the diagnosis, evaluation, prevention, and treatment of chronic kidney disease-mineral and bone disorder (CKD-MBD). *Kidney Int.* 2017;7(1):1-59. doi:10.1016/j.kisu.2017.04.001

72. Isakova T, Nickolas TL, Denburg M, et al. KDOQI US commentary on the 2017 KDIGO clinical practice guideline update for the diagnosis, evaluation, prevention, and treatment of chronic kidney disease-mineral and bone disorder (CKD-MBD). *Am J Kidney Dis.* 2017;70(6):737-751. doi:10.1053/j.ajkd.2017.07.019

73. Martinez I, Saracho R, Montenegro J, Llach F. The importance of dietary calcium and phosphorous in the secondary hyperparathyroidism of patients with early renal failure. *Am J Kidney Dis.* 1997;29(4):496-502. doi:10.1016/s0272-6386(97)90330-9

74. Andress DL. Vitamin D in chronic kidney disease: a systemic role for selective vitamin D receptor activation. *Kidney Int.* 2006;69(1):33-43. doi:10.1038/sj.ki.5000045

75. Kramer H, Toto R, Peshock R, Cooper R, Victor R. Association between chronic kidney disease and coronary artery calcification: the Dallas Heart Study. *J Am Soc Nephrol.* 2005;16(2):507-513. doi:10.1681/ASN.2004070610

76. Barsotti G, Cupisti A. The role of dietary phosphorus restriction in the conservative management of chronic renal disease. *J Ren Nutr.* 2005;15(1):189-192. doi:10.1053/j.jrn.2004.09.007

77. Uribarri J, Calvo MS. Hidden sources of phosphorus in the typical American diet: does it matter in nephrology? *Semin Dial.* 2003;16(3):186-188. doi:10.1046/j.1525-139x.2003.16037.x

78. Sullivan C, Sayre SS, Leon JB, et al. Effect of food additives on hyperphosphatemia among patients with end-stage renal disease: a randomized controlled trial. *JAMA.* 2009;301(6):629-635. doi:10.1001/jama.2009.96

79. Carrigan A, Klinger A, Choquette SS, et al. Contribution of food additives to sodium and phosphorus content of diets rich in processed foods. *J Ren Nutr.* 2014;24(1):13-19. doi:10.1053/j.jrn.2013.09.003

80. Handelman GJ, Levin NW. Guidelines for vitamin supplements in chronic kidney disease patients: what is the evidence? *J Ren Nutr.* 2011;21(1):117-119. doi:10.1053/j.jrn.2010.11.004

81. Jankowska M, Szupryczynska N, Debska-Slizien A, et al. Dietary intake of vitamins in different options of treatment in chronic kidney disease: is there a deficiency? *Transplant Proc.* 2016;48(5):1427-1430. doi:10.1016/j.transproceed.2015.11.039

82. Handelman GJ. New insight on vitamin C in patients with chronic kidney disease. *J Ren Nutr.* 2011;21(1):110-112. doi:10.1053/j.jrn.2010.11.003

83. Rafeq Z, Roh JD, Guarina P, Kaufman J, Joseph J. Adverse myocardial effects of B-vitamin therapy in subjects with chronic kidney disease and hyperhomocysteinaemia. *Nutr Metab Cardiovasc Dis*. 2013;23(9):836-842. doi:10.1016/j.numecd.2012.07.002

84. National Institute of Health. Office of Dietary Supplements website. Accessed February 8, 2021. https://.ods.od.nih.gov/Health_Information/Dietary_Reference_Intakes.aspx

85. Vamenta-Morris H, Dreisbach A, Shoemaker-Moyle M, Abdel-Rahman EM. Internet claims on dietary and herbal supplements in advanced nephropathy: truth or myth. *Am J Nephrol*. 2014;40(5):393-398. doi:10.1159/000368724

86. Osman NA, Hassanein SM, Leil MM, NasrAllah MM. Complementary and alternative medicine use among patients with chronic kidney disease and kidney transplant recipients. *J Ren Nutr*. 2015:25(6):466-471. doi:10.1053/j.jrn.2015.04.009

87. Newmaster SG, Grguric M, Shanmughanandhan D, Ramalingam S, Ragupathy S. DNA barcoding detects contamination and substitution in North American herbal products. *BMC Med*. 2013;11:222. doi:10.1186/1741-7015-11-222

88. Maryniuk MD. From pyramids to plates to patterns: perspectives on meal planning. *Diabetes Spect*. 2017;30(2):67-70. doi:10.2337/ds16-0080

89. Chiou CP, Lu YC, Hung SY. Self-management in patients with chronic kidney disease. *Hu Li Za Zhi*. 2016;63(2):5-11. doi:10.6224/JN.63.2.5

CHAPTER 4
Nutrition Management in Acute Kidney Injury

Ann Beemer Cotton, MS, RD, CNSC, and Sarita Bajpai, PhD, RDN, CD, CNSC

Introduction

Acute renal failure (ARF) has been renamed and redefined as acute kidney injury (AKI).[1] Previously, the definition of ARF was usually limited to individuals who experienced a rapid fall in the glomerular filtration rate (GFR) and eventually required kidney replacement therapy (KRT). The intensive care unit was typically the setting, and multiorgan failure (MOF) often coincided with this diagnosis. Today, with ARF renamed as AKI and staged according to specific criteria, the critically ill patient requiring KRT represents only a fraction of those with AKI.

In the last two decades, AKI is well recognized to occur across a spectrum in varying degrees or severity, with a direct impact on clinical outcomes. Levy et al,[1] and later Chertow et al,[2] found that small increases in serum creatinine, as little as 0.3 mg/dL, led to higher mortality rates, longer hospital stays, and higher costs, even when dialysis was not necessary. This growing awareness led to a new definition and classification system for ARF based on severity or staging criteria.

ACUTE KIDNEY INJURY DEFINITION AND CLASSIFICATION

The Acute Dialysis Quality Initiative was created as an initial step to define and categorize ARF by severity and outcome under the acronym RIFLE: *R*isk, *I*njury, *F*ailure, *L*oss, and *E*nd-stage (see Figure 4.1).[3-5] Under RIFLE,

AKI severity was categorized over a spectrum by Risk, Injury, and Failure. The criteria used to classify severity includes change in GFR, serum creatinine, and urine output. Outcomes under RIFLE were measured by the duration of AKI specified as Loss or duration of greater than 4 weeks and then End-stage renal or kidney disease.

FIGURE 4.1 | The RIFLE criteria

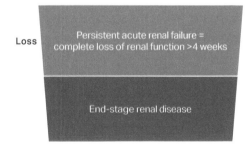

	GFR criteria	Urine output criteria	
Risk	Increased creatinine × 1.5 or GFR decrease >25%	UO <0.5 mL/kg/h × 6 h	High sensitivity
Injury	Increased creatinine × 2 or GFR decrease >50%	UO <0.5 mL/kg/h × 12 h	
Failure	Increased creatinine × 3 or GFR decrease >75% or creatinine ≥4 mg/dL (acute rise of ≥5 mg/dL)	*Oliguria* UO <0.3 mL/kg/h × 24 h or anuria × 12 h	High specificity
Loss	Persistent acute renal failure = complete loss of renal function >4 weeks		
	End-stage renal disease		

GFR = glomerular filtration rate; UO = urine output.
Adapted with permission from Macmillan Publishers Ltd. Himmelfarb J, Ikizler TA. Acute kidney injury: changing lexicography, definitions, and epidemiology. *Kidney Int.* 2007;71(10):971-976.

In 2004, the Acute Kidney Injury Network (AKIN) was established, and the term AKI was created to define the entire spectrum of acute kidney dysfunction from its earliest and mildest forms up to the need for KRT.[6] The AKIN proposed diagnostic criteria to identify the presence of AKI (Box 4.1) and then modified the RIFLE criteria to develop a three-level staging system based on newer data. These data suggested that smaller changes in serum creatinine than those utilized in RIFLE could be more sensitive in identifying AKI (Table 4.1).[6] It was anticipated that earlier identification would lead to earlier intervention and reduction of related morbidity and mortality. More recently, the 2012 Kidney Disease Improving Global Outcomes (KDIGO) AKI Guidelines acknowledged the need for an AKI definition and staging system. To facilitate use of an AKI assessment tool for clinical practice, research, and public health, the KDIGO guidelines merged the RIFLE and AKIN criteria into a single definition as shown below.

BOX 4.1 | Diagnostic Criteria for Acute Kidney Injury[7]

Acute kidney injury is defined as any of the following:

- An increase in serum creatinine (SCr) of ≥0.3 mg/dL within 48 hours
  or
- An increase in SCr to ≥1.5 times baseline that is known or presumed to have occurred within the prior 7 days
  or
- Urine volume <0.5 mL/kg/h for 6 hours

One of the main purposes of creating an AKI staging system was to permit early diagnosis that would enable rapid intervention to control worsening kidney dysfunction. The incidence of AKI varies by location with approximately 2% at community hospitals and up to 20% at large academic centers.[8] In the critical care setting, the occurrence ranges from 25% to 40% with a frequent mortality rate of greater than 50%.[9]

Knowledge of AKI staging aids in understanding the impact of AKI progression as an escalating acute inflammatory process, which spreads from the kidney to other organs, creating multisystem organ failure. Fiaccadori et al[9] refer to this progression as a kidney-centered inflammatory syndrome. AKI is observed more often in those with advanced age and with certain comorbidities to include diabetes mellitus (DM), hypertension (HTN), heart failure, and elevated baseline creatinine. These are chronic disease states often contributing to chronic malnutrition at baseline, which is then further exacerbated by the acute inflammation of AKI.

Etiology and Pathology

AKI is associated with various conditions, such as sepsis, cancer, pregnancy, pulmonary–renal syndromes, liver disease, nephrotic syndrome, and HIV infection, in addition to trauma, cardiac surgery, and post renal transplant. The etiology of AKI can be classified into the following three categories: prerenal, postrenal, and intrinsic or tubulointerstitial.[10,11] When an AKI is identified early at stage 1 or stage 2 and treated aggressively, prerenal and

TABLE 4.1 | Staging for Acute Kidney Injury[7]

Stage	Serum creatinine (SCr)	Urine output
1	1.5-1.9 times baseline or ≥0.3 mg/dL increase	<0.5 mL/kg/h for 6-12 hours
2	2.0-2.9 times baseline	<0.5 mL/kg/h for ≥12 hours
3	3.0 times baseline *or* increase in SCr to ≥4.0 mg/dL *or* initiation of kidney replacement therapy	<0.3 mL/kg/h for ≥24 hours *or* anuria for ≥12 hours

postrenal AKI are usually reversible with minimal long-term injury and limited to no requirement of nutrition intervention. If not quickly corrected, both can cause damage to the kidney parenchyma, increasing the severity of AKI and potentially advancing to AKI stage 3 with the need for short-term and possibly long-term KRT.

PRERENAL CAUSES

Prerenal AKI is most common, accounting for approximately 50% to 60% of all cases.[11] Prerenal AKI occurs from renal hypoperfusion, which can be caused by intravascular volume depletion, decreased cardiac output, early sepsis, diuretic abuse, cirrhosis, or hepatorenal syndrome.[10,12] Urine output declines, and sodium is retained with a buildup of nitrogenous waste products. Diagnostic signs include a low urinary sodium of less than 10 mEq/L, high urine osmolality of more than 350 to 500 mOsm/kg, and a blood urea nitrogen (BUN) to creatinine ratio of more than 20:1.[10,11]

Prerenal AKI has a higher prevalence in older adults because aging is associated with a general decline in kidney function, polypharmacy, increased dehydration risk (urine concentrating ability is lost with aging), impaired thirst regulation, and reduced sodium retention.[13] Early diagnosis with restoration of intravascular volume to the kidneys is essential. Prerenal azotemia should reverse within 1 to 2 days after kidney perfusion is restored, but recovery may be delayed in those with substantial decline from baseline kidney function or preexisting chronic kidney disease (CKD).[10] Limited to no specific nutrition intervention for AKI is necessary if the underlying cause is corrected and volume status is promptly restored.

POSTRENAL CAUSES

Postrenal AKI results from an obstruction of urine flow and is prevalent in approximately 5% to 15% of all patients.[12] This may be caused by prostate, gynecological, or bladder cancers; benign prostate hyperplasia; renal calculi; blood clots; or strictures.[10,12] Older adults and young individuals are most commonly affected. Often, those with severe sudden onset oliguria (urine volume of <400 mL/d) or anuria (urine volume of <50 mL/d)

are more likely to have postrenal AKI.[11,13] Other diagnostic signs may include urine osmolality of more than 400 mOsm/kg early on and approximately 300 mOsm/kg later with a BUN to creatinine ratio of 10:1 to 20:1.[11] Azotemia usually resolves by correcting the obstruction and resuming normal hydration. Again, minimal to no nutrition management is typically needed with postrenal AKI.

INTRINSIC OR TUBULOINTERSTITIAL CAUSES

Tubulointerstitial AKI, which is associated with actual tissue damage to the renal parenchyma, is prevalent in 20% to 30% of all patients.[11] Frequently, the patient will present with azotemia, hyperkalemia, and hyperphosphatemia. Urine sodium concentrations will be more than 30 to 40 mEq/L, with a urine osmolality of approximately 300 mOsm/kg. This is equivalent to the serum because the kidneys can no longer concentrate or dilute. A BUN to creatinine ratio of 10:1 to 20:1 is also seen.[10,11] The kidney's four compartments can also be used to classify causes of AKI: vascular (renal artery occlusions, atheroembolism), interstitial (often drug-induced or allergic interstitial nephritis), glomerular (glomerulonephritis, systemic disorders), and tubular (ischemic or nephrotoxic acute tubular necrosis [ATN]).[11,13] See Box 4.2 on page 52.

ATN is the most common cause of tubulointerstitial disease and can occur with prolonged systemic hypotension from excessive blood loss or prolonged clamp time during abdominal vascular surgery. Septic or hypovolemic shock and obstetric complications may also contribute. Toxicity from prescription medications, nonprescription alternative therapies and crush injury-related rhabdomyolysis are also common causes. In addition, atherosclerotic vascular disease in the expanding older population, widespread use of vasoactive agents, and the use of contrast agents for radiographic studies have led to an increased incidence of tubulointerstitial AKI. ATN is usually associated with oliguria and acute onset or worsening of azotemia, even after withdrawing the causative agent and restoring adequate

BOX 4.2 | Causes of Acute Kidney Injury[9,13,14]

TYPE OF ACUTE KIDNEY INJURY (AKI)	CAUSES
Prerenal AKI	Intravascular volume depletion: hemorrhage, vomiting, diarrhea, surgical drainage, burns, fever, third-spacing, diuretic use, inadequate volume resuscitation, hyperemesis of pregnancy, septic abortion, hypoadrenalism Decreased cardiac output: • Congestive heart failure or cardiomyopathy, valvular heart disease, pulmonary hypertension • Sepsis syndrome, cirrhosis, hepatorenal syndrome • Drugs: nonsteroidal antiinflammatory drugs (NSAIDs), angiotensin-converting enzyme inhibitors (ACE-I), calcineurin inhibitors (eg, cyclosporine or tacrolimus), radiocontrast agents, amphotericin B, cocaine, and some herbs
Postrenal AKI	Benign prostatic hypertrophy, prostate cancer, cervical cancer, colorectal cancer, intraluminal bladder or pelvic mass, retroperitoneal disorders, neurogenic bladder, urethral strictures, intratubular deposition and obstructions (uric acid and oxalate, sulfonamides, acyclovir, methotrexate)
Intrinsic or tubulointerstitial AKI	Vascular disease: atheroembolic disease, thrombotic thrombocytopenic purpura, hemolytic uremic syndrome, postpartum AKI, renal artery occlusion, thrombosis, vasculitis Interstitial nephritis: allergic reactions (antibiotics, allopurinol, NSAIDs, diuretics, ACE-I), acute pyelonephritis, infiltrative diseases (lymphoma, leukemia, sarcoidosis), infections (cytomegalovirus or candidiasis) Glomerular disease: glomerulonephritis and vasculitis (systemic lupus erythematosus), small vessel vasculitis (Wegener granulomatosis), immunoglobulin A nephropathy, post infection, radiation nephritis, scleroderma, hemolytic uremic syndrome, toxemia of pregnancy Acute tubular necrosis • Ischemia: major surgery, hypotension, cardiogenic, septic or hypovolemic shock, obstetric complications • Nephrotoxicity: acyclovir, aminoglycoside antibiotics, amphotericin B, acetaminophen, NSAIDs, radiocontrast agents/dyes, some chemotherapy and immunosuppressant agents (cisplatin, cyclosporine/tacrolimus), organic solvents (ethylene glycol and toluene), heavy metals, pigments, cocaine • Intratubular deposition and obstruction: myeloma proteins, uric acid, oxalates, acyclovir, methotrexate, sulphonamides

intravascular volume. The clinical course of ATN occurs in three phases[15]:

1. Initial Phase (time frame of hours or days)
   o the period between exposure and established kidney injury
   o usually reversible by treating the underlying disorder or removing the offending agent
2. Maintenance Phase (time frame of 10 to 16 days in oliguric patients and 5 to 8 days in nonoliguric patients)
   o established tubular epithelial cell injury
   o when urine output is at its lowest with AKI-associated complications, such as fluid overload and electrolyte imbalances (hyponatremia and hyperkalemia)
3. Recovery Phase (time frame of days to months)
   o defined by tubular epithelial cell regeneration and gradual return of GFR
   o when BUN and creatinine levels return to near baseline levels
   o may be complicated by marked diuresis with excess free water loss, volume depletion, and electrolyte imbalances (hypernatremia and hypokalemia) if not closely monitored and treated

Kidney Replacement Therapy in Acute Kidney Injury

The initiation of KRT usually occurs when overt azotemia, hyperkalemia, volume overload, or severe acidosis worsens and is resistant to conservative therapies.[7,8,11,16,17] While KRT is initiated for these AKI complications, it will also provide supportive therapy for essential functions of other organs and allow adequate nutrition support. Bellomo's first principle for nutrition support states that with AKI, nutrition should never be limited in an attempt to control azotemia, prevent volume overload, and avoid the initiation of KRT.[14] Instead, those with AKI should receive both KRT and the appropriate nutrition support.

Conventional intermittent hemodialysis (IHD) remains the standard treatment if the patient is hemodynamically stable.[10,11] When hemodynamic instability is a concern, continuous renal replacement therapy (CRRT) is initiated, providing slower, better tolerated fluid and solute removal. Access can be arteriovenous (AV), which relies on the patient's mean arterial pressure to drive the process and is rarely utilized now, or more recently venovenous (VV), which requires a pump-driven circuit that provides a more consistent and reliable blood flow rate and clearance. Types of CRRT include the following[18-20]:

- Continuous arteriovenous hemofiltration (CAVH) or continuous venovenous hemofiltration (CVVH): Solute clearance occurs through convection or movement of fluid across the semipermeable membrane of the hemofilter at a prescribed rate of 2 to 4 L/h. Most of the ultrafiltrated volume or effluent is replaced with a physiological fluid.
- Continuous arteriovenous hemodialysis (CAVHD), continuous venovenous hemodialysis (CVVHD), or sustained low-efficiency dialysis (SLED): Clearance occurs through diffusion as with IHD, in which molecules in the solvent or dialysate move from a region of higher concentration to that of a lower concentration. It provides continuous or extended hemodialysis (HD) with slower blood and dialysate flow rates. (Note: SLED is frequently delivered only in 8- to 12-hour treatments.)

- Continuous AV hemodiafiltration (CAVHDF) or continuous venovenous hemodiafiltration (CVVHDF): Clearance occurs through a mix of both convection and diffusion, as previously noted.
- Slow continuous ultrafiltration (SCUF): Clearance is limited purely to ultrafiltration without fluid replacement.

Peritoneal dialysis (PD) is another modality choice for AKI, although it is used rarely compared to IHD or CRRT. Contraindications to PD include the need for large volume removal, high solute clearance, and recent abdominal surgery.[20,21] It may still be used with severe coagulopathy, and possibly in remote rural areas where access to more advanced technology is limited.[19,20]

Regardless of the modality chosen, all replacement therapies have nutritional implications that can contribute to protein energy wasting (PEW). Nutritional needs require periodic evaluation, especially with respect to any change in KRT modality and the impact of the current modality on nutrient losses. KRT not only removes uremic waste but also protein, amino acids, and micronutrients. Each HD treatment incurs the loss of 2 to 5 g peptides and 2 to 8 g free amino acids.[22] Protein losses in PD average 10 g/d but can increase to 20 g/d or more, depending on peritoneal membrane permeability.[23] Protein loss with CRRT ranges from 1.5 to 7.2 g/d, with amino acid losses of 15 to 30 g/d directly proportional to CRRT effluent flow.[24-28] Actual amino acid loss may be estimated at 0.25 to 0.35 g/L effluent per day.[27,28] Only older data on CRRT protein and amino acid losses is available. Most studies are at least 20 years old and were conducted with replacement and dialysate flow rates of 2,000 mL/h. Practitioners should pay attention to the prescribed dialysate and replacement fluid flow rate as higher flow rates would be expected to incur greater losses of protein and amino acids.

Specific amino acids are not lost in significant quantities with CRRT and are easily replaced by nutrition support with the exception of glutamine, which is semiessential in critical illness.[25,29] The endogenous source of glutamine is muscle, which is catabolized over the course of critical illness, potentially limiting glutamine supply as muscle wasting proceeds.[30]

Frankenfield et al[25] reported glutamine losses of 2 to 4 g/d with CRRT. Although several earlier studies have demonstrated a benefit on mortality, length of hospitalization, and infectious morbidity with supplemental glutamine given in critical illness, more recent data from the well-designed Reducing Deaths due to Oxidative Stress (REDOX) study found an increase in the mortality rate with supplemental enteral or parenteral glutamine.[27,29-32] A post hoc subgroup analysis found an increase in a 28-day mortality rate among those with MOF and baseline kidney dysfunction, concluding that supplemental glutamine should not be given to patients with concomitant AKI.[33]

Peritoneal dialysate was used for many years as a dialysate and replacement fluid for CRRT and, as such, provided an energy source from the uptake of dextrose and lactate. Measured uptake from peritoneal dialysate was in the range of 140 to 355 g/d dextrose or 476 to 1,200 kcal plus approximately another 500 kcal from lactate.[34,35] Failure to account for this energy uptake could result in overfeeding.[26] The lactate load from peritoneal dialysate can also worsen hyperlactemia when lactate clearance is reduced, as in hepatic failure, or when lactate production is increased, as can occur with hemodynamic instability. Most peritoneal dialysate contains 132 mEq/L of sodium, and its use as a replacement fluid may result in hyponatremia.

Druml recommended that CRRT fluid contains a dextrose content equivalent to a serum glucose concentration of 100 to 180 mg/dL to maintain a zero glucose balance or transfer.[28] Most CRRT fluids now available contain dextrose at a physiological level of 100 mg/dL, with bicarbonate in place of lactate as the base component. These CRRT fluids separate nutrition support from CRRT mechanics and eliminate other potential metabolic derangements from excess dextrose and lactate load related to the use of peritoneal dialysate. Although when resources for CRRT are limited, as in rural or remote settings, the use of peritoneal dialysate may still be necessary.

The current recommendation for CRRT predilution or postdilution fluid is a prescribed dose of 25 to 30 mL/kg/h.[7,36] This rate may exceed the 2,000 mL/h that was used in earlier research and forms the basis for the available data on amino acid, protein, and other nutrient losses. Nutrient loss with rates greater than 2,000 mL/h during CRRT can only be approximated until further research provides additional data.

Nutrition Assessment

In 2012, the Academy of Nutrition and Dietetics and the American Society for Parenteral and Enteral Nutrition (ASPEN) standardized the process for diagnosing malnutrition, issuing a consensus statement that provided tools for identifying malnutrition in adults for all settings. This standardized process for malnutrition diagnosis adds an important and useful tool for nutrition assessment in individuals with AKI.[37]

The Academy of Nutrition and Dietetics and ASPEN created three etiology-based malnutrition diagnoses that reflect the presence or absence of inflammation. These diagnoses recognize that the inflammatory effects of disease and injury can drive malnutrition. The effects of inflammation are related to the release of proinflammatory cytokines, which can ramp up the metabolic rate and depress appetite, contributing to lean body mass wasting and weight loss. Inflammation was further delineated in the diagnoses as either chronic or acute. The etiology-based malnutrition definitions are as follows:

- Starvation-related malnutrition
- Chronic disease-related malnutrition
- Acute disease- or injury-related malnutrition

The following six characteristics were specified to identify and diagnose malnutrition: 1) insufficient energy intake, 2) weight loss, 3) skeletal muscle mass wasting, 4) subcutaneous fat loss, 5) localized or general fluid accumulation, and 6) diminished functional status as measured by handgrip strength. These characteristics should be evaluated on a continuum from admission to the hospital through the hospital stay to extended care facilities and outpatient clinics.[37]

The patient's medical history should be reviewed with attention to disease states that can contribute to a chronic inflammatory response. Some of these disease states are, but not limited to, chronic obstructive pulmonary disease, congestive heart failure (CHF), cirrhosis, DM, HTN, CKD, nonhealing wounds, periodontal disease, cancer, obesity, and neurologic disorders (eg, Parkinson's disease and multiple sclerosis). Patients with chronic diseases may present with an active, low-grade inflammatory response preexistent to the diagnosis of an AKI, especially if there is noncompliance with medical therapy or ineffective treatment. This chronic disease-related inflammation has likely created some degree of malnutrition before the development of the AKI, which should be assessed for by the registered dietitian nutritionist (RDN).

An AKI will superimpose an acute inflammatory response (also referred to as a kidney-centered inflammatory syndrome) on any preexisting chronic inflammation, accelerating and worsening lean body mass loss and subcutaneous fat wasting.[9] This process is known as PEW, with its magnitude increasing as the AKI stage moves from 1 through 3, especially when MOF ensues.[38] The incidence of PEW in AKI may be as high as 40% and requires the RDN to be vigilant to assess and then provide appropriate nutrition support to control the effects of inflammation on nutritional status.[9]

Physical Assessment

Use of actual body weight needs to be interpreted with caution during all phases of AKI, as it may reflect changes in fluid status vs actual changes in body mass. It is not uncommon for critically ill aggressively resuscitated patients with AKI to experience a volume overload of 10 to 20 L. The premorbid or edema-free weight needs to be established to determine energy and protein needs without the risk of overfeeding. Premorbid weight history is essential in order to assess for weight loss prior to the current illness and across the course of AKI. The presence of unintentional weight loss can contribute to a malnutrition diagnosis.

The presence and the resolution of edema should be evaluated through frequent physical assessments in conjunction with trending of daily and postdialysis weights.[39]

Serial reviews of daily intake and output documentation can also aid in identifying net negative or net positive fluid status. Skeletal muscle wasting and subcutaneous fat loss will likely be masked where edema is moderate to severe, complicating physical assessment efforts. However, as edema is resolved, either through diuresis and/or KRT/CRRT fluid removal, any loss of muscle mass or subcutaneous fat will become more apparent and should be documented.

Laboratory Assessment

PROTEIN

The serum proteins albumin and prealbumin have no value as laboratory nutrition markers in an acute illness or injury, including when AKI is present. Acute inflammation results in a release of inflammatory cytokines and interleukin-1, causing hepatic reprioritization of protein synthesis. This leads to increased production of acute-phase reactants, C-reactive protein, fibrinogen, ceruloplasmin, haptoglobin, and decreased synthesis of albumin and prealbumin.[40] For this reason, both albumin and prealbumin are often referred to as negative acute-phase reactants. In addition to the acute-phase response, other effects of AKI-associated critical illness will contribute to decreases in serum albumin. Sepsis can produce vascular leakage, shifting albumin from the intravascular to extravascular space; aggressive resuscitation will cause dilution of albumin; and any illness-related hepatic damage will further decrease albumin synthesis.[41] Despite these well-known limitations, depressed serum albumin has been demonstrated to be a prognostic indicator for the risk of increased morbidity and mortality.[40]

In patients with AKI, prealbumin may also act as an independent prognostic factor.[39] Low prealbumin values have been associated with a decreased chance of survival and increased mortality.[16,42-44] In a study by Perez Valdivieso et al,[41] serum prealbumin levels of less than 11 mg/dL were strongly associated with a higher risk of death and were independent of AKI severity, comorbid illnesses, serum C-reactive protein, and other confounders. The authors concluded that serum prealbumin may be an inexpensive and useful tool for evaluating the risk profiles of patients with AKI.

Nitrogen balance is a useful tool for quantifying the degree of catabolism and guiding nutrition support for critically ill patients. However, the standard method for determining nitrogen balance requires a creatinine clearance of more than 50 mL/min/1.73 m^2 for accurate interpretation, thus limiting its use in patients with oliguria and anuria. Nitrogen balance can be used to determine estimates of protein catabolism by calculating the urea nitrogen appearance (UNA) in patients with AKI, but this calculation is not without limitations in the unstable patient since it does not factor in the endogenous protein turnover.[45] UNA can be estimated during CRRT once equilibrium or steady state is reached, usually about 48 hours without any CRRT downtime. UNA is estimated from the 24-hour effluent volume and fluid removal in liters multiplied by the steady-state BUN in mg/L, then divided by 1,000 mg/L. The following equation for calculating UNA can be used for patients with AKI who are undergoing KRT such as IHD[45,46]:

Urea nitrogen appearance in g =
UUN + [(BUN2 – BUN1) × 0.6 × BW1] +
[(BW2 – BW1) × BUN2],
where UUN = urinary urea nitrogen (g/24 hour);
BUN1 = initial collection of blood urea nitrogen, post dialysis (g/L); BUN2 = final collection of blood urea nitrogen, predialysis (g/L); BW1 = postdialysis weight (kg); BW2 = predialysis weight (kg).

BUN and serum creatinine (SCr) levels with an AKI are more related to changes in kidney function and hydration status and are not reflective of nutritional status. Creatinine prior to the development of an AKI, if available, should be used to assess for change relative to baseline kidney function. SCr reflects creatinine clearance, and because muscle mass contributes to creatinine production, individuals with greater muscle mass per kilogram body weight will have a higher baseline SCr level. Similarly, in an aging population, which has lower muscle mass, a lower or normal SCr may still reflect kidney injury. A BUN to creatinine ratio can be a useful tool for evaluating kidney function vs volume status. A ratio greater than 20:1 reflects possible dehydration or an excess dietary protein intake and not a decline in kidney function. Rehydration with intravenous (IV) fluids, a liberalized fluid intake, and/or a decrease in any diuretic therapy should normalize the ratio.

SODIUM

Hyponatremia is the result of excess free water intake or the inability to excrete a free water load via the urine. Free water intake should be restricted. The medication administration record should be reviewed for infusions, including intravenous piggy backs (IVPB) of hypotonic saline or dextrose-only IV fluids, and these should be discontinued.[26]

Hypernatremia can occur if free water losses via hypotonic urine and insensible losses are not replaced or are inappropriately replaced by isonatremic or balanced crystalloid solutions. Risk of hypernatremia is greatest during the recovery or diuretic phase of AKI, when the kidney is unable to concentrate urine output and excess free water is lost in the urine. During the AKI recovery period, IV fluids may be needed to prevent hypovolemia if output greatly exceeds intake. Without adequate replacement of excess urine losses, another AKI may occur, adding further insult to kidney function.[47]

POTASSIUM

Hyperkalemia frequently occurs in AKI as urine output drops below 1 L/d. Metabolic acidosis exacerbates hyperkalemia by intracellular to extracellular redistribution of potassium. Rhabdomyolysis, tumor lysis syndrome, and gastrointestinal bleeding also can contribute to hyperkalemia. In addition, use of potassium supplements, IV fluid–containing potassium, drugs in a potassium salt form, angiotensin potassium-sparing diuretics (eg, spironolactone), and excess potassium from the diet or nutrition support must be considered and removed. Treatment of hyperkalemia may include the use of insulin and IV glucose, IV administration of sodium bicarbonate and/or calcium gluconate, potassium-binding resins (eg, sodium polystyrene sulfonate), diuretics, dialysis, or a combination of treatments.[10]

Hypokalemia may occur as a result of extracellular to intracellular shifts with refeeding syndrome in the malnourished. It can also occur during the recovery or diuretic phase of AKI or with aggressive diuretic use with insufficient potassium replacement. Magnesium deficiency may cause hypokalemia that is resistant to potassium supplementation.[48]

PHOSPHORUS

Hyperphosphatemia is an anticipated consequence of AKI. Phosphorus is the major intracellular anion, and although phosphorus excretion is often impaired during AKI, additional endogenous phosphorus may also be leaked with cellular destruction. Gastrointestinal bleeding, crush injuries causing rhabdomyolysis, and cytotoxic agents that produce tumor lysis syndrome can contribute to hyperphosphatemia as cells lyse and intracellular contents are spilled into the extracellular fluid.[48] Initiation of phosphorus binders may be necessary to correct or prevent further elevations along with removal or reduction of phosphorus sources in nutrition support.

Like hypokalemia, hypophosphatemia is infrequent but may occur with refeeding syndrome and may require repletion. Excessive or inappropriate use of phosphate binders, especially as kidney function recovers, can also contribute to lower phosphorus levels. Continuous phosphate removal occurs with CRRT and can result in hypophosphatemia usually within 48 hours after initiation of this therapy. CRRT requires frequent monitoring of serum phosphorus with IVPB or oral phosphate replacement when serum levels are less than 2.5 mg/dL.

CALCIUM

In the critical care setting, serum ionized calcium is the preferred measure of calcium status. If only serum total calcium is available, it should be corrected for hypoalbuminemia. Hypocalcemia may develop via multiple mechanisms. The loss of functional kidney mass diminishes the production of 1,25-dihydroxyvitamin D3, impairing calcium absorption in the gut. Hyperphosphate-

mia lowers calcium by binding with calcium, leading to the deposition of calcium phosphate salts in soft tissue. Calcium is lost in CRRT effluent and can result in hypocalcemia if adequate replacement is not provided.[49] Hypocalcemia also occurs as calcium is sequestered by damaged muscle tissue in rhabdomyolysis or saponified in peripancreatic fat with acute pancreatitis. Individuals with AKI related to hemorrhagic shock requiring multiple blood transfusions receive large amounts of citrate, which binds calcium and contributes to hypocalcemia. Magnesium deficiency also leads to hypocalcemia by creating parathyroid hormone resistance, inhibiting the release of calcium from bone.[48]

Hypercalcemia can develop as a result of excessive calcium supplementation, immobilization of the patient, or presence of a malignant tumor. Late-onset hypercalcemia can develop post rhabdomyolysis as the calcium initially sequestered in the damaged tissue is released.[48]

MAGNESIUM

Mild asymptomatic hypermagnesemia may occur with oliguric AKI and reflects impaired excretion. Magnesium-containing laxatives or antacids can often contribute to hypermagnesemia and need to be discontinued when oliguria or anuria is present.

Hypomagnesemia related to refeeding syndrome often coincides with hypokalemia and hypophosphatemia, especially when malnutrition is known or suspected and may become most evident in the recovery or diuretic phase of AKI. Like phosphorus, magnesium is also lost in CRRT effluent, requiring frequent monitoring and bolus repletion as an IVPB with magnesium sulfate when serum magnesium falls below 2.0 mg/dL.

MICRONUTRIENTS

Vitamin recommendations are not well defined and are typically based on healthy subjects or patients with CKD.[50] For those with AKI requiring KRT including CRRT, a renal-specific vitamin that includes 1 mg/d folate and 10 mg/d pyridoxine to replace water-soluble vitamin loss is necessary.[26] Vitamin C doses should not exceed 100 to 200 mg/d.[26,47,51] Oxalate is derived from vitamin C and is a recognized kidney toxin. When oliguria or anuria is present, oxalate accumulates in the renal tubules, incurring an additional kidney injury and lessening the likelihood of recovery.[52,53] Lactic acidosis related to thiamine depletion during CRRT has been reported.[53] During CRRT, thiamine is lost at about three to four times the Dietary Reference Intake (DRI), exceeding the dose in renal-specific vitamins and indicating a need for additional supplementation.[54] Further study is warranted to determine whether the vitamin D supplementation utilized in patients with CKD, both analogs and 25-hydroxyvitamin D, applies to patients with AKI.[50]

Conflicting reports surround vitamin A. Druml et al[50] found depressed vitamin A levels with normal retinol binding protein; however, vitamin A has an inverse relationship with C-reactive protein in inflammation. Hypercalcemia is the most common vitamin A toxicity symptom in patients with CKD and has been reported in patients with AKI as well.[54-56] Limiting vitamin A to a DRI dose range of 700 to 900 mcg/d, as recommended in patients with CKD, is also advisable in patients with AKI.[57] The standard parenteral multivitamin infusion is acceptable for use in patients with AKI if used daily as a single dose but should never be doubled or tripled.[57]

Like vitamins, trace element recommendations are not clearly defined for patients with AKI and are often derived from the DRIs or from limited research regarding trace element loss or uptake during CRRT. With CRRT, selenium loss ranges from 35 to 91 mcg/d.[58,59] This amount is at or slightly greater than the DRI. Supplementing with 100 mcg selenium daily will correct for this loss.[57] Sondheimer et al[60] reported hypercupremia in the population with CKD, which has been used as a rationale for avoiding supplementation of copper in patients with CKD. However, two studies have found that approximately 400 mcg/d copper are lost with CRRT.[58,59] This loss is well within the amount of copper provided in most commercially available enteral formulas and accounts for nearly half of the 1,000 mcg in parenteral multitrace element (MTE) preparations. If copper is omitted from parenteral nutrition (PN), as recommended when total bilirubin is greater than 3 mg/dL, it may need to be supplemented with long-

term CRRT (generally greater than 2 weeks in practice) or a deficiency state may occur.[57]

The recommended intake for zinc in patients with CKD requiring KRT is 15 mg/d and may be a starting point for dosing zinc in patients with AKI once KRT is initiated.[61] There appears to be no zinc loss with CRRT; rather, there is a positive zinc balance as zinc uptake occurs from some degree of contamination from trace elements of fluids used during CRRT.[62] Again, the standard concentration of parenteral MTE solution is acceptable for use in patients with AKI with adjustments for CRRT or a total bilirubin greater than 3 mg/dL, as previously discussed.[57]

Nutrition Needs/Nutrition Prescription

ENERGY

The goal is to provide adequate calories to meet energy requirements and minimize protein degradation without increased risk of overfeeding. Energy requirements should be based on the underlying disease state or complication, not on AKI, as this condition has limited effect on energy expenditure.

Indirect calorimetry (IC) is considered to be the gold standard method for determining energy requirements for critically ill individuals with AKI. IC identifies both hypermetabolism and hypometabolism associated with critical illness and helps match individual nutritional requirements with patient status and nutrition prescription. Many factors, however, such as the requirement of a fraction of inspired oxygen concentration greater than 60% for mechanically ventilated patients and leaking chest or endotracheal tubes, may lead to inaccurate calculation of energy requirements with IC.[45]

When direct measurement is not available, caloric requirements can be met by providing 20 to 30 kcal/kg body weight or 130% above basal energy expenditure during hypermetabolic conditions, including sepsis, multiorgan dysfunction (MOD), or use of CRRT[16,26,27] (see Box 4.3).[7,47,57,63-66]

BOX 4.3 | Daily Energy and Nutrient Recommendations for Adults With Acute Kidney Injury[7,47,57,63-66]

NUTRIENT	RECOMMENDATIONS
Energy	20 to 30 kcal/kg
Protein	0.8 to 1.0 g/kg noncatabolic, without dialysis
	1.0 to 1.5 g/kg catabolic and/or initiation of dialysis
	1.7 to 2 g/kg to a maximum of 2.5 g/kg for critically ill adults undergoing continous renal replacement therapy (CRRT)
Fat	≤1 g/kg when using parenteral nutrition
Fluid	24-hour urine output + 500 mL for insensible losses (approximately 750 to 1,500 mL/d)
	Increase fluid to prevent dehydration during diuresis or acute kidney injury resolution and, as needed, for any increased insensible losses as with fever, sepsis, or burns
Sodium	1.1 to 1.4 mmol/kg ideal body weight (IBW)
Potassium	0.9 to 2.1 mmol/kg IBW
	Requirements depend on serial laboratory values considering the need for kidney replacement therapy/CRRT, return of kidney function, and anabolism
Phosphorus	0.3 to 0.6 mmol/kg IBW
	May need to add phosphate binders with hyperphosphatemia
	Requirements may increase with CRRT/daily dialysis, return of kidney function, and anabolism

PROTEIN

Protein requirements vary across the spectrum of AKI from stages 1 through 3. When there is little to no catabolism and the AKI is short-lived, the protein need is estimated to be as low as 0.8 to 1 g/kg/d.[7,64] Once HD is required, protein intake should be a minimum of 1 g/kg/d; however, with the worsening severity of illness, increased catabolism can be expected and protein provision should be escalated to 1.5 g/kg/d. The need for CRRT further increases protein needs related to protein and amino acid losses over the CRRT filter. The 2012 KDIGO guidelines suggest an upper limit of 1.7 g/kg/d, with other guidelines and reviews pushing the protein requirement up to a range of 2 g/kg/d and 2.5 g/kg/d, with CRRT largely dependent on the degree of catabolism.[63,65,66]

FAT

The fat requirements up to 1 g/kg/d for patients with AKI are similar to those for other critically ill patients.[7,57,63] However, alterations of lipid metabolism associated with AKI can affect the dose tolerated by the patient. Triglyceride levels should be monitored at least weekly when any source of IV lipid is being given on a continuous daily basis from PN or from sedation such as propofol[63] (Box 4.4).

BOX 4.4 | Metabolic Alterations Associated With Acute Kidney Injury[57,63]

NUTRIENT	METABOLIC ALTERATIONS
Carbohydrate	Hyperglycemia, insulin resistance, accelerated hepatic gluconeogenesis despite exogenous glucose infusions
Lipid	Impaired lipolysis causing hypertriglyceridemia
Protein and amino acids	Acidosis and insulin resistance stimulating protein catabolism, skeletal muscle release of amino acids, and negative nitrogen balance; increased gluconeogenesis, ureagenesis, increased hepatic secretion of positive acute-phase proteins (ferritin, fibrinogen, and ceruloplasmin), and decreased secretion of negative acute-phase proteins (albumin, prealbumin, and transferrin)

FLUID

Fluid requirements will depend on serum sodium, volume status, presence of edema, and kidney function. During the course of AKI, fluid needs may change depending on the presence of oliguria or anuria, and in the resolution phase when polyuria occurs, additional fluid, including IV fluids, may be required. The use of HD vs CRRT may change fluid allowances based on the ability to achieve fluid removal and weight goals.

Oral Intake

A patient with AKI who is not critically ill and does not require mechanical ventilation is not an aspiration risk; this type of patient who does not have a gastrointestinal impairment requiring nil per os (npo) status should have a prescribed diet. Most of these patients will have AKI stage 1 or stage 2, and some may have had AKI stage 3 and are now in the recovery phase and just resuming an oral diet after a period of mechanical intubation. Medical comorbidities, which may preexist in patients with AKI, such as DM, CHF, HTN and cirrhosis, may require a therapeutic diet. However, if a diet is poorly tolerated, then restrictions may need to be liberalized to foster better oral intake of energy and protein. If there is a neurological disorder leading to dysphagia or the suspicion of an aspiration risk, a speech therapy evaluation may be helpful to determine the appropriate oral diet consistency or the need for an npo status.

Oral nutritional supplements may be needed to augment intake, especially if oral food intake is consistently less than 75% of estimated energy and protein needs. Choice of product will depend on hospital formulary, product composition as it compares with the patient's individual nutritional requirements, electrolytes, and fluid needs, and, of course, patient acceptance (see Chapter 18).

Nutrition Support

When patients with an AKI cannot or should not have an oral diet, specialized nutrition support, namely enteral nutrition (EN) or PN, will be necessary. The primary goal of EN and PN should be to provide adequate energy, protein, and micronutrients to mitigate the PEW of AKI and, when possible, promote wound healing, support the immune system, and reduce the risk of mortality.[9] When the gut is functional, EN should be selected as the preferred feeding route over PN. Those with AKI stage 1 and most with AKI stage 2 should be able to tolerate an oral diet; however, as the severity of an AKI escalates, especially into MOD, most patients will require mechanical ventilation and npo status. Oliguria or anuria with fluid retention, metabolic acidosis, nitrogenous waste accumulation, and electrolyte and mineral imbalances, including hyperkalemia, hyperphosphatemia, hypermagnesemia, hyponatremia, and hypocalcemia, will require either HD or CRRT to correct these abnormalities, and will also impact the prescription for EN or PN.

Continuous therapy or CRRT is often needed in patients with hemodynamic instability supported by one or more vasopressors. Advantages of this therapy include steady-state control of uremia and solute clearance with limited restrictions on the nutrition prescription. Glycemic control may become a problem when high dextrose-containing dialysate or replacement fluid is used. However, the use of fluids with high dextrose concentrations in CRRT has become very rare.[65] A high protein intake of at least 1.7 g/kg/d and up to 2.5 g/kg/d is needed with CRRT to offset treatment-related amino acid, peptide, and protein losses.[7,63-66] HD will need stricter limits on fluid and electrolyte intakes while providing at least 1.2 g/kg/d or greater of protein. Water-soluble vitamin replacement is necessary with either HD or CRRT to correct for treatment-associated losses. Close monitoring is essential to make timely adjustments in the nutrition prescription.

Due to underlying comorbid conditions contributing to chronic malnutrition and marginal to poor oral food intake prior to admission to the hospital, those with AKI are often at risk for refeeding syndrome. The hypophosphatemia, hypokalemia, and hypomagnesemia of refeeding may be further exacerbated from associated urinary losses during the polyuric phase of AKI. If refeeding syndrome is a concern, serum phosphorus, potassium, and magnesium should be monitored at least daily or more frequently and repleted via the oral, enteral, or parenteral route as appropriate to normalize levels. Neither EN nor PN should be initiated until repletion is underway. At least 100 mg thiamine should also be provided daily when refeeding syndrome is suspected, in addition to any water-soluble vitamins provided as correction for HD- or CRRT-associated losses.

ENTERAL

When EN is needed, formula selection depends on the AKI stage. Most patients requiring EN will have AKI stage 2 or stage 3. Some will be npo related to altered mental status and aspiration risk, while others will be mechanically ventilated. When urine output is adequate and electrolytes (especially potassium and phosphorus) are normal to low, a standard polymeric formula (1 to 1.5 kcal/mL) can be selected. If aggressive diuretic therapy is being used, as with AKI related to CHF or cirrhosis, a higher-calorie polymeric formula (1.5 to 2 kcal/mL) may be preferred to limit fluid delivery. The potential for refeeding syndrome should be assessed, and renal formulas, which are lower in potassium, phosphorus, and magnesium, should be avoided in favor of a standard formula to assist in repleting potassium, phosphorus, and magnesium. If hyperkalemia and hyperphosphatemia are persistent, a renal formula should be considered. This may be necessary with IHD when adjustment to a lower potassium dialysate does not adequately control hyperkalemia. With CRRT or daily HD, a renal formula is not usually needed; however, a higher protein formula should be selected to correct for the greater dialysis-

associated protein losses. Once a patient with AKI stage 3 has entered the polyuric recovery phase, low volume renal formulas should be switched out to a standard formula (1 kcal/mL) to provide additional fluid and help avoid volume depletion (see Chapter 15).

PARENTERAL

PN should only be initiated when the gut is non-functional. Indications for PN include short bowel syndrome, prolonged ileus, high output enterocutaneous fistulas (>500 mL/d), chemotherapy and/or radiation-induced enteritis, mechanical bowel obstruction, bowel ischemia, and severe malnutrition where adequate oral intake or EN is not possible.[67]

Energy is supplied using dextrose and intravenous fat emulsion (IVFE). The dextrose dosage should be limited to 3 mg/kg/min in critical illness and up to 4 mg/kg/min for more stable patients outside of critical care. The IVFE dose should not exceed 1 g/kg/d.[63] During sepsis, including peritonitis from the spillage of feculent contents into the intra-abdominal space, soy oil-based IVFE should be held for the initial 7 days of PN to avoid the proinflammatory and immunosuppressive effects of this IVFE.[63] However, if an alternative IVFE is utilized, such as an 80% olive oil/20% soy oil-based product, then IVFE may be utilized immediately on initiation of PN.[68] Protein is supplied from amino acids prescribed according to the amounts shown in Box 4.3 on page 59. See Chapter 16 for more information.

If volume overload is a concern, PN can be maximally concentrated. If the patient is not oliguric or anuric or has entered the polyuric recovery phase of AKI stage 3, the PN will need to be matched to fluid requirements to avoid volume depletion. Potassium and phosphorus are usually omitted from PN or dosed in very limited amounts when urine output is poor or HD or CRRT is needed. Any additional potassium required can be given separately as an IVPB to avoid potentiating hyperkalemia from the PN then having to discard a costly bag of PN. The dialysate or replacement fluid can be adjusted in the potassium content. Parenteral multivitamin and MTE preparations should be added, including supplemental pyridoxine, folate, and thiamine when HD or CRRT is initiated.

Summary

AKI can be extremely complex, occurring as different stages with treatment needs specific to each stage. Although nutrition support has not been demonstrated to improve outcomes consistently, the absence of nutrition support will have deleterious effects. Malnutrition is an obvious consequence, given the severity of the catabolism, metabolic alterations, and complications that occur in patients with AKI. Nutrient losses via HD or CRRT also contribute to the problem. Patients often suffer from the severity of the underlying disease and complications.[28] By being aware of all of these components, RDNs can better serve patients by developing nutrition care plans that encompass all aspects of their needs. Therefore, nutrition support for patients with AKI remains a challenge that requires a breadth of skills and knowledge.

References

1. Levy EM, Viscoli CM, Horwitz RI. The effect of acute renal failure on mortality: a cohort analysis. *JAMA*. 1996;275(19):1489-1494.
2. Chertow GM, Burdick E, Honour M, Bonventre JV, Bates DW. Acute kidney injury, mortality, length of stay, and costs in hospitalized patients. *J Am Soc Nephrol*. 2005;16(11):3365-3370. doi:10.1681/ASN .2004090740
3. Bellomo R, Ronco C, Kellum JA, Mehta RL, Palevsky P; Acute Dialysis Quality Initiative workgroup. Acute renal failure—definition, outcome measures, animal models, fluid therapy and information technology needs: the Second International Consensus Conference of the Acute Dialysis Quality Initiative (ADQI) Group. *Crit Care*. 2004;8(4):R204-R212. doi:10.1186/cc2872
4. Kellum JA. Acute kidney injury. *Crit Care Med*. 2008;36(4 suppl):S141-S145. doi:10.1097/CCM .0b013e318168c4a4
5. Himmelfarb J, Ikizler TA. Acute kidney injury: changing lexicography, definitions, and epidemiology. *Kidney Int*. 2007;71(10):971-976. doi:10.1038/sj.ki.5002224
6. Mehta RL, Kellum JA, Shah SV, et al; Acute Kidney Injury Network. Acute Kidney Injury Network: report of an initiative to improve outcomes in acute kidney injury. *Crit Care*. 2007;11(2):R31. doi:10.1186/cc5713
7. Kellum, JA, Lemeire N, Aspelin P, et al. KDIGO clinical practice guideline for acute kidney injury. *Kidney Int Suppl*. 2012;2(1):1-138. doi:10.1038/kisup.2012.1
8. Ronco C, Bellomo R, Kellum JA. Acute kidney injury. *Lancet*. 2019;394:1949-1964. doi:10.1016/S0140 -6736(19)32563-2
9. Fiaccadori E, Maggiore U, Cabassi A, Morabito S, Castellano G, Regolisti G. Nutritional evaluation and management of AKI patients. *J Renal Nutr*. 2013;23(3):255-258. doi:10.1053/j.jrn.2013.01.025
10. Mindell JA, Chertow GM. A practical approach to acute renal failure. *Med Clin North Am*. 1997;81(3):731-748. doi:10.1016/s0025 -7125(05)70543-5
11. Albright RC. Acute renal failure: a practical update. *Mayo Clin Proc*. 2001;76(1):67-74. doi:10.4065/76.1.67
12. Nally JV. Acute renal failure in hospitalized patients. *Cleve Clin J Med*. 2002;69(7):569-574. doi:10.3949 /ccjm.69.7.569
13. Rosner MH. Acute kidney injury in the elderly. *Clin Geriatr Med*. 2013;29(3):565-578. doi:10.1016/j.cger .2013.05.001
14. Bellomo R. How to feed patients with renal dysfunction. *Blood Purif*. 2002;20(3):296-303. doi:10 .1159/000047024
15. Esson ML, Schrier RW. Diagnosis and treatment of acute tubular necrosis. *Ann Intern Med*. 2002;137(9):744-752. doi:10.7326/0003-4819-137 -9-200211050-00010
16. Fiaccadori E, Lombardi M, Leonardi S, Rotelli CF, Tortorella G, Borghetti A. Prevalence and clinical outcome associated with preexisting malnutrition in acute renal failure: a prospective cohort study. *J Am Soc Nephrol*. 1999;10(3):581-593. doi:10.1681/ASN .V103581
17. Rachoin JS, Weisberg LS. Renal replacement therapy in the ICU. *Crit Care Med*. 2019;47(5):715-721. doi:10.1097/CCM.0000000000003701
18. Nystrom EM, Nei AM. Metabolic support of the patient on continuous renal replacement therapy. *Nutr Clin Pract*. 2018;33(6):754-766. doi:10.1002 /ncp.10208
19. Ronco C, Brendolan A, Bellomo R. Continuous renal replacement techniques. *Contrib Nephrol*. 2001;132:236-251.
20. Ash SR. Peritoneal dialysis in acute renal failure of adults: the safe, effective, and low-cost modality. *Contrib Nephrol*. 2001;132:210-221. doi:10.1159 /000060092

21. Mehta RL. Indications for dialysis in the ICU: renal replacement therapy vs. renal support. *Blood Purif.* 2001;19(2):227-232. doi:10.1159/000046946

22. Boxall MC, Goodship THJ. Nutritional requirements in hemodialysis. In: Mitch WE, Klahr S, eds. *Handbook of Nutrition and the Kidney.* 5th ed. Lippincott Williams & Wilkins; 2005:221.

23. Westra WM, Kopple JD, Krediet RT, Appell M, Mehrotra R. Dietary protein requirements and dialysate protein losses in chronic peritoneal dialysis patients. *Perit Dial Int.* 2007;27(2):192-195.

24. Mokrzycki MH, Kaplan AA. Protein losses in continuous renal replacement therapies. *J Am Soc Nephrol.* 1996;7(10):2259-2263.

25. Frankenfield DC, Badellino MM, Reynolds HN, Wiles CE 3rd, Siegel JH, Goodarzi S. Amino acid loss and plasma concentration during continuous hemodiafiltration. *JPEN J Parenter Enteral Nutr.* 1993;17(6):551-561. doi:10.1177/0148607193017006551

26. Marin A, Hardy G. Practical implications of nutritional support during continuous renal replacement therapy. *Curr Opin Clin Nutr Metab Care.* 2001;4(3):219-225. doi:10.1097/00075197-200105000-00009

27. Druml W. Nutritional considerations in the treatment of acute renal failure in septic patients. *Nephrol Dial Transplant.* 1994;(9 suppl 4):S219-S223.

28. Druml W. Metabolic aspects of continuous renal replacement therapies. *Kidney Int.* 1999;56(72):S56-S61.

29. Bongers T, Griffiths RD, McArdle A. Exogenous glutamine: the clinical evidence. *Crit Care Med.* 2007;35(9 suppl):S545-S552. doi:10.1097/01.CCM.0000279193.23737.06

30. Heyland D, Muscedere J, Wischmeyer PE, et al. A randomized trial of glutamine and antioxidants in critically ill patients. *N Eng J Med.* 2013;368(16):1489-1497. doi:10.1056/NEJMoa1212722

31. Wernerman J. Clinical use of glutamine supplementation. *J Nutr.* 2008;138(10):2040S-2044S. doi:10.1093/jn/138.10.2040S

32. Wischmeyer PE. Glutamine: role in critical illness and ongoing clinical trials. *Curr Opin Gastroenterol.* 2008;24(2):190-197. doi:10.1097/MOG.0b013e3282f4db94

33. Heyland DK, Elke G, Cook D, et al. Glutamine and antioxidants in the critically ill patient: a post hoc analysis of a large scale randomized trial. *JPEN J Parenter Enteral Nutr.* 2015;39(4):401-409. doi:10.1177/0148607114529994

34. Casaer MP, Mesotten D, Schetz MR. Bench-to-bedside review: metabolism and nutrition. *Crit Care.* 2008;12(4):222. doi:10.1186/cc6945

35. Frankenfield DC, Reynolds HN, Badellino MM, Wiles CE. Glucose dynamics during continuous hemodiafiltration and total parenteral nutrition. *Intensive Care Med.* 1995;21(12):1016-1022. doi:10.1007/BF01700664

36. Karkar A, Ronco C. Prescription of CRRT: a pathway to optimize therapy. *Ann Intensive Care.* 2020;10(1):32-41. doi:10.1186/s13613-020-0648-y

37. White JV, Guenter P, Jensen G, Malone A, Schofield M. Consensus statement of the Academy of Nutrition and Dietetics/American Society for Parenteral and Enteral Nutrition: characteristics recommended for the identification and documentation of adult malnutrition (undernutrition). *J Acad Nutr Diet.* 2012;112(5):730-738. doi:10.1016/j.jand.2012.03.012

38. Fouque D, Kalantar-Zadeh K, Kopple J, et al. A proposed nomenclature and diagnostic criteria for protein-energy wasting in acute and chronic kidney disease. *Kidney Int.* 2008;73(4):391-398. doi:10.1038/sj.ki.5002585

39. Sungurtekin H, Sungurtekin U, Oner O, Okke D. Nutrition assessment in critically ill patients. *Nutr Clin Pract.* 2008;23(6):635-641. doi:10.1177/0884533608326137

40. Ikizler TA, Himmelfarb J. Nutrition in acute renal failure patients. *Adv Ren Replace Ther.* 1997;4(2 suppl 1):S54-S63.

41. Perez Valdivieso JR, Bes-Rastrollo M, Monedero P, de Irala J, Lavilla FJ. Impact of prealbumin levels on mortality in patients with acute kidney injury: an observational cohort study. *J Ren Nutr.* 2008;18(3):262-268. doi:10.1053/j.jrn.2007.11.003

42. Chertow GM, Goldstein-Fuchs DJ, Lazarus JM, Kaysen GA. Prealbumin, mortality, and cause-specific hospitalization in hemodialysis patients. *Kidney Int.* 2005;68(6):2794-2800. doi:10.1111/j.1523-1755.2005.00751.x

43. Potter MA, Luxton G. Prealbumin measurement as a screening tool for protein calorie malnutrition in emergency hospital admissions: a pilot study. *Clin Invest Med.* 1999;22(2):44-52.

44. Sullivan DH, Bopp MM, Roberson PK. Protein-energy undernutrition and life-threatening complications among the hospitalized elderly. *J Gen Intern Med.* 2002;17(12):923-932. doi:10.1046/j.1525-1497.2002.10930.x

45. Goldstein-Fuchs DJ, McQuiston B. Renal failure. In: Matarese LE, Gottschlich MM, eds. *Contemporary Nutrition Support Practice: A Clinical Guide.* Saunders; 2003:460-483.

46. Butler B. Nutritional management of catabolic acute renal failure requiring renal replacement therapy. *ANNA J.* 1991;18(3):247-254.

47. McCarthy MS, Phipps SC. Special nutrition challenges: current approach to acute kidney injury. *Nutr Clin Pract.* 2014;29(1):56-62. doi:10.1177/0884533613515726

48. Canada T, Lord L. Fluids, electrolytes and acid-base disorders. In: C. Mueller, ed. *The ASPEN Adult Nutrition Support Core Curriculum.* 3rd ed. American Society for Parenteral and Enteral Nutrition. 2017.

49. Klein CJ, Moser-Veillon PB, Schweitzer A, et al. Magnesium, calcium, zinc, and nitrogen loss in trauma patients during continuous renal replacement therapy. *JPEN J Parenter Enteral Nutr.* 2002;26(2):77-92. doi:10.1177/014860710202600277

50. Druml W, Schwarzenhofer M, Apsner R, Hörl WH. Fat-soluble vitamins in patients with acute renal failure. *Miner Electrolyte Metab.* 1998;24(4):220-226. doi:10.1159/000057374

51. Druml W. Nutritional management of acute renal failure. *Am J Kidney Dis.* 2001;37(1 suppl 2):S89-S94. doi:10.1053/ajkd.2001.20757

52. Alkhunaizi AM, Chan L. Secondary oxalosis: a cause of delayed recovery of renal function in the setting of acute renal failure. *J Am Soc Nephrol.* 1996;7(11):2320-2326.

53. Nasr SH, Kashtanova Y, Levchuk V, Markowitz GS. Secondary oxalosis due to excess vitamin C intake. *Kidney Int.* 2006;70(10):1672. doi:10.1038/sj.ki.5001724

54. Cohen E, Trivedi C. Hypercalcemia from non-prescription vitamin A. *Nephrol Dial Transplant.* 2004;19(11):2929. doi:10.1093/ndt/gfh437

55. Fishbane S, Frei GL, Finger M, Dressler R, Silbiger S. Hypervitaminosis A in two hemodialysis patients. *Am J Kidney Dis.* 1995;25(2):346-349. doi:10.1016/0272-6386(95)90020-9

56. Gleghorn EE, Eisenberg LD, Hack S, Parton P, Merritt RJ. Observations of vitamin A toxicity in three patients with renal failure receiving parenteral alimentation. *Am J Clin Nutr.* 1986;44(1):107-112. doi:10.1093/ajcn/44.1.107

57. Gervasio J, Cotton AB. Nutrition support therapy in acute kidney injury: distinguishing dogma from good practice. *Curr Gastroenterol Rep.* 2009;11(4):325-331. doi:10.1007/s11894-009-0047-x

58. Berger MM, Shenkin A, Revelly JP, et al. Copper, selenium, zinc, and thiamine balances during continuous venovenous hemodiafiltration in critically ill patients. *Am J Clin Nutr.* 2004;80(2):410-416. doi:10.1093/ajcn/80.2.410

59. Story DA, Ronco C, Bellomo R. Trace element and vitamin concentrations and losses in critically ill patients treated with continuous venovenous hemofiltration. *Crit Care Med.* 1999;27(1):220-223. doi:10.1097/00003246-199901000-00057

60. Sondheimer JH, Mahajan SK, Rye DL, et al. Elevated plasma copper in chronic renal failure. *Am J Clin Nutr.* 1988;47(5):896-899. doi:10.1093/ajcn/47.5.896

61. Kalantar-Zadeh K, Kopple JD. Trace elements and vitamins in maintenance dialysis patients. *Adv Ren Replace Ther.* 2003;10(3):170-182. doi:10.1053/j.arrt.2003.09.002

62. Klein CJ, Nielsen FH, Moser-Veillon PB. Trace element loss in urine and effluent following traumatic injury. *JPEN J Parenter Enteral Nutr.* 2008;32(2):129-139. doi:10.1177/0148607108314762

63. McClave SA, Taylor BE, Martindale RG, et al. Guidelines for the provision and assessment of nutrition support therapy in the adult critically ill patient: Society of Critical Care Medicine (SCCM) and American Society for Parenteral and Enteral Nutrition (A.S.P.E.N.). *JPEN J Parenter Enteral Nutr.* 2016;40(2):159-211. doi:10.1177/0148607115621863

64. Ostermann M, Macedo E, Oudemans-van Straaten H. How to feed a patient with acute kidney injury. *Intensive Care Med.* 2019;45(7):1006-1008. doi:10.1007/s00134-019-05615-z

65. Onichimowski D, Goraj R, Jalali R, Grabala J, Mayzner-Zawadzka E, Czuczwar M. Practical issues of nutrition during continuous renal replacement therapy. *Anaesthesiol Intensive Ther.* 2017;49(4):309-316. doi:10.5603/AIT.a2017.0052

66. Fiaccadori E, Regolisti G, Maggiore U. Specialized nutritional support interventions in critically ill patients on renal replacement therapy. *Curr Opin Clin Nutr Metab Care.* 2013;16(2):217-224. doi:10.1097/MCO.0b013e32835c20b0

67. Worthington P, Balint J, Bechtold M, et al. When is parenteral nutrition appropriate. *JPEN J Parenter Enteral Nutr.* 2017;41(3):324-377. doi:10.1177/0148607117695251

68. Mirtallo JM, Ayers P, Boullata J, et al. ASPEN lipid injectable emulsion safety recommendations, part 1: background and adult considerations. *JPEN J Parenter Enteral Nutr.* 2020;35(5):769-782. doi:10.1002/ncp.10496

CHAPTER 5

Nutrition Management of the Adult Patient on In-Center Hemodialysis

Joanne Cooke, MS, RD, CSR, FAND, and Elizabeth C. Shanaman, RDN, CD, FNKF

Introduction

Kidney function is measured by glomerular filtration rate (GFR). A lower GFR results in accumulation of waste products (uremia) and fluid retention. When the GFR is less than or equal to 10 mL/min/1.73 m[2] for individuals without diabetes or 15 mL/min/1.73 m[2] for individuals with diabetes, the patient is considered to have chronic kidney disease (CKD) stage 5 and requires intervention with a transplant (see Chapter 8) or initiation of kidney replacement therapy (KRT), such as peritoneal dialysis (see Chapter 7), home hemodialysis (see Chapter 6) or in-center hemodialysis (ICHD).[1] Generally, dialysis will not be initiated until signs and symptoms of uremia are present, including loss of appetite (anorexia), nausea, vomiting, altered mental status, ammonia-like breath, hyperpigmentation, fatigue, fluid overload, shortness of breath, edema, and/or unintended solid body weight loss.[2] A simple mnemonic is used to remember the indications for dialysis; A-E-I-O-U: acid-base problems, electrolyte problems, intoxications, overload (fluid), and uremic symptoms.[3] In this chapter, the focus will be nutrition management of the adult patient who receives ICHD.

With hemodialysis (HD), an artificial kidney (dialyzer) is utilized to provide life-sustaining therapy. A dialysis machine delivers blood from the patient to the dialyzer, cleanses the blood using a prescribed bath (dialysate), and returns the blood to the patient.

Nutritional goals for patients who receive ICHD include adequate protein and energy intake; optimal fluid, weight, and blood pressure management; and acceptable laboratory values.[4] The services of a registered dietitian nutritionist (RDN) are mandated by the Centers for Medicare & Medicaid Services (CMS) guidelines to provide medical nutrition therapy, including individualized nutrition education for every patient who receives ICHD.[5]

Dialyzer, Dialysis Bath, and Access

In order to understand nutritional goals, methods of dialysis must first be explained. HD uses a dialyzer, which is a transparent cylinder that contains thousands of thin, hollow fibers. These fibers are referred to as the dialyzer membrane. There are two circuits within the dialyzer: the blood path and the dialysate path. The blood flows in one direction inside the dialyzer fibers, and the dialysate bath circulates in the opposite direction outside the fibers. The countercurrent flow allows movement of concentrated blood waste products into the dialysate bath for disposal.[1,6] Smaller molecules of urea, creatinine, potassium, phosphorus, glucose, and fluid are removed, leaving larger molecules such as red blood cells, vitamin B12, and albumin mostly intact.[6]

The movement of molecules across the membrane into the bath is due to a concentration gradient (diffusion), hydrostatic pressure (convection), and membrane pore size. Dialyzer membranes may have biocompatible properties that minimize the inflammatory response.[1,6]

Adequate dialysis is relevant in the nutrition assessment as it is adjunctive to adequate nutrient intake.[6] The adequacy of the delivered dose of dialysis is measured by a mathematical urea kinetic model (UKM) using blood urea nitrogen (BUN) before and after HD. The National Kidney Foundation's Kidney Disease Outcomes Quality Initiative (KDOQI) recommends a monthly dose measurement using single pool Kt/V (target 1.4 per session for three times weekly HD with a minimum delivered dose of 1.2), in which K is the urea clearance (mL/min), t is treatment time (min), V is body water volume (mL), and single pool is the body compartment.[6] Body mass, gender, dialyzer size, blood and dialysate flow, and time on treatment must be entered into the equation.[7] Dialysis contributes to malnutrition through nutrient losses, inflammation, and increased catabolism (during and after ICHD).[4,6,8]

Protein catabolism correlates with urea generation, which reflects protein intake in stable patients.[6] The normalized protein catabolic rate (nPCR) determined from UKM estimates irreversible nitrogen loss to urea, normalized to lean body mass.[7] A low nPCR indicates poor nutritional intake (with less urea generation) and predicts poor outcome (see Chapter 2 for more information).[6] Inadequate dialysis may be associated with increasing uremia and acidosis with frequent nausea, vomiting, altered taste (resulting in lower protein and energy intake), and less protein synthesis (hypoalbuminemia).[4,9] Barriers to adequate dialysis are multifactorial. The dose prescribed is not delivered when a patient skips treatments or shortens therapy time.[6,7,10] The postdialysis BUN sample procedure must be consistent to minimize cell urea rebound measurement.[6,7,10] Blood flow can be altered related to inadequate vascular access (stricture or central venous catheter), hypotensive episodes (reduced blood flow), or needle placement (recirculation).[6,7,10] Large patients may require increased dialysis time.[6]

Proper treatment of water used during HD is essential, as a 4-hour HD session with dialysate flow of 500 mL/minute can expose the patient to 120 L of water (more than 20 times the normal daily water exposure). Water contaminants are potentially toxic in great volume. For the patient's safety, the water for the dialysate bath is purified by reverse osmosis and may also be filtered, softened, and deionized before adding physiological serum components.[6] Dialysate is available as a ready-to-use liquid or as a concentrated powder for rehydration of base and acid components with prescribed ranges (see Box 5.1).[1,6]

BOX 5.1 | Contents of Dialysate[1,6-10]

Bicarbonate	35 to 40 mEq/L; to buffer uremic metabolic acidosis, minimize protein degradation, and achieve serum bicarbonate >22 mEq/L
Sodium	135 to 145 mEq/L; at or slightly above plasma sodium to reduce cramps and hypotension frequency by promoting vascular refilling during volume (fluid) removal
Potassium	1 to 4 mEq/L; most commonly used is 2 to 3 mEq/L, slightly lower than plasma to enhance removal; 70 to 90 mEq is removed per HD
Calcium	2.0 to 3.5 mEq/L; to maintain calcium balance and hemodynamic stability
Magnesium	0.5 to 1.0 mEq/L
Glucose (optional)	100 to 200 mg/dL; to maintain constant serum glucose during treatment
Phosphate is not included in dialysate	

To initiate HD, access to the patient's blood is essential. This access can be temporary or permanent. There are various types of vascular accesses, each with their own advantages and disadvantages.

Temporary access sites may include catheters inserted in the internal jugular, subclavian, or femoral veins. Patients with catheters have been shown to be as much as ten times more likely to become infected as those with fistulas. Catheter-related infections include exit site infection, tunnel infection, and bloodstream infection.[11] Therefore, catheters are recommended only for patients in whom arteriovenous (AV) access cannot be created or while awaiting maturation of a fistula or graft.[12]

Best practice is preemptive placement of a more permanent access, such as the AV fistula or AV graft. The preferred access for patients receiving HD is the AV fistula.[12] The AV fistula is surgically created by connecting the patient's natural artery to a natural vein and is often placed in the wrist (radial-cephalic) or elbow (brachiocephalic). According to the KDOQI guidelines, the wrist fistula is the primary choice of access because it is simple to create, protects the proximal vessels for future placement, and has fewer complications.[5] However, it can take longer for the AV fistula to mature than the AV graft.[13]

The AV graft is used when an AV fistula cannot be created.[5] A tube made from synthetic material is used to form an AV connection.[13] The advantages of the graft are short maturation time, larger surface area provided by the tube for needle placement, better ability to achieve sufficient blood flow, and ease of cannulation.[5,13] Despite the advantages, there are disadvantages which make AV grafts a poor choice in some people. An AV graft does not last as long as an AV fistula and can be more prone to clotting.

The most common KRT in the United States is HD performed in a dialysis facility. The facility's clinical staff conduct treatments during a scheduled appointment three times per week for 3 to 5 hours per session.[1,4,6,8]

Use of alternative HD treatment schedules offer additional benefits to some patients. Although rare, in-center nocturnal intermittent hemodialysis (NIHD) is performed for 7 to 8 hours, three times per week in a clinic setting, with dialysate flow rate of 400 mL/min and blood flow rate of 250 mL/min. The National Kidney Foundation KDOQI guideline for urea kinetics for NIHD is a target Kt/V of 1.4 per HD session, the same as for conventional dialysis.

Incremental HD is a relatively new way to deliver HD and may be used to assist a new patient in transitioning to HD. Residual kidney function (RKF) confers a variety of benefits to patients who receive HD, including provision of continuous clearance of middle molecules and protein-bound solutes. Since the mortality rate is highest in the first months of HD, RKF preservation may improve patient survival and quality of life (QOL).

RKF declines more rapidly with HD delivered three times a week compared to incremental HD. Incremental HD may be beneficial in reducing costs, protecting fragile vascular accesses, and optimizing resource use during the initial phase of HD.[14] Periodic monitoring of RKF is recommended in patients who receive HD through urine volume as well as residual urea clearance with dialysis adequacy and outcome markers, such as anemia, fluid gains, minerals and electrolytes, nutritional status, and QOL. Individualized dialysis prescriptions and consideration of reduced protein intake on nondialysis days are needed for individuals receiving incremental HD.[15]

Nutrition Considerations

Patients undergoing ICHD are at high risk for protein energy wasting (PEW). PEW as a result of kidney failure can affect between 25% to 60% of patients undergoing ICHD.[16,17] PEW can result from a multitude of causes including suboptimal nutrient intake, inflammatory catabolic illnesses, inflammatory processes that are not associated with specific diseases, oxidant stress, carbonyl stress, increased nutrient losses in urine (ie, proteinuria) or dialysate, decreased circulating concentrations or activities of anabolic hormones, increased levels of catabolic hormones, acidemia due to metabolic acidosis, aging, and physical deconditioning.[16] Despite the many causes, a meta-analysis of a variety of studies concludes that the early detection of malnutrition and treatment of the signs and symptoms at an early stage by increasing nutrient intake in any form are associated with improving the nutritional status in patients.[16]

It is important to adequately assess patients who are at risk for PEW. Nutrition therapy should be individualized based on various factors, such as RKF, laboratory analysis, health literacy, motivation to change, living conditions with food preparation in mind, food security issues, and overall nutritional status. Liberalization of dietary restrictions may be indicated for malnourished patients. Nutrition therapy should be reevaluated at least biannually according to the changing status of the patient.[18]

Body mass index (BMI) as a measurement of nutritional status has been used to predict mortality risk in patients who receive HD. Several studies suggest a weight paradox with dialysis showing that higher BMI, rather than lower BMI, may predict better survival among patients undergoing dialysis.[19] In patients who may begin at a normalized weight, average weight losses per year may place patients rapidly at risk for poor overall nutrition and outcomes. BMI on its own is not enough to diagnose PEW unless it is significantly low (<18 kg/m²).[20] The goal of maintaining a safer, higher weight target can be offset by the need for weight loss for transplant BMI targets (see Chapter 8 for more information).

PROTEIN

Protein recommendations are designed to compensate for free amino acid losses during the dialysis treatment. These can range anywhere from 5 to 20 g amino acids per treatment, depending on the type of dialyzer used, the length of treatment time, dialysate flow rate, and the blood flow rate.[21,22] The protein status in patients undergoing dialysis can be obtained by utilizing biochemical indicators (eg, serum albumin and nPCR), measuring various anthropometric measures, and taking dietary recalls. To measure the nutritional status of patients receiving dialysis, the KDOQI guidelines recommend using serum albumin, serial measurement of body weight, percent of usual body weight, bioelectrical impedance, dual-energy x-ray absorptiometry (DXA) scans, anthropometrics, BMI, subjective global assessment (SGA), dietary interviews, and nPCR.[20] The most common (but controversial) and widely available measure of serum protein in the population receiving dialysis is serum albumin. Baseline levels of inflammation associated with comorbidities in patients with CKD, paired with the physiology of the treatment, make albumin a marker of illness, rather than nutrition.[23] Hypoalbuminemia (low serum albumin levels) may offer an opportunity to treat an underlying disorder. Two factors influence hepatic albumin synthesis: nutritional intake and illness. Reduced protein intake slows mRNA synthesis of albumin.[24] Inflammation also lowers albumin, as does metabolic acidosis. Therefore, hypoalbuminemia is often the result of nondietary factors.[23]

For patients who are metabolically stable, KDOQI guidelines recommend protein, 1.0 to 1.2 g/kg/d (see Box 5.2). Previously, specifications indicated that protein be of high biological value, meaning meats, poultry, game, fish, eggs, soy, and dairy. The KDOQI guidelines now state that intake of vegetable or animal protein is of equal value.[20] Irrespective of the source of protein, 30% to 50% of patients receiving HD have dietary protein intakes of less than 1.0 g/kg/d, and only 35% of patients consume between 1.0 and 1.3 g/kg/d. The mean protein intake reported in the Hemodialysis Study (HEMO) was only 0.93 g/kg/d. The resulting impaired nutritional status, as reflected in daily dietary protein intakes of less than 1.0 g/kg/d and hypoalbuminemia, was associated with a higher incidence of morbidity and mortality.[17,25]

Research continues to show that without intervention, patients struggle to consume enough protein and become reliant on nutritional supplements to meet baseline needs. In recent times, finances and insurance coverage for nutritional supplements have become rare, leaving funding up to many dialysis companies. However, the risk of CMS considering provision of nutritional supplements as an enticement to come to their company for dialysis has made it harder to provide patients with needed calories and protein. Many companies now use on-dialysis supplementation, giving enteral supplements, liquid protein, and protein bars to offset the losses that occur during dialysis. The administration of nutritional supplements at the time of dialysis has shown benefit, not in the improvement of albumin but in fewer hospitalizations and a decrease in mortality rate.[26,27]

BOX 5.2 | Daily Recommended Nutrient Intakes for Adults on Hemodialysis[8,20,25,33,34,43,44]

NUTRIENT	RECOMMENDATIONS	ADDITIONAL CONSIDERATIONS
Protein **Patients who are diabetic and nondiabetic**	1.0 to 1.2 g/kg body weight	Protein level is appropriate for metabolically stable patients. Protein amount can be adjusted to maintain glycemic control in patients with diabetes mellitus.
Energy	25 to 35 kcal/kg	
Sodium (Na) and fluid	≥1 L fluid output <1 L fluid output Oliguria	<2,300 mg Na and 2 L fluid <2,300 mg Na and 1 to 1.5 L fluid <2,300 mg Na and 750 mL + 24-hour urine volume
Potassium	Adjust intake as needed per serum levels	Potassium historically limited to 2,400 mg, but no range provided in current guidelines.
Phosphorus	Adjust intake as needed per serum levels	Consider bioavailability of phosphorus sources (eg, animal, vegetable, or additives).
Calcium	800 to 1,000 mg/d (including dietary calcium, calcium supplementation, and calcium-based phosphate binders)	
Magnesium (Mg)	200 to 300 mg	Risk of high Mg comes from gastrointestinal medications, antacids or laxatives, Mg supplementation, and use of Mg-based phosphate binders.
Iron	Individualized	Consider oral vs intravenous.
Zinc	8 to 11 mg The Kidney Disease Outcomes Quality Initiative (KDOQI) guidelines suggest not routinely supplementing zinc, as there is little evidence that it improves nutritional, inflammatory, or micronutrient status.	Serum levels are low in hemodialysis (HD), but cellular levels can be high. Chronic supplementation risks copper deficiency. Zinc supplementation can help with taste issues but requires a short time frame for dosage.
Fiber	20 to 30 g	Use of soluble fiber requires increased fluid intake, which is contraindicated in patients on HD.
Vitamin A	Supplementation is not recommended.	High vitamin A levels can cause anemia and abnormal lipid and metabolism (hypercalcemia). When supplementation is warranted, patients must be monitored for toxicity.
Vitamin D	Nutritional vitamin D supplementation may be indicated based on serum levels; however, it is unknown what the desired 25 hydroxyvitamin D level should be for patients with chronic kidney disease. Active vitamin D replacement therapy is indicated to treat secondary hyperparathyroidism.	Use of active vitamin D requires close monitoring of calcium, phosphorus, and parathyroid hormone (PTH) levels.
Vitamin E	Routine supplementation is not recommended due to risks of vitamin toxicity.	Caution should be advised for patients receiving anticoagulant therapy.
Vitamin K	Unclear to supplement	Consider risks for anticoagulant therapy.
Thiamin	Recommended Dietary Allowance (RDA)	Absorption is inhibited by folate deficiency or protein–energy malnutrition. Infection, diarrhea, liver disease, surgery, or large glucose loads may increase the nutritional need for thiamin.

Continued on next page

Continued from previous page

NUTRIENT	RECOMMENDATIONS	ADDITIONAL CONSIDERATIONS
Riboflavin	RDA	Riboflavin is albumin-bound, with little stored in body tissues.
Folic acid	Recommend prescribing folate for deficiency based on clinical signs and symptoms.	Folate absorption and metabolism may be impaired in uremia or with diminished gastric acid secretion. Requirements increase in patients receiving HD and erythropoiesis-stimulating agents (ESA); and insufficiency may impair red blood cell response.
Vitamin B6	RDA	Vitamin B6 is bound to albumin and hemoglobin. Sufficient riboflavin, niacin, and zinc are necessary for B6 metabolism. Vitamin B6 is a coenzyme in amino acid and lipid metabolism and is essential for gluconeogenesis, myelin formation, and hematopoiesis. Risk of vitamin B6 deficiency increases with ESA therapy, inflammation, aging, theophylline, hydralazine, alcoholism, or tobacco smoking.
Vitamin B12	Recommend supplementation for deficiency based on clinical signs and symptoms.	Vitamin B12 is protein bound in plasma and is involved in folic acid metabolism, red blood cell formation, and synthesis of myelin and nucleic acid. Incidence of B12 deficiency increases with time spent on dialysis.
Niacin	RDA	Niacin is involved in carbohydrate, fatty acid, and amino acid metabolism and is not easily dialyzed. Pharmacological doses of nicotinic acid can lower total cholesterol and triglycerides and increase high-density lipoprotein levels (see Box 17.2). Niacinamide inhibits intestinal absorption of phosphorus for novel control of hyperphosphatemia (see Box 17.7).
Biotin	RDA	Biotin is involved in the metabolism of carbohydrates, fatty acids, and some amino acids. Clinical studies in patients undergoing incenter hemodialysis who used a pharmacological dosing of 10 mg daily reported improved hair and skin quality, relief from hiccups and improvement of restless leg syndrome. Use of high-dose biotin (1,500 to 5,000 mcg/d) may interfere with PTH enzyme-linked immunosorbent assay (ELISA), falsely depressing test results.
Pantothenic acid	RDA	Pantothenic acid is transported in red blood cells within minutes of intestinal absorption. It is necessary for metabolism of fatty acids and amino acids and for the synthesis of vitamins A and D and cholesterol.
Vitamin C	It is reasonable to consider supplementing to meet recommended intake of 90 mg/dL for males and 75 mg/dL for females	Ascorbic acid is a small, non-protein bound molecule removed by dialysis. Dietary intake is often low when vitamin C–rich fruits and vegetables are limited in diet due to potassium restriction. Peeling and twice cooking potatoes and vegetables (recommended to reduce potassium content) lowers available ascorbic acid by leaching or degradation. Risk of vitamin C deficiency increases with duration on HD with smokers and in older adults. Excessive vitamin C in oliguric patients may be metabolized to insoluble oxalate crystals that precipitate in soft tissues (hyperoxalosis).

ENERGY

For adult patients who are metabolically stable, the KDOQI guidelines recommend daily energy levels of 25 to 35 kcal/kg body weight (see Box 5.2).[20] Energy expenditure in patients who receive HD is similar to that in healthy individuals. Achieving energy intake at this level has been shown to provide neutral nitrogen balance.[17] Higher energy intakes may be indicated for patients who perform strenuous labor and those who are underweight, catabolic, or hospitalized. Adults who are sedentary and have an overall loss of lean body mass would benefit from following an exercise regimen. Improved cardiac fitness, QOL, physical function, and a decrease in levels of depression have also been shown to be benefits of exercise in the population receiving dialysis. Exercising during dialysis and on nondialysis days has been shown to be beneficial.[28] Barring the ability to exercise (eg, due to mobility or anemia), patients may benefit from the lower end of the energy recommendations.

There remains a concern about whether patients receiving HD can ingest the recommended amount of calories. In the HEMO study, 62% to 94% of patients never met the prior energy recommendations of 30 to 35 kcal/kg/d standard body weight set forth by the original KDOQI guidelines.

Intakes should be evaluated and, if insufficient, high-calorie supplements may need to be initiated. There are a variety of oral supplements available, and each should be evaluated based on individual needs and preferences (see Chapter 18).[25]

LIPIDS

Patients receiving HD are at risk for disorders of lipid metabolism based on many of their comorbid diseases. In the population undergoing dialysis, lipid-lowering medications may not show significant beneficial effects relative to the occurrence of cardiovascular events (eg, cardiovascular death, nonfatal myocardial infarction, or stroke).[29] A balance should be achieved between diet modification to targets of the Dietary Guidelines while maintaining the need for adequate calorie and protein

intake to meet the needs of patients receiving HD and prevent malnutrition. For more information about cardiovascular disease and CKD, see Chapter 11.

SODIUM AND FLUID

Hypertension in patients with CKD is usually salt-sensitive. Restricting daily sodium intake to less than 2,300 mg (<100 mEq) lowers thirst, extracellular fluid volume, weight, proteinuria, and blood pressure while enhancing the effects of antihypertensive medications (see Box 5.2).[20,30,31]

While most patients undergoing dialysis fall into the target group for the 1,500 mg sodium restriction recommended by the American Heart Association, use of this guideline may be impractical. Most Americans do not follow a low-sodium diet to a numerical value. Using numerical values such as 1,500 mg/d or 2,300 mg/d can serve as a general guide or for setting a budget (or a target) in teaching. Working with patients on small manageable changes tends to produce more realistic outcomes.[32] Adherence to sodium and fluid restrictions can be measured by intradialytic weight gain (IDWG).[1,4] An IDWG less than 5% of dry weight is desirable since an IDWG of greater than 5.7% of dry weight has been associated with an increased mortality rate of 35%.[17,33] Fluid allowance includes insensible losses (up to 1,000 mL/d) from respiration, perspiration, and fecal losses, and then includes the 24-hour urine output volume as well. General guidelines show 750 mL plus the volume of urine output can be set as a daily target.[34] Patients with RKF who receive HD generally have decreased urine output once they start HD.

POTASSIUM

As the GFR declines, the excretion rate of potassium increases through both urinary and fecal excretion. However, as kidney failure continues to worsen, this response becomes less efficient, and eventually potassium retention and hyperkalemia (high serum potassium level) will occur. The potassium allowance for a patient undergoing ICHD varies. Recommendations for potassium intake range from 2 to 4 g/d, depending on urine output.[35] Patients may develop hyperkalemia if their dietary intake of potassium is excessive or if they ingest potassium-containing oral or herbal supplements. Due to the potential for hyperkalemia, a strict dietary potassium limit may be indicated with metabolic acidosis and with use of nonsteroidal anti-inflammatory agents, potassium-sparing diuretics, angiotensin-converting enzyme inhibitors, angiotensin blockers, aldosterone receptor antagonists, or β-receptor blockers. Historically, the individual daily allowance for potassium had been 2,400 mg/d. The updated KDOQI guidelines now advise adjusting the dietary potassium intake to maintain serum potassium within the normal range (see Box 5.2.)[2,20] For educational purposes, foods are categorized as being high, medium, and low in potassium; however, frequency, portion size, and dialysis clearance all play a role in determining appropriate potassium values.

Mild hyperkalemia occurs at serum levels between 5.5 through 6.5 mEq/L. Moderate-to-severe hyperkalemia occurs at levels greater than 6.5 mEq/L. Nutrition counseling regarding avoiding high potassium sources can help patients with chronic hyperkalemia reduce potassium levels. Other measures to avoid hyperkalemia include correcting metabolic acidosis, adjusting the dialysate potassium level in the bath, and looking into other potential factors including missed treatments, constipation, access issues, and seasonal or cultural diet changes.

In certain circumstances, diet intervention alone may not resolve hyperkalemia rapidly enough, and medications may need to be given. Historically, use of an oral administration of sodium polystyrene sulfate resin may help treat hyperkalemia.[10] Use of cation exchange polymers has been the past standard, but use of the newer potassium-binding medications more often seen in patients with CKD is emerging as well. The amount of potassium in the dialysate bath ranges from 1 to 4 mEq/L and can be adjusted by the physician based on individual needs. Lowering the sodium concentration in the dialysate may also help prevent hyperkalemia in the patient receiving dialysis by preventing hyperkalemic rebound after dialysis and, therefore, preventing hyperkalemia interdialytically.[35]

Hypokalemia (low serum potassium level) in patients undergoing ICHD may be a marker of malnutrition. Patients with an inadequate intake do not ingest sufficient nutrients, including potassium. Also, patients with chronic diarrhea may exhibit hypokalemia. Moderate-to-severe hypokalemia occurs at serum levels less than 3.5 mEq/L. Patients with chronic hypokalemia may need a higher potassium dialysate bath. Dietary intake should also be evaluated.[35]

Traditionally, the HD diet has discouraged a high consumption of fruits and vegetables. The DIET-HD study examined 8,078 patients undergoing HD for 3 years and found that the average patient receiving HD consumed only two fruits and vegetables per week. When fruit and vegetable intake was increased to 17 servings per week (two to three servings daily), all-cause mortality risk was reduced by 20%. Individualized patient counseling is encouraged to help patients receiving HD safely reap the health benefits of fruits and vegetables necessary to reduce health risks and avoid over-restricting their diet.[36]

BONE METABOLISM

Calcium, phosphorus, and parathyroid hormone (PTH) are involved in bone metabolism. These laboratory results are commonly altered and are associated with greater cardiovascular calcification, morbidity, and mortality in patients undergoing HD (refer to Chapter 10 for more details).[20]

Calcium

The current guidelines for CKD recommend limiting elemental calcium intake to 800 to 1,000 mg/d in diet, supplements, and medications to avoid positive calcium balance (see Box 5.2). A serum calcium (adjusted for low albumin) of 8.4 to 10.2 mg/dL is the goal. Calcium balance is a complex interaction between bone, intestinal absorption, and kidney excretion, regulated by PTH and active vitamin D (calcitriol).[37] Laboratory results are monitored for hypercalcemia (high serum calcium level) or hypocalcemia (low serum calcium level), with calcium intake, medications, or dialysate modified as needed. Hypercalcemia may result from calcium excess (dietary, supplement, or binder), low PTH, or active vitamin D excess.[6,7] Hypocalcemia may need calcium supplementation between meals and at bedtime. Symptoms of very low or very high levels of calcium can be nonspecific complaints of anorexia, nausea, tingling in the fingers, lethargy, irritability, seizures, confusion, or weakness.

Phosphorus

Prior guidelines recommend limiting phosphorus intake to 800 to 1,000 mg/d (or <17 mg/kg body weight) to maintain serum phosphorus levels between 3.5 and 5.5 mg/dL.[20,37] Current KDOQI guidelines, however, recommend adjusting dietary phosphorus intake to maintain serum levels within normal range (see Box 5.2).[20] Phosphorus management is based on a combination of dialysis removal, intestinal binding, and diet limitations.[6] ICHD phosphorus clearance ranges from 500 to 1,000 mg per treatment (about 50% of the 2-day retention), with greater serum clearance in the first 1 to 2 hours and then a slower flux of phosphorus from cells or bone stores.[6] Phosphate binders, taken in divided doses with food at meals and snacks, intercept gastrointestinal phosphorus to form insoluble complexes, reduce absorption, and increase stool excretion.[8] To help achieve a serum albumin level of 4 g/dL, dietary counseling may recommend higher protein intakes. Protein-rich foods often have high phosphorus content, so counseling usually incorporates high protein recommendations using lower phosphorus food choices. While protein-rich foods are often high in this nutrient, the risk of lowering protein intake below goal range to achieve desired phosphorus levels outweighs the benefit.[38] Greater focus on types of foods consumed to lower intake of phosphate additives (ie, use of fresh rather than processed meats and preparation of food at home rather than dining out), ensuring adequacy of dialysis and proper use of phosphate-binding medication is preferable to improve phosphorus management.

Elevated serum phosphorus (hyperphosphatemia) is an independent risk factor for heart disease and mortality.[39] Binder use (including different classes and combinations) is associated with improved survival but is dependent on patient compliance. Food restrictions, high pill burden, cost, and new pill habits with food can be overwhelming. Meat and plant foods have less bioavailable phosphorus than phosphate additives in processed, instant, and ready-to-eat foods. Patients have difficulty quantifying phosphorus intake when food labels list content as a percent of daily value (DV) or not at all.[40] Hyperphosphatemia is seen in patient nonadherence to diet, dialysis, and medication orders, as well as in catabolism, enema use, or altered gut motility (eg, constipation or gastroparesis).[39] Uremic pruritus may occur when excessive calcium and phosphorus precipitate in the skin, leading to calciphylaxis or calcific uremic arteriopathy, which is associated with increased risk of respiratory failure and myocardial infarction.

Hypophosphatemia (low serum phosphorus level) may occur with anorexia, excessive binder or antacid use, hyperglycemia, or malabsorption (eg, celiac sprue or gastric surgery).[39] When unable to bring up phosphorus levels by righting these factors, use of phosphorus supplements may be warranted.

Parathyroid Hormone and Vitamin D

PTH is used as a marker of bone turnover. Low kidney function produces less active vitamin D (calcitriol), resulting in decreased calcium absorption and phosphorus excretion but increased PTH secretion. PTH secretion rapidly responds to hypocalcemia or hyperphosphatemia, but it is inhibited by calcitriol. Oversecretion of PTH is known as secondary hyperparathyroidism (SHPT). Active vitamin D replacement therapy is indicated to treat SHPT using first-generation calcitriol, second-generation doxercalciferol, or third-generation paracalcitriol. Studies indicate improved QOL and survival on active vitamin D replacement therapy, independent of mineral or PTH levels. Adjunctive calcimimetic therapy increases calcium sensitivity to lower serum calcium and PTH levels. Cardiovascular events account for 50% of deaths in patients on HD. When longitudinally examined, the study data demonstrate greater survival with the following ranges: 8.6 to 10.2 mg/dL calcium, 3.6 to 5 mg/dL phosphorus, less than 50 mg/dL calcium phosphorus product, and 101 to 600 pg/mL PTH.[8,37,39]

Anemia Management and Iron

There are a number of factors that lead to iron deficiency in patients receiving dialysis. These include an increased demand for iron during erythropoiesis by recombinant human erythropoietin; a decrease in iron uptake by the intestinal mucosal cells; occult gastrointestinal tract blood losses; and external blood losses, including losses resulting from blood retention in the dialyzer and bloodlines, frequent blood tests, and accidental blood losses from the vascular access. The absorption of dietary iron is also less efficient due to calcium-based phosphate binders, histamine-2 blockers, proton-pump inhibitors, and functional achlorhydria-impairing iron absorption.[41]

Because anemia is a major complication of CKD, much research has been done on correcting iron deficiency in this population. It is difficult for individuals to consume enough iron from food sources due, in part, to any concentrated sources being limited by other dietary restrictions. Several studies have supported the use of oral iron over intravenous (IV) iron, stating it is safer and equally effective as IV iron.[42] Oral supplements are less expensive than IV iron, but they may not sufficiently correct iron depletion in many patients. Supplements in the form of ferrous salts, such as ferrous fumarate, ferrous gluconate, ferrous sulfate, and iron polysaccharides, are often prescribed to correct iron deficiency. Newer phosphorus binders are iron-based with a dual-purpose goal, both replenishing iron while still binding phosphorus. The KDOQI guidelines recommend IV iron over oral iron as the route of administration for patients on HD.[41]

More data are available about vitamin status of patients receiving HD than those with CKD not requiring dialysis. The Dietary Reference Intakes (DRIs), which are developed and published by the Institute of Medicine, represent the nutrient needs of healthy populations.[45] The average patient with maintenance hemodialysis (MHD) may have low intake of vitamins C, B6, and folic acid related to reduced intake of fruits and vegetables and greater intake of processed foods.[46]

Patients using the phosphate binder sevelamer hydrochloride may have reduced vitamin B6 due to binding of the vitamin.[47] Patients undergoing MHD with nephrotic syndrome may have greater losses of vitamin C and vitamin B6, so they should be assessed and receive multivitamin supplements.[48] The European Best Practice Guidelines recommend MHD vitamin supplementation as shown in Table 5.1, but the KDOQI guidelines do not address vitamins.[49] When renal multivitamins are not available, it may be prudent to recommend the use of a daily multivitamin that meets the recommended dietary allowance (RDA) or adequate intake of the water-soluble vitamins.

Geriatric Nutrition Needs on Hemodialysis

When dialysis was first developed, resources were scarce, and geriatric patients were often excluded from treatment. In HD, older patients are now the rule rather than the exception, as older patients are now routinely dialyzed. The United States Renal Data System (USRDS) data from 2019 show that nearly one-half of patients receiving dialysis in the United States are over age 63 and that they represent the fastest growing group.[50] A consequence of the aging community undergoing HD is the emergence of new issues, including nutrient needs at advanced stages of life. Although there are no nutrition guidelines specifically for the geriatric population receiving HD, collaborative efforts between renal RDNs and providers may improve QOL and outcomes for this growing segment of the population receiving dialysis.

The prevalence of PEW is variable among seniors, and there are no age-specific guidelines for treating malnutrition. Distinguishing between the impact of CKD and the effects of aging is challenging. Older people have an inherently reduced rate of albumin synthesis related to aging, regardless of protein intake or the impact of inflammation. The Dialysis Outcomes Practice Patterns Study (DOPPS) suggested geriatric patients receiving HD had lower BMI, reduced levels of

TABLE 5.1 | Vitamin Properties

Vitamin	Standard DRIs	DRIs for patients on HD	Solubility	Protein binding in plasma	HD losses	Toxicity
A	700-900 mcg	None	Lipid	Retinol binding protein, prealbumin	None	Yes
E (alpha tocopherol)	15 IU	400-800 IU	Lipid	Lipoproteins	None	Possible
K (phylloquinone, K1)	90-120 mcg	Not available	Lipid	Lipoproteins	Unknown	No
B1 Thiamine	1.1-1.2 mg	1.1-1.2 mg	Water	Albumin	13-40 mL/min	No
B2 Riboflavin	1.1-1.3 mg	1.1-1.3 mg	Water	Albumin, IgG, weak	27-52 mL/min	No
B3 Niacin	14-16 mg	14-16 mg	Water	Weak	Minimal	No
B5 Pantothenic acid	5 mg	5 mg	Water	Unknown	30 mL/min	No
B6 Pyridoxine	1.3-1.7 mg	10 mg	Water	Albumin	54 mL/min	Yes
B7 Biotin	30 mcg	30 mcg	Water	Weak	52 mL/min	No
B9 Folic acid	400 mcg	1 mg	Water	No	135 mL/min	Yes
B12 Cyanocobalamin	2.4 mcg	2.4 mcg	Water	Transco-balamin II	Controversial	Unknown
C	75-90 mg	75-90 mg	Water	No	80-280 mg/session	Yes

DRI = dietary reference intakes | HD = hemodialysis

normalized protein nitrogen appearance, serum albumin and PTH, and elevated C-reactive protein.[51] Muscle mass appears to decline more rapidly among older adults with kidney disease.[52] Frailty, described by weakness and slowness, is associated with age, but in patients receiving HD, frailty also develops independently of age and may be associated with 25-hydroxyvitamin D deficiency and related impact on muscle target cells.[53] As stated earlier in the chapter, for those with limited movement or need for weight loss, lower end calorie goals may be appropriate. Recent European Society of Parenteral and Enteral Nutrition (ESPEN) recommendations endorse increased protein for optimal muscle

functioning with age. Renal guidelines for HD lack age-based criteria but endorse the general guideline of higher protein intake for all adults ranging from 1.0 to 1.2 g/kg/d to replete amino acid losses into the dialysate and mitigate the impact of metabolic acidosis and inflammation which increase muscle catabolism.[24]

Reduced protein and muscle stores and reduced dietary intake also impact the efficacy of medication treatment. Malnutrition results in lower serum protein (eg, albumin), which leads to a higher level of unbound drug fraction. Since only unbound drug fractions are pharmacologically active, this may result in increased drug effects, potentially causing loss of appetite and other side effects. Nutritional status reflects visceral protein level and somatic protein stores, and the biomarkers of each may not tightly correlate. No single marker of nutrition can be recommended; however, as a screening tool, albumin has the unique quality of predictive power in kidney disease. Use of a nutrition focused physical exam or other complementary approach will support the nutrition evaluation and help target nutrition therapy.

When energy and protein intake decline, the risk of nutrient deficiencies may increase. Calcium and vitamin D deficiency are more common, with greater risk of falls and fractures. Martins et al[54] compared dietary intake among geriatric patients undergoing HD to age-matched people with normal kidney function and found that the intake of protein and phosphorus was significantly lower. Although no age-based phosphorus guidelines exist, low serum phosphorus in patients receiving dialysis is associated with all-cause mortality and infection-related mortality. Overuse of medications which bind phosphorus, including phosphate binders and antacids, may cause phosphate to shift from the extracellular space into the cell and may also contribute to cardiac or respiratory arrest, neutrophil dysfunction, or lower adenosine triphosphate (ATP) content of leukocytes.[55] Careful review of dietary intake and cautious titration of phosphate binder dosage are suggested for geriatric patients. Closely monitor predialysis phosphorus levels (compared to their dietary intake and phosphate binder use) to reduce risk of hypophosphatemia. Although phosphorus rebounds within 5 hours after dialysis, geriatric patients might experience weakness and greater cardiac or respiratory risk post dialysis if they are markedly hypophosphatemic at the end of treatment. Older people are more vulnerable to circumstances and clinical factors that can precipitate malnutrition. Individualized care based on laboratory results, patient goals, and age-related needs may improve QOL. Clinicians may benefit from using a thorough nutrition evaluation with an interdisciplinary approach to individualize nutrition care for geriatric patients in the absence of nutrition guidelines for older adults receiving HD.

Summary

Nutrition is paramount for patients with CKD undergoing ICHD. Defining the nutrient needs of adults receiving ICHD is an important aspect of treatment. Assisting patients with nutritional concerns helps them better attain a higher level QOL and may improve the mortality rate in this population. It is imperative that nutrition intervention be ongoing and developed in collaboration with the interdisciplinary health care team.

References

1. Himmelfarb J. Hemodialysis. In: *Brenner and Rectors: The Kidney.* 8th ed. Saunders; 2008.
2. Daugirdas JT, Depner T, Inrig JK, et al. KDOQI Clinical Practice Guideline for Hemodialysis Adequacy: 2015 update. *Am J Kidney Dis.* 2015;66(5):884-930. doi:10.1053/j.ajkd.2015.07.015
3. Shah N. Indications for dialysis: a mnemonic and explanation. *RhoChi Post.* 2012;1(11):14.
4. Mitch WE, Ikizler TA. *Handbook of Nutrition and the Kidney.* 6th ed. Lippincott Williams & Wilkins; 2010.
5. Centers for Medicare and Medicaid Services. Measurement assessment tool: conditions for coverage for end-stage renal disease facilities. 2008. Centers for Medicare and Medicaid Services website. Accessed April 30, 2019. www.cms.gov/Medicare/Provider-Enrollment-and-Certification/GuidanceforLawsAndRegulations/Dialysis
6. Lerma E, Weir M. *Henrich's Principles and Practice of Dialysis.* 5th ed. Wolters Kluwer; 2016.
7. Miles AMV, Friedman EA. Center and home chronic hemodialysis: outcome and complications. In: Schrier RW, ed. *Diseases of the Kidney and Urinary Tract.* 8th ed. Lippincott Williams & Wilkins; 2007:2648-2670.
8. Kopple JD. Dietary considerations in patients with chronic renal failure, acute renal failure and transplantation. In: Schrier RW, ed. *Diseases of the Kidney and Urinary Tract.* 8th ed. Lippincott Williams & Wilkins; 2007:2709-2764.
9. Chiu YW, Kopple JD, Mehrotra R. Correction of metabolic acidosis to ameliorate wasting in chronic kidney disease: goals and strategies. *Sem Nephrol.* 2009;29(1):67-74. doi:10.1016/j.semnephrol.2008.10.009
10. Daugirdas JT. Chronic hemodialysis prescription. In: Daugirdas JT, Blake PG, Ing TS, eds. *Handbook of Dialysis.* 5th ed. Wolters Kluwer; 2015:192-214.

11. Momeni A, Mardani S, Kabiri M, Smiri M. Comparison of complications of arteriovenous fistula with permanent cather in hemodialysis patients: a six-month follow-up. *Adv Biomed Res.* 2017;6:106. doi:10.4103/2277-9175.213666

12. Shenoy S, Allon M, Beathard G, et al. Clinical trial end points for hemodialysis vascular access. *Clin J Am Soc Nephrol.* 2018;13(3):490-494. doi:10.2215/CJN.13321216

13. Vachharajani TJ, Wu S, Brouwer-Maier D, Asif A. Arteriovenous fistulas and grafts: the basics. In: Daugirdas JT, Blake PD, Ing TS, eds. *Handbook of Dialysis.* 5th ed. Wolters Kluwer; 2015:99-120.

14. Kalantar-Zadeh K, Unruh M, Zager PG, et al. Twice-weekly and incremental hemodialysis treatment for initiation of kidney replacement therapy. *Am J Kidney Dis.* 2014;64(2):181-186. doi:10.1053/j.ajkd.2014.04.019

15. Mathew AT, Fishbane S, Obi Y, Kalantar-Zadeh K. Preservation of residual kidney function in hemodialysis patients: reviving an old concept for contemporary practice. *Kidney Int.* 2016;90(2):262-271. doi:10.1016/j.kint.2016.02.037

16. Lodebo BT, Shah A, Kopple JD. Is it important to prevent and treat protein energy wasting in chronic kidney disease and chronic dialysis patients? *J Ren Nutr.* 2018;28(6):369-379. doi:10.1053/j.jrn.2018.04.002

17. Therrien M, Byham-Gray L, Beto J. A review of dietary intake studies in maintenance dialysis patients. *J Ren Nutr.* 2015;25(4):329-338. doi:10.1053/j.jrn.2014.11.001

18. St-Jules DE, Woolf K, Pompeii ML, Sevick MA. Exploring problems in following the hemodialysis diet and their relation to energy and nutrient intakes: the Balance Wise Study. *J Ren Nutr.* 2016;26(2):118-124. doi:10.1053/j.jrn.2015.10.002

19. Rahimlu M, Shab-Bidar S, Djafarian K. Body mass index and all-cause mortality in chronic kidney disease: a dose-response meta-analysis of observational studies. *J Ren Nutr.* 2017;27(4):225-232. doi:10.1053/j.jrn.2017.01.016

20. Ikizler TA, Burrowes JD, Byham-Gray LD, et al. KDOQI Nutrition in CKD Guideline Work Group. KDOQI clinical practice guideline for nutrition in CKD: 2020 update. *Am J Kidney Dis.* 2020;76(3)(suppl 1):S1-S107. doi:10.1053/j.ajkd.2020.05.006

21. Ikizler TA, Flakoll PJ, Parker RA, Hakim RM. Amino acid and albumin losses during hemodialysis. *Kidney Int.* 1994;46(3):830-837. doi:10.1038/ki.1994.339

22. Salame C, Eaton S, Grimble G, Davenport A. Protein losses and urea nitrogen underestimate total nitrogen losses in peritoneal dialysis and hemodialysis patients. *J Ren Nutr.* 2018;28(5):317-323. doi:10.1053/j.jrn.2018.01.016

23. de Mutsert R, Grootendorst DC, Indemans F, et al. Association between serum albumin and mortality in dialysis patients is partly explained by inflammation and not by malnutrition. *J Ren Nutr.* 2009;19(2):127-135. doi:10.1053/j.jrn.2008.08.003

24. Carrero JJ, Stenvinkel P, Cuppari L, et al. Etiology of the protein-energy wasting syndrome in chronic kidney disease: a consensus statement from the International Society of Renal Nutrition and Metabolism (ISRNM). *J Ren Nutr.* 2013;23(2):77-90. doi:10.1053/j.jrn.2013.01.001

25. Rocco MV, Paranandi L, Burrowes JD, et al. Nutritional status in the HEMO Study cohort at baseline. *Am J Kidney Dis.* 2002;39(2):245-256. doi:10.1053/ajkd.2002.30543

26. Sundell MB, Cavanaugh KL, Wu P, Shintani A, Hakim RM, Ikizler TA. Oral protein supplementation alone improves anabolism in a dose-dependent manner in chronic hemodialysis patients. *J Ren Nutr.* 2009;19(5):412-421. doi:10.1053/j.jrn.2009.01.019

27. Lacson E, Wang W, Zebrowski B, Wingard R, Hakim RM. Outcomes associated with intradialytic oral nutritional supplements in patients undergoing maintenance hemodialysis: a quality improvement report. *Am J Kidney Dis.* 2012;60(4):591-600. doi:10.1053/j.ajkd.2012.04.019

28. Johansen KL. Exercise in the end-stage renal disease population. *J Am Soc Nephrol.* 2007;18(6):1845-1854. doi:10.1681/ASN.2007010009

29. Tonelli MA, Wanner C, Cass A, et al. KDIGO clinical practice guideline for lipid management in chronic kidney disease. *Kidney Int Suppl.* 2013;3(3):274. doi:10.1038/kisup.2013.34

30. Sanghavi S, Vasolotti JA. Dietary sodium: a therapeutic target in the treatment of hypertension and CKD. *J Ren Nutr.* 2013;23(3):223-227. doi:10.1053/j.jrn.2013.01.027

31. Cobb M, Pacitti D. The importance of sodium restrictions in chronic kidney disease. *J Ren Nutr.* 2018 Sep;28(5):e37-e40. doi:10.1053/j.jrn.2018.02.001

32. Meuleman Y, Hoekstra T, Dekker FW, van der Boog P, van Dijk S, ESMO study group. Perceived sodium reduction barriers among patients with chronic kidney disease: which barriers are important and which patients experience barriers? *Int J Behav Med.* 2018;25(1):93-102. doi:10.1007/s12529-017-9668-x

33. Wiesen K. Dialysis. In: Byham-Gray LD, Burrowes JD, Chertow GM, eds. *Nutrition in Kidney Disease.* 2nd ed. Humana Press; 2014:173-195.

34. Chow JA, Kalantar-Zadeh K. Volume balance and intradialytic ultrafiltration rate in the hemodialysis patient. *Curr Heart Fail Rep.* 2017;14(5):421-427. doi:10.1007/s11897-017-0356-6

35. Karaboyas A, Zee J, Brunelli SM, et al. Dialysate potassium, serum potassium, mortality and arrhythmia events in hemodialysis: results from the Dialysis Outcomes and Practice Patterns Study. *Am J Kidney Dis.* 2017;69(2):266-277. doi:10.1053/j.ajkd.2016.09.015

36. Saglimbene VM, Wong G, Ruospo M, et al. Fruit and vegetable intake and mortality in adults undergoing maintenance hemodialysis. *Clin J Am Soc Nephrol.* 2019;14(2):250-260. doi:10.2215/CJN.08580718

37. Ketteler M, Leonard MB, Block GA, et al. KDIGO 2017 clinical practice guideline update for the diagnosis, evaluation, prevention, and treatment of chronic kidney disease-mineral bone disorder (CKD-MBD). *Kidney Int Suppl.* 2017;7(1):25-38. doi:10.1016/j.kisu.2017.04.001

38. St-Jules DE, Woolf K, Pompeii ML, Kalantar-Zadeh K, Sevick MA. Re-examining the phosphorus-protein dilemma: does phosphorus restriction compromise protein status? *J Ren Nutr.* 2015;26(3):136-140. doi:10.1053/j.jrn.2015.12.004

39. Kendrick J, Kestenbaum B, Chonchol M. Phosphate and cardiovascular disease. *Adv Chronic Kidney Dis.* 2011;18(2):113-119. doi:10.1053/j.ackd.2010.12.003

40. deFornasari MLL, Dos Santos Sens YA. Replacing phosphorus-containing food additives with foods without additives reduces phosphatemia in end-stage renal disease patients: a randomized clinical trial. *J Ren Nutr.* 2017;27(2):97-105. doi:10.1053/j.jrn.2016.08.009

41. McMurray JJV, Parfrey PS, Adamson JW, et al. KDIGO clinical practice guideline for anemia in chronic kidney disease. *Kidney Int Suppl.* 2012;2(4):292-297. doi:10.1038/kisup.2012.38

42. Roger SD. Practical considerations for iron therapy in the management of anaemia in patients with chronic kidney disease. *Clin Kidney J.* 2017;10(Suppl 1):i9–i15. doi:10.1093/ckj/sfx100

43. Bryant B. Therapeutic Research Center: Research letter #340204. February 2018. Accessed March 7, 2019. www.ospdocs.com/resources/uploads/files/Biotin%20and%20Labs.pdf

44. Kramer H, Berns JS, Choi M, Martin K, Rocco MV. 25-hydroxyvitamin D testing and supplementation in CKD: an NKF-KDOQI controversies report. *Am J Kidney Dis.* 2014;64(4):499-509. doi:10.1053/j.ajkd.2014.05.018

45. DRI. United States Department of Agriculture Dietary Reference Intakes of Vitamins and Elements. 2011. Accessed December 15, 2020. www.ncbi.nlm.nih.gov/books/NBK56068/table/summarytables.t2/?report=objectonly

46. Riberiro MMC, de Araujo ML, Netto MP, Cunha LM. Effects of customary dinner on dietetical profile of patients undergoing hemodialysis. *J Bras Nefrol.* 2011;33(1):69-77. doi:10.1590/S0101-28002011000100010

47. Takagi K, Masuda K, Yamazaki M, et al. Metal ion and vitamin absorption profiles of phosphate binder ion-exchange resins. *Clin Nephrol.* 2010;73(1):30-35. doi:10.5414/cnp73030

48. Kopple J, Massry S, Kalantar-Zadeh K. eds. *Nutritional Management of Renal Disease.* 3rd ed. American Press; 2013.

49. Fouque D, Vennegoor M, ter Wee P, et al. EBPG guideline on nutrition. *Nephrol Dial Transplant.* 2007;22(suppl 2):ii45-ii87. doi:10.1093/ndt/gfm020

50. USRDS. *US Renal Data System 2019 Atlas of Chronic Kidney Disease and End Stage Renal Disease in the United States.* National Institute of Diabetes and Digestive Kidney Diseases. 2019:706.

51. Canaud B, Tong L, Tentori F, et al. Clinical practices and outcomes in elderly hemodialysis patients: results from the Dialysis Outcomes Practice Patterns Study (DOPPS). *Clin J Am Soc Nephrol.* 2011;6(7):1651-1662. doi:10.2215/CJN.03530410

52. McIntyre CW, Selby NM, Sigrist M, Pearce LF, Mercer TH, Naish PF. Patients recieving maintenance dialysis have more severe functionally significant skeletal muscle wasting than patients with dialysis-independent chronic kidney disease. *Nephrol Dial Transplant.* 2006;21(8):2210-2216. doi:10.1093/ndt/gfl064

53. Johansen KL, Chertow GM, Jin C, Kurtner NG. Significance of frailty among dialysis patients. *J Am Soc Nephrol.* 2007;18(11):2960-2967. doi:10.1681/ASN.2007020221

54. Martins AM, Rodrigues JCD, de Oliveira Santin FG, dos Santos Barbosa Brito F, Moreira ASB, Lourenco RA. Food intake assessment of elderly patients on hemodialysis. *J Ren Nutr.* 2015;25(3):321-326. doi:10.1053/j.jrn.2014.10.007

55. Amanzadeh J, Reilly RF Jr. Hypophosphatemia: an evidenced based approach to its clinical consequences and management. *Nat Clin Pract Nephr.* 2006;2(3):136-148. doi:10.1038/ncpneph0124

CHAPTER 6

Nutrition Management of the Adult Patient on Home Hemodialysis

Lesley McPhatter, MS, RDN, CSR

Introduction

The mortality rates for patients with chronic kidney disease (CKD) undergoing dialysis in the United States are just under 20% and higher than those in other industrialized countries such as Italy, Japan, and France.[1] According to the United States Renal Data System (US-RDS) database, survival is improving slightly in all age groups since the introduction of the bundled payment system in 2011.[2] The reasons for this are multifactorial, including better monitoring and dosing of medications and an overall improved approach toward patient treatment goals.[3] However, it remains well documented that inadequate dialysis contributes to mortality. Increased treatment time and frequency, such as home hemodialysis (HHD) and nocturnal hemodialysis (NHD), continue to show a longer survival benefit as more data become available (see Box 6.1).[4-7] HHD is typically done while the patient is awake and runs 3 to 5 hours, 3 to 6 days a week (depending on residual kidney function and treatment length).[5] Currently, two types of NHD are performed in the United States. Incenter NHD is performed in dialysis facilities by the health care team. Typical treatment parameters are 8 hours per night, three times a week, or 24 hours a week, which is double the treatment time of the patient receiving usual incenter hemodialysis (ICHD).[6] Nocturnal HHD (NHHD) is performed in the patient's home by the patient or with support from a family member. Most patients perform this procedure five or six nights per week for 6 to 8 hours

BOX 6.1 | Dialysis Modality and Treatment Options

INCENTER HEMODIALYSIS (ICHD)

Location	Incenter
Frequency	3 days per week
Treatment time/ session	3 to 4 hours
Total treatment time/ week	9 to 12 hours per week

HOME HEMODIALYSIS (HHD)

Location	Home
Frequency	3 to 6 days per week
Treatment time/ session	3 to 5 hours
Total treatment time/ week	15 to 30 hours per week

INCENTER NOCTURNAL HEMODIALYSIS (NHD)

Location	Incenter
Frequency	3 days per week
Treatment time/ session	8 hours
Total treatment time/ week	24 hours per week

NOCTURNAL HOME HEMODIALYSIS (NHHD)

Location	Home
Frequency	5 to 6 days per week
Treatment time/ session	6 to 8 hours
Total treatment time/ week	30 to 48 hours per week

each night. Regardless of the modality, more frequent dialysis offers a survival benefit.[2,3]

One possible reason for decreased mortality and hospitalizations is the capacity to dialyze over 7 days, avoiding a 2-day gap between dialysis treatments. The accumulation of fluid and uremic toxins followed by the rapid removal of this buildup in the first session of the week leads to this phenomenon.[8] Uremic patients can experience decreased taste acuity and anorexia, resulting in decreased energy and protein intake. In patients who are intermittently dialyzed, dietary restrictions and fluid limitations may impair oral intake due to uncertainty about what they can or cannot eat. HHD, NHD, and NHHD provide patients with two to three times more dialysis than ICHD, which significantly improves the adequacy of dialysis. With more frequent dialysis, diet and fluid limitations are minimal or unnecessary. Studies have shown that patients have more energy, increased appetite, lower blood pressure (BP), take fewer medications, and report an improvement in overall quality of life (QOL).[9-14] Although there has been a resurgence in HHD, currently only approximately 1.8% of patients receiving dialysis undergo any type of HHD.[2] While peritoneal dialysis (PD) rates have increased by nearly 2% since the initiation of the bundled payment system in 2011, there has been no significant change in HHD.[2] Due to limited unbiased education on treatment options, patients remain fearful of self-cannulation and catastrophe at home. Newly trained nephrologists may not be educated about the benefits of HHD for the patient although surveys of nephrologists indicate HHD would be their first choice for dialysis treatment.[15,16] However, on July 10, 2019, Executive Order 13879 was signed by the US President pushing for 80% of patients with incident end-stage kidney disease (ESKD) to be on home dialysis (PD or HHD) or undergo kidney transplantation by 2025. The program, Advancing American Kidney Health, includes two notable goals: a 25% reduction in Americans developing ESKD by 2030 and a twofold increase in the number of kidney transplants by 2030.[17] This regulatory adaptation will hopefully promote public awareness and education along with significantly increasing the rates of home dialysis in the next decade.

Transitional Care Unit

In February 2016, *Nephrology News and Issues* published the first US article on an innovative patient treatment and education program.[18] The Transitional Care Unit (TCU) or Transitional Dialysis Care is designed to allow incident patients receiving dialysis an educational opportunity regarding treatment options, access, insurance, and nutrition while undergoing adequate dialysis to promote patient learning and overall well-being at the start of dialysis. The typical model involves four treatments per week, ideally without two consecutive days off from kidney replacement therapy (KRT). A detailed education schedule to promote maximum learning is shown in Box 6.2. Patients often dialyze in groups, and this setting for learning and education promotes camaraderie among patients in a stress-free environment. The patient's procedure runs at lower dialysis flow rates, and less fluid is pulled with more frequent dialysis. Appetite and overall adjustment to dialysis improve significantly. Patients active in the TCU model are provided unbiased education on all treatment modalities, and the patients, along with their intradisciplinary team, discuss the best treatment option for them.[18,19] There are currently TCUs throughout the United States offered by a variety of dialysis providers.[20] Early data from the University of Virginia have shown an increase in the number of patients choosing home therapy.[21]

Dialysis Prescription

HHD is performed by the patient or with a partner during the day and NHHD is usually performed while the patient sleeps. Due to the safety record of NHD at home, some programs have not required a partner since 2017 as one machine has Food and Drug Administration approval to be utilized without a partner. Blood flow rates (BFRs) of 200 to 350 mL/h, dialysate flow rates (DFRs) of 200 to 300 mL/h, and maximum ultrafiltration of 300 to 600 mL/h offer hemodynamic stability during treatment. In comparison, most patients receiving ICHD run BFRs of 350 to 500 mL/h and

BOX 6.2 | Transitional Dialysis Care Education and Intended Outcomes

SAMPLE HIGH-LEVEL CURRICULUM[18,19]

Week 1: Assure patient/clinical stabilization

- Emotionally support patient during the transition period
- Elicit patient's fears concerning dialysis
- Talk about the cause of the patient's kidney failure
- Explain the cost of dialysis and compensation

Week 2: Present overview of kidney failure

- Provide general review of kidney replacement therapy and access options by modality
- Review quality-of-life aspects of each modality
- Review clinical outcomes specific to each modality
- Collaboratively complete a patient-centered modality selection assessment tool such as "My Life, My Dialysis Choice"

Week 3: Provide in-depth modality education

- Provide transplantation and access education
- Present detailed peritoneal dialysis (PD) and home hemodialysis (HHD) modality education by home training team
- Present incenter education by staff about transportation, schedule, and vacation travel
- Have patients undergoing incenter hemodialysis, HHD, PD, and transplantation meet with the patient to discuss their KRT choice

Week 4: Make modality choice

- Provide final review of modality and access options
- Refer patient to transplantation center of choice
- Refer to the home training unit of choice if the patient chooses a home modality
- Finalize the access plan for the patient when transitioning out of the Transitional Dialysis Care Unit

DFRs of 600 to 800 mL/h during treatment. Patients on home dialysis dialyze 3 to 6 days per week, usually 3 to 8 hours, based on their normal preferred schedule. The BFRs and DFRs can be adjusted based on individualized patient needs.[9-11] The dialysate composition used in HHD is similar to the incenter dialysate bath, except it may be a lactate-based dialysis, and calcium and po-

tassium content of the dialysate is more limited. Newer machines may have more options for dialysate composition changes. Naturalyte is a dialysis solution that can be used with a variety of machines, including the Tablo or Fresenius 2008 home machine (Table 6.1).

TABLE 6.1 | Dialysate Concentrate Composition

Dialysate solution component	NxStage NxStage Medical, Inc[a]	Tablo Outset Medical, Inc[b]	Naturalyte Fresenius Medical Care[c]
Sodium	140 mEq/L	137 mEq/L	137 mEq/L
Potassium	1-2 mEq/L	1-3 mEq/L	1-4 mEq/L
Glucose	100 mg/dL	100 mg/dL	100 mg/dL
Magnesium	1 mEq/L	0.75 mEq/L	1.0 mEq/L
Chloride	100-101 mEq/L	105.25 mEq/L	105.5 mEq/L
Calcium	3 mEq/L	2.5 mEq/L	2-3 mEq/L
Lactate	45 mEq/L		

[a] www.nxstage.com
[b] www.outsetmedical.com
[c] https://.fmcna.com

Many patients will have improved food intake and will be able to maintain phosphorus in the lower limit of a normal range with HHD. In patients that run fewer than 30 h/wk or who take off 2 days in a row, the phosphorus levels may be higher. Also, patients with advanced renal bone disease from years of CKD may run higher than normal serum levels. An increased mortality risk has been associated with higher phosphorus and calcium levels in multiple retrospective studies. In keeping with the 2017 Kidney Disease Improving Global Outcomes (KDIGO) guidelines, goal phosphorus and calcium should be within normal limits with the caveat that an uncorrected calcium >10.2 g/dL for a 3-month rolling average is a quality improvement plan (QIP) measure.[22] Calcium in this range must be monitored closely and addressed to avoid penalty in the facility's QIP score. Reduction in the facility QIP score reduces payment to facilities that do not meet or exceed certain performance standards for identified benchmarks.[23]

Machine choice is facility specific, but newer and simpler machines are being developed that are easier to learn how to use at home. As of the writing of this chapter, in the United States, there are 9,460 patients undergoing HHD or 1.8% of the 523,513 patients on dialysis.[2] To increase those percentages and promote HHD, patients need machines that they feel comfortable using.

Any patient who can do HHD can do NHHD. Although there is debate regarding selection bias for HHD, most patients require minimal education levels and physical abilities to successfully dialyze nocturnally. One of the longest-term patients undergoing NHHD in the United States has been on dialysis since 1979 and has done NHHD the last 20 years in the University of Virginia Dialysis Program. This program, which commenced in 1997, is one of the oldest NHHD programs in the country.[13]

Diet

Kidney diet recommendations for ICHD and HHD are similar and require individualization to be clinically appropriate and acceptable to follow. Limitation of a nutrient should be based on regularly monitored laboratory values, most notably for potassium, phosphorus, and protein. Amino acid losses are estimated at 5 to 20 g per ICHD treatment.[24] Some, although not all, of the amino acid abnormalities seen during dialysis treatments may be corrected in HHD due to more efficient dialysis and improved dietary intake.[13,25]

Energy and protein requirements have yet to be established in this population. Registered dietitian nutritionists (RDNs) working with all patients receiving dialysis currently prescribe 25 to 35 kcal/kg actual or adjusted body weight and 1.0 to 1.2 g protein per kg body weight in alignment with the Kidney Disease Outcomes Quality Initiative (KDOQI) guidelines for any stable patient receiving dialysis.[26] Adjustments are made for weight changes and additional protein needs. Weight gain in this population is due to improved appetite, and increased activity and regular exercise are strongly encouraged.

Fluid restriction is not necessary in the majority of patients undergoing HHD and NHHD unless their intake exceeds the maximum fluid amount that can be removed during treatment. A typical restriction is to limit fluid removal ranging from 0.4 to 0.6 kg/h or from 400 to 600 mL/h. If a patient exceeds the amount of fluid that can be removed in one treatment (which may occur after the patient's day/night off from dialysis), the next treatment will be able to remove only the allowed amount of fluid, with the rest being removed in subsequent treatments. Fluid removal is limited to promote hemodynamic stability during treatment, and goals should not be exceeded as this will negate that benefit.[9-11] The Centers for Medicare & Medicaid Services has recognized that fluid removal at a high rate (>13 mL/kg/h) in less than 4 hours increases the risk of death and is now a monitoring factor as part of the QIP program.[23] Limiting fluid loss to <10 mL/kg/h has been shown to have the greatest impact on mortality risk.[27]

Sodium restriction is guided by the patient's blood volume and hypertensive state. Patients with low BP may benefit from increased dietary sodium, but experts recommend that patients with normal BP follow a healthy dietary recommendation of less than 2,300 mg/d.[28,29]

Potassium restriction is rarely needed. In patients who skip one night per week and have documented hyperkalemia after their longest interdialytic period, potassium restriction can be recommended. Elevated midweek serum potassium levels are rare in patients who are receiving their prescribed treatment. In patients with hypokalemia, increased oral intake of potassium should be encouraged to limit associated symptoms, such as muscle cramping.[9,10] Due to increased risk of death and poor outcomes with hyperkalemia or hypokalemia, careful monitoring and limiting or increasing dietary intake is imperative.[30]

Vitamin needs are increased due to the dialysis losses of B vitamins, and renal multivitamin supplementation should be evaluated and considered for all patients to ensure adequate vitamin replacement, in addition to dietary intake. Presently, vitamin replacement is typically the same as in ICHD: one to two renal vitamins per day after dialysis.[31] Recognizing that vitamin losses in NHHD are potentially double that of ICHD due to dialyzing twice as many days per week, future research in this area may ultimately indicate a need to further supplement these patients based on their individual needs. Vitamin supplementation recommendations in patients receiving dialysis varies widely internationally. The United States supplements approximately 79% of patients while the United Kingdom supplements fewer than 4% of patients. However, the variability in diet and the antioxidant effects of vitamin supplementation can have benefits in overall patient health.[32,33]

NHHD may also improve lipid profiles in some patients. Although additional research is needed, a small study of 11 patients showed decreased triglyceride levels and increased high-density lipoprotein levels in patients undergoing NHD, possibly due to increased activity levels. Total cholesterol and low-density lipoprotein levels were unchanged. In patients with elevated lipid levels, nutrition counseling using the dietary guidelines to limit fat and cholesterol intake may be necessary (see Chapter 11).[34]

Laboratory Data

Laboratory values should be monitored regularly according to the care team or nephrologist's protocols. Desirable levels for most laboratory values are within the normal, nonrenal reference range for the laboratory processing the specimen. Standardized weekly Kt/V and urea reduction ratios (URRs) are two to three times higher than the recommended levels for ICHD. It is important to note that a single-treatment URR may be less than the 65% recommendation for ICHD due to the lower pre– and post–blood urea nitrogen (BUN) levels. Calculating a standardized weekly Kt/V is important to determine an accurate dose Kt/V for patients using their machines with any combination of treatment schedules.

For example, a patient undergoing three ICHD treatments per week for 4 hours per session has a predialysis BUN of 75 mg/dL, a postdialysis BUN of 20 mg/dL, and a URR of 73%. A patient undergoing five NHHD

7-hour treatments per week may have a predialysis BUN of 25 mg/dL and a postdialysis BUN of 9 mg/dL, producing a single-treatment URR of 64%. However, the patient undergoing NHHD 35 hours per week vs the 12 hours per week for the patient undergoing ICHD receives three times as much dialysis as the patient undergoing ICHD. Standardized weekly Kt/V provides a better indication of the patient's true dialysis adequacy vs the one-time snapshot based on a single treatment. Serum sodium, bicarbonate, potassium, calcium, phosphorus, and albumin should be within the normal, nonrenal ranges.[7-9]

For patients dialyzing fewer than 6 days per week, slight increases may be seen in laboratory results after the patient's longest interdialytic period. Although these results do not represent the patient's true steady state, patients with hyperkalemia or hyperphosphatemia levels after a skipped treatment should be instructed to limit dietary potassium or phosphorus on the days that they do not dialyze. Patients should not skip two treatments in a row (ie, run Monday through Friday and skip weekends), as this will decrease the benefits of a regular home dialysis schedule.[9,10] Most patients take off Wednesday and Saturday nights on a five-treatment-per-week schedule.

Midweek laboratory values may indicate low potassium and phosphorus levels and require dietary intervention to improve the levels of these nutrients. Supplementation of phosphorus, either orally or in the dialysate, may be necessary if levels do not improve with dietary intervention.[7-9]

Vitamin D levels, both 25-hydroxy and 1,25-dihydroxy vitamin D levels, are increased, correlating directly with the increased dialysis dose.[34] Intact parathyroid hormone (iPTH) levels are reduced, with fewer patients requiring active vitamin D therapy for parathyroid hormone (PTH) control once they are stabilized on NHHD. Patients receiving HHD and NHHD typically run on a higher-calcium bath, which contributes to the suppression of PTH levels, along with sustained phosphorus levels in the low-normal to normal range. Most patients receiving HHD have a phosphorus level well within the 2003 KDOQI bone disease guidelines, and most patients receiving NHHD have levels approaching normal, as recommended by the KDIGO guidelines.[35] Therefore, they can be treated with active vitamin D as needed without the problems associated with hyperphosphatemia. Hypercalcemia can usually be controlled with adjustments in the calcium content of the dialysate and with calcimimetics (cinacalcet or etelcalcetide) as needed.[22] Because of the higher-calcium bath, serum calcium, when measured after treatment or midday, may run higher and does not require intervention unless the patient is symptomatic or has a value of more than 10.2 g/dL. Calcimimetics can be used in this population with or without active vitamin D and with reduced risk of hypocalcemia due to the higher calcium concentration of the dialysate when used. There is currently no specific guideline for iPTH levels in this patient population, so current recommendations for conventional hemodialysis are used.[22] Trending of individual patient data with routine monitoring of calcium, phosphorus, iPTH, alkaline phosphatase, and any additional bone testing (biopsy, dual-energy x-ray absorptiometry scan, densitometry, etc) is recommended to optimize each patient's outcome.[22]

Hemoglobin levels are well maintained in this population within the KDIGO guidelines with moderate use of erythropoietin-stimulating agents (ESA) and intravenous iron replacement (see Chapter 2).[7-9]

Other Benefits

Although difficult to quantify, HHD offers a more physiologically normal removal of uremic toxins.[9-11,36] Improvements in hemodynamic stability, decreased hypertension, and fluid removal improve cardiac output. Cardiovascular disease risk is further reduced in this population via the improvement in the calcium/phosphorus balance, reduction of serum homocysteine levels, and improved lipid profiles.[36] Furthermore, the removal of middle molecules (ie, β2-microglobulin) is improved fourfold in the NHHD population, with a concurrent reduction in plasma β2-microglobulin concentrations. Accumulation and tissue deposition of β2-microglobulin

lead to amyloidosis in patients undergoing long-term ICHD. Although unproven, this study suggests a possible delay in dialysis-related amyloidosis.[37] Additional studies are needed to determine if these phenomena can be slowed or eliminated with NHHD.

Finally, cost savings for patients receiving HHD vs those undergoing ICHD were found to be 20% greater in studies in the United States and Canada.[3,8,38-40] Although the cost of consumable products is higher, cost savings are realized with decreased personnel costs. In addition, there is a cost savings to Medicare and other insurance payers and health organizations with a reduced need for BP medications, phosphate binders, active vitamin D, and ESAs in this population, along with decreases in hospital admissions and lengths of stay.[9-11] Although no firm conclusions can be established for survival, ongoing studies show a survival benefit and decreased hospitalization rate in patients receiving HHD compared to those receiving ICHD. Five-year survival of patients receiving HHD approaches 85%. In contrast, the current 5-year survival in patients undergoing PD is 44%, and in patients on ICHD, it hovers around 25%.[2,41-44] The HHD results were positive with a decrease in left ventricular mass and improvement in perceived QOL, the two primary end points of the study.[34]

Summary

HHD is a slowly growing treatment modality in the United States.[2] A search of the Home Dialysis Central website (www.homedialysis.org) provides dialysis provider listings that offer NHHD as a home treatment option. Medicare reimbursement at adequate levels to support this modality will ultimately lead to another treatment option for more patients with CKD and allow better patient care for patients with CKD receiving dialysis. The bundling of ESKD services and the 2019 Presidential Executive Order should direct more providers to consider this cost-saving option for more patients.[17] The QIP will also continue to drive improved quality goals for better patient outcomes.[23] Furthermore, the

COVID-19 pandemic of 2020 taught invaluable lessons about the opportunities all home dialysis options offer patients. With the increased use of telehealth and during a time when stay-at-home orders were in place, the high-risk patients receiving dialysis who were at home were much better positioned to stay home and avoid exposure to the virus.

References

1. Robinson B, Zhang J, Morgenstern H, et al. Worldwide, mortality risk soon after initiation of hemodialysis. *Kidney Int.* 2014;85(1):158-165. doi:10.1038/ki.2013.252

2. US Renal Data System. USRDS 2019. Accessed April 2, 2020. www.usrds.org/reference.aspx

3. Charnow J. How 'Bundling' Changed Dialysis Care. *Nephrol News Issues.* Accessed March 2017. www.renalandurologynews.com/practice-management/dialysis-bundled-payments-trends-decreased-esa-increased-peritoneal-dialysis/article/641695

4. Pauly R, Gill J, Rose C, et al. Survival among nocturnal home haemodialysis patients compared to kidney transplant recipients. *Nephrol Dial Transplant.* 2009;24(9):2915-2919. doi:10.1093/ndt/gfp295

5. Weinhandl ED, Liu J, Gilbertson DT, Arneson TJ, Collins AJ. Survival in daily home hemodialysis and matched thrice weekly in-center hemodialysis patients. *J Am Soc Nephrol.* 2012;23(5):895-904. doi:10.1681/ASN.2011080761

6. Lacson E, Xu J, Suri RS, et al. Survival with three-times weekly in-center nocturnal versus conventional hemodialysis. *J Am Soc Nephrol.* 2012;23(4):687-695. doi:10.1681/ASN.2011070674

7. Lockridge R, Kjellstrand C. Nightly home hemodialysis: outcome and factors associated with survival. *Hemodial Int.* 2011;15(2):211-218. doi:10.1111/j.1542-4758.2011.00542.x

8. Charnow J. Longer dialysis session gap raises hospitalization, death risk. *Renal and Urology News.* 2015:9.

9. Pierratos A, Ouwendyk M, Francoeur R, et al. Nocturnal hemodialysis: three-year experience. *J Am Soc Nephrol.* 1998;9(5):859-868.

10. Pierratos A, Ouwendyk M, Francoeur R. Experience with nocturnal hemodialysis. *Home Hemodial Int.* 1997;1(1):3236. doi:10.1111/hdi.1997.1.1.32

11. McPhatter LL, Lockridge RS Jr, Albert J, et al. Nightly home hemodialysis: improvement in nutrition and quality of life. *Adv Ren Replace Ther.* 1999;6(4):358-365. doi:10.1016/s1073-4449(99)70048-8

12. McPhatter L, Lockridge R. Nutritional advantages of nightly home hemodialysis. *Nephrol News Issues.* 2002;16:31-34.

13. Lockridge R, Spencer M, Craft V, et al. Nightly home hemodialysis: five and one-half years of experience in Lynchburg, VA. *Hemodial Int.* 2004;8(1):61-60. doi:10.1111/j.1492-7535.2004.00076.x

14. Prescriber's Digital Reference. Drug Information. ww.pdrnet.gov January 2019. Accessed December 2, 2020. www.pdr.net.gov

15. Lockridge R, Pipkin M. Short and long nightly hemodialysis in the United States. *Hemodial Int.* 2008;12(suppl 1):S48-S50. doi:10.1111/j.1542-4758.2008.00296.x

16. Merighi JR, Schatell DR, Bragg-Gresham JL, Witten B, Mehrotra R. Insights into nephrologist training, clinical practice, and dialysis choice. *Hemodial Int.* 2012;16(2):242-251. doi:10.1111/j.1542-4758.2011.00649.x

17. Presidential Documents. Advancing American Kidney Health. July 10, 2019. Accessed November 5, 2020. www.govinfo.gov/content/pkg/FR-2019-07-15/pdf/2019-15159.pdf

18. Lockridge R. Using a transitional start dialysis unit to improve modality selection. *Nephrol News Issues.* 2016;30(2):22-26.

19. Lockridge R Jr, Weinhandl E, Kraus M, et al. A systematic approach to promoting home hemodialysis during end stage kidney disease. *Kidney360.* 2020;1(9):993-1001. doi:10.34067/KID.0003132020

20. Morfin J, Yang A, Wang E, Schiller B. Transitional dialysis care units: a new approach to increase home dialysis modality uptake and patient outcomes. *Semin Dial.* 2018;31(1):82-87. doi:10.1111/sdi.12651

21. Bowman B, Zhent S, Yang A, et al. Improving incident ESRD care via a transitional care unit. *Am J Kidney Dis.* 2018;72(2):278-283. doi:10.1053/j.ajkd.2018.01.035

22. KDIGO 2017 Clinical Practice Guideline Update for the Diagnosis, Evaluation, Prevention and Treatment of CKD Mineral Bone Disorder. *Kidney Int Suppl.* 2017;7(1):1-59. doi:10.1016/j.kisu.2017.04.001

23. Centers for Medicare and Medicaid Services Online. ESRD Quality Incentive Program. Centers for Medicare & Medicaid website. May 2020. Accessed April 2, 2020. www.cms.gov/Medicare/Quality-Initiatives-Patient-Assessment-Instruments/ESRDQIP/index.html

24. Ikizler T, Flakoll P, Parker R, Hakim R. Amino acid and albumin losses during hemodialysis. *Kidney Int.* 1994;46(3):830-837. doi:10.1038/ki.1994.339

25. Raj DS, Ouwendyk M, Francoeur R, Pierratos A. Plasma amino acid profile on nocturnal hemodialysis. *Blood Purif.* 2000;18(2):97-102. doi:10.1159/000014431

26. National Kidney Foundation. KDOQI clinical practice guidelines for nutrition in chronic kidney disease: 2020 Update. *Am J Kidney Dis.* 2020;76(3):18-23. doi:10.1053.j.ajkd.2020.05.006

27. Assimon MM, Wenger JB, Wang L, Flyte J. Ultrafiltration rate and mortality in maintenance hemodialysis patients. *Am J Kidney Dis.* 2016;68(6):911-922. doi:10.1053/j.ajkd.2016.06.020

28. USDA Food and Nutrition Service. *2015–2020 Dietary Guidelines for Americans.* 8th ed. Home and Garden Bulletin No. 232-CP. December 2015. Accessed November 30, 2020. www.fns.usda.gov /2015-2020-dietary-guidelines-americans

29. National Kidney Foundation KDOQI Guidelines. K/ DOQI clinical practice guidelines on hypertension and antihypertensive agents in chronic kidney disease. National Kidney Foundation website. January 2004. Accessed April 2, 2020. https://.kidneyfoundation.cachefly.net /professionals/KDOQI/guidelines_bp/guide_6.htm

30. Hung A, Hakim R. Dialysate and serum potassium in hemodialysis. *Am J Kidney Dis.* 2015;66(1):125-132. doi:10.1053/j.ajkd.2015.02.322

31. Kopple J, Swenseid M. Vitamin nutrition in patients undergoing maintenance hemodialysis. *Kidney Int Suppl.* 1975;2:79-84.

32. Kosmadakis G, Da Costa Correia E, Carceles O, et al. Vitamins in dialysis: who, when and how much? *Ren Fail.* 2014;36(4):638-650. doi:10.3109/0886022X .2014.882714

33. Fissell R, Bragg-Gresham J, Gillespie B, et al. International variation in vitamin prescription and association with mortality in the Dialysis Outcomes and Practice Patterns Study (DOPPS). *Am J Kidney Dis.* 2004;44(2):293-299. doi:10.1053 /j.ajkd.2004.04.047

34. Walsh M, Culleton B, Tonnelli M, Manns B. A systemic review of the effect of nocturnal hemodialysis on blood pressure, left ventricular hypertrophy, anemia, mineral metabolism, and health-related quality of life. *Kidney Int.* 2005;67(4):1500-1508. doi:10.1111/j .1523-1755.2005.00228.x

35. Eknoyan G, Levin A, Levin NW. Bone metabolism and disease in chronic kidney disease. *Am J Kidney Dis.* 2003;42:S1-S201. doi:10.1016/S0272 -6386(03)00905-3

36. Friedman AN, Bostom AG, Levey AS, et al. Plasma total homocysteine levels among patients undergoing nocturnal versus standard hemodialysis. *J Am Soc Nephrol.* 2002;13(1):265-268.

37. Raj DS, Ouwendyk M, Francoeur R, Pierratos A. Beta 2-microglobulin kinetics in nocturnal haemodialysis. *Nephrol Dial Transplant.* 2000;15(1):58-64. doi:10 .1093/ndt/15.1.58

38. Mohr P, Neumann P, Franco S, Marainen J, Lockridge R, Ting G. The case for daily dialysis: its impact on costs and quality of life. *Am J Kidney Dis.* 2001;37(4):777-789. doi:10.1016/s0272 -6386(01)80127-x

39. McFarlane P, Pierattos A, Redelmeier D. Cost savings of home nocturnal versus conventional in-center hemodialysis. *Kidney Int.* 2002;62:2216-2222. doi:10.1046/j.1523-1755.2002.00678.x

40. Kroeker A, Clark W, Heidenheim A, et al. An operating cost comparison between conventional and home quotidian hemodialysis. *Am J Kidney Dis.* 2003;42(1 suppl):49-55. doi:10.1016/s0272 -6386(03)00538-9

41. Pierratos A. Daily nocturnal home hemodialysis. *Kidney Int.* 2004;65(5):1975-1986. doi:10.1111/j .1523-1755.2004.00603.x

42. The FHN Trial Group. In-center hemodialysis six times per week versus three times per week. *N Engl J Med.* 2010;363(24):2287-2300. doi:10.1056 /NEJMoa1001593

43. Nesrallah G, Lindsay R, Cuerden MS, et al. Intensive hemodialysis associates with improved survival compared with conventional hemodialysis. *J Am Soc Nephrol.* 2012;23(4):696-705. doi:10.1681/ASN .2011070676

44. Mathew A, McLeggon J, Mehta N, et al. Mortality and hospitalization in intensive dialysis: a systemic review and meta-analysis. *Can J Kidney Health Dis.* 2018;5:1-18. doi:10.1177/2054358117749531

CHAPTER 7

Nutrition Management of the Adult Patient on Peritoneal Dialysis

Judith Kirk, MS, RDN, CDN, CSR, FNKF, and Meredith Larsen, MS, RDN, LD, FNKF

Introduction

Home therapies for kidney replacement therapy (KRT) are being encouraged. An Executive Order passed in 2019 set a goal for having 80% of new patients with end-stage kidney disease (ESKD) either receiving dialysis at home or receiving a transplant by 2025. One of the options for home therapy is peritoneal dialysis (PD) which utilizes the body's peritoneal membrane for dialysis. As a home therapy, PD has benefits to patients as well as being a cost-effective therapy for chronic kidney disease stage 5 dialysis (CKD 5D).[1] When choosing a home therapy such as PD, it is important to consider the following:

- Patient's self-perception, involvement, autonomy, and ability
- Impact of home dialysis on family, space to store supplies, and family support
- Patient's perception of advantages and disadvantages

The advantages of PD may include improved nutrition through better preservation of residual kidney function (RKF), personal freedom, fewer diet restrictions, improved blood pressure control, and lower infection rate. Disadvantages may include fear of clinical care role, social isolation, and disruption of lifestyle at home for the patient and family. PD has often been associated with younger adults, rather than older adults; this perception is most likely due to a concern that older adults may not be able to correctly and safely manage PD at home. A study done by Lai et al[2] did not show clinically relevant barriers to using PD for older adults over the age of 65 years but did encourage maintaining careful monitoring for nutritional and metabolic parameters.

With PD, metabolic waste products, electrolytes, and water are removed through the peritoneum, a membrane-like tissue that surrounds the abdominal cavity and covers the internal organs. The use and popularity of chronic PD have waxed and waned over the years since the treatment's inception. As of 2017, the United States Renal Data System (USRDS) reported that approximately 10.4% of patients on dialysis in the United States were using PD, which reflects an 8.3% increase from 2000.[3] Approximately 11% of patients receive PD worldwide, with a dramatic difference in the use of PD among various countries. Between 1997 and 2008, the proportion of all patients on dialysis treated with PD did not change in developing countries but significantly declined by 5.3% in developed countries. The proportion of patients receiving PD on automated peritoneal dialysis (APD) has been steadily increasing. In developed countries like the United States, the percentage of patients receiving PD on APD has steadily increased by approximately 30%. The use of APD has increased by 14.5% in developing countries.[4,5]

History of Peritoneal Dialysis

According to early clinical experience with infusion and removal of a saline solution described in 1923, health care practitioners noted that after 1 hour of dwell time, the urea nitrogen concentration of the infused fluid increased to nearly the same level as the urea nitrogen concentration of blood in a guinea pig.[6,7] Over the next 50 years, numerous researchers explored the use of "peritoneal dialysis" with varying degrees of success. In the early days of PD, the ability to access the peritoneal cavity was cumbersome and prone to contamination, often resulting in peritonitis and adhesions. Indwelling catheters were abandoned for a technique that allowed the catheter to be removed after each dialysis session.[7] The repeated puncture technique was successful but very time consuming.

In the mid- to late 1960s, catheter materials were improved, and in 1968, Tenckhoff's indwelling silicone rubber catheter was widely accepted. This indwelling catheter, along with strict aseptic technique, increased the successful use of PD.[8] In 1976, Popovich, a biomedical engineer, and Moncrief, a nephrologist, announced the development of a new form of PD where ambulatory patients were continuously treated with 2 L of dialysate in the peritoneal cavity, which was exchanged four times per day. This treatment was called continuous ambulatory peritoneal dialysis (CAPD).[8] Within 2 years, CAPD fluid was available in flexible plastic bags, along with other necessary equipment and supplies that made the PD process more convenient. Today, dialysis fluid is available in different volumes to accommodate a patient's peritoneal capacity.[9]

The next major development was APD, in which a simple pump console performs all exchanges, typically while the patient sleeps. The two forms of APD currently in use are continuous cyclic peritoneal dialysis (CCPD) and tidal peritoneal dialysis (TPD) with the former being most commonly prescribed. APD offers certain benefits for some patients and reportedly has a lower incidence of peritonitis, better small solute clearances, and a reduced incidence of hernias. APD is also more suitable for patients who have a rapid rate of solute transfer across their peritoneal membrane because of the rapid, frequent exchanges with shorter dwell times (see Box 7.1).[10]

BOX 7.1 | Types of Peritoneal Dialysis[9,11,12]

Continuous ambulatory peritoneal dialysis (CAPD)

Continuous therapy, using manual exchanges. Gravity infusion of dialysate into the peritoneal cavity, allowed to dwell, and then drained. Repeated four to five times per day; typically longer dwell at night. This dwell stays in throughout the night and is drained in the morning.

Automated peritoneal dialysis (APD)
Continuous cyclic peritoneal dialysis (CCPD)

Machine-assisted, cyclic infusion of dialysate into the peritoneal cavity with shorter dwell times; usually done at night. CCPD can include daytime manual dwell(s) as needed, otherwise nighttime exchanges with a dry day, at which time neither dialysis nor ultrafiltration (fluid removal) is taking place.

Tidal peritoneal dialysis (TPD)

Machine-assisted, cyclic infusion of dialysate into the peritoneal cavity. TPD is a variant of APD that is meant to optimize solute clearance by leaving a portion of the dialysis fluid in the peritoneal cavity throughout the dialysis session. This therapy is used primarily for patients who have poor catheter function, low drain alarms, and drain discomfort. High-volume TPD can improve clearances but can be costly and inconvenient.

Doing APD overnight may offer some psychosocial and physical benefits over CAPD because of fewer connections and a dry day, which can help minimize body image issues and reduce intra-abdominal pressure and pain. For patients who can achieve adequate dialysis with a dry day, nighttime APD may make it easier to work or go to school. For patients who work a night shift, APD can be performed during the day with a dry night.

Process of Peritoneal Dialysis

PD involves the transport of solutes and fluid across the peritoneal membrane, which separates the blood in the peritoneal capillaries from the dialysis solution in the peritoneal cavity. During the time the PD solution dwells in the peritoneal cavity, three processes occur: diffusion, ultrafiltration (UF), and absorption. Uremic solutes and potassium diffuse from the blood into the dialysis solution. Glucose, lactate or bicarbonate, and some calcium diffuse in the opposite direction. Diffusion depends on the concentration gradient and molecular weight of the solute, the effective peritoneal membrane surface area, and the peritoneal membrane resistance. The following factors influence solute diffusion:

- peritoneal membrane surface area and dwell time
- peritoneal membrane permeability
- concentration gradient
- temperature of dialysis solution
- blood flow—patient vascular system
- dialysis solution volume in 24 hours

UF depends on the concentration gradient for the osmotic agent (dextrose, icodextrin, or amino acids), the peritoneal membrane surface area and characteristics, the ability of the osmotic agent to maintain the gradient, hydrostatic and oncotic pressure gradients, and sieving. Sieving occurs when a solute is carried along with water across the membrane by convection. Fluid absorption occurs through the lymphatics at a relatively constant rate and counteracts both solute and fluid removal to a small degree.[9,13,14] The following factors influence UF:

- peritoneal membrane surface area
- peritoneal membrane permeability
- pressure gradients—glucose creates a colloidal osmotic gradient between blood and the PD solution, removing water from the blood

Patients are taught to use a sterile technique to perform the connection and disconnection to the indwelling catheter during an exchange. After instilling fluid and allowing it to dwell in the peritoneal cavity, the fluid is drained to either the original bag or an empty drain bag. A new bag is connected and fresh PD fluid is instilled. Several aids have been developed to minimize breaches in sterility, including complex tubing sets that allow a "flush before fill" process. All drained PD fluids, with metabolic waste and extra water, are discarded.[9,13,14] With cycler machines, a drain is performed at the start of therapy as a safety measure to avoid overfill (see Figure 7.1).

FIGURE 7.1 | Peritoneal dialysis

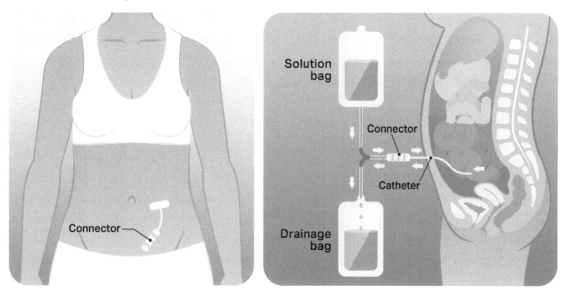

With CAPD, a sterile hypertonic solution of dextrose and electrolytes is instilled via gravity flow into the peritoneal cavity through an indwelling catheter. Each CAPD exchange requires a connection to instill and drain.[9,13,14] This process is typically repeated four times per day. The dialysate partially equilibrates with the solutes in the plasma by shifting body solutes into the dialysate. At the same time, plasma water is removed by UF as a result of the osmotic gradient created by the dialysate. The dialysate is drained after 4 to 5 hours (except at night, when the dwell is lengthened to 9 to 11 hours to accommodate sleep), and the process is repeated. This process of instilling and draining the dialysate is called an exchange. An exchange usually takes 20 to 30 minutes and is performed by patients at home or work after 1 to 2 weeks of training.

With APD, there are fewer connections. The patient uses a machine to instill fluid, and cycles of dialysate are achieved without disconnecting for each of the exchanges. Essentially, the patient connects before going to sleep, and typically if their prescription requires a daytime dwell, the cycler machines can be programmed for a last fill before they disconnect. There are several line connections on the cycler machine, so the mixing of dialysate needed for the cycles can be programmed and tailored to meet the patient's individual needs for each night. Some patients, especially those with significant RKF, can skip the last fill and allow the peritoneum to be dry during the day.

Access to the peritoneum is typically via a permanent, double-cuff Tenckhoff or alternative design catheter, which is a length of silicone tubing with side holes at the internal end, a mesh flange at the skin line, and connector fittings on the exposed end.[11] The catheter is inserted via a simple surgical procedure and allowed to heal for 1 to 2 weeks prior to use. In certain circumstances, urgent PD can be initiated sooner with medical supervision.[9,13-15] Sterile PD fluid is provided in various-sized bags, depending on the manufacturer, the solution chosen, and the method of PD being employed.[15] The traditional PD fluid consists of potassium-free lactated Ringer's solution with the pH reduced to approximately 5.5 to prevent caramelization during heat sterilization.

Newer solutions are bicarbonate or bicarbonate–lactate mixtures, which have a more normal pH and are reported to minimize discomfort on infusion. While bicarbonate solutions are theoretically more biocompatible, the long-term benefit to patient outcomes is still being determined.[9,13,14] The 15 to 42.5 g of glucose monohydrate (sometimes labeled as "dextrose monohydrate") acts as the osmotic agent in typical PD fluids, although other osmotic agents are available. Osmotic agents used in PD fluids include glucose monohydrate (1.5%, 2.5%, and 4.25%) commonly used in the US population, anhydrous glucose (1.36%, 2.27%, and 3.86%) more routinely used outside the United States, amino acids (1% to 2%), and icodextrin (7.5%). Table 7.1 provides a quick estimate of dextrose contained in PD fluid per volume.

TABLE 7.1 | Peritoneal Dialysis Fluids Quick Estimate[16,17]

Solution concentration, %	Grams monohydrous dextrose per				
	1 L	1.5 L	2 L	2.5 L	3 L
1.5	15.0	22.5	30.0	37.5	45.0
2.5	25.0	37.5	50.0	62.5	75.0
4.25	42.5	63.8	85.0	106.3	127.5

Peritoneal Membrane

The peritoneal membrane has the primary physiological function of lining the walls of the abdominal cavity and encapsulating the internal organs (eg, stomach, liver, spleen, pancreas, and parts of the intestines). The adult peritoneal surface area is approximately 1.75 ± 0.5 m^2 and is estimated to be equal to an individual's skin surface area.[9,13,14] The peritoneum has three physical characteristics: a visceral portion that covers the internal organs (approximately 80%), a parietal portion that overlays the abdominal walls, and a folded mesentery that connects the two. The top layer that is exposed to dialysate during PD is composed of a single layer of mesothelial cells. Next is a thick layer of interstitium that is perfused with a network of capillaries through which the blood flows to portal and systemic venous circulations.[9,13,14] Clinical observations indicate that there are three pore sizes in the peritoneal capillaries. Large pores allow macromolecules (eg, protein) to be transported by convection. Small pores are responsible for transport of small solutes like urea, creatinine, sodium, and potassium, along with water. Ultrapores are responsible for transporting fluid only and for the sieving of solutes along with water across the semipermeable membrane.[9,13,14] Characteristics of the peritoneal membrane transport affect dry weight in the first year; changes are greater in non–fast transporters.

Removal of Solutes and Fluid

The rate at which solutes are removed during PD depends primarily on the rate of equilibration between the dialysate and the blood. This is described graphically as "D over P curves," or the ratio of dialysate to plasma concentration as a function of dwell time. Smaller solutes equilibrate more quickly than large ones because the diffusion coefficient varies inversely to the square root of a solute's molecular weight. Small solutes such as urea equilibrate almost completely. Equilibration rates vary considerably from patient to patient. The characteristics of the peritoneal membrane are distinguished by the peritoneal equilibration test (PET). The PET measures equilibrium of solutes between dialysis and plasma, absorption of dextrose from the peritoneal cavity, and UF at 4 hours. Patients are classified as high transporters, low transporters, high-average transporters, or low-average transporters (see Box 7.2).[9,13,14] Knowledge of a patient's membrane category can assist in ensuring that a patient receives adequate treatments by predicting clearance and UF response to the prescription. While membrane characteristics should be considered, it is possible to manage patients carefully and allow them to use the therapy that best fits their lifestyle.

BOX 7.2 | Peritoneal Membrane Classifications[9,13,14]

HIGH	**Predicted solute clearance**	Rapid
	Predicted ultrafiltration (fluid removal)	Poor
	At risk for albumin loss	High
	Preferred dialysis regimen	Nocturnal intermittent peritoneal dialysis (cycler night + dry day)
		Continuous cyclic peritoneal dialysis (CCPD) (cycler night and avoid long day dwells with dextrose)
HIGH-AVERAGE	**Predicted solute clearance**	Good
	Predicted ultrafiltration (fluid removal)	Good
	At risk for albumin loss	High-average
	Preferred dialysis regimen	CCPD or continuous ambulatory peritoneal dialysis (CAPD) standard dose peritoneal dialysis (PD)
LOW-AVERAGE	**Predicted solute clearance**	Adequate/slower
	Predicted ultrafiltration (fluid removal)	Good
	At risk for albumin loss	Low-average
	Preferred dialysis regimen	CCPD or CAPD standard dose PD
LOW	**Predicted solute clearance**	Slow/inadequate
	Predicted ultrafiltration (fluid removal)	Excellent
	At risk for albumin loss	Low
	Preferred dialysis regimen	CAPD or high-dose PD
		Avoid short dwells

Peritoneal membrane transport testing should be repeated when clinically indicated. Some clinical indications for repeat PET testing are as follows: unexplained volume overload, decreasing drain volume, increasing clinical need for hypertonic dialysate dwells to maintain drain volume, worsening of hypertension (HTN), change in measured peritoneal solute removal (Kt/V urea), and unexplained signs or symptoms of uremia.[11]

Adequacy of Dialysis

The peritoneal clearance of solutes is measured to ensure the patient's individualized dialysis prescription is adequate. It represents the net result of diffusion plus UF minus lymphatic absorption. It can be calculated as quantity of solute removed over a period of time divided by the plasma concentration.[9,13,14] Clearance is highest at the start of a PD dwell when both the blood urea concentration and the PD fluid glucose osmotic gradients are high. Clearances can be increased by maximizing the total daily time on treatment (fewer or no dry periods), maximizing the effective peritoneal membrane surface area with larger dwell volumes, and maximizing UF with higher glucose concentrations or other osmotic agents.[9,13,14] Adequacy of dialysis should be measured on a regular basis, and treatment should be adjusted when measures of adequacy drop below the recommended targets (see Box 7.3). A common standard is to check for adequacy of dialysis quarterly and repeat, as needed, whenever adequacy drops below target range or the effectiveness of a prescription change needs to be assessed.

BOX 7.3 | Peritoneal Dialysis Adequacy Targets[16]

Experts recommended that peritoneal dialysis (PD) Kt/V (effluent and urine) be measured within 1 month of treatment initiation and at least every 4 months thereafter. Quarterly measurements may be more easily scheduled and tracked.

Continuous ambulatory peritoneal dialysis (CAPD)

Target   Weekly Kt/V ≥1.7[a]

This approach requires 24-hour dialysate collection. The urea content of effluent (drained dialysate after an exchange) is divided by the average plasma urea during the same 24-hour period to calculate the peritoneal clearance of urea. Concomitant plasma sampling for CAPD is not critical since urea is relatively constant.

Residual kidney Kt (K is clearance of solute and t is time) is calculated for the same time period. Peritoneal and residual urine urea clearances are added to determine a total Kt.

If the patient is anuric, an aliquot sample is used from the dialysate drain jug after it is agitated to avoid solute precipitating out of solution.

The total Kt is normalized to the patient's estimated body water (V) for a total daily Kt/V and then multiplied by 7 to obtain the weekly Kt/V. Note: Normalization to ideal body weight is standard for some of the computer calculations of Kt/V. Clinical judgment of physical signs and symptoms of uremia should be considered along with the calculated dialysis Kt/V in patients who are underweight or obese.

Automated peritoneal dialysis (APD)

Target   Weekly Kt/V ≥1.7[a]

The same approach is applied, except that the blood urea nitrogen (BUN) is variable. An average BUN is best estimated from a sample between 1 PM and 5 PM on a noncycling day although this is not often possible as many patients on peritoneal dialysis will receive daily dialysis.

Target   Creatinine clearance

A similar calculation is performed but using effluent and blood creatinine levels. This calculation is no longer considered necessary to measure adequacy.

---

[a] If the individual has more than 100 mL/d of residual urine volume and residual clearance is being considered as part of the total weekly urea clearance goal, a 24-hour urine collection for urine V and urea clearance should be obtained at least every 2 months.

Various interventions, as shown in Box 7.4, may be undertaken to improve and maintain adequacy, depending on the type of PD being used and the characteristics of the peritoneal membrane.[9,13,14] The Kidney Disease Outcomes Quality Initiative (KDOQI) has published clinical practice guidelines for PD adequacy. These guidelines are summarized in Box 7.5.[18] Calculations of Kt/V and the normalized protein equivalent of nitrogen appearance (nPNA) in PD are now almost always calculated using computer programs.[19]

BOX 7.4 | Achieving Peritoneal Dialysis Adequacy Targets[9,13,14]

Continuous ambulatory peritoneal dialysis (CAPD)	
Ways to improve Kt/V	Increase exchange volume. A 25% increase in fill volume will typically increase Kt/V by 18% to 20%. May increase patient's sense of fullness or cause back pain, abdominal distention, and has the potential for leaks or a hernia.
	Increase frequency or number of exchanges. Exchanges need to be well spaced to best maintain urea equilibration. Added exchanges will decrease dwell time and can decrease creatinine clearance. Increased frequency of exchanges may interfere with the patient's lifestyle and add to the cost of therapy.
	Increase osmotic pressure of dialysate. This strategy increases both clearance and ultrafiltration, but additional dextrose load can lead to or aggravate obesity, hypertriglyceridemia, may worsen diabetic control, and over time may also damage the peritoneal membrane.
Automated peritoneal dialysis (APD)	
Ways to improve Kt/V	Add a daytime dwell to improve both urea and creatinine clearance. Long daytime dwell may cause net fluid resorption. Multiple, short daytime dwells would help prevent fluid resorption.
	Increase dwell volumes on the cycler. This is usually tolerated since the patient is supine while dialyzing.
	Increase time on cycler. This increases clearance but is limited by the time the patient is willing to spend on the cycler.
	Increase frequency of cycles to maximize the concentration gradient. Need to balance benefit of increased frequency with lost dialysis time during cycling.
	Increase osmotic strength of dialysate. Same benefits and potential problems as in continuous ambulatory peritoneal dialysis.

BOX 7.5 | Summary of Kidney Disease Outcomes Quality Initiative (KDOQI) Peritoneal Dialysis Adequacy Guidelines[16]

The standard target is to initiate dialysis incrementally to maintain a total Kt/V of at least 1.7 and normalized protein nitrogen appearance (nPNA) of at least 0.8 g/kg.

Peritoneal dialysis (PD) adequacy testing should be performed within 1 month and at least one additional time between months 2 and 6 (depending on consistency from initial results), and then every 4 months; quarterly is standard.

Nutritional status of patients on PD should be assessed at least every 4 months using subjective global assessment, and protein nitrogen appearance or nPNA.

Identifying and correcting patient or staff errors are important for meeting the minimum targets (ie, body size and severe malnutrition).

Regular measurements of clinical outcomes should be performed (eg, patient survival, technique survival, hospitalization rates, patient-based quality of life, albumin, hemoglobin/hematocrit, and nPNA).

The following are indications for PD: patient preference, medical complications, and no assistant for home hemodialysis (HD).

The following are contraindications for PD: loss of peritoneal function, inability to perform and no assistant, and mechanical defects/leaks.

The following are potential contraindications for PD: diverticular/bowel disease, severe malnutrition, and body size.

Reasons to consider changing to HD include the following: consistent adequacy failure, unmanageable hypertriglyceridemia, recurrent peritonitis/complications, technical/mechanical problems, and severe malnutrition.

Nutrition Assessment

Nutrition was identified as a critical part of successful PD therapy early after its inception.[7,9] Nutrition assessment methods for PD are similar to those for any patient with chronic kidney disease (CKD). There is no single measure that consistently and accurately assesses nutritional status. Assessment techniques are reviewed thoroughly in Chapter 2, but for PD they may include assessment of appetite, history of dietary intake, body weight and body mass index (BMI), biochemical data, anthropometric measurements, and nutrition focused physical findings.[20,21] Subjective global assessment (SGA) is an independent predictor of all-cause mortality in the patient population with CKD undergoing dialysis, and the 7-point SGA is recommended as a valid and reliable tool for assessing nutritional status in adults with CKD stage 5D.[18,22,23]

Peritoneal protein losses and calorie load from dialysis fluids add to the complexity in determining oral nutrient needs for individuals receiving PD.[24] Furthermore, the incidence of protein–energy malnutrition (PEM) and protein energy wasting (PEW) is significant in patients receiving PD and requires provision of adequate calories and protein without creating other nutrient imbalances. Transporter status may play a role as well in a patient's ability to clear waste products and, thus, may have an impact on nutritional status.[9,13,14] Nutrition recommendations should be made in close collaboration with the physician or other provider (nurse practitioner or physician assistant) with the goal of optimizing nutritional status. Practitioners should pay attention to assessing energy needs and addressing malnutrition, inflammation, appetite, vitamins/minerals, as well as the importance of mineral and bone management.[25,26]

In the assessment of protein nutrition, mortality risk increased in patients with CKD stage 5D, low serum albumin, and high C-reactive protein (CRP) but not with low serum albumin and normal CRP.[25] The inflammatory status of the patient should be considered when using serum albumin for nutrition risk assessment. Another indicator, the normalized protein catabolic rate (nPCR), reflects daily protein intake in stable patients receiving dialysis. There are inconsistent reports in patients receiving PD; however, a study showed that lower nPCR is associated with poorer nutritional status and increased risk of all-cause mortality in patients receiving PD who were monitored for 11 years.[19]

Nutrient Recommendations

Nutrient requirements for individuals on PD are somewhat different than for those receiving hemodialysis (HD), although the nutrients that are tracked and potentially modified are the same. PD nutrient recommendations remain heavily influenced by landmark balance studies from the early 1980s. The studies were conducted in eight clinically stable men undergoing CAPD. Nitrogen, potassium, magnesium, phosphorus, and calcium balances were measured to determine dietary protein requirements and mineral balances.[27] Macronutrient recommendations have been defined by the KDOQI Clinical Practice Guidelines for Nutrition in CKD: 2020 Update.[18] The KDOQI nutrition guidelines recommend prescribing an energy intake of 25 to 35 kcal/kg body weight per day based on age, gender, level of physical activity, body composition, weight status goals, and concurrent illness or presence of inflammation to maintain normal nutritional status. Appropriate nutrient modifications are then made, depending on the response of the individual patient.

Nephrology registered dietitian nutritionists (RDNs) avail themselves of varied, ongoing, and progressive nutrition interventions to help patients undergoing PD meet nutrient needs.[22,25,28] In the United States, most patients receiving PD are seen at least monthly with a review of laboratory results and nutrition education. Additional dietary intervention is by clinical judgment for a face-to-face or telehealth meeting. Discussion of goals related to dietary modification or weight management may be reviewed, particularly when preparing a patient receiving PD for transplant listing. Newer studies have shown a positive relationship regarding the role of dietary intervention and nutrition counseling with respect to outcomes.[29]

PROTEIN

Many early studies of protein losses during PD have provided the basis for protein intake recommendations. A balance study by Blumenkrantz et al[30] used two levels of protein intake—1.44 g/kg and 0.98 g/kg—supported by high-energy diets. This group found that nitrogen balance was strongly positive on the higher protein intake and neutral on the lower protein intake. Numerous other studies confirm a relationship between dietary protein intake and protein-related nutritional parameters, such as albumin, total body protein, and nitrogen balance.[18,24,30,31] The current recommendation for patients who are metabolically stable is for 1.0 to 1.2 g/kg body weight. Dietary protein intakes (DPIs) of 1.2 g/kg/d or more are almost always associated with neutral or positive nitrogen balance.[18] While metabolically stable patients on PD are able to maintain adequate protein stores with slightly lower intakes, a DPI of 1.2 to 1.3 g/kg/d is likely to provide insurance for maintaining good protein nutrition and replacing the losses of albumin and amino acids in the majority of patients undergoing PD.[19,32] For patients at risk of hyperglycemia and hypoglycemia, higher levels of dietary protein may need to be considered to maintain glycemic control.[9,13,14,24] Muscle wasting, decreased serum proteins, increased susceptibility to infection, and delayed wound healing are associated with insufficient DPI.[9,13,14,25,28]

Protein losses through the peritoneal membrane can vary by tenfold among patients; however, they are fairly consistent in an individual patient.[9,13,14] The most rapid loss of protein is in the initial 2 hours of an exchange and during the first exchanges of the day, but long dwell exchanges also have significant protein losses.[9,13,14,33] Of the 5 to 15 g protein lost in a day, 50% to 80% is albumin.[9,13,14] Protein losses are affected by the size and molecular weight of the protein, the composition of the dialysate, the permeability of the peritoneal membrane, the frequency and the duration of dialysis, body surface area, and the patient's characteristics (eg, clinical status and serum protein levels, specifically albumin). Protein losses have been reported to be higher in patients with

diabetes mellitus (DM) and patients with acute peritonitis.[33-35] In addition to whole protein losses, amino acids are lost during the dialysis process. The amount of amino acids lost during PD approximate the amount removed during HD.[9,13,14]

More recent studies carried out by Westra et al[24] measured 24-hour protein losses to dialysate in stable patients on APD. This group found average protein losses were 10 ± 0.6 g/d, similar to losses published in previous CAPD balance studies. Furthermore, 24-hour protein losses were higher with increased numbers of exchanges and longer dwell times. Nearly two-thirds of the protein losses on APD were during nighttime cycling, primarily because of the large volume of dialysate that is exchanged. Dialysate protein and amino acid losses were equivalent to approximately 15% of dietary nitrogen intake. This study confirmed the increased dietary protein requirements of patients undergoing PD.

Despite education and encouragement, some patients on PD are unable to eat adequate protein with conventional foods.[32] Nutritional supplements, enteral feedings, or special protein-containing dialysate may be utilized to enhance nutrient intake, especially of protein.[9,13,14,18] See Box 7.6 on page 96 for suggested nutrition interventions based on a patient's nPNA. nPNA is sometimes used interchangeably with nPCR. While it does not provide insight into visceral or somatic growth to assess change in lean body mass, it is an effective indicator to assess DPI in stable patients receiving dialysis.[18,19]

ENERGY

Energy levels are prescribed to allow the patient receiving PD to achieve and maintain a reasonable body weight and are calculated based on age, gender, activity levels, body composition, weight status goals, and concurrent illness. Adequate energy intake is critical for the efficient utilization of dietary protein. Total calorie recommendations are 25 to 35 kcal/kg body weight per day. Body weight, whether ideal, actual, or standard, can be determined by the clinical judgment of an RDN. The total energy should include kilocalories that are absorbed from peritoneal fluids.[18,36] As part of the nutrition

BOX 7.6 | Suggested Nutrition Intervention Based on Normalized Protein Equivalent of Nitrogen Appearance[a]

Normalized protein equivalent of nitrogen appearance (nPNA) is calculated from measures of urea in blood and dialysate. In stable patients, the nPNA should reflect the intake of protein in g/kg. It is important to validate nPNA with reported intake, protein stores, and nutritional status. Anabolism or catabolism will cause nPNA to be different from reported intake as described here.

nPNA	POSSIBLE SIGNIFICANCE	NUTRITIONAL INTERVENTION
>1.5	Excessive protein intake, excessive low biological value protein or catabolism	Assess dietary intake; consider reducing protein intake if excessive and patient is well nourished. **Note:** In a catabolic state (weight loss/decreased protein status), nPNA will be higher than expected and higher than actual intake.
1.2 to 1.3	Ideal; includes added measure of safety beyond usual needs	Encourage patient to continue current intake if protein status/weight are acceptable and stable.
1.1 to 1.2	Marginal; some patients may maintain nutritional status at this level but not most	Evaluate agreement of nPNA and reported intake; counsel patient to increase protein consumption as appropriate for findings.
<1.1	Potentially inadequate protein intake, especially in unstable patients or patients with increased needs Increased risk for morbidity and mortality	Assess dietary intake; counsel patient to increase protein/calorie intake as appropriate. If the patient is unable to increase intake of conventional foods, advise oral nutrition supplement. **Note:** In an anabolic state (weight increase/improved protein status), nPNA may be lower than expected and lower than actual protein intake.
<0.8	Inadequate in nearly all patients	Same as above but strongly consider adding an oral nutrition supplement as tolerated; encourage increased intake of conventional foods and easy-to-eat proteins.
<0.6	Very unlikely to sustain acceptable nutritional status	Increasingly aggressive and progressive nutrition support as accepted by the patient, including enteral feeding, intraperitoneal nutrition, and total parenteral nutrition.

[a] Routinely assess adequacy; inadequate dialysis may hinder patient's ability to eat the recommended amounts of nutrients, especially protein. Consider increasing the adequacy level in any patient who has an unexplained decrease in appetite and signs of malnutrition.

assessment, clinicians must approximate the calories absorbed from the PD dialysate either by a simple estimate based upon dextrose concentrations, volume and estimated absorption rate (see Box 7.7), use of one of several predictive equations or a direct measure of dextrose concentration change from infused PD fluid and that of drained PD fluid (see Box 7.8).[16,33] Dextrose is the most common osmotic agent in PD solutions. In North America, these solutions are labeled as containing 1.5%, 2.5%, and 4.25% dextrose (monohydrate glucose). Multiply the grams monohydrate glucose concentration by 3.4 to estimate kilocalories. The true anhydrous glucose concentrations (1.36%, 2.27%, and 3.86%) are listed on PD solutions in Europe. Multiply the grams anhydrous glucose by 3.7 to estimate calories.

Patients receiving PD can absorb as much as 20% to 30% of their daily needs from the dialysis fluids, depending on the dextrose concentration, membrane characteristics, and volume and frequency of exchanges.[16,17] Despite this calorie load, many patients undergoing PD do not reach the recommended calorie levels. Fewer calories are absorbed with short, more frequent exchanges, such as the exchanges performed in APD, where the contact between blood and dialysis fluid is minimized and the osmotic gradient is preserved. Osmotic agents such as icodextrin (a high-molecular-weight, starch-derived glucose polymer) or amino acids have the ability to maintain the osmotic gradient and help minimize the calorie load.[36,37] Burkart[21] measured calories absorbed in CAPD and APD with various dextrose levels and ico-

BOX 7.7 | Simple Estimate of Calories Absorbed From Dialysate[16,17]

The following values are only a rough estimate of calories as this calculation does not consider peritoneal membrane characteristics or dwell time.

DEXTROSE, %	DEXTROSE, g/L	g × 3.4 = kcal AVAILABLE	CAPD kcal ABSORBED (60%-70% ABSORBED)	APD kcal ABSORBED (40%-50% ABSORBED)
1.5	15	51	31-36 kcal/L	20-26 kcal/L
2.5	25	85	51-60 kcal/L	34-43 kcal/L
4.25	42.5	145	87-102 kcal/L	58-73 kcal/L

CAPD = continuous ambulatory peritoneal dialysis; APD = automated peritoneal dialysis

Estimated kcal absorbed = Dialysate volume in L × g dextrose/L × 3.4 kcal/g × % absorption where absorption is calculated at 40% to 50% with APD and 60% to 70% with CAPD

Continuous ambulatory peritoneal disease example:

Regimen: three 2-L exchanges of 1.5% dextrose and one 2-L exchange of 2.5% dextrose

6 L of 1.5% dextrose = 6 L x 15 g dextrose/L

= 90 g dextrose x 3.4 kcal/g

= 306 kcal x 0.6 absorption

= 184 kcal absorbed

2L of 2.5% dextrose = 2 L x 25 g dextrose/L

= 50 g dextrose x 3.4 kcal/g

= 170 kcal x 0.6 absorption

= 102 kcal absorbed

Total calories absorbed for 24 hours = 184 kcal + 102 kcal

= 286 kcal

BOX 7.8 | Suggested Formulas to Estimate Caloric Absorption From Peritoneal Dialysis Solutions[16,17]

Grodstein formula
Note: Does not consider peritoneal membrane transport characteristics. Cannot be used for automated peritoneal dialysis.

Glucose absorbed = $(11.3x - 10.9) \times$ Total L of dialysate

where x = average glucose concentration infused

Example: Patient is receiving 4 L of 1.5% dextrose and 4 L of 2.5% dextrose solution.

Average glucose concentration = Dextrose solution/Total liters

= (4 × 1.5) + (4 × 2.5)/8

= (6 + 10)/8

= 2

Glucose absorbed = [(11.3 × 2) − 10.9] × 8

= (22.6 − 10.9) × 8

= 11.7 × 8

= 93.6 g

Calorie contribution = 93.6 g × 3.4 kcal/g

= 318 kcal

Continued on next page

Continued from previous page

D/D₀ formula
Note: Considers modality and membrane transport characteristics

Glucose absorbed = (1 – D/D0)xi

where D/D_0 is the fraction of glucose remaining and xi is the initial glucose infused (total g of dextrose).

Example: D/D_0 from peritoneal equilibration test (PET) curve is 0.4
Initial glucose infused from 4 L of 1.5% dextrose and 4 L of 2.5% dextrose.

Initial glucose infused = (4 x 15 g) + (4 x 25 g)
= 60 g + 100 g
= 160 g

Glucose absorbed = (1 – 0.4) x 160 g
= 96 g

Calorie contribution = 96 g x 3.4 kcal/g
= 326 kcal

Direct measure
If the D/D_0 PET curve is not available, then directly measure the glucose absorbed using glucose in the 24-hour spent dialysate. Formula requires volume of exchange and glucose in 24-hour spent dialysate.

Glucose absorbed = glucose infused – glucose remaining

Example: Instilled 4 L of 4.25% of dextrose and 4 L of 1.5% dextrose
24-hour dialysate volume = 11,000 mL (11 L)
Glucose level in 24-hour dialysate collection (from laboratory)[a] = 1,281 mg/dL (12.81 g/L)

Glucose infused = (4 x 42.5 g) + (4 x 15 g)
= 170 g + 60 g
= 230 g

Glucose remaining = glucose in dialysate collection × volume
= 12.81 g/L × 11 L
= 140.9 g

Glucose absorbed = 230 g – 140.9 g
= 89.1 g

Calorie contribution = 89.1 g x 3.4 kcal/g
= 303 kcal

[a] To convert mg/dL to g/L: mg/dL × 1 g/1,000 mg × 10 dL/1 L = g/L

---

dextrin. His estimation of calories absorbed from peritoneal fluids is similar to that reported in other studies and shows that icodextrin exchanges decrease the calorie load as only approximately 25% or the carbohydrate (approximately 150 calories) is absorbed during an 8 hour dwell compared to much higher percentages of carbohydrate being absorbed from dextrose based fluids.

The disadvantages of glucose as an osmotic agent include absorption of calories, potential for anorexia, rapid loss of UF capabilities, and metabolic abnormalities, such as hyperglycemia, hyperinsulinemia, hyperlipidemia, and obesity.[33,38,39] A balance of oral and dialysate calories is needed to prevent undesired weight gain. While calorie absorption from PD fluids can be estimated, it is important for practitioners to monitor patients for weight changes and metabolic abnormalities. In addition to adjusting the oral calorie intake, changes in the dialysis prescription and even the osmotic agent may be required.[33,38]

SODIUM

Sodium balance and blood pressure control are important to the success of PD. Early reports of good sodium removal on CAPD led to liberalized dietary sodium recommendations.[7,39,40] Over time, experts have recognized that many patients receiving CAPD have subclinical volume expansion that can be associated with HTN, cardiovascular abnormalities, and poor survival.[41,42] Although opinions differ, excessive dietary sodium likely contributes to HTN and volume overload, especially once RKF is lost.[39]

Sodium removal in PD depends mainly on convection and diffusion, although diffusion is limited because of the small concentration gradient between the PD fluid (132 mEq/L) and the plasma concentration (140 mEq/L).[9,13,14] Sodium clearance is higher in CAPD than in APD. The two main determinants of sodium removal are UF and the mode of PD. Limiting dietary sodium can help control thirst and minimize the frequency with which hypertonic exchanges must be used to maintain fluid balance. The KDOQI recommendations are to limit sodium intake to less than 2,300 mg/d to help with volume control and HTN.[18] Obviously, the balance between salt restriction and the patient's ability to ingest and enjoy foods is important, so dietary modification must be individualized.

Volume control is also enhanced with dialysate solutions that use an alternative osmotic agent. Icodextrin offers the potential for more UF than 1.5% or 2.5% dextrose solutions during long dwell dialysis exchanges. Icodextrin is also effective in restoring UF in patients who lose their UF capability with dextrose.[36] Commercial solutions with amino acids that serve as an effective nonglucose osmotic agent and as a source of protein are available outside the United States. In the United States, amino acid-containing solutions are available only in individually compounded solutions used for treating inadequate protein intake.

FLUIDS

Fluid balance in patients receiving PD should be maintained primarily through modification of dietary sodium intake. Patients on PD are taught to vary the concentration of dialysate based on the fluctuations in their weight and volume status. While varying the dextrose concentrations of the dialysate allows removal of excess fluid, consistent, long-term use of hypertonic solutions can be detrimental to the peritoneal membrane. Modifying dietary sodium and fluid intake can help maintain fluid balance, allow achievement of dry weight (ie, edema-free body weight), and minimize the use of hypertonic exchanges. Fluid allowance is dependent on PD UF and residual urine output.[43] Fluid intake of 1 to 3 L/d is commonly considered, depending on urine output, UF capacity, cardiac status, and blood pressure. The goal is to maintain fluid balance and minimize hypertonic exchanges. Ongoing monitoring is recommended.

POTASSIUM

PD clears potassium at a rate similar to urea. With 10 L of ultrafiltrate, approximately 1,400 to 1,800 mg/d is cleared.[9,13,14] Most patients tolerate a normal daily potassium intake of 3 to 4 g, similar to what might be found in a general diet that does not contain excessive amounts of dairy products, fruits, and vegetables. Current KDOQI recommendations suggest adjusting dietary potassium intake to maintain serum potassium within the normal range. In the classic balance studies, Kopple and Blumenkrantz[44] estimated dietary potassium intake from 2,500 to 3,200 mg/d based on the protein intake and serum levels that were well within the normal range. They also found that fecal excretion of potassium was significantly increased to as much as 800 mg/d in patients undergoing CAPD, making hyperkalemia uncommon. In cases of hyperkalemia, potassium binders may be an option. To address either hyperkalemia or hypokalemia, clinical judgment should be used for patients who may need dietary adjustments to lower potassium levels or potassium supplementation if they are unable to increase dietary intake enough to correct low serum levels.[18,45]

Hypokalemia can result from different causes, including abnormal cellular redistribution after inadequate dietary intake, excessive restriction, or disproportionate dialysis clearance. Blood potassium levels may also be depleted with prolonged gastrointestinal (GI) losses (eg, diarrhea, vomiting, or gastric suction) and with certain diuretics. Diabetic acidosis, which draws potassium into the intracellular fluid, may also result in hypokalemia.

CALCIUM

Current recommendations suggest adjusting calcium intake (including dietary calcium, calcium supplements, and calcium-based binders) with consideration of concurrent use of vitamin D analog and calcimimetic medications in order to avoid hypercalcemia. Calcium removal by PD depends on the calcium content of the PD fluids and the patient's serum levels.[18] Current recommendations are to limit the total elemental calcium to avoid hypercalcemia, with no more than 1,500 mg from calcium-based phosphate binders.[18] This recommendation is based on the increased soft tissue calcification in patients with CKD, which may contribute to the higher incidence of cardiovascular disease (CVD) in patients with CKD. Although the full mechanisms of soft tissue calcification are still being investigated, it seems prudent to avoid excessive calcium loads above the daily recommended intake. Studies recommended that serum calcium be maintained in the low-normal range for the laboratory being used or as close to normal as possible.[9,13,14,18]

PHOSPHORUS

Observational studies have shown that high serum phosphorus is associated with the potential for increased cardiovascular events and higher mortality rates. Clearance of phosphorus by APD/CAPD is about 300 mg/d with four 2-L exchanges.[13,14,16] Most patients will require phosphate binders and dietary modification of phosphorus. The United States commentary regarding the Kidney Disease Improving Global Outcomes (KDIGO) Clinical Practice Guidelines for Bone Metabolism and Disease recommends adjusting dietary phosphorus intake to maintain serum phosphorus in the normal range.[18,46] Limiting dietary phosphorus is difficult to accomplish, considering the increased protein levels needed with APD/CAPD because high-protein foods are also high in phosphorus. Kopple and Blumenkrantz[44] showed an average dietary phosphate intake of 1 to 1.9 g/d with their low- and high-protein diets. Dietary phosphorus intake should be limited but individualized to the patient's needs.

In addition to the phosphorus that is naturally found in food, there are more than 60 phosphate-containing food additives. Foods containing phosphate additives can increase total phosphorus intake by up to twofold. Phosphorus from additives is nearly entirely absorbed, whereas only approximately 60% of naturally occurring phosphorus is absorbed.[47] The inadvertent consumption of phosphate additives hinders attempts to reduce dietary phosphorus intake, particularly in patients who rely heavily on processed foods. Incorporating plant-based proteins may help to reduce phosphorus intake because the phosphorus absorption from these foods is less.

In addition to dietary phosphorus limits, phosphate binders are employed to help control serum phosphorus levels. Available binders and their uses are detailed in Chapter 10. In general, serum phosphorus levels should be kept as close to normal as possible.[18,46]

CHOLESTEROL AND TRIGLYCERIDES

Lipid abnormalities are common in patients receiving PD, particularly low levels of high-density lipoproteins (HDL), elevated very low-density lipoproteins, and elevated triglyceride levels.[48] The pathogenesis of this lipid profile is not fully understood, but both peritoneal protein loss and glucose absorption may contribute.[49] The relationship between low serum cholesterol and mortality risk found in patients receiving HD is not observed in patients undergoing PD, possibly due to the high-energy intake and hypertriglyceridemia that are common in PD. Higher cholesterol levels—greater than 250 mg/dL—are also associated with increased mortality risk in patients undergoing PD.[13,14,18] Dietary modifications in patients on PD have minimal effect on lipid profiles; however, patients receiving PD should be educated on minimizing intakes of simple carbohydrates, saturated fats, and cholesterol. It is reasonable to not routinely prescribe long-chain n-3 polyunsaturated fatty acids (PUFA), including those derived from fish or flaxseed and other oils, to lower the mortality risk or incidence of cardiovascular events. However, it is reasonable to consider prescribing 1.3 to 4 g/d long-chain n-3 PUFA to improve the lipid profile. Priority should be given to meeting protein requirements, with guidance on how to minimize saturated fat. Often, the protein-rich foods that are higher in cholesterol or saturated fats (eg, eggs and cheese) are most desirable to patients.[10] Alternative osmotic agents can reduce the glucose load, but long-term effects on lipid profiles have been mixed.[13,14,18]

VITAMINS AND MINERALS

Vitamin and mineral recommendations for patients on PD are similar to those for patients on HD. Water-soluble vitamins are lost to the peritoneal dialysate and must be replaced. In addition, vitamin deficiencies can occur with poor intake, interference of absorption by multiple medications, and altered metabolism.[18,50-52] Nutritional vitamin D and active vitamin D analogs are prescribed based on the needs of the patient and in response to surrogate markers of bone and mineral health, such as serum calcium, phosphorus, alkaline phosphatase, and parathyroid hormone (PTH) (see Chapter 10). A summary of nutrient recommendations is provided in Box 7.9.[18,46]

FIBER

The pressure of PD fluids on the intestinal tract can make bowel regularity challenging. Fluid limitations and some medications, such as oral iron, can also cause or exacerbate constipation. Constipation is often cited as

---

BOX 7.9 | Recommended Nutrient Intakes for Individuals Treated With Peritoneal Dialysis[18,46]

Nutrient recommendations vary slightly depending on the source of information, but the general levels here provide a starting point for nutrient prescription. As a patient adjusts to the dialysis regimen and stabilizes on peritoneal dialysis (PD), patient-specific modifications should be made in response to changes in body weight or composition, protein stores, and other metabolic or clinical indicators.

NUTRIENT	RECOMMENDATIONS
Protein (g/kg)	1.2 to 1.3 g/kg body weight
	1.0 to 1.2 g/kg body weight in patients who are metabolically stable
Calories (kcal/kg)	25 to 35 kcal/kg body weight in patients who are metabolically stable
	Clinical judgment by the registered dietitian nutritionist or international equivalent to maintain normal nutrition
	Dialysate calories are included in the total daily recommendation
Sodium	2,300 mg/d; maintain fluid balance, minimize hypertonic exchanges
Potassium	2 to 4 mg/d; individualize for maintenance of serum levels within normal range
Calcium	Adjustment of calcium intake to avoid hypercalcemia or calcium overload (includes dietary calcium, calcium supplements, calcium-based binders)
	Consideration of concurrent use of vitamin D analogs and calcimimetics
Phosphorus	Adjustment of dietary intake to maintain serum phosphorus level in normal range
	Addition of plant-based proteins and avoidance of processed foods (ie, phosphorus additives) to minimize dietary phosphorus load
Fluids	1 to 3 L/d or depending on urine output, ultrafiltration capability, cardiac status, and blood pressure; maintain fluid balance; minimize hypertonic exchanges
Vitamins	Monitoring for clinical signs/symptoms of deficiency
Pyridoxine	10 mg/d or as needed to correct for deficiency/insufficiency
Ascorbic acid	90 mg/d for males, 75 mg/d for females
Thiamine	1 to 5 mg/d or as needed to correct for deficiency/insufficiency
Folic acid	1 to 10 mg/d or as needed to correct for deficiency/insufficiency
Vitamin A	Not routinely needed

Continued on next page

Continued from previous page

NUTRIENT	RECOMMENDATIONS
Vitamin E	Not routinely needed
Vitamin K	Avoidance in patients receiving anticoagulant medicines known to inhibit vitamin K activity (ie, warfarin compounds)
Minerals	
Iron	Supplementation often required in patients on PD, generally given by IV because oral iron may contribute to constipation and is not well absorbed
Selenium	Not routinely supplemented
Zinc	Not routinely supplemented
1,25-dihydroxyvitamin D/analogs	Individualized administration to maintain normal bone turnover and avoidance of secondary hyperparathyroidism
Vitamin D2 or D3	Insufficient knowledge of absolute needs, but nutritional supplements are likely to be beneficial, especially if blood levels are less than 30 mg/dL

the most common reason for poor PD drainage and—in extreme conditions—may create risk for fecal peritonitis. Ikizler et al[18] recommended that patients undergoing PD ingest at least 20 to 25 g fiber per day. Research suggests that a diet higher in fiber reduces all-cause mortality risk. In a study by Xu et al,[20] higher fiber intake correlated to 13% reduction in all-cause mortality risk and appeared to have a protective effect for patients without DM undergoing PD. While PD allows a more liberal intake of fruits and vegetables than HD, it may still be difficult to achieve this goal without fiber supplements.

Special Considerations for Chronic Peritoneal Dialysis

OBESITY

Obesity is an important consideration for patients on PD. Although obesity presents challenges, barriers can be overcome; this should not exclude a patient from trialing PD.[53] To be successful, the focus of care needs to be addressed via an interdisciplinary approach, which includes the patient, physician, RDN, nurse, and social worker.

Weight management and adherence to diet are key factors to consider. Concerns include weight gain from dialysate fluid (refer to Box 7.7) and ability to achieve and maintain adequacy of dialysis (Kt/V >1.7 mini-

mum). Weight changes in patients receiving PD can be influenced by dextrose absorption from the dialysate.[54] High fluid gains lead to selection of higher dextrose solutions and further weight gain.

Increases in BMI in patients on PD may be associated with fluid overload as well. Both a high BMI and high waist circumference have been independently associated with an increased mortality rate.[55,56] Although paradoxically, a BMI identified as overweight may be protective and may be a factor for a reduced mortality risk. Generally, extremes of high and low weight present the greatest risk for mortality.

Fluid management and adequacy of dialysis are critical. As the standard dialysate fluid available in the United States is dextrose based, weight gain can be minimized with the use of fewer hypertonic exchanges. An alternative to dextrose, icodextrin, is a polymer-based option that does not contribute to the caloric load like the standard dextrose containing dialysis fluid. This choice is prescribed for patients with obesity as well as DM for caloric and glycemic controls. Although it reduces dextrose load, the icodextrin infusion requires a longer dwell time, typically 5- to 10-hour dwells, and daytime dwells for patients on APD. As dwell time progresses, fluid is collected in the peritoneum, which can contribute to abdominal distention and GI symptoms such as bloating and decreased appetite. In addition to GI symptoms, shortness of breath is reported by patients. Another concern of icodextrin can be an allergic reaction. If symptoms of an allergic reaction occur (often severe rash), icodextrin should be discontinued immediately. In some cases, a second trial of icodextrin at a later date may be a consideration for a patient with obesity or DM.

A patient with obesity and PD can do well with weight management, fluid management, and ability to meet adequacy of dialysis.[57-59] However, when these factors are not effectively achieved, a change to HD or home HD is pursued.

DIABETES MELLITUS

PD is considered to be a good method of KRT in patients with DM because of a steadier biochemical state, fluid balance, lack of vascular compromise, absence of heparin therapy, and the simplicity of the technique for patients with vision or sensory limitations. When compared to HD, some research suggests that PD offers an equal or lower risk of death across all subgroups, including people with DM, in the first 1 to 2 years of dialysis.[13,14,60,61] The improved outcomes are thought to result from a lower prevalence of infections and congestive heart failure and better preservation of RKF.

PD requires close monitoring of blood glucose levels and the potential increased use of insulin or other glucose-lowering agents.[62] When the glucose in the PD fluid diffuses into the circulation, it exacerbates poor glycemic control and increases the risk of vascular complications. Nutrient modification, minimizing the use of hypertonic exchanges, and weight control remain the primary PD management methods for individuals with DM. Subcutaneous administration of insulin is acceptable in patients receiving PD. Intraperitoneal (IP) administration of insulin is no longer a practice in patients on PD due to the inability to quickly adjust the insulin dose.

Patients receiving PD are affected by dextrose load and can "burn out" their peritoneal membrane. A sustained use of hypertonic solutions can have a detrimental effect on the peritoneal membrane. The prolonged exposure of the membrane to high glucose concentrations can diminish the effectiveness of the membrane to clear toxins and can potentially produce membrane failure in a patient requiring a need to convert to HD or home HD. Membrane failure can occur in any patient on PD, but there is more risk and prevalence for the patient with DM and obesity. Fluid management is a primary goal for avoiding hypertonic solutions and minimizing the risk for membrane failure.

Patients on PD, particularly those with DM, are likely to benefit from the use of modern PD solutions that contain the glucose polymer, icodextrin, or amino acids as the osmotic agent, instead of glucose. These non-glucose PD fluids may help improve glycemic control for individuals with DM. It is important to note that icodextrin increases blood maltose levels and may cause a falsely high glucose reading if the correct glucometer is not used for glucose monitoring. See Chapter 9 for additional information in this regard.

GASTROINTESTINAL CONCERNS

GI symptoms are common for patients undergoing PD.[63,64] Symptoms often include, but are not limited to, loss of appetite, feeling of fullness or bloating, nausea, and constipation. GI symptoms are often less prevalent during overnight therapy when the patient is horizontal and sleeping. This gives the patient the daytime hours to be "dry" (no dialysis fluid in their peritoneum) and, thus, meals are generally better tolerated. For patients who need dialysis fluid in their peritoneum during the day (daytime dwells), GI symptoms may be more frequent. These symptoms can be reduced by planning meals after a PD dwell is drained or before a PD exchange fill is performed. This can create challenges for patients with regard to quality of life (QOL) and burden of PD on patient, family, and caregivers.

GI symptoms are also associated with medications. Phosphate binders can have significant GI side effects related to nausea and constipation. Sometimes, patients will reduce their binder use due to these side effects with resulting hyperphosphatemia. Assessing phosphate binder utilization and tolerance is important on an ongoing basis. Calcimimetics are another class of medications that can have an effect on the GI tract. Adjustments in medications relating to calcium, phosphorus, and PTH balance is an ongoing challenge. For patients on PD, anemia is an ongoing concern. Iron infusions are administered regularly for anemia management. Oral iron can be a cause of constipation for many patients, so intravenous (IV) iron infusion is the intervention of choice. Some patients cannot tolerate IV iron infusions, in which case oral iron is administered. Attention to bowel function is important and should be reviewed with patients monthly. Constipation can adversely affect the effectiveness of PD and requires close monitoring.

There is accumulating evidence that dialysis results in a number of unique factors that can alter both the microbiota and the integrity of the intestinal barrier. This results in increases of circulatory toxic metabolites, endotoxin, indoxyl-sulfate and p-cresyl-sulfate, and is associated with systemic inflammation, CVD risk, and mortality. To date, there have been several systematic reviews and meta-analyses that have investigated the effects of prebiotics, probiotics, and symbiotic interventions on circulating toxic metabolites and inflammation in the population receiving dialysis, including patients on PD. Supplementation was found to reduce these circulatory toxic metabolites and had a favorable effect on GI symptoms. Limitations of the reviews and meta-analysis included a high bias risk and a lack of documentation regarding side effects. Further high-quality trials would be appropriate to define the role of prebiotics, probiotics, and symbiotic therapy.

MALNUTRITION

One of the most important factors affecting the QOL of patients with CKD is nutrition.[14,29,39,65] Prevention of malnutrition increases the patient's QOL and life span. The goal is for early diagnosis and treatment for at-risk patients.

For a variety of reasons, a significant number of patients receiving PD are malnourished.[57] Studies vary in their comparison of rates of malnutrition between HD and PD because of differing definitions of malnutrition and variety in patient populations. A complex of malnutrition inflammation, PEM, and PEW is common in individuals with CKD.

An increased incidence of malnutrition in PD is correlated with lower RKF, older age, and DM.[2,29,39,57] Underweight status based on BMI can be used as a predictor of higher mortality. There are several causes of PEM and PEW in individuals with CKD. Causes specific to PD include increased protein losses and anorectic factors (eg, abdominal discomfort due to dialysate volume), absorption of glucose from dialysate, inadequate dialysis, and increased circulating anorexigens (eg, cholecystokinin, leptin, glucagon, tumor necrosis factor, glucose-dependent insulinotropic peptide, and other cytokines).[13,14]

Several confounding factors make identification of malnutrition more challenging in patients receiving PD. Albumin is the primary protein lost to dialysate, and albumin is abnormally distributed between the extravascular and intravascular spaces. Increased plasma volume and PD fluid loads can lead to dilutional alterations. Albumin, as an acute-phase reactant, is also negatively affected by inflammation and infection. Serum albumin, while not a clinically useful measure of protein energy status for patients on dialysis, may be used as a predictor of hospitalization and mortality with lower levels associated with higher risk. The ability to use weight change as a sign of malnutrition is limited because many patients on PD have body composition changes without actual body weight changes. Patients receiving PD may waste muscle stores and yet maintain weight with increased body fat. Females and persons with DM are prone to increased body fat when undergoing PD.[60-62] Monthly weight tracking and addressing nutrition utilizing a 7-point SGA or malnutrition–inflammation score tool are recommended. Food records, 24-hour recalls, food frequency, nPCR, and nondietary factors (eg, medication use, access to food, depression, cognitive function, and social/cultural) should also be considered as methods for assessing dietary intake.[18]

Appetite is a key indicator to track for nutrition; a decreased appetite is a symptom often found in patients with CKD.[66] A disruption in appetite should be assessed and addressed as soon as possible to prevent a decline in nutritional status. Appetite is an important marker preceding nutrition decline. A poor appetite can lead to decreased intake and eventually increase PEW. Nutrition counseling regarding appetite has been found to be effective in stabilizing nutrition. The Appetite and Food Satisfaction Questionnaire, developed by Melo et al,[25] is a valid, easy-to-use tool that is applied as an initial screening to identify patients on PD with potential risk of malnutrition. Several considerations regarding the role of appetite include the following:

- altered metabolism—comorbidities, age
- psychosocial factors—anxiety, lack of support system
- inflammation cytokines—potential suppression of appetite
- mobility difficulty—impact on food procurement and preparation, whereby a study showed 64% patients with mobility problems had low albumin levels[67]
- income—reliance on a fixed income (not just low income) shown as a predictor for inadequate protein, poor appetite, and malnutrition
- anorexia—cause for infection, peritonitis, inadequate dialysis resulting in uremia, comorbid conditions, effects of dialysate solutions resulting in increased glucose absorption, higher blood glucose levels, and increased insulin response

The treatment of malnutrition in patients receiving PD is complex. Methods include traditional progressive interventions such as increased counseling and education regarding needs, oral nutrition supplements, appetite stimulants, enteral feeding, intraperitoneal nutrition (IPN), and parenteral nutrition (PN). With the burden of dialysis treatments, some patients and clinicians are reluctant to add the burden of aggressive nutrition support, but it is critical to reduce morbidity and mortality.

While increased calorie and protein intake may be encouraged for malnourished patients, many find this difficult.[13,14,18] Consumption of nutritional supplements may be limited by the same lack of appetite and inability to increase intake. Appetite stimulants have been used to treat undernutrition with some success. Megestrol acetate has been shown to improve nutritional status by increasing appetite and intake when given at about half the conventional dose. However, side effects of megestrol acetate such as diarrhea, confusion, hyperglycemia, and increased fat mass have been reported.[68,69]

Tube feeding is commonly employed in pediatric patients receiving PD. Tube feeding is possible in adult patients on PD, but reports of its use are few. PN may be considered for use in patients with PD, but the burden of the combined therapies would probably limit the duration of use.

Of the more aggressive support methods, IPN is the least burdensome because it is incorporated as part of the dialysis process.[18,70] Outside the United States, commercial, shelf-stable amino acid solutions are available for use as a supplemental protein source, with 22 g protein per 2-L exchange of 1.1% amino acids. In the United States, various home care companies will qualify patients and provide IPN with compounded solutions that include amino acids with varying levels of dextrose to supplement oral intake. The results of research with IPN have been varied, but logically, solutions that can help replace protein and amino acid losses in patients on PD should benefit individuals who have low nutritional intake and become malnourished.[13,14,18] IPN has the potential for increasing lean body mass and handgrip strength and improving protein synthesis.

Malnutrition in patients on PD is much more complicated than simple inadequate nutrient intake. All available progressive interventions should be considered to treat malnutrition, but their application depends on the willingness, ability, and specific needs of each patient.

PERITONITIS

Peritonitis remains a serious complication in patients on PD and can lead to death. In the majority of cases, peritonitis is due to either contamination during the PD exchange or an exit site infection. For the most part, peritonitis is effectively treated with IP antibiotics. Although the incidence of peritonitis has declined substantially with new connection systems and techniques, it still has the potential to exacerbate poor nutritional status due to added protein losses. Protein losses are reported to increase by 50% more than normal during peritonitis. Poor nutritional status may increase the risk for developing peritonitis, and peritonitis may hinder protein and energy intake.[62,71] Peritonitis and malnutrition are interrelated because poor nutritional status may increase the risk for development of peritonitis, which increases protein losses and hinders UF. Practitioners should pay special attention to nutrition support during episodes of peritonitis;

BOX 7.10 | Common Side Effects of Peritoneal Dialysis and Potential Interventions

ISSUES	INTERVENTIONS
Weight gain, hypertriglyceridemia, hyperglycemia	Increase exercise as tolerated and allowed by physician. Limit sodium and fluid to minimize hypertonic exchanges. Use solutions with alternate, non-glucose osmotic agents. Modify energy intake to facilitate weight maintenance/loss. Modify intake of sugars and fats, especially saturated fats.
Protein losses, malnutrition, wasting	Educate/continually follow-up regarding protein goals and ways to meet those goals. Eat protein foods first and limit fluids at mealtime. Eat frequent, smaller portions of protein and easy-to-eat proteins, such as eggs, yogurt, and cottage cheese. Strive to build up protein intake slowly to reach optimal amount. Educate/follow-up on sterile technique to avoid peritonitis. Use nutrient-tailored supplements. Use amino acid peritoneal dialysis (PD) fluids if available; refer for supplemental intraperitoneal nutrition if the nutrient intake is inadequate with conventional foods. Use renal-specific water-soluble vitamin daily/nutritional vitamin D. Identify, avoid, or treat sources of inflammation.
Fullness, abnormal gastrointestinal (GI) function, constipation, satiety	Eat frequent, smaller meals. Limit fluid intake with meals but allow adequate total fluids. Eat while draining or when the peritoneum is empty. Increase dietary fiber to avoid constipation. Limit use of hypertonic exchanges. Use more frequent, smaller-volume exchanges. Treat gastroparesis with appropriate medications.
Hypokalemia, potassium depletion	Increase intake of higher potassium fruits and vegetables. Supplement potassium if serum levels are significantly low and/or the patient is unable to adequately increase dietary intake.
Hyperkalemia	Limit ingestion of high potassium foods. Maintain normal bowel function. Evaluate for signs of gastrointestinal bleeding and hyperglycemia. Ensure adequate dialysis.
Hypotension or hypotensive symptoms	Adjust the PD fluids for less ultrafiltration. Consult with physician regarding antihypertensive medications. Adjust salt and fluid intake if over restricted.
Hypertension	Reduce sodium and fluid intake. Perform dialysis exchanges as prescribed. Evaluate antihypertensive medications.
Ultrafiltration loss	Maintain strict adherence to sterile procedure and avoidance of peritonitis. Limit the use of hypertonic exchanges. Moderate intake of sodium and water. Use alternative osmotic agents (icodextrin or amino acids). Use more biocompatible solutions.

the maintenance of good nutritional status may help patients on PD avoid or minimize the risk of this type of infection.[12,13,17] See Box 7.10 for common side effects related to PD and potential interventions.

Summary

Nutrition is a critical part of successful PD treatment. The differences in nutrient requirements for CAPD vs those for APD are thought to be minimal. The balance of nutrients must consider protein needs, protein losses, and energy sources, including those from PD fluids. The recognition of the potential for chronic volume overload as well as the possible negative impacts of frequent hypertonic exchanges are consistent with the recommendation for a moderate sodium restriction for those on PD, even with the availability of non-glucose dialysis fluids.

Patients receiving PD are likely to benefit from diet modification to reduce cardiovascular and bone and mineral abnormalities. Currently, studies are being assessed for the efficacy of prebiotic, probiotic, and synbiotic supplementation in modulating gut-derived circulatory particles associated with CVD.[72] The continuous nature of PD allows somewhat more freedom in dietary choices, especially in relation to potassium. All dietary modification must start with the goals of maintaining good nutritional status and meeting nutrient needs, especially in malnourished patients. Individualized meal patterns and a variety of food choices are essential for optimizing nutritional status, ease of adherence, and QOL. The nutrition plan should restrict nutrients no more than absolutely necessary and may need continual adjustment over the course of the patient's life while on dialysis. Modifications should be made for changes in nutritional status, comorbid conditions, mode of therapy, acute illness, and psychosocial state.

The type of PD therapy should consider the individual patient and lifestyle; a structured education intervention could help patient choice. An interdisciplinary team approach is a must with the patient, RDN, physician, nurse, and social worker all working together. Telemonitoring systems for nutritional intake tracking for patients on PD are now being developed and may play a role in future considerations for home dialysis therapies like PD.[73]

References

1. Chang Y, Hwang J, Hung S, et al. Cost-effectiveness of hemodialysis and peritoneal dialysis: a national cohort study with 14 years follow-up and matched for comorbidities and propensity score. *Sci Rep.* 2016;6:30266. doi:10.1038/srep30266

2. Lai S, Amabile MI, Bargagli MB, et al. Peritoneal dialysis in older adults: evaluation of clinical, nutritional, metabolic outcomes, and quality of life. *Medicine (Baltimore).* 2018;97(35):e11953. doi:10.1097/MD.00000000000119531

3. USRDS 2019 Annual Data Report: Atlas of End-Stage Renal Disease in the United States, National Institutes of Health, National Institute of Diabetes and Digestive and Kidney Diseases, Bethesda, MD. US Renal Data System website. 2019. Accessed September 2020. www.usrds.org/annual-data-report

4. Oreopoulos DG, Ossaeh S, Thodis E. Peritoneal dialysis: past, present, and future. *Iran J Kidney Dis.* 2008;2(4):171-182.

5. Jain AK, Blake P, Cordy P, Garg AX. Global trends in rates of peritoneal dialysis. *J Am Soc Nephrol.* 2012;23(3):533-544. doi:10.1681/ASN.2011060607

6. Twardowski ZJ. History of peritoneal access development. *Int J Artif Organs.* 2006;29(1):2-40. doi:10.1177/039139880602900102

7. Gokal R. History of peritoneal dialysis. In: Gokal R, Khanna R, Krediet RT, Nolph KD, eds. *Textbook of Peritoneal Dialysis.* Springer; 2000:1-17.

8. Popovich RP, Moncrief JW, Decherd JF, Bomar JB, Pyle WK. The definition of a novel portable/wearable equilibrium peritoneal dialysis technique (abstract). *ASAIO Trans.* 1976;5:64.

9. Daugirdas JT, Blake PG, Ing TS. *Handbook of Dialysis.* 5th ed. Lippincot Williams & Wilkins; 2014.

10. Boen ST. History of Peritoneal Dialysis. In: Nolph KD, ed. *Peritoneal Dialysis.* Klower Academic Publishers; 1989:1-12.

11. Lysaght MJ, Moran J. Peritoneal dialysis equipment. In: Bronzino JD, ed. *Tissue Engineering and Artificial Organs*. 3rd ed. Taylor & Francis Group, CRC Press; 2006:68-1–68-13.

12. Blumenkrantz MJ, Kopple JD, Moran JK, Coburn JW. Metabolic balance studies and dietary protein requirements in patients undergoing continuous ambulatory peritoneal dialysis. *Kidney Int.* 1982;21(6):849-861. doi:10.1038/ki.1982.109

13. Kopple J, Massry S, Kalantar-Zadeh K, Fouque D (eds). *Nutritional Management of Renal Disease*. 4th ed. Academic Press; 2021.

14. Mitch W, Ikizler TA (eds). *Handbook of Nutrition and Kidney Disease*. 7th ed. Lippincott Williams & Wilkins; 2017.

15. Hernández-Castillo JL, Balderas-Juárez J, Jiménez-Zarazúa O, et al. Factors associated with urgent-start peritoneal dialysis catheter complications in ESRD. *Kidney Int Rep.* 2020;5(10):1722-1728. doi:10.1016/j.ekir.2020.07.025

16. McCann L (ed). *Pocket Guide to Nutrition Assessment of the Patient with Kidney Disease*. 6th ed. National Kidney Foundation, Inc; 2021.

17. Podel J, Hodelin-Wetzel R, Saha DC, Burns G. Glucose absorption in acute peritoneal dialysis. *J Ren Nutr.* 2000;10(2):93-97. doi:10.1016/s1051-2276(00)90006-2

18. Ikizler TA, Burrowes JD, Byham-Gray LD, et al. KDOQI Nutrition in CKD Guideline Workgroup. KDOQI clinical practice guideline for nutrition in CKD: 2020 update. *Am J Kidney Dis.* 2020;76(3)(suppl 1):S1-S107. doi:10.1053/j.ajkd.2020.05.006

19. Fein PA, Weiss S, Avram MM, et al. Relationship of normalized protein catabolic rate with nutrition status and long-term survival in peritoneal dialysis patients. *Adv Perit Dial.* 2015;31:45-48.

20. Xu X, Li Z, Chen Y, Liu X, Dong J. Dietary fibre and mortality risk in patients on peritoneal dialysis. *Br J Nutr.* 2019;122(9):996-1005. doi:10.1017/S0007114519001764

21. Burkart J. Metabolic consequences of peritoneal dialysis. *Semin Dial.* 2004;17(6):498-504. doi:10.1111/j.0894-0959.2004.17610

22. Dai L, Mukai H, Lindholm B, et al. Clinical global assessment of nutritional status as predictor of mortality in chronic kidney disease patients. *PLoS One.* 2017;12(12):e0186659. doi:10.1371/journal.pone.0186659

23. Vogt BP, Borges MCC, de Goes CR, Caramori JCT. Handgrip strength is an independent predictor of all-cause mortality in maintenance dialysis patients. *Clin Nutr.* 2016;34(6):1429-1433. doi:10.1016/j.clnu.2016.03.020

24. Westra WM, Kopple JD, Krediet RT, Appell M, Mehrotra R. Dietary protein requirements and dialysate protein losses in chronic peritoneal dialysis patients. *Perit Dial Int.* 2007;27(2):192-195.

25. Melo TL, Meireles MS, Kamimura MA, Cuppari L. Concurrent validity of an appetite questionnaire in peritoneal dialysis. *Perit Dial Int.* 2020;40(1):41. doi:10.1177/0896860819879878

26. Alves FC, Sun J, Qureshi AR, et al. The higher mortality associated with low serum albumin is dependent on systemic inflammation in end-stage kidney disease. *PLoS One.* 2018;13(1):e0190410. doi:10.1371/journal.pone.0190410

27. Kopple JD, Blumenkrantz MJ. Nutritional requirements for patients undergoing continuous ambulatory peritoneal dialysis. *Kidney Int Suppl.* 1983;16:S295-S302.

28. Musso CG, Jauregui JR, Macias Nunez JF. Frailty phenotype and chronic kidney disease: a review of the literature. *Int Urol Nephrol.* 2015;47(11):1801-1807. doi:10.1007/s11255-015-1112-z

29. Gunalay S, Ozturk YK, Akar H, Mergen H. The relationship between malnutrition and quality of life in haemodialysis and peritoneal dialysis patients. *Revista da Associacao Medica Brasileria.* 2018;64(9):845-852. doi:10.1590/1806-9282.64.09.845

30. Blumenkrantz MJ, Kopple JD, Moran JK, Coburn JW. Metabolic balance studies and dietary protein requirements in patients undergoing continuous ambulatory peritoneal dialysis. *Kidney Int.* 1982;21(6):849-861. doi:10.1038/ki.1982.109

31. Bergstrom J, Furst P, Alvestrand A, Lindholm B. Protein and energy intake, nitrogen balance and nitrogen losses in patients treated with continuous ambulatory peritoneal dialysis. *Kidney Int.* 1993;44(5):1048-1057. doi:10.1038/ki.1993.347

32. Sutton D, Higgins B, Stevens JM. Continuous ambulatory peritoneal dialysis patients are unable to increase dietary intake to recommended levels. *J Ren Nutr.* 2007;17(5):329-335. doi:10.1053/j.jrn.2007.02.003

33. Caron-Lienert RS, Poli-de-Figueiredo CE, Prado Lima Figueiredo AE, et al. The influence of glucose exposure load and peritoneal membrane transport on body composition and nutritional status changes after 1 year on peritoneal dialysis. *Perit Dial Int.* 2017;37(4);458-463. doi:10.3747/pdi.2016.00265

34. Prasad N, Gupta A, Sharma RK, Sinha A, Kumar R. Impact of nutritional status on peritonitis in CAPD patients. *Perit Dial Int.* 2007;27(1):42-47. doi:10.1177/089686080702700110

35. Whaley-Connell A, Pavey BS, Satalowich R, et al. Rates of continuous ambulatory peritoneal dialysis-associated peritonitis at the University of Missouri. *Adv Perit Dial.* 2005;21:72-75.

36. Chen CH, Perl J, Teitelbaum I. Prescribing high-quality peritoneal dialysis: the role of preserving residual kidney function. *Perit Dial Int.* 2020;40(3):274-281. doi:10.1177/0896860819893821

37. Rodriquez-Carmona A, Fontan MP, Lopez EG, Falcon TG, Cambre HD. Use of icodextrin during nocturnal peritoneal dialysis allows sustained ultrafiltration while reducing the peritoneal glucose load: a randomized crossover study. *Perit Dial Int.* 2007;27(3):260-266.

38. Bodnar DM, Busch S, Fuchs J, Piedmonte M, Schrieber M. Estimating glucose absorption in peritoneal dialysis using peritoneal equilibration tests. *Adv Perit Dial.* 1993;9:114-118.

39. Avram MM, Mittman N, Fein PA, et al. Dialysis vintage, body composition, and survival in peritoneal dialysis patients. *Adv Perit Dial.* 2012;28:144-147.

40. Fine A, Fontaine B, Ma M. Commonly prescribed salt intake in continuous ambulatory peritoneal dialysis patients is too restrictive: results of a double-blind crossover study. *J Am Soc Nephrol.* 1997;8(8):1311-1314.

41. Khandelwal M, Kothari J, Krishnan M, et al. Volume expansion and sodium balance in peritoneal dialysis patients. Part I: Recent concepts in pathogenesis. *Adv Perit Dial.* 2003;19:36-43.

42. Khandelwal M, Kothari J, Krishnan M, et al. Volume expansion and sodium balance in peritoneal dialysis patients. Part II: Newer insights in management. *Adv Perit Dial.* 2003;19:44-52.

43. Tzamaloukos A, Raj D, Onime A, Servilla KS. The prescription of peritoneal dialysis. *Semin Dial.* 2008;21(3):250-257. doi:10.1111/j.1525-139X.2007.00412.x

44. Kopple JD, Blumenkrantz MJ. Nutritional requirements for patients undergoing continuous ambulatory peritoneal dialysis. *Kidney Int Suppl.* 1983;16:S295-S302.

45. Factor KF. Potassium management in pediatric peritoneal dialysis patients: can a diet with increased potassium maintain normal serum potassium without a potassium supplement? *Adv Perit Dial.* 2007;23:167-169.

46. Isakova T, Nickolas TL, Denburg M, et al. KDOQI US commentary on the 2017 KDIGO clinical practice guideline update for diagnosis, evaluation, prevention, and treatment of chronic kidney disease-mineral and bone disorder (CKD-MBD). *Am J Kidney Dis.* 2017;70(6):737-751. doi:10.1053/j.ajkd.2017.07.019

47. Sarathy S, Sullivan C, Leon JB, Sehgal AR. Fast food, phosphorus-containing additives and the renal diet. *J Ren Nutr.* 2008;18(5):466-470. doi:10.1053/j.jrn.2008.05.007

48. Heimburger O, Stenvinkel P, Berglund L, Tranoeus A, Lindholm B. Increased plasma lipoprotein(a) in continuous ambulatory peritoneal dialysis is related to peritoneal transport proteins and glucose. *Nephron.* 1997;76(2):239-241. doi:10.1159/000188831

49. Kanbay M, Baybek N, Delibasi T, et al. Effect of peritoneal dialysis solution type on serum lipid levels in end-stage renal disease. *Ren Fail.* 2007;29(3):309-313. doi:10.1080/08860220601166545

50. Blumberg A, Hanck A, Sander G. Vitamin nutrition in patients on continuous ambulatory peritoneal dialysis (CAPD). *Clin Nephrol.* 1983;20(5):244-250.

51. Boeschoten EW, Shriiver J, Krediet RT, Schreurs WH, Arisz L. Deficiencies of vitamins in CAPD patients: the effects of supplementation. *Nephrol Dial Transplant.* 1988;3(2):187-193.

52. Alhosaini M, Leehey DJ. Magnesium and dialysis: the neglected cation. *Am J Kidney Dis.* 2015;66(3):523-531. doi:10.1053/j.ajkd.2015.01.029

53. Lee MB, Bargman JM. Myths in peritoneal dialysis. *Curr Opin Nephrol Hypertens.* 2016;25(6):602-608. doi:10.1097/MNH.0000000000000274

54. Lo WK. Metabolic syndrome and obesity in peritoneal dialysis. *Kidney Res Clin Pract.* 2016;35(1):10-14. doi:10.1016/j.krcp.2015.12.007

55. Castro ACM, Bazanelli AP, Nerbass FB, Cuppari L, Kamimura MA. Waist circumference as a predictor of mortality in peritoneal dialysis patients: a follow-up study of 48 months. *Br J Nutr.* 2017;117(9):1299-1301. doi:10.1017/S0007114517001179

56. Sayed-Foad A, Zahmatkesh G, Streja E, et al. Association of body mass index with mortality in peritoneal dialysis patients: a systemic review and meta-analysis. *Perit Dial Int.* 2016;36(3):315-325. doi:10.3747/pdi.2015.00052

57. Kennedy C, Bargman J. Peritoneal dialysis in the obese patient. *Clin J Am Soc Nephrol.* 2020;15(2):276-278. doi:10.2215/CJN.10300819

58. Amer M, Tan E, Waters G. The effect of large body weights on peritoneal dialysis outcomes. *Nephrology.* 2017;22(suppl 3):14. doi:10.1111/nep.13103

59. Ananthakrishnan S, Elias RM, Sekercioglu N, et al. Peritoneal dialysis outcomes in overweight patients: analysis of a modern cohort. *Am J Kidney Dis.* 2011;57(4):A21. doi:10.1053/j.ajkd.2011.02.021

60. Dasgupta MK. Strategies for managing diabetic patients on peritoneal dialysis. *Adv Perit Dial.* 2004;20:200-202.

61. Chung SH, Noh H, Ha H, Lee HB. Optimal use of peritoneal dialysis in patients with diabetes. *Perit Dial Int.* 2009;29(suppl 2):S132-S134.

62. Obi Y, Streja E, Mehrotra R, et al. Impact of obesity on modality longevity, residual kidney function, peritonitis, and survival among incident peritoneal dialysis patients. *Am J Kidney Dis.* 2018;71(6):802-813. doi:10.1053/j.ajkd.2017.09.010

63. Dong R, Guo Z, Ding J, Zhou Y, Wu H. Gastrointestinal symptoms: a comparison between patients undergoing peritoneal dialysis and hemodialysis. *World J Gastroenterol.* 2014;20(32):11370-11375. doi:10.3748/wjg.v20.i32.11370

64. Hasanzamani B, Naderzadeh A, Miri M, Ahadi M. Gastrointestinal symptoms in patients undergoing peritoneal dialysis. *J Renal Inj Prev.* 2020;9(4):e31. doi:10.34172/jrip.2020.31

65. Garibotto G, Saffioti S, Russo R, et al. Malnutrition in peritoneal dialysis patients: causes and diagnosis. *Contrib Nephrol.* 2003;140:112-121. doi:10.1159/000071431

66. Aguilera A, Cirugeda A, Amair R, et al. Ghrelin plasma levels and appetite in peritoneal dialysis patients. *Adv Perit Dial.* 2004;20:194-199

67. Young V, Balaam S, Orazio L, et al. Appetite predicts intake and nutritional status in patients receiving peritoneal dialysis. *J Ren Care.* 2016;42(2):123-131. doi:10.1111/jorc.12156

68. Costero O, Baio MA, del Peso G, et al. Treatment of anorexia and malnutrition in peritoneal dialysis patients with megestrol acetate. *Adv Perit Dial.* 2004;20:209-212.

69. Rammohan M, Kalantar-Zadeh K, Liang G, Ghossein C. Megestrol acetate in moderate dose for the treatment of malnutrition-inflammation complex in maintenance dialysis patients. *J Ren Nutr.* 2005;15(3):345-355. doi:10.1016/j.jrn.2004.10.006

70. Park MS, Choi SR, Song YS, Lee SY, Han DS. New insight of amino acid-based dialysis solutions. *Kidney Int Suppl.* 2006;103:S110-S114. doi:10.1038/sj.ki.5001925

71. Piraino B. Insights on peritoneal dialysis-related infections. *Contrib Nephrol.* 2009;163:161-168. doi:10.1159/000223795

72. March DS, Jones AW, Bishop NC, Burton JO. The efficacy of prebiotic, probiotic, and synbiotic supplementation in modulating gut-derived circulatory particles associated with cardiovascular disease in individuals receiving dialysis: a systematic review and meta-analysis of randomized controlled trials. *J Ren Nutr.* 2020;30(4):347-359. doi:10.1053/j.jrn.2019.07.006

73. Oliveres-Gandy HJ, Dominguez-Isidro S, Lopez-Dominguez E, et al. A telemonitoring system for nutritional intake in patients with chronic kidney disease receiving peritoneal dialysis therapy. *Comput Biol Med.* 2019;109:1-13. doi:10.1016/j.compbiomed.2019.04.012

CHAPTER 8

Nutrition Management of the Adult Kidney Transplant Patient

Hannah Norris, RDN, CSR, and Carolyn C. Cochran, RDN, LD, MS, CDCES, FNKF

Introduction

Kidney transplantation is the preferred modality of kidney replacement therapy (KRT) for many patients with end-stage kidney disease (ESKD) and it is the most common solid organ transplant. Kidney transplantation is economically advantageous, costing less than long-term dialysis, which is an important factor in today's health care economy.[1] In 2019, according to the United Network for Organ Sharing (UNOS), 23,401 kidney transplants (the highest number in the United States to date) and 872 kidney/pancreas transplants were performed.[2,3] Paired donation affords another option for living kidney donation. The UNOS organization defines paired donation as "two or more pairs of living donors swapping to make a compatible match."[2] Living-related and non-related donation (including paired donation) afford options for a preemptive transplant in some recipient cases, which avoids the need for dialysis.[3]

Nutrition care of the kidney transplant recipient is a dynamic process. It involves integrating knowledge of the patient's complex medical condition, chronic kidney disease (CKD), and the impact of ongoing therapeutic interventions on the patient's nutritional status. Personally tailored approaches to nutrition management have been associated with longer life and possibly improved graft survival.[4] Continual reassessment of the nutrition goals and efficacy of therapy allow for adjustment of nutrition priorities.

Three phases of care have been identified for organ transplant recipients: pretransplantation phase, acute posttransplantation recovery period, and chronic posttransplantation phase or maintenance phase. In the pretransplantation period, the goal is to meet current education and nutrition needs, optimize the patient's nutritional status, and assist the patient in meeting body weight (BW) criteria for transplantation (as per transplant facility guidelines). During the work-up phase, potential nutrition concerns that may occur post transplant should be introduced.

In the acute posttransplant period (usually 6 to 8 weeks after transplantation or longer, if complications ensue), the goal is to support the patient's increased metabolic demands of surgical recovery using current nutrition guidelines with consideration given to high-dose immunosuppressive therapy. A plan for nutritional rehabilitation to facilitate the patient's recovery is formulated and initiated.[5,6] During the chronic posttransplantation period, nutritional rehabilitation can be realized despite the presence of multiple comorbidities that may also require nutrition interventions. In addition to preexisting comorbid conditions, complications related to long-term immunosuppressive therapy may emerge in individuals genetically predisposed to problems such as diabetes mellitus (DM) and cardiovascular disease (CVD).[5-8]

Pretransplantation Period

A complete evaluation of the patient's nutritional status before transplantation is imperative to identify deficits and, when possible, to correct them before surgery. Registered dietitian nutritionists (RDNs) must keep in mind that the transplant candidate has been subjected to the deleterious effects of a chronic disease with organ failure and that not all deficiencies identified can be corrected without organ replacement.[5,6] The baseline data gathered during initial nutrition assessment are used to develop a plan of care for that candidate. A more detailed nutrition assessment of the patient with CKD is discussed in Chapter 2.

The pretransplantation evaluation should include a medical history, diet history (including social, financial, and support systems), anthropometric data, biochemical indexes of nutritional status, evaluation of gastrointestinal (GI) abnormalities, food allergies, medications affecting nutrition parameters, use of nutrition supplement(s), vitamins, minerals, herbal/botanical product use, nutrition focused physical exam (NFPE), and information about current KRT, if any.[5] If the candidate is already on KRT, it is helpful to receive input from the dialysis facility's RDN. The dialysis RDN can provide insight not only into nutritional issues but also social situations, food insecurity, health literacy, and compliance concerns that may not otherwise be evident during the evaluation process with the transplant team. The transplant RDN can then assess nutrition needs and other factors that may impact transplant outcomes and formulate recommendations. For the severely malnourished patient, specialized nutrition support before surgery may be indicated.

In addition to the standard nutrition assessment, many transplant centers are now assessing patients for frailty since this condition is frequently observed in patients with CKD and is associated with an increased risk of adverse outcomes.[9-14] Researchers have determined that frailty is associated with less of a chance of being listed for transplant and more frequent death while waiting for a transplant. Linda P. Fried, MD, MPH,[9] defined frailty as:

a biologic syndrome of decreased reserve and resistance to stressors, resulting from cumulative declines across multiple physiologic systems, and causing vulnerability to adverse outcomes. This concept distinguishes frailty from disability. There is a growing consensus that markers of frailty include age-associated declines in lean body mass, strength, endurance, balance, walking performance and low activity and that multiple components must be present clinically to constitute frailty.

There are multiple tools for assessing frailty; however, the Fried Frailty Index is widely accepted and has been validated in the kidney transplant population.[10] In some transplant centers, this test is performed by the RDN at the same time as the nutrition assessment. Other centers may have other staff members perform all or part of the frailty assessment, while still other transplant centers may not be assessing for frailty status at all. Frailty pre–kidney transplant is associated with higher risk of mortality post transplant, increased risk of delayed graft function (DGF), longer length of hospitalization, and early hospital readmission post transplant.[10-12] The Fried Frailty Index consists of a 5-point assessment that includes slowness, exhaustion, physical activity, unintentional weight loss, and weakness. Each category has a specific criterion that must be met, and a score of three or more points indicates frailty (see Box 8.1). Transplant centers may have their own criteria regarding frailty that shows how each factor fits into their selection criteria. Assessing for frailty is helpful during the patient's transplant evaluation process and should be considered along with the patient's medical and psychosocial evaluation. Frailty is a potentially modifiable risk factor via rehabilitation that can improve outcomes in this vulnerable population.[10]

Obesity is an important consideration in assessing patient suitability for kidney transplantation. Although obesity appears to provide a survival benefit in patients receiving dialysis, it remains unclear to what degree obesity contributes to poor transplant outcomes, such as lower rates of graft and/or patient sur-

BOX 8.1 | Fried Frailty Assessment[9]

FRIED FRAILTY CRITERIA	
Slowness	4-meter walk test. **Criterion:** • 7 seconds or more for people of normal stature scores 1 point • 6 seconds or more for short statured (≤173 cm for males and ≤159 cm for females) scores 1 point
Exhaustion	How many days in the last week did you feel this way? • Everything I did was an effort. • I could not get going. **Criterion:** 3 days or more for either question scores 1 point.
Physical activity	Based on the Minnesota Leisure Time Activity questionnaire, patients will be asked about their activity over the last 4 weeks. Inpatients will be asked about activity in the 4 weeks before their hospitalization. **Criterion:** Less than 383 kcal expended per week for males and less than 270 kcal expended per week for females scores 1 point.
Unintentional weight loss	Self-reported weight loss of more than 10 lb or measured weight loss of more than 5% of total body weight in the previous year scores 1 point.
Weakness	Mean value of three tests of maximum grip strength with the dominant hand will be calculated. **Criterion:** If below cutoffs, 1 point is scored.

Body mass index (male)	Grip strength, male (kg)	Body mass index (female)	Grip strength, female (kg)
<24	≤29	≤23	≤17
24.1-26	≤30	23.1-26	≤17.3
26.1-28	≤30	26.1-29	≤18
>28	≤32	>29	≤21

vival, and higher rates of DGF and infection.[15,16] One group of researchers found that greater pretransplant muscle mass, reflected by higher pretransplant serum creatinine level, is associated with higher survival rates for both transplanted grafts and patients.[17] Other research indicates that central obesity, measured as waist-to-hip ratio, is a stronger predictor of all-cause and cardiovascular death than body mass index (BMI) in the general population and those with kidney transplantation.[18,19] While evaluation of BMI has shortcomings (fluid vs fat vs muscle mass, presence of polycystic organs, weight distribution per body type, etc), it remains a commonly used indicator. At this time, national guidelines for BMI status for candidacy have not been established, and each transplant center

determines guidelines and criteria (usually BMI of 30 to 40) for identifying the level of obesity that would serve as a contraindication for transplant. Some patients may agree to undergo bariatric surgery to lose weight to meet the criteria for kidney transplant. Notably, having an altered digestive process as a result of bariatric surgery may necessitate care in the selection of medications that the patient is able to absorb and tolerate after transplant.[20]

A low BMI may place the patient at risk for posttransplant complications, but there are limited studies that address this issue. In one study, a clear disadvantage was shown in terms of long-term graft survival for transplant patients with a low BMI.[21] It was assumed that these patients had reduced nutrient availability, thus leading to an immunomodulatory effect of caloric restriction to mitigate T-cell activation.[21] Low serum albumin levels and serum markers of protein status are predictors of surgical risk and infection. Transplant centers may or may not utilize eligibility standards for underweight/undernourished transplant candidates, but aggressive nutrition intervention is indicated and may improve transplant outcomes.[21]

Due to the limited availability of organs, the selection of transplant candidates who are likely to have a positive outcome remains an important issue. Both deceased and living-related or living-unrelated transplant recipients should meet center-specific criteria, including BMI guidelines, prior to transplantation. Future studies should investigate whether weight adjustment can favorably impact posttransplant outcomes in patients who are underweight or obese and if pharmacological agents or surgical treatment for obesity should be more seriously considered for the pretransplant population with ESKD.

Acute Posttransplant Period

IMMUNOSUPPRESSIVE THERAPY

The goals of pharmacological immunosuppression are to prevent acute and chronic rejection, minimize the toxicities of the agents, and lessen rates of infection and malignancy while achieving the highest possible rates of patient and graft survival. Two types of immunosuppressive therapy are generally used: induction therapy and antirejection therapy. Induction therapy utilizes antilymphocyte antibody medications that are administered for a short duration immediately post transplant to minimize risks of early rejection episodes. Their adverse effects are usually minimal and do not pose any major nutritional consequences. Antirejection therapy is also utilized in the immediate posttransplant phase but is continued indefinitely. Four classes of immu-

nosuppressive medications are commonly utilized for antirejection therapy: corticosteroids, calcineurin inhibitors (CNI), antimetabolites, and mammalian target of rapamycin inhibitors.[22-24]

In multidrug therapy, each class of drug mediates the immunocompetence cascade at a different point. The goal of any immunosuppressive regimen is to inhibit the adaptive immune response while allowing nonspecific immune functions to remain intact. There is no consensus as to the optimal immunosuppressive regimen, and each transplant program utilizes combinations of agents differently.[23] Immunosuppressive agents also have nonimmunologic adverse effects. Multitherapy regimens are commonly used to lower doses of individual agents in order to minimize associated adverse effects. Some of the currently used agents are listed in Box 8.2.

Cyclosporine A

Cyclosporine A (CsA) revolutionized solid organ transplantation in the 1980s because it dramatically reduced the incidence of acute rejection episodes and increased kidney graft survival from approximately 50% to 80% at 1 year.[25] CsA and its successors are cyclic polypeptides extracted from the fungus *Tolypocladium inflatum* gams. CsA selectively inhibits adaptive immune responses but also has some nonimmunologic adverse effects, which may include gingival hyperplasia, GI disturbances, hyperglycemia, hyperkalemia, hypertension (HTN), hyperlipidemia, hypophosphatemia, hypomagnesemia, hepatotoxicity, and nephrotoxicity. This agent is absorbed in the upper small intestine and can be affected by food, drug–drug interactions, bile flow, and the patient's lipoprotein and hematocrit status. Due to the nephrotoxic adverse effects, CsA peak and trough levels and kidney function are closely monitored. Neoral is a microemulsion preparation of CsA and has better absorption because it is not dependent on bile. Therefore, it is preferred over CsA in patients with gastroparesis, diarrhea, biliary diversion, cholesta-

BOX 8.2 | Potential Adverse Effects of Immunosuppressants With Nutritional Implications[23-29]

AGENT (BRAND NAMES)	ADVERSE EFFECTS	INTERVENTIONS
Cyclosporine A (Sandimmune, Neoral)[a]	Hyperkalemia	Restrict potassium intake. Support use of potassium binders and changes in patient's pharmaceutical regimen.
	Hyperglycemia	Monitor blood glucose levels. Address carbohydrate load and distribution. Support use of appropriate agents to improve glycemic control.
	Gingival hyperplasia	Practice good oral hygiene.
	Hypertension	Restrict sodium intake.
	Hypomagnesemia	Suggest magnesium supplements if diarrhea is not present. Support a magnesium-rich diet if patient is not hyperkalemic.
	Gastrointestinal distress	Provide nutrient-dense foods patient tolerates and accepts. Ensure adequate protein and fluid intake.
	Hyperlipidemia	Support therapeutic lifestyle changes, including nutrition and exercise. Support use of appropriate pharmaceutical interventions.
	Hypophosphatemia	Encourage high phosphorus foods. Suggest phosphorus supplements as appropriate.
Azathioprine (Imuran)[b]	Infection	Address increased nutrient demands.
	Mouth ulcers	Evaluate diet texture and medications.
	Folate deficiency	Suggest folate supplements.
	Gastrointestinal distress	Provide nutrient-dense foods patient tolerates and accepts.
		Recommend adequate protein and fluids. Consider lactose intolerance.
Corticosteroids (Prednisone,[c] **Prednisolone,**[c] **Solumedrol**[d]**)**	Cushingoid appearance	Address carbohydrate load and distribution. Provide intervention if patient is hyperglycemic.
	Sodium retention, bilateral edema	Restrict sodium intake.
	Enhanced appetite	Advise weight reduction, if appropriate. Suggest low-calorie meals/snacks and eating behavior modification. Encourage exercise, as medically advised.
	Hyperlipidemia	Limit fat intake to less than 30% of calories during long-term phase. Encourage therapeutic lifestyle changes: nutrition, exercise, soluble fiber. Support appropriate pharmaceutical interventions.
	Hyperglycemia	Monitor blood glucose levels. Address carbohydrate load and distribution. Support use of appropriate pharmaceutical interventions.
	Protein catabolism	Increase protein provision.
	Gastrointestinal ulceration	Limit/restrict caffeine, if sensitive.
	Bone loss	Ensure adequate calcium and vitamin D intake. Support appropriate use of bisphosphonates, calcitriol, and estrogen/testosterone.
		Encourage exercise per medical limits.

Continued on next page

Continued from previous page

AGENT (BRAND NAMES)	ADVERSE EFFECTS	INTERVENTIONS
Tacrolimus (Prograf, FK506)[e]	Hypertension	Restrict sodium intake.
	Hyperglycemia	Monitor blood glucose levels and address carbohydrate load and distribution. Support appropriate pharmaceutical interventions.
	Hyperlipidemia	Limit fat intake to less than 30% of calories during long-term phase. Encourage therapeutic lifestyle changes: nutrition, exercise, soluble fiber. Support appropriate pharmaceutical interventions.
	Hyperkalemia	Restrict potassium intake from diet and supplements. Support use of potassium binders as appropriate.
	Hypokalemia	Encourage intake of potassium-rich foods. Support use of potassium supplements, if needed.
	Hypomagnesemia	Suggest magnesium supplements. Monitor for diarrhea.
	Hypophosphatemia	Encourage high phosphorus foods. Suggest phosphorus supplements as appropriate.
	Gastrointestinal distress	Provide nutrient-dense foods patient tolerates and accepts. Ensure adequate protein and fluid intake. Consider lactose intolerance.
Mycophenolate mofetil (CellCept, RS-61443)[f] **Antithymocyte globulin (ATG)**[g] **Muromonab CD3 (Orthoclone OKT3)**[h] **Daclizumab (Zenepax)**[f] **Basiliximab (Simulect)**[a]	Gastrointestinal distress	Provide nutrient-dense foods patient tolerates and accepts. Ensure adequate protein and fluid intake. Suggest small frequent meals/snacks. Consider oral nutrition supplements. Consider lactose intolerance.
Sirolimus (Rapamune)[i]	Hyperlipidemia	Limit fat intake to less than 30% of calories during long-term phase. Support therapeutic lifestyle changes with nutrition, exercise, and soluble fiber. Support appropriate pharmaceutical interventions, if needed.
	Hypertension	Restrict sodium intake.
	Delayed wound healing	Suggest vitamin supplementation and increased protein intake.
	Hypokalemia	Encourage selection of high potassium foods. Suggest potassium supplements, if needed.

[a] Novartis Pharmaceuticals
[b] Bedford Laboratories
[c] Rixabe Laboratories
[d] Pfizer
[e] Astellas Pharma US, Inc.
[f] Novartis Pharmaceuticals Corp.
[g] Upjohn Co.
[h] Otho Biotech
[i] Wyeth Pharmaceuticals

sis, and malabsorption. Compared to CsA, there are usually fewer adverse effects with neoral.[25]

Tacrolimus/Everolimus

Tacrolimus was approved as an immunosuppressive agent in kidney transplantation in 1997. Whereas both tacrolimus and CsA inhibit interleukin (IL)-2 synthesis and release, each reacts differently at the cellular level. The ingestion of food with tacrolimus affects the rate and the extent of the drug's absorption. It is absorbed primarily from the small intestine, and there is a large interpatient and intrapatient variability, especially for patients with GI disease. Gastric emptying of solids is faster in patients taking tacrolimus vs patients taking CsA, and this secondary effect may be beneficial for patients with gastric motility disorders. Adverse effects include insulin resistance, HTN, hyperlipidemia, hyperkalemia or hypokalemia, hypophosphatemia, hypomagnesemia, and GI distress, including anorexia, nausea, vomiting, and diarrhea or constipation.[25]

Mycophenolate Mofetil

Mycophenolate mofetil (MMF) became available for use in kidney transplantation in 1995 and has proven more effective than azathioprine for preventing acute rejection when used in combination with CsA and prednisone. It is a prodrug, which serves to improve MMF's oral bioavailability, and it is not nephrotoxic.[25] It is mainly used as an adjunctive agent in multitherapy protocols with CsA, corticosteroids, or tacrolimus. Its primary effect on the immune system is to inhibit T-cell proliferation. This agent has several adverse effects, but the most common is GI distress, including diarrhea (up to 30% incidence), nausea, dyspepsia, bloating, and vomiting (up to 20% incidence). The distribution of dosages throughout the day has been shown to be helpful in minimizing symptoms.[25]

Sirolimus

Sirolimus, which was approved for use in transplantation in 1999, is a macrolide antibiotic that is structural-ly similar to tacrolimus and inhibits the proliferation of immune cells. It has been shown to reduce significantly the incidence of acute rejection in the early posttransplant period, when compared to either azathioprine or placebo supplementation. Unlike CNI, sirolimus does not cause nephrotoxicity unless it is used in combination with standard doses of CNI. Reduced doses of CNI have been used safely in combination with sirolimus.[25] Potential adverse effects include dyslipidemia (hypertriglyceridemia and hypercholesterolemia), which is due to its inhibition of lipoprotein lipase or reduced catabolism of apoB100-containing lipoproteins. Other adverse effects include increased liver enzymes, delayed wound healing, anemia, HTN, and hypokalemia. When sirolimus is used in combination therapy with CsA and corticosteroids, the dyslipidemias can be further exacerbated.[23-25]

Azathioprine

Azathioprine, initially prescribed as standard immunosuppressive therapy in the 1960s, is an antimetabolite that was used as an adjunctive agent until the introduction of MMF, which has caused its discontinuation in most transplant programs. Adverse effects include thrombocytopenia and leukopenia. Common GI adverse effects include diarrhea and cholestasis.[25]

Corticosteroids

Corticosteroids, which became available in the 1960s, are used to reverse kidney transplant rejection.[21] The most commonly prescribed corticosteroids used in transplant programs include prednisone and methylprednisolone. Corticosteroids have antiinflammatory properties and inhibit the production of lymphokines. This class of immunosuppressants can be administered in high oral or parenteral doses for acute rejection or in oral pulse doses, which are then tapered to maintenance levels or in some cases discontinued.[23,25]

Protocols incorporating rapid discontinuation of prednisone (RDP) after kidney transplantation have been associated with no difference in short- and long-term graft survival when compared to chronic maintenance prednisone.[27,28] Some programs may only use steroids during the transplant hospitalization and not as long-term treatment. Associated adverse effects are believed to be dose-dependent and may include impaired wound healing, avascular necrosis of long bones, upper GI ulceration, protein catabolism, HTN, steroid-induced DM, cataract formation, and stimulation of appetite with resultant weight gain.[27,30] These adverse effects have been reduced with steroid-minimization protocols, especially with significantly lower incidences of hyperlipidemia and posttransplant DM.[28] Corticosteroids can also potentially retard growth in the pediatric population undergoing transplant.

Other Agents

Monoclonal antibodies (muromonab-CD3) and anti-thymocyte globulin (ATG) are examples of immunosuppressants used either perioperatively for induction therapy or for acute rejection episodes. These agents may cause GI distress and flu-like symptoms in the first few days of administration, but these are usually short-lived.[23,25] Daclizumab is a genetically engineered monoclonal antibody that is an IL-2 receptor antagonist. This agent can be combined with traditional immunosuppressive therapy. It is an intravenous (IV) preparation administered in one to five doses within the first 8 weeks postoperatively.[25] Basiliximab is another IL-2 antagonist that is used in combination therapy, usually with CsA and corticosteroids. This medication is administered preoperatively and then given on the fourth postoperative day. There are no known nutritional adverse effects with daclizumab or basiliximab.[25] Several immunosuppressive agents are currently being investigated in clinical trials. RDNs are challenged to stay informed about the various nutrition-related adverse effects of each agent and assist patients in appropriate management.

NUTRITIONAL REQUIREMENTS

Currently accepted practices regarding nutrition recommendations for adult kidney transplantation are shown in Box 8.3.[31] Nutrient requirements are increased during the acute posttransplantation phase, which usually lasts 6 to 8 weeks. This period may be extended when rehospitalization or other complications are present.

Protein

The acceleration of the transplant recipient's protein catabolic rate (PCR) is related to the administration of large doses of corticosteroids and postoperative stress.[30] This increase in PCR seems to persist at least through the third postoperative week and increases again if rejection therapy is needed. Maintenance of protein balance during this period is a formidable task, and negative protein balance will ensue if the protein intake does not equal the PCR. During the acute posttransplantation phase, the present recommendation for protein intake is a range of 1.2 to 2 g/kg standard BW or adjusted BW.[31,32]

Energy

Energy requirements are increased in the acute posttransplantation phase due to high-dose corticosteroid therapy and surgical stress. Energy requirements can be estimated by calculating 30 to 35 kcal/kg standard or adjusted BW or by using the Harris-Benedict equation multiplied by 1.3 to 1.5.[31,32] Due to CKD prior to transplant patients may display protein energy wasting and negative nitrogen balance, with loss of lean body mass.[33] Energy needs may be further increased in the posttransplant period in the presence of fever and infection. Long-term posttransplant energy needs are estimated by calculating 23 to 35 kcal/kg standard or adjusted BW in stable patients with functioning grafts. The goal is to maintain a desirable, healthy BW.[31] The Academy of Nutrition and Dietetics Evidence Analysis Library Guidelines for CKD do not support less than 23 kcal/kg.[26]

Carbohydrate

Glucose intolerance postoperatively can result from immunosuppression, surgical stress, genetic predisposition, obesity, increased age, and infection. CNI, CsA,

BOX 8.3 | Daily Recommended Nutrient Intakes for Adult Kidney Transplantation[26,31,32]

NUTRIENT	ACUTE PERIOD	CHRONIC PERIOD
Protein	1.2 to 2.0 g/kg[a]	0.6 to 0.8 g/kg[a] (without diabetes mellitus)
		0.8 to 0.9 g/kg[a] (with diabetes mellitus)
		Adjust with chronic graft dysfunction.
Energy	30 to 35 kcal/kg[a] or basal energy expenditure (BEE) × 1.3 to 1.5	23 to 35 kcal/kg[a]
	May increase with postoperative complications.	Adjust calories to maintain desirable body weight.
Carbohydrate	Limit simple carbohydrate intake with elevated blood glucose levels and unwanted weight gain.	Emphasize complex carbohydrate intake and distribution.
Fat	Remainder of calories (30% of total calories); emphasize polyunsaturated fatty acid (PUFA) and monounsaturated fatty acid (MUFA) sources in place of saturated fat	Less than 30% total calories; emphasize PUFA and MUFA sources in place of saturated fat
Sodium	Restrict if blood pressure/fluid status dictates. Aim for 2 to 4 g with delayed graft function.	2.3 g
		Individualize with hypertension or edema.
Potassium	2 to 4 g, if hyperkalemic	Individualize to maintain normal serum levels.
Calcium	Individualize to maintain normal serum levels.	800 to 1,500 mg; maintain normal serum levels
Phosphorus	Individualize to maintain normal serum levels.	Individualize to maintain normal serum levels.
Other vitamins	Dietary Reference Intake (DRI)[b,c]	DRI[c]
Other minerals	DRI[c]	DRI[c]
Trace elements	DRI[c]	DRI[c]
Fluid	Limited only by graft function; generally unrestricted and encouraged.	Limited only by graft function; generally unrestricted.

[a] Based on standard or adjusted BW. Use clinical judgment.

[b] Dietary Reference Intake is based on recommended dietary allowance or adequate intake.

[c] Due to lack of research, no specific recommendations are available for this population and the DRI is used.

and tacrolimus have also been associated with increased risk for DM after transplantation. However, tacrolimus is five times more diabetogenic than CsA.[34] New-onset DM after transplantation (NODAT) increases the risk of graft loss, infection, and CVD.[35] Hyperglycemia should be aggressively managed with insulin and hypoglycemic agents, a carbohydrate-controlled diet (amount and distribution), and appropriate exercise per medical clearance. A high-fiber diet is also recommended to assist with glucose control and lipid management.[31]

Fat

During the acute postoperative period, dietary fat is used to supply the remainder of the total energy after calculating the amount provided by protein and carbohydrate. As in the chronic posttransplant phase, every effort should be made to follow the National Heart, Lung, and Blood Institute Adult Treatment Panel III Guidelines, as dyslipidemia and CVD are often preexisting risk factors. Temporary liberalization may be necessary to meet increased energy needs if the patient is unable to sustain adequate intake.[22]

Sodium and Fluids

Sodium intake should be restricted in the acute postoperative period in the presence of poor allograft function, bilateral edema, or posttransplant HTN. Some immunosuppressive medications can cause HTN and fluid retention (see Box 8.2), which may necessitate sodium restriction. Blood pressure (BP) and fluid status should be closely monitored to determine whether sodium restriction is indicated.[31] Fluid requirements can vary depending on volume status. Fluid intake should be restricted only in the posttransplant period in the presence of poor allograft function with poor urine output.[6,31,32] In cases of low serum sodium, liberalization of dietary intake may be appropriate. During the long-term maintenance phase, sodium control guidelines for patients mirror healthy adults at 2.3 g/d. Dietary sodium adjustments may be needed to manage HTN or maintain fluid balance.

Potassium

Individualized potassium intake is recommended unless hyperkalemia or hypokalemia is present. With hypokalemia, a diet rich in high potassium foods that the patient tolerates is usually sufficient; however, supplementation may be needed. Adoption of the Dietary Approach to Stop Hypertension (DASH) diet or Mediterranean diet could result in increased potassium intake. If serum potassium is elevated, dietary restriction is indicated. Poor graft function, suppression of aldosterone levels, impaired potassium excretion associated with CNI use, and use of potassium-sparing diuretics may contribute to hyperkalemia.[36] Certain drugs (eg, Bactrim) can also cause retention of potassium.[37] The prevalence of hyperkalemia post transplant is estimated to be as high as 44% to 73% for patients on CNI.[38] In patients with uncontrolled hyperglycemia, the effect of elevated blood glucose may also result in an elevated serum potassium.[38] If the patient has metabolic acidosis, correction of this problem can resolve hyperkalemia. Hypokalemia has also been reported in kidney transplant recipients due to potassium-wasting diuretics and requires treatment.[39]

Vitamins and Minerals

A multivitamin product that provides 100% of the Dietary Reference Intake (DRI) is usually recommended in the stable posttransplant patient.[31] However, based on test results or diagnosis, some vitamins and minerals may need to be given in therapeutic doses.

Calcium and vitamin D supplementations are indicated to treat bone loss due to osteoporosis, pretransplant renal osteodystrophy, and posttransplant corticosteroid therapy. Experts recommend long-term calcium supplementation of 800 to 1,500 mg/d with total calcium intake not to exceed 2,000 mg/d.[32] Vitamin D deficiency continues to be an issue, even in the presence of stable transplanted graft function. Cholecalciferol supplementation significantly increases serum 25-hydroxyvitamin D levels and decreases parathyroid hormone (PTH) levels. Active vitamin D metabolites may have additional benefits in reducing hyperparathyroidism after kidney transplantation.[40,41] If hypercalcemia is present, vitamin D and calcium supplements should be discontinued, and some facilities institute a low calcium diet. Although currently an off-label use, cinacalcet has also been prescribed to treat tertiary hyperparathyroidism.

Posttransplant anemia, defined by abnormal hematocrit and hemoglobin levels, has been shown to occur in approximately 20% to 51% of all stable posttransplant patients.[42] Of those patients, about 10% required erythropoietin therapy. Multivariate analyses revealed that female gender, lower kidney function, the dose of angiotensin-converting enzyme inhibitors, and the immunosuppressive drugs MMF and tacrolimus were associated with lower red blood cell counts.[42] All causes for ongoing anemia should be investigated, and appropriate supplementation should be provided, such as iron, folate, and vitamin B12.

Zinc deficiency is associated with corticosteroid therapy, and early studies have shown that posttransplant patients with subnormal plasma and hair zinc levels during the pretransplantation period did not show normalization of these parameters until 1 year after transplantation.[43] Further studies have not been found to confirm this phenomenon, especially in the current era of steroid minimization. When faced with wound complications, zinc status should be considered, with supplementation if dietary zinc intake is insufficient.

Hypomagnesemia has been reported in kidney transplant recipients treated with CNI, CsA, and tacrolimus. Serum magnesium should be monitored regularly and supplemented, if indicated. Symptoms of magnesium deficiency may not be present. Dietary sources of magnesium are usually not adequate to correct hypomagnesemia.[22]

Herbals and Botanicals

Herbal products and botanicals have an enormous presence in the US health care system. The Dietary Supplement Health and Education Act, which became a law in 1994, established a formal definition for dietary supplements.[44] Unfortunately, no proof of efficacy, safety, or quality-control standards is required, thus increasing the risks of adverse effects from these products.[45] Some herbal preparations are advertised to enhance the immune

system (eg, ginseng, echinacea, astragalus, and noni juice), which theoretically may increase the risk of organ rejection.[22] Others, like St John's wort, can cause drug–drug interactions, which may affect drug absorption and affect trough levels of immunosuppressant medications.[22,44] Green tea, dong quai, ginseng, milk thistle, and ginger have varying effects on in vitro immune assays and should be avoided or used with extreme caution.[22] Until adequate research is available, herbals and botanicals in the transplant population will continue to be contraindicated. Because patients frequently inquire about reasons for avoiding specific herbs and botanicals, Table 8.1 gives an overview of some items.[46]

TABLE 8.1 | Transplant Herbs and Botanicals[a]

Herb/botanical/fruit	CYP 450 3A4 absorption pathway	Known to improve immune function	Advertised to improve immune function	Comments*	Reference
A Andrographis paniculata (Green chiretta)	●[47]	●	●	May ↓ BP, slow blood clotting; May contribute to AKI[48]	47, 48
Astragalus	●[49]	●		May affect BG and BP[50]	51
B Berberine	●[52]			May ↓ BG, BP, and cholesterol[50]; May ↓ inflammation, antioxidant properties[53]	52-55
Bitter orange (Seville)	○				54
Bergamot (flavor in teas; topical uses; aromatherapy) *See also:* grapefruit	●[56]			May ↓ BG; May interfere with photosensitizing drugs[50]	55, 56
Black currant			○	May ↓ BP and cholesterol[50]	55
Black mulberry	●			May ↓ BG	55, 57
Black raspberry	●				58, 59
C Carambola (Star Fruit)	●[60]		●	High in vitamin C	60
Cat's claw (uncaria tomentosa)	●[54]				54
Chamomile tea	●[54]			Essential oil may inhibit CYP450 3A4	54, 61
Chilean tea (peumus boldus, or Boldo)				For gallstones and gastrointestinal disorders; interferes with warfarin	62
Chrysanthemum	●[63]		○		63
Chlorella			○		
Cranberry extracts and supplements	● (for juice)[64]				64
Corn silk				May ↓ BG, BP, potassium	55

*BG = blood glucose | BP = blood pressure | ↑ = increase | ↓ = decrease;
● Indicates a strong correlation; ○ indicates a weaker correlation. Only supplements with correlation were included. See Chapter 19.

Continued on next page

Continued from previous page

Herb/botanical/fruit	CYP 450 3A4 absorption pathway	Known to improve immune function	Advertised to improve immune function	Comments*	Reference
D Dandelion	○			Diuretic effect	63
Dang gui	○				65
Dang shen (ginseng substitute)	No effect[66]		○		66
Danshen	●[66]			For CVD, HTN, stroke	66
Dong quai (angelica dahurica)	●[54]				54
E Echinacea	●	○		Affects intestinal and hepatic CYP 450 3A4[18]	67
Elderberry	No effect[68]	○[69]	○		68, 69
Embilica officinalis (gooseberry)		Possible immune-modulator[70]		May ↓ BG[71]	70, 71
Evening primrose (oenothera species)	●[54]			Bleeding risk	54
Evodia Rutaecarpa (Wuzhuyu, Wu Zhu Yu, Wu Zhu Yu Tang, Evodiae Fructae/us)	○[72]		○	Antioxidant and antiinflammatory agent; to ↓ body fat (not to be taken with caffeine)	72
F Feverfew (tanacetyn parthenium)	●[54]				54
Frankincense (boswellia species)	●[54]				54
G Garlic	No effect[67]	●	●	Minimal quercetin	54, 67
Ginger	○[73]				73
Ginko biloba	No effect[67]			Antioxidant properties	54, 67
Ginseng (Panax ginseng)	○[74]	○[75]	○		54, 74, 75
Goldenseal	●[67]			Used for URI, contains berberine	54, 67
Grape, wild (grape seed extract)	○[66]			Used for antioxidant and anticancer properties	66
Grapefruit (bergamottin)	○[76]			Fruit, juice, and juice blends	54, 76
Green tea	○[77]	○[78]			77, 78
Guggul	○[79]			Contains quercetin	54, 79
K Kava (piper methysticum)	●[54]				54
L Licorice (glycyrrhiza glabra)	●[54]			For cough, antiinflammatory	54
M Mandelo	○				
Melatonin	○				80
Milk thistle	No effect[67]			Used for liver function	54, 67
Minneola	○				

*BG = blood glucose | BP = blood pressure | ↑ = increase | ↓ = decrease;
● Indicates a strong correlation; ○ indicates a weaker correlation. Only supplements with correlation were included. See Chapter 19.

Continued on next page

Continued from previous page

Herb/botanical/fruit	CYP 450 3A4 absorption pathway	Known to improve immune function	Advertised to improve immune function	Comments*	Reference
O Oldenlandia diffusa (Bai Hua She Cao)	● Inducer[66]			For autoimmune disease, tumors, and infection	66
Oroblanco	○			Grapefruit hybrid	
P Piperine (black pepper)	○[81]			<1 g inhibited CYP450 3A4	81
Phellodendron species	●[54]				54
Pomegranate	○				
Pomelo, pummelo (pamplemousse, shaddock)	○			Related to grapefruit	54
Q Quercetin					82
R Rhodiola root		○			
S Saw palmetto	No effect[83]			Study dose: 320 mg cap 1 qd × 14 days	54, 83
Schisandra	●			Used for weight loss	
Sheng di huang (Rehmannia glutinosa)	Minimal effect[66]	●	●	To ↑ immune function and improve memory	66
Soda beverages: Fanta (various grapefruit flavors) Fresca (black cherry citrus, original citrus, peach citrus) Squirt Sun Drop	●			Contain grapefruit	84
St John's Wort	● Inducer[67]			May ↑ BP May be in some brands of oat teas used for gout	54, 67
T Tangelo	●			Grapefruit hybrid	
U Uva ursi (Arctostaphylos uva ursi, bearberry, bear's grape, foxberry, crowberry, kinnikinnick, tinnick)	○[85]			Used to treat UTIs	85
V Valerian	Minimal effect[66]			Used for sleep disorders; study dose: 1 g dry root extract each evening for 14 days	86
W Wine, red (Resveretrol)	●[54]				54

*BG = blood glucose | BP = blood pressure | ↑ = increase | ↓ = decrease;
● Indicates a strong correlation; ○ indicates a weaker correlation. Only supplements with correlation were included. See Chapter 19.

CVD = cardiovascular disease; HTN = hypertension; URI = upper respiratory infection; qd = every day | UTI = urinary tract infection

aThe authors would like to extend their appreciation to Rebecca Chrasta, MCN, RDN, LD, for assistance in the preparation of this chart.

COMMON POSTTRANSPLANT NUTRITION CONCERNS

Hyperglycemia

The development of hyperglycemia after kidney transplant is common with increased risk and incidence.[87] Prednisone causes insulin resistance, and CNI impair insulin secretion. Prior personal or family history of DM, age, and obesity also increase the risk of developing hyperglycemia. The incidence of elevated glucose levels is greater when high-dose steroids are given during the initial postoperative days or during treatment for acute rejection. The frequency of hyperglycemia is reduced in posttransplant recipients with steroid-free protocols and use of lower tacrolimus doses in some transplant programs.[88,89] Postoperative glucose monitoring should begin immediately. Development of hyperglycemia causes increased graft loss and reduced patient survival after transplant.[89,90] Nutrition therapy should balance the increased need for calories and protein with carbohydrate consistency and distribution. Oral or injectable hypoglycemic agents or various insulin therapies in conjunction with nutrition counseling and exercise may be appropriate to achieve glycemic control. Studies completed among persons diagnosed with DM have shown a 1% to 2% decrease in hemoglobin A1c levels after medical nutrition therapy (MNT) intervention.[91,92] The Comparing glycaemic benefits of Active Versus passive lifestyle Intervention in kidney Allograft Recipients (CAVIAR) trial showed that active lifestyle intervention performed by a renal RDN post–kidney transplant did not change markers of glucose metabolism compared to the group who received passive lifestyle intervention. Active intervention included lifestyle advice provided by the RDN using behavior change counseling techniques, whereas passive intervention included receiving written information only. However, the active intervention group did have a lower incidence of NODAT and some improvement in weight and fat mass.[93]

Gastrointestinal Issues

A wide range of GI symptoms, including diarrhea, nausea, and vomiting, are associated with various immunosuppressive agents. Complications may also be secondary to infection, mucosal injury, and ulceration, which can manifest anywhere in the GI tract. These can vary in severity from mild and manageable to severe. Adverse GI events are common in transplantation, occurring in up to 20% of kidney transplant recipients.[94,95] Preexisting GI issues should also be considered, such as history of gastroparesis.

Viral infections such as cytomegalovirus (CMV) are common in the immunocompromised patient. CMV can affect any portion of the GI tract and may lead to ischemic colitis and toxic megacolon.[96] Symptoms may include dysphagia, odynophagia, nausea, vomiting, abdominal pain, diarrhea, GI bleeding, or gut perforation. It is imperative to minimize any delay in diagnosis because CMV can quickly spread to other organs. Herpes simplex virus (HSV), another common viral infection, can affect any region of the GI tract but most often affects the oral cavity and esophagus. One study of 221 patients with kidney transplants found HSV esophagitis in only five patients, an incidence of 2.2%, over an 8-year period.[97]

Fungal infections are also common in the early posttransplantation phase and usually present as *Candida* esophagitis with or without thrush. One study showed decreased survival rates in patients with this complication.[98] Transplant programs typically prescribe prophylactic antifungal agents to prevent fungal infections.[97]

Bacterial infections of the gut are frequently diagnosed in the transplant recipient and include *Clostridium difficile* colitis. Symptoms include diarrhea and abdominal tenderness. Colitis usually responds to appropriate pharmacological treatment.[95] Several factors can be responsible for posttransplantation ulcer formation, including the administration of corticosteroids or a prior history of peptic ulcer disease. One study showed that the prevalence of *Helicobacter pylori* was

70% in kidney transplant recipients and that gastritis was present in 65% of recipients.[99] Transplant candidates need to be evaluated for *Helicobacter pylori* if there is no other obvious indication for peptic ulcer disease. Most transplant programs initially prescribe prophylactic histamine-2 receptor blockers.

Although the incidence of ulceration is low, the stress of surgery, nonsteroidal anti-inflammatory agents, corticosteroids, and other immunosuppressive agents may impact the formation of ulcers after kidney transplantation.[100] Prophylaxis for posttransplantation ulceration may complicate immunosuppression.[94] Due to the decrease in gastric secretions, the GI flora may be altered, increasing overgrowth of undesirable organisms and resulting in an infection. In a 3-year study of kidney transplant recipients, Logan et al[101] found a low frequency of upper GI tract complications and no difference in the frequency of complications between patients on tacrolimus and patients on CsA-based immunosuppression. The complication rates were similar in patients receiving omeprazole and those receiving ranitidine as antiulcer prophylaxis.

Other causes of diarrhea include development of lactose intolerance after a period of time with minimal or no milk intake (as may occur with CKD and dialysis) or due to intake of mineral supplements to replete low serum magnesium or phosphorus (or both). Lactose malabsorption may also have secondary causes, such as infection or conditions causing changes in the mucosal integrity of the small intestine.[102,103]

Altered Electrolytes

Hypophosphatemia Hypophosphatemia is common immediately following a kidney transplant, as a patient's glomerular filtration rate (GFR) normalizes. Preexisting hyperparathyroidism contributes to low phosphorus levels.[104] This problem may persist up to a year post transplant. Many patients, whether coming from dialysis or not, have been accustomed to restricting phosphorus and may inadvertently continue a low-phosphorus diet or continue routine phosphate

binders or calcium supplements given with meals. A patient may also be experiencing upper GI symptoms and taking an over-the-counter (OTC) calcium carbonate after eating, which also binds phosphorus in that meal. Abnormalities can occur even with a stable, functioning allograft. Intracellular phosphorus shifts are also associated with high levels of dextrose provision.

Repletion of phosphorus can be achieved through the administration of oral supplements and the encouragement of foods and beverages high in phosphorus. Some patients may even require IV phosphorus. Certain phosphorus supplements contain significant amounts of potassium when given in high doses and require close monitoring of serum potassium levels. If persistent hyperkalemia is present, switching to a sodium phosphate preparation is preferred. See Table 8.2 for a list of phosphorus-containing preparations.[105] Oral phosphorus supplements should be discontinued once normal phosphorus levels are achieved and maintained (see Chapter 17).

TABLE 8.2 | Oral Phosphorus Supplements[a]

Product name	Phosphorus	Potassium	Sodium
Phos-NaK Powder (OTC)[b]	250 mg/ 8 mmol	280 mg/ 7.1 mEq	164 mg/ 6.9 mEq
K-Phos Original dissolvable tablets (RX)[c]	114 mg/ 3.7 mmol	144 mg/ 3.7 mEq	0
K-Phos MF (RX)[c]	124 mg/ 4 mmol	43 mg/ 1.1 mEq	67 mg/ 2 mEq
K-Phos No.2 (RX)[c]	250 mg/ 8 mmol	88 mg/ 2.3 mEq	134 mg/ 5.8 mEq
Phospha 250 Neutral (RX)[d]	250 mg/ 8 mmol	45 mg/ 1.1 mEq	298 mg/ 13 mEq
K-Phos Neutral (RX)[c]	250 mg/ 8 mmol	45 mg/ 1.1 mEq	298 mg/ 13 mEq
Virt-Phos 250 Neutral (OTC)[c]	250 mg/ 8 mmol	0	0

[a] Potassium and sodium phosphate powder (Neutra-Phos), potassium phosphate powder (Neutra-Phos K), and sodium phosphate oral solution have been removed from the market.

[b] Cypress Pharmaceuticals, Madison, MS 39130

[c] Beach Pharmaceuticals, Tampa, FL 33681

[d] Rising Pharmaceuticals, Allendale, NJ 07401

Hyperkalemia Posttransplant hyperkalemia may be a result of poor graft function, CNI therapy, or cell lysis related to the catabolic effect of surgery and corticosteroid use or damage during laboratory testing. Certain phosphorus supplements used to treat posttransplant hypophosphatemia contain potassium and require close monitoring of serum potassium levels, especially if given in higher doses. If persistent hyperkalemia is present, switching the phosphorus supplement to a sodium phosphate preparation is preferred (see Table 8.2 on page 125).[105] Patients should be counseled about minimizing intake of high potassium food choices, including avoidance of potassium chloride salt substitutes. If the patient takes a multivitamin, the product should be evaluated for potassium content and held until the problem is resolved or switched to a potassium-free product. Hyperkalemia may also occur when a patient has an unusually excessive intake of a food or beverage considered low in potassium. A high dietary phosphorus or magnesium intake, commonly encouraged in the treatment of hypophosphatemia or hypomagnesemia, may also contribute to a higher potassium load. Treatment includes dietary potassium restriction and provision of adequate calories and protein to minimize catabolism of endogenous tissue.[106] If hyperkalemia continues to persist, a binding medication can be considered.

Hypomagnesemia Hypomagnesemia is often seen in posttransplant patients as an adverse effect of CNI, CsA, and tacrolimus. A diet liberal in magnesium may be instituted; however, since a diet rich in magnesium is also high in potassium, caution is needed if serum potassium is elevated. Often, the provision of oral magnesium supplements is required. The chemical composition of magnesium compounds differs with variable absorption potential. Magnesium supplements may cause diarrhea, especially when taken in higher dosages. IV supplementation provides rapid normalization of serum value but is not useful on a routine basis. Magnesium supplements should be taken apart from MMF so as not to interfere with absorption.

Food Safety

Food-borne infections are a common and possible life-threatening problem for millions of individuals in the United States and around the world.[107] According to the Centers for Disease Control and Prevention,[108] "foodborne pathogens cause up to 48 million illnesses, 128,000 hospitalizations, and 3,000 deaths in the US each year." There are at least 250 known food-borne diseases, but information on the risk of infection from food sources in the immunosuppressed patient is limited.[107,108] Individuals infected with food-borne microorganisms exhibit symptoms ranging from mild intestinal distress to severe dehydration, which could jeopardize adequate immunosuppression and renal perfusion.

Given the increased prevalence of food-borne outbreaks, it is prudent to reinforce all food safety guidelines as published by the US Department of Agriculture Food Safety and Inspection Service. The booklet *Food Safety: A Need-To-Know Guide for Those at Risk* is available free of charge and can be ordered by calling 1-888-674-6854 or emailing the US Department of Agriculture Meat and Poultry Hotline at mphotline@usda.gov. This new booklet replaces the former one titled *Food Safety for Transplant Recipients*, which continues to be available online.

Food handling guidelines apply not only to meal preparation in the home but are also appropriate for other family members, care providers, friends, and even organizations such as church groups, who may be participating in the patient's postsurgical recovery. Practitioners should note that transplant recipients are immunosuppressed for the life of the graft and should remain mindful about safety issues for the duration of their transplant.

Drug–Nutrient Interactions

Some foods and herbal supplements can interfere with the absorption of certain medications, including certain immunosuppressants, calcium channel blockers, and antilipidemics. There is a high degree of individual variability in the general population, which makes response unpredictable. Any transplant recipient taking

CsA, tacrolimus, everolimus, sirolimus, or other drugs affected by potential absorption issues should avoid intake of any fruit or supplement that inhibits the cytochrome P450 isoenzyme CYP3A4 in the gut wall. The pharmacokinetics of CsA showed variability when administered with grapefruit.[109] Bailey et al,[110] Kim et al,[111] and Sorokin et al[112] reported that the duration of the effect of grapefruit juice can last 24 hours and that repeated intake can have a cumulative effect. In addition to grapefruit and grapefruit juice, pomegranate and pomegranate juice blends, Seville (bitter) oranges, and star fruit interfere with absorption. Table 8.1 includes some beverages known to contain grapefruit.[113]

Nutrition Support Considerations

Inadequate nutrient intake can complicate the kidney transplant patient's postoperative course. Some patients experience a temporary loss or slow return of appetite. Others may suffer from gastroparesis or other altered GI function. Oral supplementation to achieve adequate protein and calories is a priority in the immediate postoperative phase.

For patients who are unable to meet their nutrition needs orally, enteral nutrition may be required. Tube feedings are not often needed after transplant, but when they are used, a standard polymeric, high-nitrogen formula is recommended. Other formulas may be necessary, depending on the patient's graft function. The appropriate enteral route (gastric vs small bowel) will depend on the patient's GI symptoms. See Chapter 15 for additional information.

Parenteral nutrition (PN) is rarely required after kidney transplant but is perhaps more likely seen after kidney/pancreas transplant. If PN is necessary, it is primarily used in patients with a prolonged ileus, intractable diarrhea, unresolved gastroparesis, or other nonfunctional GI problems. Allograft function as determined by urine output, electrolytes, blood urea nitrogen (BUN)/creatinine levels, fluid balance, and dialysis status also must be considered. See Chapter 16 for additional information.

Long-Term Posttransplant Period

Nutrition needs are largely stabilized 4 to 8 weeks after a kidney transplant. At this point, clinicians should begin monitoring patients for signs and symptoms of obesity, dyslipidemia, hyperglycemia, and osteoporosis. The nutritional objectives of the long-term posttransplantation phase are the provision of adequate nutrients and the management of long-term nutritional complications. RDNs who provide MNT for transplant recipients in the first 3 years post transplant will receive reimbursement for the nutritional services provided with a current Medicare provider number. Patients only need to obtain an order from their physician to access this MNT service. RDNs should be encouraged to obtain their provider number for their work with posttransplant recipients because these opportunities are not being realized to their full potential.

NUTRITION GOALS

Recommendations for the long-term posttransplant recipient are the same as those for any healthy person: maintain a healthy weight as well as normal serum glucose, lipid, and BP levels. Overall, a heart-healthy diet, one that is moderate in sodium and fat, should be followed. Many recipients with kidney transplant have DM and will benefit from a controlled carbohydrate intake.

Basal calorie requirements can be estimated for weight maintenance or for attainment of a desirable weight using the Mifflin-St. Jeor or Harris-Benedict equations. Recommendations vary from 1.1 to 1.3 times the basal energy expenditure to 23 to 35 kcal/kg BW.[32,114-116] Adjustment should be individualized to support a healthy body weight. Protein intake of 0.6 to 0.8 g/kg is generally recommended for recipients without diabetes mellitus during this phase while protein goals for individuals with diabetes mellitus are 0.8 to 0.9 g/kg. (see Box 8.3).[32,117]

There is a lack of evidence indicating whether routine vitamin supplementation is beneficial after transplant. Some programs do recommend a multivitamin immediately after transplant, whereas others do not.

OBESITY

Weight gain ranging between 20 and 40 lb in the first 6 months after transplant is not uncommon.[118,119] The causes of posttransplantation obesity are multifactorial and include the elimination of the cachectic effects of dialysis, the discontinuation of most dietary restrictions, the lack of physical activity, and an increased appetite and improved sense of taste from resolution of uremia and steroid administration.[120,121]

Management of obesity is as challenging in this population as in any other. Lifestyle changes involving diet, behavior modification, and physical activity are the cornerstones of successful treatment. Small studies have shown that early intensive RDN intervention can reduce weight gain in this population.[118] Reducing portion sizes, keeping food records, and setting realistic goals can help the recipient focus on weight loss. An idea for future studies includes investigating whether weight loss favorably affects long-term outcomes. Some patients have shown positive results from gastric surgery; however, this therapy is not without its own potential side effects.[118]

HYPERGLYCEMIA

The development of NODAT is another long-term complication, one that is a predictor of increased mortality in recipients.[122-125] Increased glucose levels put patients at risk for infection and overall decreased graft survival.[126] The incidence of DM post transplant is reported to be from 12% to 46%.[127,128] The etiology is primarily from the diabetogenic effects of CNI and corticosteroids, with long-term use of CNI resulting in gradual β cell dysfunction. It has been proposed that "resting" of the β cells could be done using basal insulin in the immediate posttransplant period.[129] As steroid dose is decreased or discontinued, normalization of glucose levels may occur. Long-term use of CNI may result in gradual β cell dysfunction. For patients with a family history of DM, predisposing ethnicity, advancing age, and undesired weight gain, precipitation of type 2 DM can occur.

MNT should focus on carbohydrate, both quantity and distribution. Depending on the type of medication(s) used and the patient's activity level, sources of carbohydrate may be needed at specific times to minimize instances of hypoglycemia.

Patients should be treated in accordance with guidelines published by the American Association of Clinical Endocrinology and the American Diabetes Association. Additional guidelines recommend a hemoglobin A1c target of 7% to 7.5% due to risk of hypoglycemia and the frequent presence of CVD.[128,130]

Medications for glycemic control should be evaluated for each patient's situation. Oral and/or injectable hypoglycemic agents or various combinations of insulin therapy may be required for treatment, particularly in the first year after surgery. Practitioners should consider the potential for fluid retention with thiazolidinedione therapy as a complicating factor, especially in patients who have this concern. Sodium-glucose cotransporter two inhibitors can result in volume depletion, and patients have shown a higher risk of genitourinary infection; both are to be avoided in the posttransplant immunosuppressed population. Assurance of graft function is an unknown factor, so use of metformin may not be an ideal choice because it is not recommended when estimated GFR is less than 30 mL/min/1.73 m^2 due to the potential for lactic acidosis. Referral to an endocrinologist for long-term management is often recommended.

For posttransplant patients with chronic graft dysfunction, care may be needed to avoid the potential for low blood glucose levels with use of glycemic agents due to the extended activity of insulin with decreased renal insulin clearance (see Chapter 3).

DYSLIPIDEMIA

The occurrence of dyslipidemia in posttransplant recipients has been reported to be as high as 60% to 79%.[131] Dyslipidemia can lead to CVD, which is the leading cause of mortality in patients with kidney transplant.[132,133] Other factors that can precipitate dyslipidemia include immunosuppressive therapy, obesity, age, gender, history of DM, and sedentary lifestyle. Patients are encouraged to lose weight, modify dietary fat intake, and quit smoking. These lifestyle modifications should be considered as the first step in treatment. Reducing saturated fat, trans fat, and cholesterol while attaining a healthy weight is key to reducing lipid levels.

Lipid profiles of patients with CVD can improve by adding fiber, nuts, and plant stanols to the diet. Fiber has been shown to lower cholesterol levels by 2% to 3% and also lower low-density lipoprotein (LDL) cholesterol levels up to 7%. Nuts have been shown to lower cholesterol levels by 4% to 21% and LDL levels by up to 29%.[134-137] Plant stanols have shown the greatest lipid-lowering effect; a 2 g/d regimen, if consistently adhered to, can lower cholesterol/LDL levels by 9% to 15%.[138,139] However, no studies have been conducted in posttransplant recipients.

In studies on patients with kidney transplant taking CsA, some benefit was shown when reducing triglyceride levels and platelet aggregation.[140] A Cochrane Review showed that fish oils provide a slight improvement in high-density lipoprotein (HDL) cholesterol and diastolic BP in kidney transplant recipients. There appeared to be no harmful effects of taking fish oil, but there was not enough information to show any benefit in preventing heart disease or improving kidney function.[141,142] More studies are needed before regular use of fish oil can be recommended. Compliance with fish oil administration can be difficult, as many patients report "fishy burps" or a lingering bad taste. Clinicians should suggest that patients freeze the capsules, which often eliminates this problem. Prescription n-3 supplements are also available and can be an option for patients.

Hyperhomocysteinemia in posttransplant recipients has been reported, although the exact mechanism is unknown. Elevation of homocysteine levels was thought to be a risk factor for CVD, but there has been no evidence to link reduction in homocysteine levels to reduction in cardiac events or mortality rate.[143,144]

OSTEOPOROSIS

Osteoporosis is a problem for many posttransplant kidney recipients. Long-term corticosteroid therapy results in inhibition of bone formation and high bone turnover. Stimulation of bone resorption also leads to bone loss.[145] Prednisone decreases the intestinal absorption of calci-

um and increases the amount of calcium excreted in the urine, which adds to the loss. Even in patients who are weaned off prednisone, some bone damage may have already occurred.[145] Posttransplant patients are already at risk because of preexisting hyperparathyroidism and abnormalities in vitamin D metabolism. Other factors (eg, cigarette smoking, a sedentary lifestyle, excess alcohol consumption, and chronic diuretic use) also increase osteoporosis risk. For these reasons, a higher level of calcium and vitamin D may be indicated. Patients should consume adequate vitamin D and calcium or include supplements, if needed.

After kidney transplant, PTH function usually returns to normal. In some patients with long-standing kidney failure, the abnormal parathyroid function due to hypertrophied glands has occurred for an extended period and does not return to normal. To protect the transplanted kidney from negative effects that excess PTH may have (eg, kidney stones, decreased function, and effects of hypercalcemia), patients may be referred for parathyroid surgery. Although controversial, posttransplant hypercalcemia due to elevated PTH (tertiary hyperparathyroidism) has been treated with calcimimetics.[146] In addition, this is an off-label use, so therapy may not be a financially viable option for the patient. A moderate dietary calcium intake may be recommended for hypercalcemia, but experts do not know if it is effective in this scenario. If instituted, practitioners should inquire into any OTC supplements containing calcium that the patient may be taking, as well as possible treatment of upper GI complaints with calcium-based antacids.

PHYSICAL ACTIVITY

The Academy of Nutrition and Dietetics Evidence Analysis Library regarding nutrition management of patients with CKD, including post transplant, supports exercise with medical clearance as tolerated. The National Kidney Foundation's A to Z Health Guide offers general advice on physical fitness for kidney transplant recipients. A systematic review of 24 studies of exercise training after kidney transplant was performed. The results showed that in mid-age transplant patients, without major comorbidities, an aerobic or resistance supervised exercise program lasting 3 to 6 months could be suggested within the comprehensive treatment of kidney transplantation.[147] In addition to improved strength and balance, another goal is to lessen the impact of immunosuppressive drugs, such as osteoporosis, hyperglycemia and other issues. Weight bearing and resistance exercise help to maintain bone density and strengthen bones and muscles.[148] The Exercise in Renal Transplant (ExeRT) trial found that both aerobic and resistance training were beneficial in kidney transplant recipients, improving measures, such as VO2 peak, isometric muscle force, and sit-to-stand performance.[149]

OTHER COMORBID AND COMPLICATING ISSUES

As in the general population, each transplant recipient presents with an ever-changing array of issues that may have nutrition implications. Intervention recommendations may range from a temporary liquid diet after dental surgery to various avenues of nutrition support during cancer therapy.

Anemia

Anemia after kidney transplant is more common in recipients over 60 years and those taking certain medications. Compared to White patients, anemia occurs more prevalently in Black patients and is less common in patients with Hispanic ethnicity. Iron supplementation may be clinically warranted in some patients exhibiting indexes of low serum iron. Oral iron supplements may have poor GI absorption. If needed, IV supplementation is an efficient and rapid route for iron repletion. With adequate iron stores present, use of erythropoietin supplement could be approved. If the patient remains nonresponsive, assay of vitamin B12 and folate could indicate need for supplementation.[150,151]

Cancer

A variety of types of cancer may occur after transplantation, each presenting a challenge in dealing with immunosuppressive therapy.[152] Given the prevalence of cancer therapy, collaboration with the RDN and oncology staff is recommended to best meet the needs of the patient and caregivers.

Pregnancy

For women of child-bearing age who have had a kidney transplant and hope to become pregnant, chances are improved as compared to CKD. However, the incidence of complications is increased, including gestational DM and HTN, preeclampsia, and preterm delivery. Pregnancies are usually considered high risk (see Chapter 12).[153,154]

The Academy of Nutrition and Dietetics Evidence Analysis Library guidelines for macronutrient and micronutrient requirements during pregnancy should be used, with consideration of the patient's individual comorbid conditions and laboratory results. Food safety guidelines for pregnant mothers comply with recommendations post transplant. Breastfeeding has been a controversial topic over the years. Many transplant facilities do not recommend breastfeeding due to risk of ongoing exposure to drugs potentially present in breast milk. Some studies have shown minimal transfer and encourage this practice.[155] One study suggested that the potential benefit of immune enhancement through breast milk may be negated for the infant. With the polypharmacy presence in transplant recipients, the potential of each drug's transfer to the infant via breast milk should be evaluated.

Hyperuricemia

Incidence of hyperuricemia increases with CKD and with the use of immunosuppressive drugs post–kidney transplant. Newer medications for gout therapy have become more effective in treating the symptoms. A patient may have interest in nutrition interventions, such as a purine-controlled diet or cherry supplementation. However, weight reduction may be the single most effective lifestyle approach.[156]

Nephrolithiasis

Presence of kidney stones may have been a precipitating factor in the evolution of a patient's CKD or may be occurring de novo in the posttransplant period. Based on a 2016 meta-analysis, the incidence of nephrolithiasis after transplant is approximately 1% with calcium oxalate and calcium phosphate stones being most common, followed by struvite stones and urate stones. Of interest is the possible presence in the allograft when transplanted.[157]

When stone composition is known, appropriate MNT can be recommended to compliment pharmaceutical interventions (see Chapter 14).

Chronic Allograft Nephropathy

The expected duration of a transplanted organ is unknown. The slow, gradual decline in graft function over years may be a result of scarring. Although research is limited, there is evidence that a moderate protein restriction may improve perm-selectivity.[158] With the progression of chronic kidney dysfunction, the guidelines for MNT for CKD could be applied (see Chapter 3).

Summary

Nutrition interventions for the patient with a kidney transplant vary, depending on the phase of transplant, medications prescribed, and the patient's health status. During the acute posttransplantation phase, the goals are to provide adequate calories and protein for wound healing, infection prevention, and normalization of electrolyte imbalance. The goals for the long-term posttransplantation phase are to achieve and maintain ideal BW, manage any nutrition-related condition, and prevent or minimize immunosuppressive adverse effects, particularly obesity, hyperglycemia, dyslipidemia, and bone loss. The RDN is an invaluable member of the transplant health care team and provides MNT to have a positive impact on nutrition-related posttransplant medical outcomes and enhance the transplant recipient's quality of life.

References

1. Goodman W, Danovitch G. Options for patients with kidney failure. In: Danovitch G, ed. *Handbook of Kidney Transplantation.* 4th ed. Lippincott Williams & Wilkins; 2005:19.
2. United Network of Network Sharing: Kidney Paired Donation. September 2020. Accessed September 27, 2020. https://.unos.org/transplant/kidney-paired -donation
3. Organ Procurement and Transplantation Network: Data Reports. September 2020. Accessed September 20, 2020. https://.optn.transplant.hrsa .gov/data/view-data-reports/national-data/#
4. Sabbatini M, Ferreri L, Pisani A, et al. Nutrition management in renal transplant recipients: a transplant team opportunity to improve graft survival. *Nutr Metab Cardiovasc Dis.* 2019;29(4):319-324. doi:10.1016/j.numedc.2019.01.002
5. Hasse JH, Matarese LE. Solid organ transplantation. In: Mueller CM, Lord LM, Marian M, McClave S, Millar S, eds. *The A.S.P.E.N. Nutrition Support Core Curriculum.* 3rd ed. American Society for Parenteral and Enteral Nutrition; 2017:603-618.
6. Kent PS. Transplantation. In: Byham-Gray LD, Burrowes JD, Chertow GM, eds. *Nutrition and Kidney Disease.* Humana Press; 2008:263-286.
7. Fazelzadeh A, Mehdizadeh A, Ostovan M, Raiss-Jalali G. Predictors of cardiovascular events and associated mortality of kidney transplant recipients. *Transplant Proc.* 2006;38(2):509-511. doi:10.1016/j .transproceed.2006.02.004
8. Sezer S, Bilgic A, Uyar M, Arat Z, Ozdemir F, Haberal M. Risk factors for development of posttransplant diabetes mellitus in renal transplant recipients. *Transplant Proc.* 2006;38(2):529-532. doi:10.1016/j .transproceed.2005.12.066
9. Fried LP, Tangen CM, Walston J, et al. Frailty in older adults: evidence for a phenotype. *J Gerontol A Biol Sci Med Sci.* 2001;56(3):46-56. doi:10.1093/Gerona /56/3/m146
10. Haugen CE, Chu NM, Ying H, et al. Frailty and access to kidney transplantation. *Clin J Am Soc Nephrol.* 2019;14(4):576-582. doi:10.2215/CJN.12921118
11. McAdams-DeMarco MA, Ying H, Olorundare I, et al. Individual frailty components and mortality in kidney transplant recipients. *Transplantation.* 2017;101(9):2126-2132. doi:10.101097 /TP0000000000001546
12. Alfaadhel TA, Soroka SD, Kiberd BA, Landry D, Moorhouse P, Tennankore K. Frailty and mortality in dialysis: evaluation of a clinic frailty scale. *Clin J Am Soc Nephrol.* 2015;10(5):832-840. doi:10.2215/CJN .07760814

13. McAdams-DeMarco MA, King EA, Luo X, et al. Frailty, length of stay, and mortality in kidney transplant recipients: a national registry and prospective cohort study. *Ann Surg.* 2017;266(6):1084-1090. doi:10.1097/SLA.0000000000002025

14. McAdams-DeMarco MA, Law A, Salter ML, et al. Frailty and early hospital readmission after kidney transplantation. *Am J Transplant.* 2013;13:2091-2095. doi:10.1002/ajt.12300

15. Armstrong K, Campbell S, Hawley C, Johnson D, Isbel N. Impact of obesity on renal transplant outcomes. *Nephrology.* 2005;10(4):405-413. doi:10.1111/j.1440-1797.2005.00406.x

16. Hasse J. Pretransplant obesity: a weighty issue affecting transplant candidacy and outcomes. *Nutr Clin Pract.* 2007;5:494-504. doi:10.1177/0115426507022005494

17. Streja E, Molnar MZ, Kovesdy CP, et al. Associations of pretransplant weight and muscle mass with mortality in renal transplant recipients. *Clin J Am Soc Nephrol.* 2011;6(6):1463-1473. doi:10.2215/CJN.09131010

18. Postorino M, Marino C, Tripepi G, et al. Abdominal obesity and all-cause and cardiovascular mortality in end-stage renal disease. *J Am Coll Cardiol.* 2009;53(15):1265-1272. doi:10.1016/j.jacc.2008.12.040

19. Orazio L, Armstrong K, Banks M, Johnson D, Isbel N, Hickman I. Central obesity is common in renal transplant recipients and is associated with increased prevalence of cardiovascular risk factors. *J Nutr Diet.* 2007;64(3):200-206. doi:10.1111/j.1747-0080.2007.00151.x

20. Stein J, Stier C, Raab H, Weiner R. Review article: the nutritional and pharmacological consequences of obesity surgery. *Aliment Pharmacol Ther.* 2014;40(6):582-609. doi:10.1111/apt.12872

21. Rettkowski O, Weinke A, Hamza A, Osten B, Fornara P. Low body mass index in kidney transplant recipients: risk for long-term graft function? *Transplant Proc.* 2007;39(5):1416-1420. doi:10.1016/j.transproceed.2006.11.031

22. Guichard S. Nutrition in the kidney transplant recipient. In: Danovitch G, ed. *Handbook of Kidney Transplantation.* 4th ed. Lippincott Williams & Wilkins; 2005:475-494.

23. Kaufman D. Kidney Transplantation. In: Stuart F, Abecaiss M, Kaufman D, eds. *Organ Transplantation.* 2nd ed. Landes Bioscience; 2003:138-143.

24. Leichtman A. Balancing efficacy and toxicity in kidney-transplant immunosuppression. *N Engl J Med.* 2007;357(25):2625-2627. doi:10.1056/NEJMe078181

25. Danovitch G. Immunosuppressive medications and protocols for kidney transplantation. In: Danovitch G, ed. *Handbook of Kidney Transplantation.* 4th ed. Lippincott Williams & Wilkins; 2005:72-110.

26. The Academy of Nutrition and Dietetics Evidence Analysis Library. EAL-KDOQI (CKD) Guideline: 2020. November 2020. Accessed November 1, 2020. www.andeal.org/topic.cfm?menu=5303&cat=5557

27. Rajab A, Pelletier RP, Henry ML, Ferguson RM. Excellent clinical outcomes in primary kidney transplant recipients treated with steroid-free maintenance immunosuppression. *Clin Transplant.* 2006;20(5):537-546. doi:10.1111/j.1399-0012.2006.00521.x

28. Matas AJ. Minimization of steroids in kidney transplantation. *Transpl Int.* 2009;22(1):38-48. doi:10.1111/j.1432-2277.2008.00728.x

29. Pirsch J, Simmons W, Sollinger H. Appendix I. In: Stuart F, Abecaiss M, Kaufman D, eds. *Organ Transplantation.* 2nd ed. Landes Bioscience; 2003:589-612.

30. Seagraves A, Moore EE, Moore FA, Weil R III. Net protein catabolic rate after kidney transplantation: impact of corticosteroid immunosuppression. *JPEN J Parenter Enteral Nutr.* 1986;10(5):453-455. doi:10.1177/0148607186010005453

31. Blue LS. Adult Kidney Transplantation. In: Hasse JM, Blue LS, eds. *Comprehensive Guide to Transplant Nutrition.* American Dietetic Association; 2002:49.

32. McCann L. Transplantation. In: Special populations with chronic kidney disease. In: *Pocket Guide to Nutrition Assessment of the Patient With Kidney Disease.* 6th ed. National Kidney Foundation; 2021:11-48–11-54.

33. Teplan V, Valkovsky I, Teplan V Jr, Stollova M, Vyhnanek F, Andel M. Nutritional consequences of renal transplantation. *J Ren Nutr.* 2009;19(1):95-100. doi:10.1053/j.jrn.2008.10.017

34. Vincenti F, Jensik S, Filo R, Miller J, Pirsch J. A long-term comparison of tacrolimus (FK506) and cyclosporine in kidney transplantation: evidence for improved allograft survival at five years. *Transplantation.* 2002;73(5):775-782. doi:10.1097/00007890-200203150-00021

35. Davidson J, Wilkinson A. New-onset diabetes after transplantation 2003 international consensus guidelines. *Diabetes Care.* 2004;27(3):805-812. doi:10.2337/diacare.27.3.805

36. Leventhal J, Schlueter W. Early medical problems common to many recipients. In: Stuart F, Abecassis M, Kaufman D, eds. *Organ Transplantation.* 2nd ed. Landes Bioscience; 2003:426-436.

37. Horn J, Hansten P. Trimethoprim and potassium-sparing drugs: a risk for hyperkalemia. *Pharmacy Times.* February 2011. Accessed August 20, 2020. www.pharmacytimes.com/publications/issue/2011/February2011/DrugInteractions-0211

38. Christie E, Okel J, Gowrishankar M. Hyperkalemia in the early post transplant period. *Transplantation.* 2018;102:S597. doi:10.1097/01.tp.0000543485.27703.d0

39. Farina N, Anderson C. Impact of dextrose dose on hypoglycemia development following treatment of hyperkalemia. *Ther Adv Drug Saf.* 2018;9(6):323-329. doi:10.1177/2042098618768725

40. Courbebaisse M, Thervet E, Souberbielle JC, et al. Effects of vitamin D supplementation on the calcium-phosphate balance in renal transplant patients. *Kidney Int.* 2009;75(6):646-651. doi:10.1038/ki.2008.549

41. Ebeling P. Approach to the patient with transplantation-related bone loss. *J Clin Endocrinol Metab.* 2009;94(5):1483-1490. doi:10.1210/jc.2009-0205

42. Winkelmayer WC, Kewalramani R, Rutstein M, Gabardi S, Vonvisger T, Chandraker A. Pharmacoepidemiology of anemia in kidney transplant recipients. *J Am Soc Nephrol.* 2004;15(5):1347-1352. doi:10.1097/01.asn.0000125551.59739.2e

43. Mahajan SK, Prasad AS, Rabbani P, Briggs WA, McDonald FD. Zinc deficiency: a reversible complication of uremia. *Am J Clin Nutr.* 1982;36(6):1177-1183. doi:10.1093/ajcn/36.6.1177

44. Allen D, Bell J. Herbal medicine and the transplant patient. *Nephrol Nurs J.* 2002;29(3):269-274.

45. Colson CR, DeBroe ME. Kidney injury from alternative medicines. *Adv Chron Kidney Dis.* 2005;12(3):261-275. doi:10.1016/j.ackd.2005.03.006

46. Brown AC. Herb and dietary supplements related to kidney toxicity case reports in PubMed. *Renal Nutrition Forum.* 2017;36(4):7-16.

47. Qiu F, Hou XL, Takahashi K, Chen LX, Azuma J, Kang N. Andrographolide inhibits the expression and metabolic activity of cytochrome P450 3A4 in the modified Caco-2 cells. *J Ethnopharmacol.* 2012;141(2):709-713. doi:10.1016/j.jep.2011.09.002

48. Zhang WX, Zhang ZM, Zhang ZQ, Wang Y, Zhou W. Andrographolide induced acute kidney injury: analysis of 26 cases reported in Chinese Literature. *Nephrology (Carlton).* 2014;19(1):21-26. doi:10.1111/nep.12172

49. Lau C, Mooiman KD, Maas-Bakker RF, Beijnen JH, Schellens JH, Meijerman I. Effect of Chinese herbs on CYP3A4 activity and expression in vitro. *J Ethnopharmacol.* 2013;149(2):543-549. doi:10.1016/j.jep.2013.07.014

50. National Library of Medicine. Pub Med. National Institute of Health website. Accessed January 2018. June 4, 2018. www.ncbi.nlm.nih.gov/pubmed

51. National Center for Complimentary and Integrative Health. National Institute of Health website. September 2019. Accessed June 4, 2018. https://.nccih.nih.gov

52. Guo Y, Chen Y, Tan ZR, Klaassen CD, Zhou HH. Repeated administration of berberine inhibits cytochromes P450 in humans. *Eur J Clin Pharmacol.* 2012;68(2):213-217. doi:10.1007/s00228-011-1108-2

53. Li Z, Geng YN, Jiang JD, Kong WJ. Antioxidant and anti-inflammatory activities of berberine in the treatment of diabetes mellitus. *Evid Based Complement Alternat Med.* 2014;2014:289264. doi:10.1155/2014/289264

54. Nowack, R. Review Article: Cytochrome P450 enzyme, and transport protein mediated herb-drug interactions in renal transplant patients: grapefruit juice, St John's Wort – and beyond! *Nephrology (Carlton).* 2008;13(4):337-347. doi:10.1111/j.1440-1797.2008.00940.x

55. Vitamin & Supplement Center. Web MD website. January 2020. Accessed June 4, 2020. www.webmd.com/vitamins/index

56. He K, Iyer KR, Hayes RN, Sinz MW, Woolf TF, Hollenberg PF. Inactivation of cytochrome P450 3A4 by bergamottin, a component of grapefruit juice. *Chem Res Toxicol.* 1998;11(4):252-259. doi:10.1021/tx970192k

57. Hsu PW, Shia CS, Lin SP, Chao PD, Juang SH, Hou YC. Potential risk of mulberry-drug interaction: modulation on P-glycoprotein and cytochrome P450 3A. *J Agric Food Chem.* 2013;61(18):4464-4469. doi:10.1021/jf3052384

58. Kim H, Yoon YJ, Shon JH, Cha IJ, Shin JG, Liu KH. Inhibitory effects of fruit juices on CYP3A activity. *Drug Metab Dispos.* 2006;34(4):521-523. doi:10.1124/dmd.105.007930

59. Dreiseitel A, Schreier P, Oehme A, Locher S, Hajak G, Sand PG. Anthocyanins and their metabolites are weak inhibitors of cytochrome P450 3A4. *Mol Nutr Food Res.* 2008;52(12):1428-1433. doi:10.1002/mnfr.200800043

60. Zhang JW, Liu Y, Cheng J, et al. Inhibition of human liver cytochrome P450 by star fruit juice. *J Pharm Pharm Sci.* 2007;10(4):496-503. doi:10.18433/j30593

61. Ganzera M, Schneider P, Stuppner H. Inhibitory effects of the essential oil of chamomile (Matricaria recutita L.) and its major constituents on human cytochrome P450 enzymes. *Life Sci.* 2006;78(8):856-861. doi:10.1016/j.lfs.2005.05.095

62. Izzo AA. Interactions between herbs and conventional drugs: overview of the clinical data. *Med Princ Pract.* 2012;21(5):404-428. doi:10.1159/000334488

63. Dufay S, Worsley A, Monteillier A, et al. Herbal tea extracts inhibit Cytochrome P450 3A4 in vitro. *J Pharm Pharmacol.* 2014;66(10):1478-1490. doi:10.1111/jphp.12270

64. Srinivas NR. Cranberry juice ingestion and clinical drug-drug interaction potentials; review of case studies and perspectives. *J Pharm Pharm Sci.* 2013;16(2):289-303. doi:10.18433/j3ng6z

65. Stargrove MB, Treasure J, McKee DL. *Herb, Nutrient and Drug Interactions: Clinical Implications and Therapeutic Strategies.* Mosby/Elsevier. 2008.

66. Wanwimolruk S, Phopin K, Prachayasittikul V. Cytochrome P450 enzyme mediated herbal drug interactions (Part 2). *EXCLI J.* 2014;13:869-896.

67. Wanwimolruk S, Prachayasittikul V. Cytochrome P450 enzyme mediated herbal drug interactions (Part 1). *EXCLI J.* 2014;13:347-391.

68. Sprouse AA, van Breemen RB. Pharmacokinetic interactions between drugs and botanical dietary supplements. *Drug Metab Dispos.* 2016;44(2):162-171. doi:10.1124/dmd.115.066902

69. Roschek Jr B, Fink RC, McMichael MD, Li D, Alberte RS. Elderberry flavonoids bind to and prevent H1N1 infection in vitro. *Phytochemistry.* 2009;70(10):1255-1261. doi:10.1016/j.phytochem.2009.06.003

70. Srikumar R, Parthasarathy NJ, Manikandan S, Narayanan GS, Sheeladevi R. Effect of Triphala on oxidative stress and on cell-mediated immune response against noise stress in rats. *Mol Cell Biochem.* 2006;283(1-2):67-74. doi:10.1007/s11010-006-2271-0

71. Sabu MC, Kuttan R. Anti-diabetic activity of medicinal plants and its relationship with their antioxidant property. *J Ethnopharmacol.* 2002;81(2):155-160. doi:10.1016/s0378-8741(02)00034-x

72. Ueng YF, Don MJ, Jan WC, Wang SY, Ho LK, Chen CF. Oxidative metabolism of the alkaloid rutaecarpine by human cytochrome P450. *Drug Metab Dispos.* 2006;34(5):821-827. doi:10.1124/dmd.105.007849

73. Li M, Chen PZ, Yue QX, et al. Pungent ginger components modulates human cytochrome P450 enzymes in vitro. *Acta Pharmacol Sin.* 2013;34(9):1237-1242. doi:10.1038/aps.2013.49

74. Malati CY, Robertson SM, Hunt JD, et al. Influence of Panax ginseng on cytochrome P450 (CYP)3A and P-glycoprotein (P-gp) activity in healthy subjects. *J Clin Pharmacol.* 2012;52(6):932-939. doi:10.1177/0091270011407194

75. Kang S, Min H. Ginseng, the 'Immunity Boost': The effects of Panax ginseng on immune system. *J Ginseng Res.* 2012;36(4):354-368. doi:10.5142/jgr.2012.36.4.354

76. Bailey DG, Malcolm J, Arnold O, Spence JD. Grapefruit juice-drug interactions. *Br J Clin Pharmacol.* 1998;46(2):101-110. doi:10.1046/j.1365-2125.1998.00764.x

77. Satoh T, Fujisawa H, Nakamura A, Takahashi N, Watanabe K. Inhibitory effects of eight green tea catechins on Cytochrome P450 1A2, 2C9, 2D6, and 3A4 activities. *J Pharm Pharm Sci.* 2016;19(2):188-197. doi:10.18433/J3MS5C

78. Kim YH, Won YS, Yang X, et al. Green tea catechin metabolites exert immunoregulatory effects on CD4(+) T cell and natural killer cell activities. *J Agric Food Chem.* 2016;64(18):3591-3597. doi:10.1021/acs.jafc.6b01115

79. Brobst DE, Ding X, Creech KL, Goodwin B, Kelley B, Staudinger JL. Guggulsterone activates multiple nuclear receptors and induces CYP3A gene expression through the pregnane X receptor. *J Pharmacol Exp Ther.* 2004;310(2):528-535. doi:10.1124/jpet.103.064329

80. Hardeland R. Aging, melatonin and the pro- and anti-inflammatory networks. *Int J Mol Sci.* 2019;20(5):1223. doi:10.3390/ijms20051223

81. Bhardwaj RK, Glaeser H, Becquemont L, Klotz U, Gupta SK, Fromm MF. Piperine, a major constituent of black pepper, inhibits human P-glycoprotein and CYP3A4. *J Pharmacol Exp Ther.* 2002;302(2):645-650. doi:10.1124/jpet.102.034728

82. Elbarbry F, Ung A, Abdelkawy K. Studying the inhibitory effect of quercetin and thymoquinone on the human cytochrome P450 enzyme activities. *Pharmacogn Mag.* 2018;13(suppl 4):S895-S899. doi:10.4103/0973-1296.224342

83. Markowitz JS, Donovan JL, Devane CL, et al. Multiple doses of saw palmetto (Serenoa repens) did not alter cytochrome P450 2D6 and 3A4 activity in normal volunteers. *Clin Pharmacol Ther.* 2003;74(6):536-542. doi:10.1016/j.clpt.2003.08.010

84. The Coca Cola Company. Product Information. Coca Cola Company USA web site. January 2020. Accessed June 4, 2020. www.coca-colaproductfacts.com/en/home-page

85. Chauhan B, Yu C, Krantis A, et al. In vitro activity of uva-ursi against cytochrome P450 isoenzymes and P-glycoprotein. *Can J Physiol Pharmacol.* 2007;85(11):1099-1107. doi:10.1139/Y07-106

86. Donovan JL, DeVane CL, Chavin KD, et al. Multiple night-time doses of valerian (Valeriana officinalis) had minimal effects on CYP3A4 activity and no effect on CYP2D6 activity in healthy volunteers. *Drug Metab Dispos.* 2004;32(12):1333-1336. doi:10.1124/dmd.104.001164

87. Annual Report of the U.S. Organ Procurement and Transplantation Network and the Scientific Registry of Transplant Recipients: Transplant Data 1996-2005. Scientific Registry of Transplant Recipients website. January 2020. Accessed August 17, 2020. www.srtr.org/reports-tools/srtroptn-annual-data-report

88. Crutchlow MF, Bloom RD. Transplant-associated hyperglycemia: a new look at an old problem. *Clin J Am Soc Nephrol.* 2007;2(2):343-355. doi:10.2215/CJN.03671106

89. Haririan A, Sillix DH, Morawski K, et al. Short-term experience with early steroid withdrawal in African-American renal transplant recipients. *Am J Transplant.* 2006;6:2396-2402. doi:10.1111/j.1600-6143.2006.01477.x

90. Kasiske BL, Snyder JJ, Gilbertson D, Matas AJ. Diabetes mellitus after kidney transplantation in the United States. *Am J Transplant.* 2003;3(2):178-185. doi:10.1034/j.1600-6143.2003.00010.x

91. Pastors JG, Franz MJ, Warshaw H, Daly A, Arnold M. How effective is medical nutrition therapy in diabetes care? *J Am Diet Assoc.* 2003;103(7):827-831. doi:10.1016/s0002-8223(03)00466-8

92. Pastors JG, Warshaw H, Daly A, Franz M, Kulkarni K. The evidence for the effectiveness of medical nutrition therapy in diabetes management. *Diabetes Care.* 2002;25(3):608-613. doi:10.2337/diacare.25.3.608

93. Wilcox J, Waite C, Tomlinson L, Driscoll J, Karim A, Day E, Sharif A. Comparing glycaemic benefits of Active Versus passive lifestyle Intervention in kidney Allograft Recipients (CAVIAR): study protocol for a randomised controlled trial. *Trials.* 2016;17(1):417. doi:10.1186/s13063-016-1543-6

94. Helderman JH, Goral S. Gastrointestinal complications of transplant immunosuppression. *J Am Soc Nephrol.* 2002;13(1):277-287.

95. Ponticelli C, Passerini P. Gastrointestinal complications in renal transplant recipients. *Transpl Int.* 2005;18(6):643-650. doi:10.1111/j.1432-2277.2005.00134.x

96. Bardaxoglou E, Maddern G, Ruso L, et al. GI surgical emergencies following kidney transplantation. *Transpl Int.* 1993;6(3):148-152. doi:10.1007/BF00336358

97. Mosimann F, Cuenoud PF, Steinhauslin F, Wauters JP. Herpes simplex esophagitis after renal transplantation. *Transpl Int.* 1994;7(2):79-82. doi:10.1007/BF00336466

98. Schmidt A, Oberbauer R. Bacterial and fungal infections after kidney transplantation. *Curr Opin Urol.* 1999;9(1):45-49. doi:10.1097/00042307-199901000-00008

99. Özgür O, Boyacioğlu D, Özdoğan M, Gür G, Telatar H, Haberal M. Helicobacter pylori infection in haemodialysis patients and renal transplant recipients. *Nephrol Dial Transplant.* 1997;12(2):289-291. doi:10.1093/ndt/12.2.289

100. Troppman C, Papalois BE, Chiou A, et al. Incidence, complications, treatment and outcome of ulcers of the upper gastrointestinal tract after renal transplantation during the cyclosporine era. *J Am Coll Surg.* 1995;180(4):433-443.

101. Logan A, Morris-Stiff G, Bowrey D, Jurewicz W. Upper gastrointestinal complications after renal transplantation: a 3-yr sequential study. *Clin Transplant.* 2002;16(3):163-167. doi:10.1034/j.1399-0012.2002.01012.x

102. Misselwitz B, Butter M, Verbeke K, Fox MR. Update on lactose malabsorption and intolerance: pathogenesis, diagnosis and clinical management. *Gut.* 2019;68(11):2080-2091. doi:10.1136/gutjnl-2019-318404

103. Szilagyi A, Ishayek N. Lactose intolerance, dairy avoidance, and treatment options. *Nutrients.* 2018;10(12):1994. doi:10.3390/nu10121994

104. Torres A, Lorenzo V, Salido E. Calcium metabolism and skeletal problems after transplantation. *J Am Soc Nephrol.* 2002;13(2):551-558.

105. *Drug Facts and Comparisons 2017.* Lippincott Williams & Wilkins; 2017.

106. Beto J, Bansal VK. Hyperkalemia: evaluating dietary and nondietary etiology. *J Ren Nutr.* 1992;2(1):28-29.

107. United States Department of Agriculture. Foodborne Illness and Disease. November 2020. Accessed November 29, 2020. www.fsis.usda.gov/wps/portal/fsis/topics/food-safety-education/get-answers/food-safety-fact-sheets/foodborne-illness-and-disease

108. US Food and Drug Administration. Center for Food Safety and Applied Nutrition. Foodborne Pathogenic Microorganisms and Natural Toxins Handbook. *Bad Bug Book.* 2nd ed. June 2012. Accessed March 15, 2019. www.fda.gov/files/food/published/Bad-Bug-Book-2nd-Edition-%28PDF%29.pdf

109. Hollander A, Van Rooij J, Lentjes E, et al. The effect of grapefruit juice on cyclosporine and prednisone metabolism in transplant patients. *Clin Pharmacol Ther.* 1995;57(3):318-324. doi:10.1016/0009-9236(95)90157-4

110. Bailey DG, Malcolm J, Arnold O, et al. The effect of grapefruit juice on cyclosporine and prednisone metabolism in transplant patients. *Br J Clin Pharm.* 1998;46:101-110.

111. Kim H, Yoon YJ, Shon JH, Cha IJ, Shin JG, Liu KH. Inhibitory effects of fruit juices on CYP3A activity. *Drug Metab Dispos.* 2006;34(4):521-523. doi:10.1124/dmd.105.007930

112. Sorokin AV, Duncan B, Panetta R, Thompson P. Rhabdomyolysis associated with pomegranate juice consumption. *Am J Cardiol.* 2006;98(5):705-706. doi:10.1016/j.amjcard.2006.03.057

113. Auten AA, Beauchamp LN, Taylor J, Hardinger KL. Hidden sources of grapefruit in beverages: potential interactions with immunosuppressant medications. *Hosp Pharm.* 2013;48(6):489-493. doi:10.1310/hpj4806-489

114. Blue LS. Nutrition considerations in kidney transplantation. *Top Clin Nutr.* 1992;7(3):7-23.

115. Hasse JM. Recovery after organ transplantation in adults the role of postoperative nutrition therapy. *Top Clin Nutr.* 1998;13:15-26.

116. The Academy of Nutrition and Dietetics Evidence Analysis Library. Chronic Kidney Disease Guidelines: CKD Energy Intake. November 2019. Accessed September 15, 2020. http://.andevidencelibrary.com/template.cfm?template=guide_summary&key=2410

117. Lopes IM, Martin M, Errasti P, Martinez JA. Benefits of a dietary intervention on weight loss, body composition and lipid profile after renal transplantation. *Nutrition.* 1999;15(1):7-10. doi:10.1016/s0899-9007(98)00137-3

118. Parikh CR, Klem P, Wong C, Yalavarthy R, Chan L. Obesity as an independent predictor of post-transplant diabetes mellitus. *Transplant Proc.* 2003;35(8):2922-2926. doi:10.1016/j.transproceed.2003.10.074

119. Clunk J, Lin C, Curtis J. Variables affecting weight gain in renal transplant recipients. *Am J Kidney Dis.* 2001;38(2):349-353. doi:10.1053/ajkd.2001.26100

120. Patel MG. The effect of dietary intervention on weight gains after renal transplantation. *J Ren Nutr.* 1998;8(3):137-141. doi:10.1016/s1051-2276(98)90005-x

121. Hines L. Can low fat/cholesterol nutrition counseling improve food intake habits and hyperlipidemia of renal transplant patients? *J Ren Nutr.* 2000;10(1):30-35. doi:10.1016/s1051-2276(00)90020-7

122. Cosio FG, Pesavento TE, Kim S, Osei K, Henry M, Ferguson R. Patient survival after renal transplantation: IV. impact of posttransplant diabetes. *Kidney Int.* 2002;62(4):1440-1446. doi:10.1111/j.1523-1755.2002.kid582.x

123. Jarieoo MS. Post-transplant diabetes: incidence, relationship to choice of immunosuppressive drugs and treatment protocol. *Adv Ren Replace Ther.* 2001;8(1):64-69. doi:10.1053/jarr.2001.21703

124. Basri N, Aman H, Adiku W, Baraqdar A, Bonatero I, Nezamuddin N. Diabetes mellitus after renal transplantation. *Transplant Proc.* 1992;24(5):1780-1781.

125. Shivaswamy V, Boerner B, Larsen J. Post-transplant diabetes mellitus: causes, treatment, and impact on outcomes. *Endocr Rev.* 2016;37(1):37-61. doi:10.1210/er.2015-1084

126. Hasse JM. Diet therapy for organ transplantation. *Nurs Clin North Am.* 1997;32(4):863-880.

127. Baron P, Waymack JP. A review of nutrition support for transplant patients. *Nutr Clin Pract.* 1999;8(1):12-18. doi:10.1177/011542659300800112

128. American Diabetes Association. Standards of medical care in diabetes—2007. *Diabetes Care.* 2007;30(suppl1):S4-S41. doi:10.2337/dc07-S004

129. Chakkera HA, Weil EJ, Pham PT, Pomeroy J, Knowler WC. Can new-onset diabetes after kidney transplant be prevented? *Diabetes Care.* 2013;36(5):1406-2067. doi:10.2337/dc12-2067

130. Kobashigawa JA, Kasiske BL. Hyperlipidemia in solid organ transplantation. *Transplantation.* 1997;63(3):331-338.

131. Hricik ED. Hyperlipidemia in renal transplant recipients. *Graft.* 2000;4:11-19.

132. Ojo AO, Hanson JA, Wolfe RA, Leichtman AB, Agodoa LY, Port FK. Long-term survival in renal transplant recipients with graft function. *Kidney Int.* 2000;57(1):307-313. doi:10.1046/j.1523-1755.2000.00816.x

133. Van Horn L, Liu K, Gerber J, et al. Oats and soy in lipid-lowering diets for women with hypercholesterolemia: is there synergy? *J Am Diet Assoc.* 2001;101(11):1319-1325. doi:10.1016/s0002-8223(01)00317-0

134. Brown L, Rosner B, Willett WW, Sacks FM. Cholesterol-lowering effects of dietary fiber: a meta-analysis. *Am J Clin Nutr.* 1999;69(1):30-42. doi:10.1093/ajcn/69.1.30

135. Kris-Etherton PM, Zhao G, Binkoski AE, Coval SM, Etherton TD. The effects of nuts on coronary heart disease risk. *Nutr Rev.* 2001;59(4):103-111. doi:10.1111/j.1753-4887.2001.tb06996.x

136. Lovejoy JC, Most MM, Lefevre M, Greenway FL, Rood JC. Effect of diets enriched in almonds on insulin action and serum lipids in adults with normal glucose tolerance or type 2 diabetes. *Am J Clin Nutr.* 2002;76(5):1000-1006. doi:10.1093/ajcn/76.5.1000

137. Christiansen LI, Lahteenmaki PLA, Mannelin MR, Seppanen-Laakso TE, Hiltunen RV, Yliruusi JK. Cholesterol-lowering effect of spreads enriched with microcrystalline plant sterols in hypercholesterolemic subjects. *Eur J Nutr.* 2001;40(2):66-73. doi:10.1007/s003940170017

138. Tikkanen MJ, Hogstrom P, Tuomilehto J, Keinanen-Kiukaanniemi S, Sundvall J, Karppanen H. Effect of a diet based on low-fat foods enriched with nonesterified plant sterols and mineral nutrients on serum cholesterol. *Am J Cardiol.* 2001;88(10):1157-1162. doi:10.1016/s0002-9149(01)02053-7

139. Van der Heide JJ, Bilo HJ, Donker JM, Wilmink JM, Tegzess AM. Effect of dietary fish oil on renal function and rejection in cyclosporine-treated recipients of renal transplants. *N Engl J Med.* 1993;329(11):769-773. doi:10.1056/NEJM199309093291105

140. Lim AK, Manley KJ, Roberts MA, Fraenkel MB. Fish oil for kidney transplant recipients. *Cochrane Database Syst Rev.* 2007;18(2):CD005282. doi:10.1002/14651858.CD005282.pub2

141. Lindeman RD, Romero LJ, Yau CL, Koehler KM, Baumgartner RN, Garry PJ. Serum homocysteine concentrations and their relation to serum folate and vitamin B12 concentrations and coronary artery disease prevalence in an urban, bi-ethnic community. *Ethn Dis.* 2003;13(2):178-185.

142. Lim AKH, Manley KJ, Roberts MA, Fraenkel MB. Fish oil for kidney transplant recipients. *Cochrane Database Syst Rev.* 2007;18(2): CD005282. doi:10.1002/14651858.CD005282.pub2

143. Schnyder G, Roffi M, Flammer Y, Pin R, Hess OM. Effect of homocysteine-lowering therapy with folic acid, vitamin B12, and vitamin B6 on clinical outcome after percutaneous coronary intervention: the Swiss Heart study: a randomized control trial. *JAMA.* 2002;288(8):973-979. doi:10.1001/jama.288.8.973

144. Massari PU. Disorders of bone and mineral metabolism after renal transplantation. *Kidney Int.* 1997;52(5):1412-1421. doi:10.1038/ki.1997.469

145. Epstein S, Shane E, Bilezikian JP. Organ transplantation and osteoporosis. *Rheumatology.* 1995;7:255-261.

146. Henschkowski J, Bischoff-Ferrari HA, Wuthrich RP, Serra AL. Renal function in patients treated with cinacalcet for persistent hyperparathyroidism after kidney transplantation. *Kidney Blood Press Res.* 2011;34(2):97-103. doi:10.1159/000323902

147. Greenwood SA, Koufaki P, Mercer TH, et al. Aerobic or resistance training and pulse wave velocity in kidney transplant recipients: a 12-week pilot randomized controlled trial (the Exercise in Renal Transplant [ExeRT] Trial). *Am J Kidney Dis.* 2015;66(4):689-698. doi:10.1053/j.ajkd.2015.06.016

148. Walker M, Wells CL. Side effects of immunosuppressant medications as they affect physical fitness: a physical therapist's point of view. National Kidney Foundation website. Accessed October 16, 2020. www.kidney.org/atoz/content/sideeffects

149. Calella P, Hernandez-Sanchez S, Garofalo C, Ruiz J, Carrero J, Bellizzi V. Exercise training in kidney transplant recipients: a systematic review. *J Nephrol.* 2019;32(4):567-579. doi:10.1007/s40620-019-00583

150. Chang Y, Shah T, Min DI, Yang JW. Clinical risk factors with the post-transplant anemia in kidney transplant recipients. *Transpl Immunol.* 2016;38:50-53. doi:10.1016/j.trim.2016.07.006

151. Kamar N, Rostaing L, Ignace S, Villar E. Impact of post-transplant anemia on patient and graft survival rates after kidney transplantation: a meta-analysis. *Clin Transplant.* 2012;26(3):461-469. doi:10.1111/j.1399-0012.2011.01545.x

152. Cheung CY, Tang SCW. An update on cancer after kidney transplant. *Nephrol Dial Transplant.* 2019;34(6):914-920. doi:10.1093/ndt/gfy262

153. Deshpande NA, James NT, Cucirka LM, et al. Pregnancy outcomes in kidney transplant recipients: a systematic review and meta-analysis. *Am J Transplant.* 2011;11(11):2388-2404. doi:10.1111/j.1600-6143.2011.03656.x

154. Yoshikawa Y, Uchida J, Akazawa C, Suganuma N. Perspective on pregnancy counseling for kidney transplant recipients. *Transplantation.* 2018;102:S70. doi:10.1097/01.tp.0000542648.56866.24

155. Bramham K, Chusney G, Lee J, et al. Breastfeeding and tacrolimus: serial monitoring in breast-fed and bottle-fed infants. *Clin J Am Soc Nephrol.* 2013;8(4):563-567. doi:10.2215/CJN.06400612

156. Effective Health Care Program. Management of gout. Comparative Review #176. November 2016. Accessed September 17, 2020. https://.effectivehealthcare.ahrq.gov/sites/default/files/related_files/gout_executive.pdf

157. Cheungpasitporn W, Thongprayoon C, Mao M, et al. Incidence of kidney stones in kidney transplant recipients: a systematic review and meta-analysis. *World J Transplant.* 2016; 6(4):790-797. doi:10.5500/wjt.v6.i4.790

158. Chadban S, Chan M, Fry K, et al. Protein requirement in adult kidney transplant recipients. *Nephrol.* 2010;15:568-571. doi:10.1111/j.1440-1797.2010.01238.x

Other Conditions and Special Populations With Kidney Disease

CHAPTER 9

Nutrition Management of Diabetes in Chronic Kidney Disease

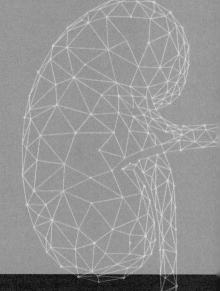

Sharon R. Schatz, MS, RD, CSR, CDCES, Pamela S. Kent, MS, RD, CDCES, LD, and Victor Yu, PhD, RD, BC-ADM

Introduction

Managing diabetes mellitus (DM) is critical to the prevention of its related complications, especially kidney and cardiovascular disease (CVD), as they all impact one another. Medical nutrition therapy (MNT) is part of a multidimensional approach in DM treatment that can delay or prevent the progression of chronic kidney disease (CKD) from reaching the need for kidney replacement therapy (KRT). Individuals who reach CKD stage 5 due to DM have the poorest outcomes, worse rehabilitation potential, greater hospitalization rates, and more costly medical expenses.[1-3] The presence of both DM and CVD with CKD is associated with a higher death risk, although having DM alone does not increase the mortality risk.[4] Due to the complexity of DM in CKD, the registered dietitian nutritionist (RDN) needs a thorough understanding of DM-related complications, the management of such complex situations, and their cross interactions to provide comprehensive nutritional care.

DM is the most common etiology for patients with CKD, and it is the reported leading cause of end-stage kidney disease (ESKD) cases in the United States.[3,5] In 2017, DM was the primary cause of ESKD in 46.9% of incident patients, while only 38.6% of prevalent patients with ESKD had DM as the primary cause of kidney failure.[3] The discrepancy in the rates of total incidence vs total prevalence could be attributed to a lower survival rate in patients with DM. In these incident patients with DM, KRT was as follows: 89.7% hemodialysis (HD), 9.5% peritoneal dialysis (PD), and 0.8% kidney transplantation.[3] The rates of kidney failure in Whites have increased annually since 2011, whereas, in contrast, the rates of kidney failure in Blacks with DM have fallen each year since 2007.[6]

DM as the primary cause of ESKD requiring dialysis may be overreported, as the majority of diagnoses are not confirmed by renal biopsy.[6] In people with long-standing type 1 diabetes mellitus (T1DM) and history of albuminuria, ESKD is almost solely due to diabetic nephropathy with diabetic kidney disease (DKD) typically developing after a 5- to 10-year duration.[7-9] However, DKD may be present at the time of diagnosis of type 2 diabetes mellitus (T2DM); and kidney disease could also be due to hypertensive or renovascular disease or a combination of these factors plus diabetic nephropathy, although other causes of CKD may be present.[7-9] Furthermore, those with DM are at higher risk of developing acute kidney injury (AKI) than those not having DM.[8]

Overview of Diabetes Classifications and Screening

The four classification categories for DM are as follows: 1) T1DM (due to autoimmune β-cell destruction), 2) T2DM (due to a progressive loss of β-cell insulin secretion frequently on the background of insulin resistance [IR]), 3) gestational diabetes mellitus (GDM), and 4)

specific types due to other causes, including chemical-induced diabetes mellitus (such as glucocorticoid use or after organ transplantation). Diagnostic tests do not necessarily detect DM in the same individuals, and blood glucose criteria should be used to diagnose DM in conditions associated with increased red blood cell (RBC) turnover, HD, or erythropoietin therapy.[10] The American Diabetes Association (ADA) advocates DM screening for all adults starting at age 45 or at any age for those who are overweight or obese (body mass index [BMI] of ≥25 or ≥23 in Asian Americans) and have one or more risk factors, such as a first-degree relative with DM, a high-risk race or ethnicity, history of CVD, hypertension (HTN), a high-density lipoprotein cholesterol (HDL-C) level less than 35 mg/dL and/or a triglyceride (TG) level greater than 250 mg/dL, or physical inactivity. Certain medications (eg, glucocorticoids, thiazide diuretics, some HIV medications, and atypical antipsychotic agents) are known to increase the risk of DM and should be considered a screening factor.[10] Boxes 9.1 and 9.2 outline the criteria for diag-

nosing DM and identifying individuals at high risk for development of DM.

Presently, there is a diabesity epidemic. Youth onset of T2DM is attributed to being overweight, family history of DM, race, and ethnicity with more prevalence in Blacks, Hispanics, Asian Pacific Islanders, and Indigenous Americans.[11,12] There are greater long-term risks of premature ESKD and CVD due to high rates of HTN and microalbuminuria, and the development of DKD and other complications advancing more rapidly. Progressive DKD in this population is more than that of youth with T1DM or T2DM in adults with similar disease duration.[11] Youth onset of T2DM is associated with higher mortality than T1DM, and it may be more aggressive and treatment resistant than T2DM in adults.[12] Risk-based screening for T2DM or prediabetes in asymptomatic children and adolescents is now recommended based on obesity, maternal history of DM or GDM during the child's gestation, family history of T2DM, race/ethnicity, and signs of IR or associated conditions.[10] This subgroup needs more careful monitoring and treatment.[11]

BOX 9.1 | Criteria for Diagnosis of Diabetes[10]

Hemoglobin A1c *or*	≥6.5% (≥48 mmol/mol) performed in a laboratory using a National Glycohemoglobin Standardization Program–certified method and standardized to the Diabetes Control and Complications Trial assay (only plasma blood glucose criteria should be used to diagnose diabetes mellitus)
Fasting plasma glucose (no caloric intake for ≥8 hours) *or*	≥126 mg/dL (≥7.0 mmol/L)
2-hour plasma glucose *or*	≥200 mg/dL (≥11.1 mmol/L) using 75 g anhydrous glucose dissolved in water per the World Health Organization description
Random glucose	≥200 mg/dL (≥11.1 mmol/L) in a patient with classic symptoms of hyperglycemia

BOX 9.2 | Prediabetes or Increased Risk for Developing Diabetes[10]

Hemoglobin A1c *or*	Between 5.7% and 6.4% (39 to 47 mmol/mol)
Impaired fasting glucose *or*	100 to 125 mg/dL (5.6 to 6.9 mmol/L)
Impaired glucose tolerance	2-hour plasma glucose between 140 and 200 mg/dL (7.8 to 11.0 mmol/L) during 75 g oral glucose tolerance test per World Health Organization description

PREDIABETES AND INSULIN RESISTANCE

IR is an underappreciated metabolic aspect of CKD that is seldom labeled as prediabetes in the kidney literature. Impaired fasting glucose (IFG) and impaired glucose tolerance are hallmarks of prediabetes and are associated with IR, which has also been labeled as metabolic syndrome (MS), dysmetabolic syndrome, or previously as syndrome X. MS is additionally linked to intra-abdominal or visceral obesity, HTN, and dyslipidemia. The American Association of Clinical Endocrinologists (AACE) prefers the term "insulin resistance syndrome" (IRS), as this more accurately pinpoints the underlying pathophysiology and the compensatory hyperinsulinemia that unites these conditions.[13] Having IR does not equate to having each of the abnormalities; however, having one component raises the likelihood of IRS diagnosis (see Box 9.3).[13]

BOX 9.3 | Insulin Resistance Syndrome Components[13]

Glucose intolerance: impaired glucose fasting or impaired glucose tolerance

Abnormal uric acid metabolism

Dyslipidemia: triglycerides, high-density lipoprotein cholesterol, low-density lipoprotein cholesterol, particle size (small, dense)

Hemodynamic changes: including renal sodium retention and blood pressure (~50% with hypertension have insulin resistance)

Prothrombotic factors

Markers of inflammation, such as C-reactive protein and white blood cell count

Endothelial dysfunction

All components defining MS are involved in the development of CKD, and each entity has been associated with both CKD incidence and progression, although causality is unproven.[14,15] Significant relationships were found between MS, the presence and number of its elements (and their combinations), and CKD; having more features increased the odds of having CKD.[15,16] Nevertheless, IR may be the most important related etiological factor for CKD as insulin is an anti-inflammatory

hormone and is an independent predictor of CVD mortality in patients with ESKD without DM.[14,17,18]

The degree of IR contributes significantly toward enhanced protein catabolism. Although pathogenesis and exact sites have not been elucidated, possible mechanisms of IR include increased hepatic gluconeogenesis, decreased hepatic and/or skeletal muscle glucose uptake, impaired intracellular glucose metabolism, metabolic acidosis, and chronic inflammation. The most likely site of IR is muscle tissue.[19,20] Hyperactivation of the renin-angiotensin aldosterone system with angiotensin II and aldosterone are implicated in both HTN and IR. There is increasing evidence for the important roles of the parathyroid hormone (PTH) and vitamin D; uremic toxins and oxidative stress may also contribute to IR. Modification of intestinal flora and activation of inflammation pathways have been implicated in the pathogenesis of IR in patients with obesity and those with DM and correcting some uremia-associated factors by modulating flora may improve insulin sensitivity.[21]

Impaired tissue sensitivity to insulin occurs in nearly all patients with uremia and is largely responsible for the abnormal glucose metabolism seen in this setting. Decreases in insulin clearance may mask IR, and normoglycemia is maintained at the expense of hyperinsulinemia. Mild glucose elevations may precede dyslipidemia. Hyperglycemia is a late manifestation of IR, and most patients without DM do not develop persistent hyperglycemia unless a genetic predisposition to DM exists.[22] However, IFG may play an important role in inflammation, malnutrition, and short-term mortality in patients receiving HD who do not have DM.[23] IR may improve with weight reduction and/or pharmacologic treatment of hyperglycemia but is seldom restored to normal.[10] Limited physical activity may potentiate IR, and exercise may improve insulin signaling and build up muscle tissue in individuals with CKD.[20] Therefore, dietary and lifestyle interventions may be warranted. The ADA also recommends consideration of metformin therapy for prevention of T2DM in those with prediabetes, especially for those with a BMI of greater than 35, those under 60 years of age, and women with prior GDM.[24] Monitoring plasma glucose levels can be construed as important in those without DM undergoing dialysis, given the potential development of DM with dialysis due to a bidirectional association.[1,25]

TYPE 1 AND TYPE 2 DIABETES

As mentioned earlier, DM is characterized by hyperglycemia resulting from defects in insulin secretion, insulin action, or both. T1DM is usually due to an autoimmune destruction of pancreatic β cells, leading to absolute insulin deficiency. These individuals present with markedly elevated blood glucose levels and acute symptoms of DM, with ketoacidosis often being the first disease manifestation in children and adolescents. Patients with T1DM will require insulin therapy, and insulin pumps are becoming more commonly used for management.

T2DM reflects having relative vs absolute insulin deficiency with the presence of IR; it frequently goes undiagnosed for many years, as insulin secretion is defective and insufficient to compensate for the IR.[10] Hyperglycemia develops gradually, so patients often do not recognize the classic symptoms until complications appear. The risk of developing T2DM increases with age, obesity, and lack of physical activity. Certain ethnicities or races, especially Indigenous Americans, Alaska Natives, Asians, Blacks, and Hispanics, are more predisposed.[10,26]

As with CKD, DM (especially T2DM) needs to be viewed as a progressive disease with clinical practice guidelines that provide a basis for the continuum of care realizing that needs and treatment goals are subject to change. Blood glucose becomes more difficult to control with disease advancement, and pharmacologic management may be needed in addition to lifestyle interventions.[27-30] Unless specifically contraindicated, metformin is the initial pharmacological therapy in patients with T2DM because of its effect on glycemia, absence of weight gain or hypoglycemia, generally low level of side effects, high level of acceptance, and relatively low cost.[27,30,31]

Metformin can be used safely in people with a reduced estimated glomerular filtration rate (eGFR). The Food and Drug Administration (FDA) in 2016 revised the drug's label to reflect its safety in those with an

eGFR of equal to or greater than 30 mL/min/1.73 m², indicating that it should not be initiated with an eGFR of less than 45 mL/min/1.73 m².[8,27] The risks and benefits of continuing metformin treatment require monitoring and reassessment when the eGFR level falls to less than 45 mL/min/1.73 m².[27] Per the Kidney Disease: Improving Global Outcomes (KDIGO) recommendations, metformin dose reduction is indicated for patients whose eGFR is less than 45 mL/min/1.73 m² or for those people who are at risk of AKI having an eGFR of 45 mL/min/1.73 m² to 59 mL/min/1.73 m².[30] Vitamin B12 deficiency can occur with metformin, and B12 levels should be monitored in patients with long-term use (>4 years).[27,30] If gastrointestinal (GI) intolerance occurs with metformin, it can be mitigated by gradual dose titration.

The addition of other glucose-lowering medications should be considered with persistent symptomatic hyperglycemia, taking into consideration established atherosclerotic CVD or CKD as well as the compelling need to minimize hypoglycemia.[7,29,30] For those with T2DM and CKD, using a sodium-glucose cotransporter inhibitor (SGLT2i) when eGFR is more than 30 mL/min/1.73 m² should be considered or, if contraindicated or not preferred, a glucagon-like peptide-1 (GLP-1) receptor agonist (when eGFR is >30 mL/min/1.73 m²), as both have been shown to reduce CKD progression with proven CVD benefits.[27,29,30,32,33] However, according to the newest KDIGO Diabetes Management in CKD Guidelines, most patients with T2DM, CKD, and eGFR equal to or greater than 30 mL/min/1.73 m² would benefit from treatment with both metformin and a SGLT2i.[30]

Professional organizations have recently updated and published antidiabetic medication guidelines and adjustments for DM and CKD. These include the newly available KDIGO Diabetes in CKD Guidelines,[30] the Management of Hyperglycemia in Type 2 Diabetes Consensus Report by the ADA and the European Association for the Study of Diabetes,[29] the ADA Standards of Medical Care in Diabetes 2021,[8,27] and the 2020 Consensus Statement by the AACE and the American College of Endocrinology (ACE) on the Comprehensive Type 2 Management Algorithm.[34] As pharmacology treatments emerge and more studies are conducted, these recommendations and guidelines are subject to change with many of the DM and endocrinology organizations providing annual updates. With such a diverse and heterogeneous population with DM, RDNs need to be familiar with the variety of available medical treatments and determine where the patient is along the continuum of care in order to individualize education and meal plans accordingly. Concordantly, patients need to better understand the mechanisms of diabetic medications being employed. Refer to Chapter 17 for additional medication information.

AADE7 Self-Care Behaviors

DM is a complex condition that requires an interdisciplinary approach, coordination of care, and patient commitment to the plan of care. Interventions aimed at promoting *healthy behavior* changes can prevent or delay DKD. Diabetes self-management education and support provide the foundation to help people with DM navigate these decisions and activities and can improve health outcomes.[35]

The Association of Diabetes Care & Education Specialists (ADCES), formerly known as the American Association of Diabetes Educators (AADE), updated the AADE7 Self-Care Behaviors to provide an evidence-based model for assessment, intervention, and evaluation of individuals and populations living with diabetes.[36] The seven key areas align with AADE's vision of "optimal health and quality of life for persons, with, affected by, or at risk for diabetes and chronic conditions" and shifted the focus away from educational content delivery to an outcome-driven practice incorporating patient-centric care and self-determined goals.[36] The AADE7 Self-Care Behaviors are as follows:

- healthy coping
- healthy eating
- being active
- taking medication
- monitoring
- reducing risk
- problem-solving

The AADE7 was revised into a diagram emphasizing the interrelatedness of these behaviors (see Figure 9.1). The core model brings together the key focus areas that overlap in nature with healthy coping at

FIGURE 9.1 | Transformation of the AADE7

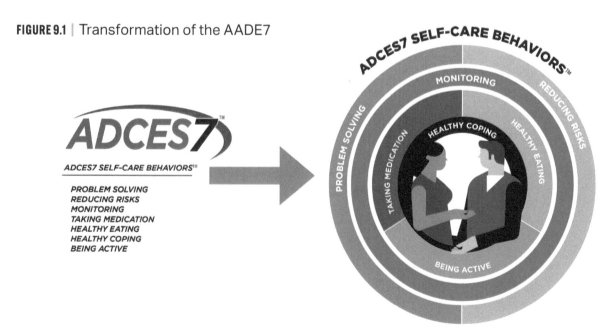

the center as the critical first step in sustainable DM self-management. The next inner rings of healthy eating, being active, and taking medications serve as the basis for individualized care plans and the key areas individuals with DM regularly undertake to self-manage their condition. The monitoring ring encircles the previous three self-care behaviors and healthy coping, as this area provides information to enhance knowledge and drive behavior change. The outermost ring contains the self-care behaviors of reducing risk and problem-solving which influence motivation and actionable goals.

The AADE7 incorporates digital technology and the changing health care landscape. Providers can use this model to guide the health care team in effective patient-centric collaboration and goal setting to achieve health-related outcomes and improved quality of life. Box 9.4 provides examples for the AADE7.

BOX 9.4 | American Association of Diabetes Educators Self-Care Examples for Diabetes and Kidney Disease

SELF-CARE FOR DIABETES AND KIDNEY DISEASE	MANAGEMENT OF KIDNEY DISEASE PROGRESSION
Healthy coping	Assess for depression and diabetes distress.
	Support the patient and family/caregivers.
	Discuss treatment options which align with goals and lifestyle.
	Discuss concerns and early intervention for vascular access placement.
Healthy eating	Recommend carbohydrate intake to achieve glycemic control.
	Limit dietary sodium to 2,300 mg/d.
	Recommend protein intake of 0.8 g/kg/d.
	Limit dietary potassium intake if serum level is elevated.
	Manage mineral bone disease per stage of chronic kidney disease (CKD).
	Manage dyslipidemia with lifestyle management.
	Treat vitamin deficiency.
Being active	Physical activity is recommended under physician supervision.
Taking medication	Antidiabetic agents may need adjustment with advancing kidney disease.
	Medications may increase risk of hyperkalemia.
	Medications may be needed to manage dyslipidemias.
	Phosphate-binding medication and vitamin D analogs may be prescribed.
Monitoring	A hemoglobin A1c goal of less than 7% may delay the onset or progression of diabetic kidney disease (DKD).
	An unexplained improvement in blood sugar levels may indicate DKD progression.
	Review and monitor estimated glomerular filtration rate and, urine albumin to creatinine ratio.
Problem-solving	Treat hypoglycemia with low potassium options.
	Medication management may need adjustment with advancing CKD.
	Educate on sick day management.
	Educate on CKD symptoms as indicated.
	Address social determinants of health.
Reducing risks	Encourage smoking cessation and education.
	Treat blood pressure to achieve goal.
	Manage risk factors for cardiovascular disease.
	Treat CKD–mineral bone disease.

The AADE7 Self-Care Behaviors dovetail with the newest KDIGO Diabetes Management in CKD Guidelines regarding approaches to management of patients with DM and CKD.[30] The KDIGO guideline recommends that a structured self-management educational program be implemented for the care of these patients. Their key objectives are as follows:

- Improve DM-related knowledge, beliefs, and skills.
- Improve self-management and self-motivation.
- Encourage adoption and maintenance of healthy lifestyles.
- Improve vascular risk factors.
- Increase engagement with medication, glucose monitoring, and complication screening programs.
- Reduce risk to prevent (or better manage) DM-related complications.
- Improve emotional and mental well-being, treatment satisfaction, and quality of life.

Diabetic Kidney Disease and Predialysis

DKD occurs in 20% to 40% of people with DM, yet these individuals are less likely to have pre-ESKD nephrology care when compared to those with cystic kidney disease and glomerulonephritis. The ADA specifically addresses DKD when referral to a nephrologist is indicated.[4,8,37] Risk factors for DKD can be conceptually classified as susceptibility factors (eg, older age, male sex, race/ethnicity, and family history), initiation factors (eg, hyperglycemia and AKI), and progression factors (eg, HTN, dietary factors such as high protein intake, and obesity).[38] DKD is usually a clinical diagnosis based on the presence of albuminuria and/or reduced eGFR in the absence of signs or symptoms of other primary causes of kidney damage.[8] The classical presentation of DKD includes long-standing DM, retinopathy, albuminuria, and gradually declining eGFR. In patients with T2DM, signs of CKD may be present at the time of diagnosis or without retinopathy, and diminished eGFR without albuminuria is being more frequently reported in patients with both T1DM and T2DM.[8]

Recent epidemiological studies have disclosed a wide heterogeneity of DKD. In addition to the classical albuminuric phenotype, two new albuminuria-independent phenotypes have emerged (ie, "nonalbuminuric renal impairment" and "progressive renal decline"), suggesting that DKD progression toward ESKD may occur through two distinct pathways, albuminuric and nonalbuminuric.[39] Although ESKD may be the most noticeable consequence of DKD, the majority of patients actually die from CVD complications prior to requiring KRT.[38]

Mogensen[40] originally reported that microalbuminuria predicted clinical proteinuria and increased mortality. The earliest clinical manifestation of diabetic nephropathy is the appearance of microalbuminuria (≥30 mg/d). Persistent microalbuminuria in the range of 30 to 300 mg/d is an established risk factor for the development of overt nephropathy (urine excretion rate of >300 mg in 24 hours).[41] Hyperglycemia, a well-known driver of microalbuminuria, is modifiable and reduces the risk of DKD. The original Kidney Disease Outcomes Quality Initiative (KDOQI) Clinical Practice Guideline for DM and CKD recommended a target hemoglobin A1c (HbA1c) of approximately 7.0% to prevent or delay the progression of microvascular complications of DM, including DKD.[42]

The landmark Diabetes Control and Complications Trial (DCCT) demonstrated that intensive glycemic control in patients with T1DM decreased the risks of microalbuminuria and macroalbuminuria, compared with conventional treatment.[43] The beneficial effects continued with long-term follow-up in the Epidemiology of Diabetes Interventions and Complications (EDIC) study. The intensively managed group continued to demonstrate lower rates of both microalbuminuria and macroalbuminuria.[44] Similar benefits of intensive glycemic control on the development of elevated albuminuria were observed in patients with T2DM.[45-47]

In the United Kingdom Prospective Diabetes Study (UKPDS), the incidence of microalbuminuria in patients with T2DM was 2% per year and the prevalence was 25% 10 years after diagnosis.[48] Proteinuria develops more frequently in patients with T1DM (15% to 40%) usually after 15 to 20 years of DM duration, but in patients with T2DM, the prevalence varies between 5% to 20% due to timing of diagnosis.[37,49]

Although a kidney biopsy is required to definitively diagnose DKD, careful screening can identify this without the need for a biopsy; and DKD is unlikely in patients with T1DM without diabetic retinopathy (DR).[7,43,50] Annual urine testing for microalbuminuria is essential to detect kidney disease at its earliest and most treatable stages. Those with T1DM for equal to or greater than 5 years, all people with T2DM, and all people with DM with comorbid HTN should be assessed every year for urinary albumin (spot urinary albumin:creatinine ratio) and eGFR. Patients with DM and urinary albumin greater than 300 mg/g creatinine and/or an eGFR rate of 30 to 60 mL/min/1.73 m[2] should be monitored twice annually to guide therapy.[8] Albuminuria is a marker of greatly increased CVD morbidity and mortality risks for patients with either T1DM or T2DM.[51] Although evidence is lacking that intensive glycemic control slows progression to the clinical end point of ESKD, the clinical course of DKD can be modified by interventions impacting earlier manifestations of the disease course.

ROLE OF OPTIMIZING GLYCEMIC CONTROL AND DIABETIC KIDNEY DISEASE

Glycemic control is a major focus to prevent or delay the progression of microvascular complications of DM. Intensive glycemic control with the goal of achieving near-normoglycemia has been shown to delay the onset and the progression of albuminuria and reduced eGFR in people with T1DM and T2DM.[8] There is a lag time of at least 2 years in T2DM to more than 10 years in T1DM for the effects of intensive glucose control to manifest as improved eGFR outcomes.[8] The results from clinical trials have suggested that intensive glycemic control is accompanied by an increase in hypoglycemia and a potential in all-cause mortality.[45-47,52] The presence of CKD affects the risks and the benefits of intensive glycemic control, and individuals with prevalent CKD and substantial comorbidities may have target HbA1c goals that are not as low.[8]

Fluctuations in blood glucose levels can occur due to alterations in insulin metabolism with deteriorating kidney function.[22] The kidney plays a vital role in both the clearance and the degradation of insulin, resulting in lower insulin requirements once the eGFR is less than 60 mL/min/1.73 m[2].[53] With less kidney mass, patients with CKD may experience reduced renal gluconeogenesis.[54] Patients with CKD may also develop suboptimal nutrition, leading to a reduction in glycogen stores.[55] Drug-dosing requirements need to be adjusted, if antidiabetic agents are renally excreted and have a prolonged half-life in patients with CKD predisposing them to episodes of hypoglycemia. These factors may contribute to a greater risk for hypoglycemia among patients with CKD and may be an unintended consequence of therapy to treat hyperglycemia. As insulin lasts longer in people with kidney disease, one must expect worsening of CKD when the patient has improved glycemic control without changes in medication, weight, or physical activity. Patients need to be educated on the signs and symptoms of hypoglycemia and proper management. Target HbA1c levels may need to be modified because of the risk of hypoglycemia and mortality with declining kidney function. As both patient and disease factors influence the target HbA1c, the benefits of glycemic control must be individualized.

DIRECT KIDNEY EFFECTS OF GLUCOSE-LOWERING MEDICATIONS

Some antidiabetes medications have direct effects on the kidney in addition to lowering glucose, and the newest recommendations from the ADA include specific guidelines for their use.[8] SGLT2i reduce renal tubular glucose reabsorption, may lessen oxidative stress in the kidney by 50%, and slow GFR loss through mechanisms that appear to be independent of glycemia.[8,27,32] GLP-1 receptor agonists are a newer class of antihyperglycemic agents that have been reported to improve kidney outcomes.[8,27,33] GLP-1 receptor agonists have been shown to prevent the onset of macroalbuminuria and reduce the decline of GFR in those with DM; and they may exert their beneficial actions on the kidneys through blood pressure (BP)-lowering effects, reduction of insulin levels, and weight loss in addition to decreasing blood glucose levels.[33,56]

PROTEIN, ENERGY, AND DIABETIC KIDNEY DISEASE PROGRESSION

The effect of dietary protein intake on kidney disease progression has been a topic of controversy.[57,58] A meta-analysis of several small studies showed that protein restriction may be beneficial in some patients whose nephropathy was progressing despite optimal glucose and BP control.[59] In 2007, the National Kidney Foundation (NKF) KDOQI Clinical Practice Guidelines for the Nutritional Management for Diabetes and Chronic Kidney Disease were initially introduced.[42] These guidelines recommended a dietary protein intake of 0.8 g/kg body weight per day with CKD stages 1 through 4 (equating to approximately 10% of daily caloric intake), which is the current adult Dietary Reference Intake for protein. In 2012, the KDIGO expert panel recommended a dietary protein intake of 0.8 g/kg body weight per day while avoiding levels above 1.3 g/kg body weight per day. This group also reported that there was insufficient evidence to demonstrate that long-term restriction of dietary protein intake below 0.8 g/kg body weight per day was beneficial to patients with DKD.[60]

The newest 2020 KDIGO Diabetes Management in CKD Guidelines[30] recommend maintaining the 0.8 g/kg body weight per day for those with DM and CKD without dialysis. These guidelines indicate that protein needs should be calculated by normalizing weight to the median weight for height in those who are significantly overweight. Alternatively, in overweight patients, clinicians may use an ideal weight rather than the patient's actual weight to avoid excessively high protein intake estimation. The guidelines note that neither lower nor higher protein intake appears beneficial and that each is associated with potential harm. They acknowledge that patients with CKD and DM often have multiple comorbid diseases, which may complicate an already complex diet regimen, and also address other

psychosocial factors that may influence the person's ability to do this, emphasizing the need for patient-centered care.

The ADA still recommends approximately 0.8 g protein per kg body weight per day for those with CKD not dependent on dialysis. The ADA also advises against higher levels of protein (>20% of daily calories from protein or >1.3 g/kg body weight per day) due to increased albuminuria, more rapid loss of kidney function, and CVD mortality.[8] Furthermore, protein intake of less than 0.8 g/kg body weight per day is not advocated, as this does not alter glycemic measures, CVD risk measures, or the course of GFR decline.[8]

The 2020 KDOQI Clinical Practice Guideline for Nutrition in Chronic Kidney Disease opinion is as follows: For "the adult with CKD 3–5 and who have diabetes, it is reasonable to prescribe a dietary protein intake of 0.6–0.8 g/kg body weight per day to maintain a stable nutritional status and optimize glycemic control."[61] This view is concurred by the 2020 Academy of Nutrition and Dietetics Evidence Analysis Library (EAL).[62] These guidelines do not include a statement regarding protein prescription for people without close clinical supervision. Adjustments that might be needed in patients with DM or lipid profile management to accommodate this protein level were not addressed. Attaining the lower protein goal could necessitate a higher ingestion of carbohydrates and fat skewing the metabolic profile and requiring other treatment modifications. When indicated, the protein restriction should not be at the expense of glycemic control nor promote a catabolic state. This restriction needs to be balanced with the possibility of undernutrition on low-protein diets in those with DM because insulin deficiency stimulates gluconeogenesis and increases protein degradation.[51,63-65] The differences in recommendations underscore the importance of individualizing the nutrition prescription for each person. Protein intake levels for nephrotic syndrome were not mentioned in the new KDOQI guidelines.

If DKD progresses and patients require KRT, the 2020 KDOQI nutrition guidelines, the 2020 Academy of Nutrition and Dietetics EAL, and KDIGO provide an opinion consensus statement that it is reasonable to prescribe a dietary protein intake of 1.0 g/kg body weight per day to 1.2 g/kg body weight per day to maintain a stable nutritional status. For patients at risk of hyperglycemia and hypoglycemia, higher levels of dietary protein intake may need to be considered to maintain glycemic control.[61,62]

Energy guidelines are based on age, gender, level of physical activity, body composition, weight status goals, CKD stage, and concurrent illness or presence of inflammation to maintain normal nutritional status. The 2020 KDOQI and 2020 Academy of Nutrition and Dietetics EAL nutrition guidelines both provide opinion statements with a recommended energy intake of 25 to 35 kcal/kg body weight per day for patients with metabolically stable CKD stages 1 through 5D.[61,62] The energy needs for those not metabolically stable were not indicated. The RDN should use clinical judgment and closely monitor individual patient intakes and outcomes when making energy recommendations with counseling.

HYPERTENSION MANAGEMENT AND DIABETIC KIDNEY DISEASE

The prevalence of HTN among US adults with DM was 77.1% and 66.3% according to the American College of Cardiology (ACC)/American Heart Association (AHA) and ADA definitions, respectively, compared to an overall 29.1% prevalence in adults according to the data from the 2013–2014 National Health and Nutrition Examination Survey (NHANES).[66,67] In patients with T1DM, HTN often occurs subsequently to diabetic nephropathy; however, HTN often presents with other components of the MS in patients with T2DM. HTN increases the risk of both macrovascular and microvascular complications, including stroke, peripheral vascular disease (PVD), coronary artery disease (CAD), DR, and diabetic nephropathy.[68-70]

Initial treatment should focus on lifestyle changes that target smoking and eliminating tobacco products, diet modifications, exercise, and weight loss with the ultimate goal of reducing both CVD risk and DKD progression. Reduced sodium intake has been shown to reduce BP, proteinuria, and volume status.[71] Dietary

sodium recommendations for individuals with DKD and those with CKD do not currently differ, and the recommended range for individuals with DKD is less than 2,300 mg sodium per day.[8,72] The KDIGO guidelines, however, recommend that sodium intake be less than 2 g/d or less than 5 g sodium chloride in patients with DM and CKD.[62]

Management of HTN contributes significantly to the reduction of CVD burden in DKD, although professional organizations differ in their recommendations. The 2017 ACC/AHA Guideline for High Blood Pressure in Adults recommends a target BP of less than 13/80 mm Hg in patients with CKD, with or without DM.[69] Older patients with CKD and frailty have been shown to be at higher risk of adverse effects from intensive BP control.[70] The ADA recommends treating patients to maintain BP levels less than 140/90 mm Hg to reduce CVD mortality and slow CKD progression with a lower BP target, less than 130/80 mm Hg, as appropriate for individuals at high risk of CVD, if achievable without undue treatment burden.[8,70] The AACE recommends less than 130/80 mm Hg for BP.[34] Therapy for HTN and DM should be part of a shared decision-making process based on comorbidities, anticipated benefit for reduction in progressive DKD, atherosclerotic cardiovascular disease, heart failure (HF), DR, and risk of adverse events.[48] Those with DKD are at increased risk of CKD progression (particularly those with albuminuria) and CVD, and in some cases may be suitable for lower BP targets.[8]

The 2014 expert panel and newest KDIGO and ADA clinical guidelines all support using angiotensin-converting-enzyme inhibitors (ACE-Is) or angiotensin II receptor blockers (ARBs) at maximally tolerated doses as first-line therapy for the treatment of HTN in patients with DKD.[48,62,70,73] The ADA has specific recommendations regarding their use.[8] Large, prospective randomized studies in patients with T1DM and T2DM have demonstrated that ACE-Is or ARBs are the drugs of choice for treating HTN to delay the clinical progression of microalbuminuria and slow the decline in eGFR.[74] Several studies and a meta-analysis concluded that both drug classes are equally safe and effective in managing HTN and reducing proteinuria.[75-77] Use of

ACE-Is or ARBs may elevate serum creatinine levels and exacerbate hyperkalemia in patients with advanced kidney disease; so serum potassium should be monitored routinely. It is likely that the patient will also be on a diuretic for BP and/or fluid control, which may cause potassium wasting. The treatment of HTN in patients with DKD should address lifestyle, pharmacotherapy, and patient education to improve self-management to reduce risk factors.

Kidney Replacement Therapy

Upon initiation of dialysis, patients with DM have more comorbid conditions and a notable incidence of complications. They often require more time from health care professionals than patients without DM. Distinguishing patient complaints related to long-standing DM vs those of uremia might be difficult.[78] Although it is recommended that dialysis initiation criteria be the same for those with and without DM, people with DM in both the United States and Europe tend to have dialysis initiated at a higher mean eGFR, more so in the United States.[3,78,79] Those who start dialysis due to volume overload or HTN are more likely to have DM.[80] Priority should be given to the patient's general status and preference in selecting KRT, as evidence is lacking as to the superiority of one modality over another.[78] Having DM does not generally alter the dietary recommendations for patients with HD and PD (see Chapters 5, 6, and 7).

HEMODIALYSIS

HD is the most common form of KRT used in patients with DM. A study done in veterans showed that higher HbA1c levels (>8) and random glucose levels (≥200 mg/dL) during the pre-ESKD period were associated with greater 1 year post-ESKD mortality.[81] There is an escalating risk of all-cause mortality along with CVD and cardiac mortality, demonstrating that the burden of DM heightens over time among patients with HD.[82] DM may affect HD treatments by compromising dialysis delivery due to vascular access management problems and a patient's greater frequency of intradia-

lytic hypotension related to autonomic nervous system dysfunction, cardiac diastolic dysfunction, and susceptibility to overhydration. Stability during treatment is influenced by removal of large fluid volumes, especially when done too rapidly; and there is greater difficulty in achieving targeted weights leading to poorer BP control and cardiovascular accidents. Additional HD sessions may be indicated to safely remove excessive weight gains. Weight status needs to be closely evaluated to deter accumulated volume overload, as lean body mass may decline and go undetected, resulting in elevated postdialytic weights.

Glucose can be dialyzed out during treatments when the dialysate content is lower than the patient's blood sugar level. HD solutions customarily contain glucose levels of 200 mg/dL to keep the patient's blood sugar stable during treatment, but the effect of the dialysis industry, having lowered the dialysate glucose concentration to 100 mg/dL, has had insufficient data.[19] Furthermore, hemodynamic changes during dialysis induce stress hormones and inflammatory cytokines that can influence blood glucose homeostasis.[83] Frequent episodes of intradialytic hypotension and hypoalbuminemia are powerful clinical predictors of hypoglycemia in patients with DM undergoing HD.[83]

Pretreatment and posttreatment blood glucose testing may be needed for a patient with volatile glycemia. There may also be a need for additional or enhanced glucose monitoring in patients who are prone to hypoglycemia several hours after leaving the dialysis center, with an increased risk for such up to 24 hours.[84] Use of snacks with 15 to 30 g carbohydrates either before treatment or after treatment or both before and after treatment may be beneficial when hypoglycemia is a problem; and nutritional supplements or 100-calorie snacks offer convenient choices. HD-associated hyperglycemia can further complicate the scenario, as it is similar to the Somogyi effect or rebound hyperglycemia that occurs in response to prolonged hypoglycemia.[19] In addition, insulin might be dialyzed in the presence of an especially high gradient, and insulin clearance is dependent on the type of dialyzer membrane contributing to hyperglycemia.[19]

HD treatment schedules may also have an influence on glycemic control when the carbohydrate-to-medication balance is disturbed, resulting in either hyperglycemia or hypoglycemia. Fluctuations in blood glucose due to changes in eating patterns and/or administration of medications may occur, and there could be inconsistencies as to what the patient does on treatment vs nontreatment days. For individuals who use insulin, this could potentiate having either too much insulin on board, compounded by the extended duration of exogenously administered insulin, or too little circulating insulin against varying amounts of food. Use of neutral protamine Hagedorn (NPH) and regular human insulins may be of particular concern given their lack of sufficiently predictable time mechanisms.[85] The patient may also experience problems with hypoglycemia with other antidiabetic agents, although this is less likely. Eating during treatment may be medically contraindicated or prohibited by a state's department of health regulations. Posttreatment fatigue may alter the amount of intake as well as the food choices, and transportation factors may further compound the situation due to time away from home. The patient's nutritional status can ultimately be impacted. Therefore, it is crucial to determine what the patient is actually doing regarding food and medications on dialysis days, nontreatment days, and weekends. Regular, consistent habits for food intake and medication administration should be encouraged as much as possible. Medications employed for DM may need adjustment, such as using more flexible insulin-dosing regimens, altering insulin dosing on treatment days, or using a sliding scale for insulin to minimize overlap or gaps.

Consequences of hyperglycemia in patients receiving HD are increased thirst, excessive fluid intake with higher interdialytic weight gains, hyperkalemia, shifts in serum osmolality, anorexia, nausea, vomiting, weakness, headache, confusion, drowsiness, lethargy, tremors, seizures, and unconsciousness as well as cardiac-related consequences (eg, angina, silent myocardial infarction [MI], and higher systemic BP).[1,86] Furthermore, dialysis-associated hyperglycemia during its development can cause changes exclusively in the internal balance of body solute (hypertonicity) and fluids (intracellular volume contraction and extracellular volume expansion) without affecting the external balance of water or solute.[87]

PERITONEAL DIALYSIS

PD results in more steady-state serum chemistries and fluid balance. Survival with DM is better with PD during the initial 2 years of ESKD treatment and in younger patients, which may be related to the integrity of the peritoneal membrane.[1] Multiple preexisting risk factors and comorbid diseases, especially CVD, influence the survival of patients with DM receiving PD.[88] The infrequent occurrence of hypotension is the greatest advantage with PD. There is a superior preservation of residual kidney function and a sustained daily ultrafiltration (UF).[89] Not needing to create an arteriovenous fistula lessens cardiac overload and acceleration of HF, in addition to avoiding possible peripheral and coronary steal syndromes.[1,89] There may be fewer episodes of progressive DR.[89] PD, therefore, may be used as the first approach for KRT in patients with DM before transitioning to HD, which is done in many other countries. This modality recently has become more encouraged in the United States. Strict blood glucose control, tight regulation of BP with ACE-I or ARBs, and other therapies may improve the survival of patients with DM undergoing PD, although the simple correction of a single cardiovascular risk factor is not likely to be effective.[88] Continued use of statins may be beneficial, although initiation of such once KRT has begun may not be without risk.[90] See Chapter 17 for more information on medications.

Nevertheless, the underlying diabetic state may compound or exacerbate the side effects related to intraperitoneal (IP) exposure to high glucose concentrations. These ensuing problems include an inflammatory state, hyperlipidemia, fibrosis, generalized intra-abdominal fat accumulation, increased risk of CVD, weight gain, obesity, fluid overload, hyperinsulinemia, aggravated dysregulated metabolic response to glucose, acute hyperglycemia, and faster transport membrane status.[1,89]

The protein loss into dialysate is significantly greater with DM, possibly due to high permeability of the peritoneal membrane.[1,89] There is no greater occurrence of encapsulating peritoneal sclerosis, peritonitis, or exit-site infection with DM, although another study showed that poor glycemic control is a consistent predictor of subsequent risk of catheter tunnel and exit-site infection among patients starting PD.[91-94]

Ultimately, the long-term glucose exposure increases peritoneal small-solute transport and decreases UF, with the glucose either directly or indirectly contributing to the peritoneal membrane alteration through generation of glucose degradation products or advanced glycation end products (AGEs).[1] High transporters can have large glucose loads from rapid peritoneal glucose absorption and will benefit from nocturnal automated PD.[95] The osmotic gradient between dialysis and blood lessens, resulting in reduced UF, diminished urea removal, and fluid retention; and a vicious cycle could develop with generalized edema, requiring frequent use of higher percent dextrose dialysate contributing to further hyperglycemia.[95] Carbohydrate-sparing dialysate solutions are amino acids (presently unavailable in the United States) and icodextrin.[95]

The absorption mechanism and the metabolism of icodextrin differ from glucose.[96] The benefits are better glycemic control, less weight gain, increased UF volume and solute clearance, enhanced membrane preservation, decreased concerns with hyperlipidemia, and not increasing insulin sensitivity.[1,95,96] Although icodextrin is a 7.5% solution, its carbohydrate absorption is equivalent to a 2.5% dextrose bag and is associated with the UF of a 4.25% solution. The extent of icodextrin absorption depends on the dwell time of the solution, and the mean carbohydrate absorption for icodextrin is 29.5 ±5 g vs 62 ±5 g for a 4.25% solution glucose per 12-hour dwell.[97] It is often used as a last fill option for daytime dwell in the peritoneal cavity. Icodextrin increases blood maltose levels, which may interfere with glucose dehydrogenase-based blood glucose meters giving false readings. Test strips that use glucose oxidase or hexokinase methods should be used (for detailed information, refer to the manufacturer's guidelines).

Glycemic control with PD is multifaceted in that the amount of glucose that is absorbed is dependent on the tonicity, dwell times, and volume of the solutions in conjunction with the patient's peritoneal equilibration test (PET) characteristics. Measuring blood glucose concentration at various levels of glucose absorption from the abdominal cavity during a PET may help determine the proper insulin dose. The glucose absorption in patients on PD aggravates insulin-stimulated glucose uptake by muscle.[98] In patients with T2DM, the remaining β-cell function deteriorates with time, further affecting insulin requirement. The risk for hypoglycemia needs to be offset against the glucose absorption, and there is potential for fluctuating hypoglycemia and hyperglycemia.

The timing of continuous ambulatory peritoneal dialysis (CAPD) exchanges is another factor influencing blood sugars.[95] It is important to evaluate the timing of the exchanges performed and whether they are done consistently each day. Their relationship to meals and carbohydrate consumption will also affect glycemic response. These factors need to be considered and coordinated with DM medications.

Use of either IP or subcutaneous insulin and other antidiabetic medications can help achieve good glycemic control, although IP insulin is not prescribed by many nephrologists.[95] Total insulin dose may be higher with IP administration with some activity being lost due to the dilutional consequence of delayed absorption and/or adsorption to the plastic surface of the dialysate delivery system, resulting in greater cost.[99] The frequency of peritonitis during IP insulin administration increases slightly only in CAPD, possibly due to the frequent handling of equipment and supplies. Various insulin regimens can be employed with PD. Continuous cycling PD is one place where use of NPH insulin could be considered due to its peak action and duration. Only treating with sliding scale insulin may not adequately cover the carbohydrate influx, and some type of basal insulin is usually designated for coverage. However, the importance of adequate patient education and frequent monitoring needs to be emphasized, and medication alone is insufficient to improve glycemic control.[100]

Prior KDOQI nutrition guidelines for the stable maintenance of chronic patients on PD recommended including absorbed glucose from the peritoneal dialysate as part of the total caloric intake, but this was not discussed in the most recent version.[62,101] This still seems applicable, as the amount can be significant accounting for 10% to 30% of daily energy, or as much as 100 to 300 g glucose per day.[1] Optimization of sodium and fluid intakes lessen the frequency of using higher dextrose concentrations that are needed for UF, resulting in fewer problems with hyperglycemia, hyperlipidemia, and excess weight gain. Exposure to the dextrose load can cause a lack of hunger that adversely influences intake adequacy. Calories absorbed from PD may allow maintenance of body weight (BW), while gastrointestinal issues negatively impact protein consumption. PD is associated with more gastroesophageal reflux disease (GERD) symptoms and eating dysfunction.[102] Severely slowed gastric emptying may be present even when patients are tested with an empty peritoneal cavity.[103] Reducing fill volume may be helpful if gastroparesis is present or there are expressed patient complaints of "feeling too full."[104]

TRANSPLANTATION AND HYPERGLYCEMIA

Hyperglycemia is common following kidney transplantation and is detectable in 90% of kidney allografts in the first few weeks post transplantation.[10,105,106] Hyperglycemia may develop from immunosuppressive medications, infections, or other medical complications. The term *posttransplantation diabetes* (PTDM) includes newly diagnosed DM post transplant, whether or not it was present or undetected prior to surgery with ongoing hyperglycemia.[107] This diagnosis should be reserved for patients who are clinically stable on antirejection therapy with adequate kidney function in the absence of acute infection.[10] The term *new-onset DM after transplantation* (NODAT) was originally used to describe newly diagnosed DM, but there is no standard definition due to differences in follow-up, diagnostic criteria, and medical management.[105,108-110] NODAT excludes patients with undiagnosed pretransplant DM as well as PTDM that resolves by the time of hospital discharge.[10] Any form of abnormal glycemic control heightens the risk for posttransplant CVD.

The standard for diagnosing PTDM is an oral glucose tolerance test (OGTT) compared to a fasting glucose test alone.[10,111] OGTTs are not typically used in transplant programs as the test is impractical and time consuming. Screening patients using fasting glucose and/or HbA1c can identify high-risk patients requiring further assessment and may reduce the number of overall OGTTs required.[10] The International Consensus on Posttransplantation Diabetes Mellitus Expert Committee recommends the use of an elevated HbA1c to diagnosis PTDM; however, conditions that change RBC turnover (such as anemia) and allograft function need to be considered.[107] Risk factors may be modifiable or nonmodifiable, including antirejection therapies, older age, obesity, being Black or having Hispanic ethnicity, history or presence of hepatitis C virus or cytomegalovirus (CMV), prediabetes, male sex, and a strong family history of DM.[10,110,112] Therefore, the pretransplant assessment should include screening for risk factors and an MNT referral as needed. Sharif and colleagues[113] reported the benefit of lifestyle management in reducing the progression of PTDM. These factors merit additional attention in dialysis units for patients seeking transplantation. Studies have reported that transplant patients with hyperglycemia and PTDM after transplantation have higher rates of rejection, infection, and rehospitalization.[10] Posttransplant monitoring for hyperglycemia and weight gain is indicated. Choosing a maintenance immunosuppression regimen based on hepatitis C virus or CMV serology may modify the risk of PTDM.[110] Nutrition management is essentially the same for the well-functioning simultaneous pancreas–kidney transplant and the solitary kidney transplant for patients with DM. See Chapter 8 for information about adult transplantation.

Glycemic Control: Measurement and Monitoring, Management, and Goals

Hyperglycemia defines DM, and glycemic control is fundamental to the management of DM.[114] Therefore, it is useful to understand some of the terminology and principles. Glycemia, the concentration of glucose in the blood, can be either direct (denoting a single point in time without information) or indirect (having been influenced). Glycation (based on the nonenzymatic addition of sugar to amino acid groups to produce an amine) is continuous over the life of a protein reflecting average blood glucose. Self-monitoring of blood glucose (SMBG) and HbA1c are available to health care providers and patients to assess the effectiveness and safety of a management plan with regard to glycemic control. SMBG reflects a direct measure of glycemia, whereas HbA1c is indirect and a form of glycation.

Research is ongoing as to the clinical markers of glycemic control and how to best determine this in regard to CKD. Caution should be observed due to assay methodology, testing standardization, and study design which can complicate the comparison of results with different glycemia measures. In addition, countries display large differences in characteristics of patients receiving HD and related practices implicating a need for domestic guidelines.[115] It is important to comprehend what the different indicators do and what the utilization of each can be in this population. Understanding these complex issues will enable the RDN to make appropriate recommendations and counsel accordingly.

Epidemiological analyses suggest that the greatest number of complications will be averted by taking patients from very poor control to fair/good control.[114] The presence of DKD affects the risks and the benefits of intensive glycemic control and requires detailed knowledge of which and how medications can be safely used.[27,116] Poorer glycemic control is associated with a worse prognosis and higher death risk in patients receiving dialysis.[117-120] U-shaped relationships between HbA1c levels and mortality have been shown in studies of patients with CKD as well as those on dialysis, although some study results did not concur regarding ESKD.[115,121-123] Low HbA1c may be a surrogate of poor nutritional status with under 6% warranting additional workup.[124] Glycemic control can still impact vision, neurological outcomes, nutritional status, infection, fluid and electrolyte balance, and rate of hospitalizations.[122]

Patients without glycosuria may be prone to wide fluctuations as well as rapid increases in blood sugar. While most attention is on hyperglycemia, hypoglycemia is of significant concern in this population. Risk for hypoglycemia is influenced by prolonged action and decreased metabolism of hypoglycemic agents (particularly sulfonylureas and insulin), longer duration of DM, compromised renal gluconeogenesis due to reduction in functioning renal mass, impaired sympathetic counterregulatory responses due to autonomic neuropathy (AN), presence of liver disease, alcohol consumption, poor dietary intake, chronic malnutrition, problems linked to dialysis, fewer glycogen stores with advanced age, chronic inflammation, and drug–drug interactions.[1,19,83,117,125] Weight loss occurring before initiation of dialysis makes the body more sensitive to the action of insulin. Acidosis limits the liver's ability to compensate via hepatorenal reciprocity.[125] DM medications may not be properly adjusted as eGFR declines or needs change afterward. Physician ownership as to who makes these adjustments needs to be established to facilitate referrals and coordinate care. CKD itself is now seen as an independent risk factor for hypoglycemia, and it is experienced with more than twice the incidence to those with DM without CKD.[125] Cognitive decline has also been associated with increased risk of hypoglycemia.[126]

MEASUREMENT AND MONITORING

Present comprehensive DM–related monitoring is lacking in patients with ESKD. In 2015, 86.5% of patients with DM and ESKD received at least one HbA1c test, 71.8% received a lipid test, and 46.9% received a dilated eye exam.[4] The ADA recommends assessment of glycemic status (HbA1c or other glycemic testing) at least twice a year for patients who are meeting treatment goals and have stable glycemic control and quarterly for patients not meeting glycemic goals or who have a change in management, such as medication type and/or dosage.[30,62,114] The patient's specific needs and goals should dictate SMBG frequency and timing although it may be needed four times per day with insulin to avoid hypoglycemia and deter hyperglycemia.[114,127]

HEMOGLOBIN A1C AND OTHER GLYCEMIC CONTROL MARKERS

HbA1c reflects mean glycemia over the preceding 2 to 3 months, with the most recent 30 days having the greatest influence. It has been used as a surrogate for risk of DM-related complications since 2003 when the DCCT trial was published. In 2010, HbA1c became a diagnostic measure for DM with the National Glycohemoglobin Standardization Program (NGSP) forming standardized results to those of the DCCT trials.[128] Attaining the target goal may not reflect having consistently met preprandial and postprandial glucose goals. Recent infection could skew the value higher, and poor food intake could lower the number. Thus, HbA1c may signal a need for change in management, although not what kind, being unable to predict both glycemic variation and incidence of hypoglycemia. HbA1c has been strongly correlated ($r = 0.92$) with mean blood glucose levels and established estimated average glucose (eAG) values, equating to 7% with an eAG of 154 mg/dL, although some studies have shown higher HbA1c levels in Blacks than in Whites at a given mean glucose concentration.[114] The use of eAG may facilitate patient understanding due to expression in a more familiar measure, although the values may not be exactly the same for patients undergoing dialysis.

HbA1c is the most consistent index of circulating glucose. However, there are accuracy limitations and interpretation concerns regarding its use in patients with CKD, especially those on dialysis. The onset of anemia with advancing CKD is linked to iron, folate, and erythropoietin deficiencies with each able to influ-

ence HbA1c.[95,117] As eGFR falls, erythrocyte survival time becomes 20% to 50% shorter with less exposure for glycation, resulting in a lower value.[117,129] Recent transfusions, accelerated erythropoiesis due to erythropoietin use, administration of iron or vitamin B12, and metabolic acidosis can also decrease HbA1c.[1,117] Conversely, the HbA1c value could be raised due to uremic acidosis, urea dissociation caused by carbamylated hemoglobin formation, hypertriglyceridemia, splenectomy, hyperbilirubinemia, chronic alcoholism, large salicylate ingestion, opiate addiction, and iron or vitamin B12 deficiency.[1,78,117] Carbamylation of hemoglobin is more of a past concern as there is no interference based on most modern studies although use of older studies might suggest this problem.[130] Laboratories should only use NGSP-certified assay methods whose performance for HbA1c is excellent.[114,117] Although there is potential for some differences when compared to patients not receiving dialysis, trends emerge over time as to the stability, worsening, or improvement of glycemic control when HbA1c is monitored quarterly. HbA1c is deemed as providing valid, reliable results for patients on dialysis with appropriate methodology, and is the current marker for recognized organization guidelines and recommendations.[7,30,42,78,114,131,132] The KDIGO HbA1c recommendation places a higher value on potential accrued benefits through accurate assessment of long-term glycemic control (which may optimize antihyperglycemic treatment) while placing a lower value on the inaccuracy of HbA1c measurement as compared with directly measured blood glucose levels in patients with advanced CKD.[30] HbA1c values should be interpreted with the limitations in mind at lower levels of eGFR, particularly with kidney failure.[30]

Due to the aforementioned concerns, other glycated protein markers such as glycated albumin (GA) and fructosamine (FA), which measure glycemic control over shorter periods of time, have been studied for use in patients with CKD and for those requiring dialysis. GA and FA are not the same and cannot be used interchangeably. FA is the name for all extracellular glycated proteins independent of RBCs, whereas GA is protein specific and expressed as a percentage of total albumin.

Most of the research has been done in Asia which differs in patient demographics, dietary habits, and HD therapeutic regimens, especially regarding erythropoietin use; these factors can influence study results.[115,133]

FA testing is available in the United States, but accuracy is low with different methodologies lacking specificity and having no standardization.[128,130,134] FA may be biased by hypoalbuminemia and other factors.[30] High-protein turnover and influences by all proteins are considerations when using FA.[30,78,128,134] In patients with CKD, FA is viewed as unreliable, especially in patients receiving PD.[1,30,128]

GA, presently used in Japan, awaits FDA approval in the United States for commercial availability.[128,135] In observational studies, GA is associated with all-cause and cardiovascular mortality in patients treated with chronic HD.[30] It can be useful in starting or modifying drug therapy and can be used reliably in patients with CKD.[128,129,135,136] GA, however, may not be applicable in disorders with protein loss, clinical conditions involving wide variability in albumin metabolism, and disease states with albumin turnover (such as massive proteinuria, nephrotic syndrome, and PD where albumin is low and there are high protein losses) as well as in other medical conditions.[1,30,78,128,135,136] High BMI, body fat mass, and visceral adipose tissue may have a negative influence on serum GA, which may be more relevant in the United States.[1,78,128,129,136] Whether GA should replace HbA1c is controversial, and standardization is an issue along with how frequently it should be measured.[127] The literature consensus suggests that additional studies are warranted for GA use in patients with CKD.

BLOOD GLUCOSE MONITORING

Patients undergoing dialysis should be encouraged to perform SMBG, as many do not test once they start KRT. Monthly and random blood glucose testing done at dialysis treatments is not a substitute for home testing, especially as there is lack of standardization among dialysis clinics. SMBG, particularly in individuals using insulin, is an important adjunct to HbA1c, as it can distinguish among fasting, preprandial, and postprandial hyperglycemia; detect glycemic variability; identify hypoglycemia; and provide immediate feedback about the effects of food choices, activity, and medication.[137] With multiple-dose insulin use or insulin pump therapy, SMBG may be indicated before meals, snacks, and bedtime to detect variations in blood glucose levels, especially asymptomatic hypoglycemia and hyperglycemia that may require insulin adjustments.[137] It may also be necessary to check glucose before, during, and after exercise depending on the intensity. Changes in insulin routine, activity, or travel as well as intercurrent illness and stress may require additional monitoring.[137,138] Intensive insulin therapy for tight control may require checking up to six to ten times daily, although tight control may not necessarily be indicated for patients with ESKD or advanced complications.[137] The optimal frequency and timing of SMBG for patients with less frequent insulin injections, noninsulin therapies, or MNT alone are unknown, but the feedback can still be instrumental.[137]

A reasonable approach would be to monitor fasting blood glucose and then vary a second blood check by rotating different days and times to see if a pattern emerges prior to certain meals, such as 2 hours postprandial or at bedtime. Only checking the fasting level is insufficient; however, for those using basal insulin, it can help determine dosing decisions in order to lower HbA1c.[137] Postprandial glucose monitoring is advocated for by AACE guidelines and may significantly impact HbA1c and also lower CVD risk, which has been shown in epidemiological but not intervention trials.[1,34] Health care providers need to initially and routinely evaluate each person's monitoring technique for accuracy.

SMBG alone does not lower blood glucose levels, and the information must be integrated into clinical and self-management plans to be useful.[137] SMBG requires acting on results and pattern management, with patients being taught how to use the data to adjust food intake, exercise, and/or pharmacologic management to achieve specific glycemic goals. Justification may need to be provided for Medicare and other insurance providers regarding the monthly quantity of test strips being ordered, as Medicare presently only covers three test strips daily if using insulin.

Glycemic control has been best evaluated by monitoring both SMBG and HbA1c.[114] This combined approached allows better trend analysis. HbA1c may indicate adequate overall control, but insight from SMBG enables determination of the contributing effects from hypoglycemic and hyperglycemic events, some of which could be deleterious to the patient. Again, it is emphasized that glycemic goals need to be individualized for patients with DM and CKD. An extensive set of algorithms is available from the AACE and ACE to manage patients with T2DM with lifestyle therapy, glycemic control, antidiabetic medications, and other factors. Detailed charts are available in the ADA and European Association for the Study of Diabetes Type 2 Management consensus report.[28,34] Health care providers rely on trustworthy glucose information to make informed decisions to prescribe and adjust their patients' medication dosage. Continuous glucose monitoring (CGM) may possibly provide this need.

CGM provides information about the direction, magnitude, duration, frequency, and causes of fluctuations in blood glucose levels and can help identify and prevent unwanted periods of hypoglycemia and hyperglycemia.[139] There are three categories of CGM systems: 1) retrospective CGM—generates a report for evaluation after the CGM is removed; 2) real-time CGM devices—refer to sensor transmitting and displaying the data automatically throughout the day so that the person can review glucose levels and adjust treatment as needed; and 3) intermittent or "flash" scanned CGM—have glucose levels that can be seen while the device is worn when they are queried.[30] Time frequencies for CGM may be more often as newer devices are developed, and each type has its pros and cons. Time in range, a metric derived from CGM that assesses the percentage of a CGM reading within a certain range, may serve as an appropriate treatment target in addition to or instead of HbA1c with commonly accepted ranges being 70 to 180 mg/dL at greater than 70% of readings.[30] The ADA has standardized CGM metrics for clinical care.[114] A glucose management indicator derived from CGM data can be used to index glycemia for individuals in whom HbA1c is not concordant with directly measured blood glucose levels or clinical symptoms.[30] Technology in this area is quickly advancing. The health care provider and patient must evaluate each system carefully to make the best selection. Ultimately, financial considerations and reimbursement would steer the decision process. Many commercial payers, Medicare and Medicaid, are providing coverage for CGM.[140] Manufacturer guidelines also need to be checked for suitability of use with CKD and dialysis.

GOALS

Glycemic control needs to be individualized in patients with advanced DKD. Multiple factors including age, life expectancy, BW, duration of DM, stage of CKD, and other comorbidities need to be considered when determining risks and benefits of intensive control.[30,121,141] Hypoglycemia is the major limiting factor in the glycemic management of both T1DM and T2DM.[114] Intensive glycemic control may be inappropriate for many frail older people with advanced CKD, and most trials and studies have excluded this population and not specifically addressed the issue despite the number of older people receiving dialysis.[142,143] The ADA recommendation is to avoid hypoglycemia and symptomatic hyperglycemia in older adults with DM.[126] Hypoglycemia increases the risk of cognitive decline, and severe hypoglycemia has been linked to increased risk of dementia.[126] The ADA recommends HbA1c less than 8.0% for older adults with multiple coexisting chronic illnesses, including CKD stage 3 or worse.[126] The presence of CKD requiring dialysis places older adults in the category of very complex/poor health with limited remaining life expectancy making the benefit of glycemic control uncertain.[126] Reliance on HbA1c is to be avoided, and there are guidelines for higher fasting, preprandial, and bedtime glucose levels.[126]

Specific targets must consider both overtreatment and undertreatment.[117] The ADA goals of care are preventing complications and optimizing quality of life.[144] The 2012 update to the KDOQI guidelines regarding glycemic control goals are as follows: 1) aiming to reach a target HbA1c of approximately 7.0% to prevent or delay the progression of microvascular complications of DM, including DKD; 2) not treating to reach an HbA1c target of less than 7.0% in patients at risk of hypoglycemia; and 3) suggesting that target HbA1c be extended above 7.0% in individuals with comorbidities or limited life expectancy and risk of hypoglycemia.[122] These are similar to but differ slightly from the ADA goals of HbA1c less than 7% for many nonpregnant adults and less stringent HbA1c goals (such as <8%) being appropriate for patients with a history of severe hypoglycemia, limited life expectancy, advanced microvascular or macrovascular complications, extensive comorbid conditions, or long-standing DM in whom the goal is difficult to achieve.[114] Canadian and British DM goal targets are set a bit higher, again expressing concerns regarding hypoglycemia, with additional delineations that include dependence, frailty, dementia, and end-of-life care.[131,132]

The exact HbA1c targets for the best outcomes in patients with CKD and receiving dialysis historically were not established. Suggested treatment goals were 7% to 7.5% for patients 50 years of age or less without significant comorbid conditions and 7.5% to 8.0% for older patients (>50 years of age) who have multiple comorbid conditions with a range of 7% to 8% being reasonable for most patients.[95,127] However, in 2020, the KDIGO guidelines released factors specifically address-ing HbA1c use in patients with CKD to guide decisions with a range of individualized targets as low as under 6.5% up to as high as under 8%. Refer to Figure 9.2.[30] This was done, considering the increasing availability of treatments for T2DM unassociated with hypogly-cemia, allowing more aggressive glycemic targets for appropriate patients. The need for individualization is again underscored.

Preprandial and postprandial blood glucose targets need to be individualized.[127] Both are directly correlat-ed to the risk of complications with some evidence that postprandial glucose might constitute a stronger independent risk factor for CVD complications.[131] There are controversies as to whether mean glycemia or glycemic variability (GV) is the main determining factor for chronic damage in DM, and the additional therapeutic goal of glucose variability has recently been gaining support.[131,134] A recent study in China con-cluded that higher GV is associated with an increased mortality risk among patients with DM receiving HD and that future studies are needed to explore wheth-er decreasing GV would reduce that risk.[145] The ADA recommends preprandial blood glucose values of 80 to 130 mg/dL and peak postprandial blood glucose less than 180 mg/dL for many nonpregnant adults with DM while acknowledging more or less stringent goals being appropriate for individual patients. Postprandial glucose may be targeted if HbA1c goals are not met

FIGURE 9.2 | Glycemic targets in patients with diabetes and chronic kidney disease

< 6.5%	HbA1c	< 8.0%
CKD G1	Severity of CKD	CKD G5
Absent/minor	Macrovascular complications	Present/severe
Few	Comorbidities	Many
Long	Life expectancy	Short
Present	Hypoglycemia awareness	Impaired
Available	Resources for hypoglycemia management	Scarce
Low	Propensity of treatment to cause hypoglycemia	High

G1 = eGFR ≥90 mL/min per 1.73 m²; G5 = eGFR <15 mL/min per 1.7 m².

Reproduced with permission from Kidney Disease: Improving Global Outcomes (KDIGO) Diabetes Work Group. KDIGO 2020 Clinical Practice Guideline for Diabetes Management in Chronic Kidney Disease. *Kidney Int.* 2020;98(4S):S1-S115.[30]

despite reaching preprandial glucose goals; blood glucose values should be checked 1 to 2 hours after the beginning of the meal.[114] Reasonable goals for glycemic control in patients on dialysis are a fasting serum glucose of less than 140 mg/dL and a postprandial value of less than 200 mg/dL, but this was not addressed in the KDOQI Diabetes Update.[122,146] See Table 9.1.[147]

Medical Nutrition Therapy

AMERICAN DIABETES ASSOCIATION GENERAL GOALS OF MEDICAL NUTRITION THERAPY

MNT has an essential role in overall DM management, and each person who has DM should be engaged in education, self-management, and treatment planning with the health care team.[148] Understanding the nutritional needs for earlier stages of CKD and KRT will help guide the decision-making for these adjustments while incorporating the basic principles for good DM management. The ADA general goals of MNT are as follows: 1) promote and support healthful eating patterns to improve overall health by achieving and maintaining BW goals, individualized glycemic control, BP, and lipid goals, and delaying or preventing complications; 2) address individual nutrition needs based on personal and cultural preferences, health literacy and numeracy, access to healthful foods, willingness and ability to make behavioral changes, and barriers to change; 3) maintain the pleasure of eating by providing nonjudgmental messages about food choices; and 4) provide the practical tools for developing healthy eating

patterns, rather than focusing on individual macronutrients, micronutrients, or single foods.[148,149]

The challenge is integrating these goals with nutrient modification for CKD. Practitioners should also pay attention to the following:

- balance of food intake, exercise, and available insulin with kidney function and/or dialysis to achieve glycemic goals
- adequate energy intake to promote optimal nitrogen utilization
- achievement of acceptable biochemical parameters and fluid status
- prevention and treatment of acute and long-term complications of DM and their potential impact on nutritional well-being
- improvement in overall health through appropriate food choices and physical activity
- consideration of psychosocial support system, including financial constraints, while respecting the individual's willingness to make changes

Monitoring glucose, HbA1c, lipids, BP, and kidney status is essential to evaluating nutrition-related outcomes. If the goals are unmet, changes must be made in the overall management plan. The RDN's role is to help patients learn a problem-solving approach that includes diet as one of many factors that will impact these goals.

MACRONUTRIENT DISTRIBUTION

Macronutrient distribution needs to be individualized based on current eating patterns, preferences, and metabolic goals as well as physical activity, food preferences, and availability.[149] There is no ideal percentage of calories

TABLE 9.1 | Glycemia Therapy Goals for Diabetes and Kidney Disease[114,146,147]

	Chronic kidney disease stages 1 through 5	Hemodialysis	Peritoneal dialysis
Fasting plasma glucose (mg/dL)	80-130	<140	"Fasting" PG[a]: <160
2-hour postprandial glucose (mg/dL)	150-180	<200	<200
Random blood glucose (mg/dL)	Avoid hypoglycemia <70	Avoid hypoglycemia <70	Avoid hypoglycemia <70

[a] Patients on peritoneal dialysis are never truly "fasting" as patients have glucose-rich dialysate dwelling overnight in their peritoneal cavity from which glucose is continuously absorbed. The fasting plasma glucose can be influenced even if this dwell is a minimal amount.

from protein, fat, and carbohydrate for people with DM that is supported by research.[148-150] Regardless of macro-nutrient mix, total energy intake should be appropriate to attain weight management goals.[149] Although there are implications for protein intake and DKD, research is inconclusive regarding an ideal amount of protein to optimize either glycemic or CVD risk.[148]

The ADA Guidelines refer to the National Academy of Medicine acceptable distribution of 20% to 35% of total caloric intake from fat for all adults, although reported consumption has been 36% to 40%.[148-150] Differing amounts of fat intakes (27% to 40% of total energy), independent of weight loss, did not have a significant effect on HbA1c.[150] The types or quality of fats in the eating plan may influence CVD outcomes beyond the total amount of fat.[149]

The most evidence for improving glycemia for those with DM has been demonstrated by reducing the overall carbohydrate intake.[148] The Dietary Guidelines for Americans recommend carbohydrate intake from a variety of different foods which compromises roughly 45% to 65% of calories, but this can help be fulfilled by the body's physiological processes.[72,149] A variety of studies with differing amounts of carbohydrate (39% to 57% of energy), independent of weight loss, reported no significant effect on HbA1c. Most individuals with DM report a moderate intake of carbohydrate (44% to 46%), and efforts to modify habitual eating patterns are often unsuccessful in the long term.[150] Interpreting the research for low-carbohydrate diets is complicated due to the wide range of definitions, and long-term sustainability is challenging. Although low-carbohydrate diets show promise to improve glycemia for up to a year for those with T2DM or prediabetes, they are inappropriate for some groups, including those with kidney disease.[148] Furthermore, they need to be used with caution for those on SGLT2i therapy due to the risk of ketoacidosis.[148,149]

DIETARY STRATEGIES FOR CARBOHYDRATE MANAGEMENT

Achieving blood glucose goals is largely dependent on reducing postprandial glucose excursions. Dietary car-bohydrates are the major determinant of postprandial glucose levels, so food and nutrition interventions are crucial to improve outcomes. As both the amount and source of carbohydrates will influence glycemic control, the issue is one of degree. The quality of carbohydrate foods should be addressed as part of the individualized eating plan.[149] Lowering glycemic index or glycemic load may or may not have a significant effect on glycemic control and more research is warranted, as the literature is complex and often yields mixed results.[148,150,151] The AACE and ACE, however, advocate limiting high glycemic index foods for those with T2DM.[34] Refer to Figure 9.3 on page 160.[152]

A variety of eating patterns (combinations of different foods or food groups that represent all foods and beverages consumed) are acceptable for DM management.[149] An eating plan is a guide as to what, when, and how much should be eaten on a daily basis which applies to the person's individually selected eating pattern.[149] A whole-diet approach considers the synergistic effects of nutrients, resulting in cumulative effects on health and disease.[62] Until more evidence about comparative benefits of different eating patterns is strengthened, the focus is on the following common factors among the patterns: 1) emphasize nonstarchy vegetables, 2) minimize added sugars and refined grain, and 3) choose whole foods over highly processed foods to the best extent possible.[148] The Mediterranean diet is one such approach, although other diets high in fruits and vegetables have been considered applicable, while bearing in mind the need to make adjustments for micronutrient content.[62,149] There is inadequate research about dietary patterns to promote one over the other for persons with T1DM.[149] Nevertheless, the AACE and ACE advise consistency for day-to-day carbohydrate intake for patients with T2DM and note the importance of eating a healthy high-fiber breakfast and not skipping meals to decrease the risk of unhealthy eating at night.[34] The KDIGO Guideline advises that people with DM and CKD should consume an individualized diet high in vegetables, fruit, whole grains, fibers, legumes, plant-based proteins, unsaturated fats, and nuts while lower in processed meats, refined carbohydrates, and sweetened beverages.[30]

FIGURE 9.3 | Determinant of carbohydrate absorption

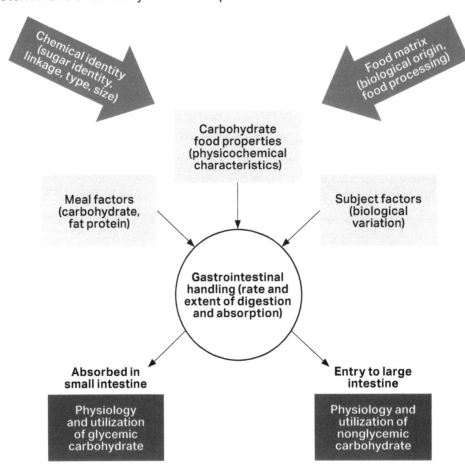

Adapted with permission from Schatz SR. Glycemic index and glycemic load: a new look at an old topic. *The Cutting Edge Newsletter.* 2014;35.

A simple and effective approach to glycemia and weight management that emphasizes portion control and healthy food choices may be considered for those with T2DM who are not taking insulin, who have limited health literacy or numeracy, or who are older and prone to hypoglycemia.[149] Evidence is strong and consistent that weight reduction can delay the progression of prediabetes and T2DM. All patients who are overweight and obese should be advised of the health benefits of weight loss and encouraged to engage in a program of intensive lifestyle management.[29,34] This has additional significance for those on dialysis who seek transplant listing.

Careful management of carbohydrate intake and available insulin is integral for achieving glycemic control in any meal-planning approach, and the RDN is best qualified to match the appropriate method to each person's lifestyle and capabilities. This involves understanding therapy intricacies for patients with T1DM and T2DM, knowing how much and when carbohydrate should be consumed, and balancing the effects from DM medications; many strategies can be employed. Those who take insulin at mealtimes require education to couple its administration with the carbohydrate intake; or if meal schedule or carbohydrate consumption is variable, the person needs to understand the importance of the relationship between carbohydrate intake and insulin.[148]

Carbohydrate counting (carb counting) is recommended for those with T1DM using intensive insulin therapy or those with T2DM who are prescribed a flexible insulin therapy program to determine mealtime insulin dosing.[148-150] Patient motivation and a higher literacy level are required for carb counting. This involves use of insulin:carbohydrate ratios, and careful record keeping is essential until an accurate ratio is established. These ratios can assist in effectively modifying insulin dosing from meal to meal, and the insulin dosage must also consider exercise and current blood glucose levels. It is highly recommended that blood glucose be checked 2 hours after a meal to determine if additional insulin adjustments are needed.[148] Protein and fat intakes should be relatively constant, with carbohydrate consumption not varying widely to avoid excess energy intake and undesired weight gain at the expense of glycemic control.

Carbohydrate consistency based on timing and amount is advised for fixed insulin dose use or insulin secretagogues to improve glycemic control and reduce risk of hypoglycemia.[148-150] This can be achieved by the following: carb counting alone (without use of ratios); plate method, portion control, and a simplified meal plan; or food lists and carbohydrate choices.[150] The modified plate method uses measuring cups and portion control and can provide a more visual approach (which is preferred, because descriptions of the concept can be confusing when unfamiliar).[148] Food choices may need modification to accommodate sodium, potassium, and phosphorus restrictions. The Academy of Nutrition and Dietetics has educational tools including Dish Up a Kidney Friendly Meal (for dialysis as well as earlier stages of CKD) and Making Choices Meal Planning for Diabetes and CKD (www.eatrightstore.org/product-subject/kidney-disease) for use with patient care.

HYPOGLYCEMIA TREATMENT

Hypoglycemia treatment requires ingestion of fast-acting carbohydrate at the alert value of 70 mg/dL, and the acute response correlates better with the glucose content of food than with its carbohydrate content.[114] Foods with added fat or high in protein are not indicated as the glycemic response will be slower.[114] Use of car-

bohydrate foods high in protein should also be avoided to treat hypoglycemia due to potential concurrent rise in endogenous insulin.[148] The 15/15 rule is usually employed to treat hypoglycemia: take 15 g carbohydrate, wait 15 minutes, and retest to determine the blood sugar levels or evaluate relief of symptoms.[138] If necessary, repeat with another 15 g carbohydrate, continue the process until the blood sugar level improves, and then when normalized, the person should eat a meal or snack to deter recurrence. Commonly used agents (such as orange or other fruit juices and regular soda) may result in fluid overload and/or hyperkalemia in the oliguric patient with DM. Better 15 g carbohydrate choices to suggest are: commercially formulated specialty glucose products such as tablets, gel, spray, or 2-oz shots; 1 tablespoon sugar, honey, or corn syrup; or hard candies, jellybeans, or gumdrops (see food label to determine 15 g equivalent).[138] The patient's ability to chew or swallow can sometimes be compromised during a hypoglycemic episode, so items more easily dissolved or absorbed may be preferred. Patients experiencing hypoglycemia sometimes tend to overtreat the episode, resulting in hyperglycemia. Glucagon administration, which requires special instruction for use, may be indicated for people who are unable or unwilling to consume carbohydrate by mouth or if the hypoglycemia is too severe.[114,138] Patients need to be educated about the symptoms, causes, and prevention of hypoglycemia.

DIETARY PROTEIN

The protein requirements are those that are appropriate for the stage of CKD or the mode of KRT. In an opinion statement, the recent KDOQI guidelines for protein requirements for patients receiving HD suggest 1.0 g/kg to 1.2 g/kg BW/d and for patients at risk of hypo- and hyperglycemia, higher levels of dietary protein may need to be considered to maintain glycemic control.[62] The KDIGO guideline adds that higher protein may help avoid hypoglycemia when given to those on dialysis with DM who have a decreased ability for gluconeogenesis.[30] A review article indicated that 20% to 30% of energy as protein might improve glucose control and aid in satiety.[153] The amount of protein might need to be increased due to infection, wound healing, or the need to replenish depleted visceral protein stores. Protein (ranging from 0.8 g/kg/d to 2.0 g/kg/d) does not seem to have a significant effect on fasting glucose levels, HbA1c, or insulin requirements in adults with T1DM and T2DM.[150]

Controversy exists regarding the role of plant-based protein and benefit with DKD.[150] The AACE and ACE advocate a primarily plant-based meal plan for patients with T2DM in general, without mention of DKD.[34] Vegetable protein diets may have beneficial effects on overall health, and in patients with CKD, there may be positive biological actions as well as clinical benefits.[62] However, the recent KDOQI guideline opinion is that there is insufficient evidence to recommend a particular type of protein as comparison, randomized, control trials regarding vegetable protein and animal protein diets in patients with CKD are limited.[62] The KDIGO guideline concurs indicating that although observational studies reported that high consumption of red and processed meat is associated with increased risk of CKD progression and mortality and that fruit and vegetable intake were associated with a decline in the progression of CKD, the benefits have not been corroborated in clinical trials; thus, no recommendation was made for the type of protein in patients with DM and CKD.[30] Fish and other low-fat protein sources, such as egg whites, egg substitutes, and skinless poultry, can be encouraged as well as the use of soy products (with adjustment for phosphorus and potassium content). Protein powders and nutritional supplements could be employed when intake of other protein sources is inadequate.

Metabolic acidosis also needs to be corrected to maintain positive nitrogen balance because acidosis reduces albumin synthesis and increases amino acid oxidation. Interventional studies correcting serum bicarbonate without changes in protein intake typically have not resulted in improved serum albumin levels, suggesting that the benefit of adequate protein intake in maintaining serum albumin exceeds the potentially deleterious effect of the associated higher acid loads on reducing albumin synthesis.[154]

DIETARY FAT

RDNs should encourage consumption of a cardioprotective eating pattern with the recommended energy intake.[150] Recommendations to improve the lipid profile in patients with DM include the reduction of saturated fat, avoidance of *trans* fat, and cholesterol intake; increase of dietary omega-3 fatty acids, viscous fiber, and plant stanols/sterols intake; and increased physical activity.[70,148] The AACE and the ACE advocate a diet high in polyunsaturated and monounsaturated fatty acids with a limited intake of saturated fat and avoidance of *trans* fats.[34] The Dietary Guidelines for Americans advise limiting saturated fat to 10% of total calories.[72] As saturated fats are progressively decreased, they should be replaced with unsaturated fats and not with refined carbohydrate.[148] The emphasis seems to be more on eating patterns. Consuming foods rich in long-chain omega-3 fatty acids, such as fatty fish, nuts, and seeds, is recommended to prevent or treat CVD (although adjustments may be needed for phosphorus content).[148] Evidence does not support a beneficial role for the routine use of omega-3 dietary supplements.[62,148] See Chapter 11 for more information about CVD.

SUGAR AND NONNUTRITIVE SWEETENERS

Nonnutritive sweeteners, when substituted isocalorically for other carbohydrates, will not have a significant effect on HbA1c, insulin levels, or glycemic management, but they can reduce overall energy and carbohydrate intake.[148,150] They are an acceptable substitute for nutritive sweeteners when consumed in moderation, but excessive intake could displace nutrient-dense foods.[148,150] Sugar-sweetened beverages should be avoided and replaced by water to control glycemia and weight and reduce risk for CVD and fatty liver disease.[148] Sugar-sweetened beverages are perceived to be contributors to increased risk of T2DM, heart disease, kidney disease, and nonalcoholic liver disease.[148] The AACE and the ACE advise against the use of sucrose- and high-fructose–containing foods.[34] Their use could be of particular concern in patients on PD, given the absorption of sugar and subsequent calories from the dialysate. The nonnutritive sweeteners are generally safe to use with the regulatory agency-defined acceptable daily intake levels, although their use is being evaluated for other potential adverse health effects.[148] Sugar alcohols can have gastrointestinal effects in sensitive individuals.[149]

DIETARY FIBER

The ADA recommends carbohydrate intake from vegetables, fruits, legumes, whole grains, and dairy products, with an emphasis on foods higher in fiber and minimally processed as being preferred over other sources, especially those containing added sugars.[148] Choosing a variety of fiber-containing foods is encouraged as they provide vitamins, minerals, phytochemicals, and antioxidants important for good health. However, in patients with CKD and DM, there are numerous potential barriers to achieving high-fiber intakes, such as palatability, limited food choices, phosphorus restrictions, potassium control, and gastrointestinal side effects with potential fluid restrictions. As such, priority should be given toward encouraging fiber intakes set for the general population—14 g/1,000 kcal.[72,149] Adequate fiber intake is of particular concern for those on PD to help deter constipation. Inclusion of viscous fiber (such as in oats, legumes, and citrus) intake is advised as part of lifestyle management for lipid control but may require adaption with CKD dietary constraints.[70]

SODIUM AND FLUID CONSIDERATIONS

Issues of sodium and fluid control can be more complicated with DM. There is a 94% higher risk of greater fluid retention in patients with DM on HD.[119] Hyperglycemia may contribute to thirst; and sweetened beverages should be avoided, as they are not thirst quenching and can compound the existing hyperglycemia. Dry mouth may be more of a thirst trigger than hyperglycemia, and this problem may be predisposed by neuropathy as well as the contributing factors of decreased salivary flow rates and effects of xerogenic agents.[155,156] Artificial saliva products and alcohol-free mouthwash may help to ease dry mouth, and good oral hygiene is essential.

Sodium-related increased thirst may be due to sodium modeling or hypertonic saline treatment for orthostatic hypotension during HD, although these practices are changing. Diminished taste sensation in the elderly may result in higher salt use to season food and increase the desire to drink more. Fluid intake may also be greater with severe gastroparesis when solid food is not well tolerated. If chewing or swallowing problems exist, excessive fluids may be consumed. However, people with orthostatic hypotension may need their sodium intake to be guided by their health care provider, just as in some rare cases with excess sodium sweat losses during high temperatures and high levels of physical activity.[30]

POTASSIUM CONSIDERATIONS

Patients with DM who receive HD may be prone to hyperkalemia due to factors other than excessive potassium intake. These include insulin deficiency and IR, aldosterone deficiency, acidosis, use of ACE-I and ARBs, and intracellular to extracellular fluid shifts attendant to hyperglycemia (whether or not acidosis is present).[86,157,158] Closer monitoring of potassium may be needed if plant-based diets are employed, as the intake of more fruits and vegetables could increase the potassium load. It may be advisable to emphasize portion sizes and items lower in potassium when trying to increase total fruit and vegetable consumption to maintain normal potassium levels. It is important to instruct patients on low potassium methods to treat hypoglycemia to deter the development of hyperkalemia. Hypokalemia may be a problem with PD due to enhanced dialysate losses; use of lower-calorie, lower-carbohydrate, and high-potassium foods may need to be encouraged. Use of some diuretics, even when concomitant with dialysis, has the potential to predispose patients to hypokalemia.

COUNSELING CONSIDERATIONS

Shared decision-making should be a cornerstone of patient-centered nutrition management in patients with DM and CKD, and it enables patients to make informed decisions about their nutrition intake and dietary choices.[30] Understanding and integrating the rationale and basic concepts of nutritional goals for both DM and CKD are fundamental for successful dietary acceptance, adherence, and management. Too often, the diets are seen as two separate entities instead of a combined cohesive approach, and the patient may feel overwhelmed by the multiple restrictions or recommendations. Many previously enjoyed foods may no longer be routinely advised, and the kidney diet at times may seem "unhealthy" as the potassium and phosphorus controls limit intake of many fruits, vegetables, high-fiber foods, and dairy products. It is a challenge to dispel a patient's preconceived notions, and patients may resist changing current practices. Additionally, it is ill advised to assume a preexisting good understanding of what DM control and its management involve, despite a long-standing history of DM. It is important to understand that patients may be accustomed to feeling hyperglycemic and fearing potential hypoglycemia. Probing, open-ended questions may be needed to ascertain current practices and beliefs regarding the use of foods, intake and timing of meals and snacks; medication administration, timing, and most recent dosing adjustments; and frequency of foot care and vision exams.

How we speak with patients matters and influences their perception. The use of empowering language in DM care and education can help inform and motivate while language that shames and judges may undermine this effort.[144] The ADA recommends language that 1) is neutral and based on facts, actions, or physiology; 2) stigma free; 3) maintains strength-based, respectful, and imparting hope; 4) fosters collaboration between patients and providers; and 5) remains person centered.[144] This has additional pertinence and potential impact when combined with the needs of CKD self-management.

Diabetes-Related Complications, Comorbidities, and Concerns

Complications and comorbidities due to DM influence the MNT care plan and ultimately impact the patient's nutritional and metabolic status. Microvascular and macrovascular complications increase the risk of four common disabilities in patients with ESKD: blindness, amputation, paresis or paralysis of one or more limbs, and dementia. Gastrointestinal issues can severely compromise intake adequacy. The presence of DM places patients in the highest-risk group for future CVD events, even without previous history for such.

DIABETIC RETINOPATHY AND VISUAL PROBLEMS

DM is the leading cause of blindness among adults aged 20 years to 74 years in developed countries, while DR is the most common microvascular diabetic complication existing globally in approximately two-thirds of patients with T1DM and a quarter of patients with T2DM.[8,159,160] The risk factors are extended duration of DM, advanced age, hyperglycemia, hyperlipidemia, proteinuria, severe obesity, and alcohol use.[161-163] Optimized glycemic, BP, and lipid control will reduce the risk or slow the progression of DR.[8] Similar pathological features exist in both DKD and DR.[160] CKD has been associated with a higher rate of DR with elevated urine albumin: creatinine ratio having a greater influence than decreased eGFR in T2DM, although diminishing eGFR can be a predictor of DR even without albuminuria.[159,161] Cranial neuropathy involves the oculomotor nerve, and microvascular nerve palsy can cause double vision and other problems with eyesight.[162] Glaucoma, cataracts, and other eye disorders may develop earlier and more frequently in people with DM.[8] Dilated and comprehensive eye examinations should be done annually if any level of DR exists, and every 1 to 2 years if there is no evidence of DR for one or more annual eye exams and well-controlled DM.[8] Patients may be considered legally blind, which differs from total blindness. Loss of vision can negatively impact the performance of activities of daily life, as well as food preparation and shopping; appreciation of food presentation, which can affect appetite and intake; the ability to adhere to the proper diet; medication administration; and self-care management of DM. Adaptive equipment, alternate teaching tools, voice blood glucose meters, and additional social service resources may need to be employed.

DIABETIC NEUROPATHY

Diabetic neuropathy (DN), the most common type of neuropathy, presents the most prevalent and troublesome chronic complications of DM in perhaps 8% of those newly diagnosed and in greater than 50% with long-standing DM with an unknown true prevalence.[8,162-165] DN is generally classified as peripheral or autonomic, although there are other types. It is a set of clinical syndromes that involve distinct regions of the nervous system (either singly or combined) with diverse manifestations affecting both small fibers and large fibers that may cause numbness and loss of protective sensation.[8,164,166] Different forms of DN often coexist in the same person.[164] Multiple organ systems are impacted including the cardiac, gastrointestinal, genitourinary, and integumentary. DN is often diagnosed by exclusion as other causes of neuropathy could exist.[8,164,166]

Sensorimotor Neuropathy

Distal symmetric polyneuropathy (DSPN) is the most common form of DN, accounting for up to 75% of DN.[165,166] Although T2DM is more common, it has a 45% incidence of neuropathy compared with the 54% to 59% associated with T1DM.[165] As with DKD, DSPN is seen after longer duration of T1DM and may be present at the time of diagnosis with T2DM, with rates increasing after a shorter duration.[166] Sensorimotor neuropathy results in sensory loss, resulting in the inability to feel, identify, or manipulate smaller objects.[166] Patients may experience frequent burning pain, electrical or stabbing sensations, paresthesia, hyperesthesia, and deep aching pain; and the symptoms are usually worse at night, disturbing sleep with symptoms varying according to the class of sensory fibers involved.[162,167] Focal neuropathies can also cause carpal tunnel syndrome, already a concern in HD, and foot drop, which can affect weight bearing. Mobility and dexterity issues can adversely impact daily activities, with potential consequences on provision and intake of food. Peripheral neuropathy in individuals with T2DM can have loss of handgrip strength when comparing measurements over time which bears consideration when completing the physical assessment.[62]

Hyperglycemia is the primary risk factor, in addition to independent causes including age, duration of DM, cigarette smoking, HTN, elevated TGs, higher BMI, alcohol consumption, and taller height.[162] Owing to a growing understanding of the association between MS and DSPN, more emphasis has been placed on obesity (particularly visceral adiposity), dyslipidemia, and HTN in T2DM.[165] Treatment is geared toward glycemic control and neuropathic pain management with either pregabalin or duloxetine recommended as the initial drug treatment while nothing specific is currently available for the underlying nerve damage.[8,167] Gabapentin, an anticonvulsant, has shown efficacy for pain control in DN, but it is not FDA approved for this indication.[8] A variety of drug therapies have been trialed, including antidepressants; and many of these may have adverse effects that are anticholinergic, such as dry mouth (xerostomia), constipation, and exacerbation of slow stomach emptying and/or other potential side effects (diarrhea, nausea, vomiting, fatigue, anorexia, increased appetite, weight gain, dizziness, and peripheral edema). Topical treatments, such as capsaicin and lidocaine, have been used for DSPN, but these also do not have FDA approval for this indication.[8,168] Oxidative stress, thought to be the key pathological process inducing nerve damage, may be related to hyperglycemia or possibly triggered by vascular abnormalities; therapies are currently under investigation.[162,164,168]

There is a higher incidence of diabetic foot disease with concurrent CKD in all stages, especially those on dialysis; and dialysis itself is an independent predictor.[8,169] Foot ulcers and amputation are consequences of DN and/or peripheral artery disease (PAD).[8] Risk factors for foot disease in those with DM and CKD are peripheral neuropathy (that could be due to uremia itself); susceptibility to infection; reduced ability to perform foot self-care or inspection (related to visual impairment, reduced mobility and manual dexterity); anemia which impairs wound healing and tissue oxygenation; time demands of treatment; and depression.[80,169] Poor glycemic control, foot deformities, preulcerative callus or corn, and cigarette smoking are additional factors.[8,170] Loss of protective sensation is a major component, with patients being unaware of or ignoring early foot lesions, wearing damaging footwear, and failing to report foot problems at an early stage to deter the need for lower-extremity amputation (LEA).[8,171] Recommendations made by the ADA are applicable to the care of patients with DM on dialysis, including comprehensive foot evaluation at least annually and more frequently if there are histories of ulcers or amputations, foot deformities, insensate feet, and PAD which requires screening and assessment.[8] In 2005, the KDOQI guidelines recognized the importance of preventive foot care as a part of patient education and advocated for foot examination at the initiation of dialysis to help reveal high-risk conditions requiring further regular examinations and referrals.[172] A multidisciplinary approach is recommended; and patient education is warranted regarding risk factors and appropriate management, including selection of proper footwear.[8,173] The significance of good foot care cannot be emphasized enough, given the potential for LEA, immobility limiting the person's ability to perform activities of daily living, and the presence of foot ulcers, which increase metabolic requirements for wound healing. These patients should be advised to wear socks with shoes and not go barefoot to minimize the incidence of potential foot injuries that could predispose the patients to infection.

Autonomic Neuropathy

Cardiovascular autonomic neuropathy Cardiovascular autonomic neuropathy (CAN), the most clinically important form of AN, is a CVD risk factor and is associated with mortality independent of other cardiovascular risk factors.[8] Another bidirectional relationship exists as renal insufficiency is a risk factor for CAN, and CAN independently predicts the progression of DKD.[166,174] Damage occurs to the autonomic nerve fibers that innervate the heart and blood vessels, resulting in abnormalities in heart rate control and vascular dynamics, with clinical manifestations of abnormal BP regulation, resting tachycardia, orthostatic hypotension, orthostatic tachycardia or bradycardia, exercise intolerance, and silent MI.[1,8,167] Symptoms of CAN may have special significance during HD treatments.

Gastrointestinal autonomic neuropathy (GAN) Up to 75% of people with DM may experience gastrointestinal symptoms.[175] AN can affect the entire gastrointestinal system involving any organ in the digestive system: esophagus, stomach, gallbladder, pancreas, and small and large intestines. This encompasses gastric function abnormalities (sensor and motor modality) and impairs gastrointestinal hormonal secretion resulting in the following[8,156,166,175-178]:

- *Gastroparesis (GP)*: most important manifestation which may be 50%, although the actual documented prevalence by radiological testing is lacking; nonobstructive delayed gastric emptying, with impaired gastric acid secretion and motility that is linked to disruption of vagal nerve function and dysfunction of intrinsic enteric neurons. Signs and symptoms include nausea, early satiety, postprandial fullness, anorexia, epigastric discomfort, abdominal pain described as burning or cramping, bloating, belching, and emesis of undigested food that had been consumed hours or days prior.

- *GERD*: 30% or more prevalence; esophageal dysfunction, with disordered peristalsis and abnormal lower-esophageal sphincter function; results in heartburn and dysphagia for solid foods. Limiting intake of caffeine, peppermint, pepper, spicy foods, alcohol, and fried and fatty foods may help minimize the symptoms. Individuals should remain in an upright position for 2 hours after eating and also consider elevating the head of the bed when sleeping.

- *Diabetic diarrhea*: 20% prevalence; profuse, watery, and often nocturnal, alternating with constipation; due to decreased gastrointestinal motility, reduced fluid absorption, bacterial overgrowth, pancreatic exocrine insufficiency, reduced insulin-growth factor 1 resulting in smooth muscle atrophy, coexistent celiac disease, abnormal bile salt metabolism, and depression.

- *Fecal incontinence*: related to anal sphincter incompetence or diminished rectal sensation, can often be nocturnal.

- *Constipation*: could affect up to 60% of people with long-standing DM; dysfunction of intestinal neurons, and, if severe, can cause fecal impaction or bowel perforation.
- *Gallbladder disease*: IR implicated in gallbladder dysmotility contributing to gallstone formation or acalculus cholecystitis. Cholecystitis is more common with DM, and biliary obstruction can develop.

GP has far-reaching effects and consequences and is mainly found in patients with long-standing DM.[166] Scoring systems have been developed, including one by the FDA (originally designed for clinical trials but also useful to document symptoms), the Gastroparesis Cardinal Symptom Index for patient-reported outcomes, and another based on the GP severity of illness.[177] Symptoms, however, do not necessarily correspond with its severity.[167] Organic causes and some medications, especially opioids and other pain management agents, can alter gastric emptying and need to be ruled out.[166-168] Pyloric dysfunction is an overlooked aspect in the pathogenesis of GP with evidence of pylorospasm with DM, and extragastric delays in small bowel and colonic transit may exist in 40% of the patients with GP.[178]

Food, especially higher in fat content, stays in the stomach longer, causing unpredictable glucose levels and late insulin reactions; and erratic blood sugar control may precede the actual diagnosis of GP. There is ultimately the potential for fermentation with bacterial overgrowth or bezoar development, causing possible obstruction and blocking passage to the small intestine. Furthermore, nutrient delivery to the small bowel will be impeded, meal-related protein synthesis is probably decreased, and medication absorption can be affected.[156] These effects can have an impact on phosphate binder absorption, and timing of use may need to be adjusted to compensate.

Glycemia and GP influence each other. Hyperglycemia slows gastric emptying, whereas hypoglycemia can accelerate gastric emptying. Poor glycemic control worsens symptoms of early satiety, fullness, and nausea.[1,167,175] Euglycemia may improve gastric emptying; however, having GP complicates balancing insulin

doses with food absorption, and hypoglycemia may be a result of mismatched exogenous insulin administration and glucose absorption.[1,167] There is potential for hyperglycemia emergencies, including DM ketoacidosis and hyperosmolar hyperglycemia syndrome.[177] More frequent monitoring of blood glucose levels will help determine insulin requirements and needed adjustments. Rapid-acting insulin may not be appropriate with GP.[179] Changing insulin types, doses, and/or the timing of injections is often indicated to improve blood glucose control. For some patients, injecting insulin after meals may be warranted, especially with a rapid-acting form. The insulin needs to be matched with the availability of the carbohydrate considering all of the different factors. CGM and insulin pumps may be useful in those with GP.

Patients with GP should eat small, frequent meals of low-fat, low-fiber foods with liquids. Eating high-protein foods first and limiting filling or high-volume foods may help combat early satiety. Foods that have small particles or are blenderized may also be beneficial. Carbonated beverages should probably be avoided to decrease bloating, as they can worsen proximal gastric distention. When symptoms are severe, only liquids may be tolerated. Patients should chew food thoroughly and maintain an upright posture for at least 30 minutes after each meal.

Medication therapy for GP includes the following[8,177,178,180,181]:

- metoclopramide: a prokinetic agent that also has an antiemetic effect, is intended for only short-term use due to adverse central nervous system side effects, whose benefits may not outweigh its risks
- domperidone: a prokinetic that is available for use only under a special program administered by the FDA (It does not cross the blood-brain barrier nor induce central nervous system effects but has similar efficacy to metoclopramide.)
- erythromycin: a motilin receptor agonist to increase stomach muscle contractions that has the disadvantages of being an antibiotic; effective for short-term use due to tachyphylaxis

- antiemetics to help relieve nausea and vomiting
- certain antidepressants to help relieve nausea and vomiting
- pain medicines that do not contain narcotics to reduce abdominal pain

It may be beneficial to withdraw medications with adverse effects on GI motility, such as opioids, anticholinergics, tricyclic antidepressants, some DM medications, or even renal-related prescriptions.[8] Drug–drug interactions are a concern as patients may be taking a combination of antiemetics, prokinetic agents, and pain modulators.[178] Additional therapies are oral or nasal tube feeding, jejunostomy tube feeding, parenteral nutrition, venting gastrostomy, laparoscopic pyloroplasty, and gastric electrical stimulation.[168,177,178,180,181]

Diabetic enteropathy can complicate nutritional status and cause limited food intake, potential weight loss, alteration of fluid and electrolyte balance, and hypoglycemia. Treatment may include gluten-free or lactose-free diets, limiting soluble fiber, or adding cholestyramine, somatostatin, and pancreatic enzymes. Intermittent and even potentially long-term administration of selective antibiotics (rifaximin has been most extensively studied) might be employed to combat intestinal bacterial overgrowth.[175] Use of loperamide hydrochloride (Imodium) can be helpful to decrease bowel motility, especially in fecal incontinence.[175,181] Diphenoxylate hydrochloride/atropine sulfate (lomotil) is also effective in the management of diarrhea. Osmotic laxatives may be preferable to bulking agents and fiber supplementation for slow transit constipation. See Chapter 17 for more detailed medication information.

CARDIOVASCULAR DISEASE

Issues related to CVD and DM go beyond dyslipidemia, although cholesterol abnormalities have a more pronounced CVD risk in patients with DM when compared to patients without DM. Patients with DM on dialysis were more likely to have a past history of HTN, MI, PVD, and cerebrovascular disease.[182] Nontraditional risk factors for HF include IR and urine albumin: creatinine ratio; and independent of CAD, CKD and DM increase the risk of HF.[183] DM is a risk factor for congestive heart failure (CHF) and ischemic heart disease, often due to the combined effect of volume overload and left ventricular hypertrophy (LVH).[1,70] Patients on dialysis with CHF, pulmonary edema, or fluid overload have very poor survival rates compared to patients with CHF and DM without kidney failure; and the elderly have the worst outcomes.[184] Those with DN, even in the absence of HTN or CAD, are likely to present a distinct pathological condition, defined as diabetic cardiomyopathy, although the pathogenesis is not fully known.[183] Patients with T2DM on HD, who have poor glycemic control, have a higher risk of sudden cardiac death, although studies have yet to be initiated on whether tight glycemic control will decrease this risk.[185]

Coronary and peripheral artery calcifications are prevalent at earlier stages of DKD, occurring prior to any dialysis, use of calcium-containing phosphate binders, or initiation of vitamin D therapy. This suggests that DM itself plays a role, possibly due to the deposition of advanced glycation end products (AGEs) and dyslipidemia related to HTN and accelerated by uremia.[1] Predictors for peripheral vascular calcification in HD for individuals with DM were higher values of HbA1c and longer duration of dialysis.[186] Produced AGEs stiffen structural collagen backbones that can increase inflammation and tissue fibrosis, promoting diastolic dysfunction and atherosclerosis.[187]

MINERAL AND BONE DISORDERS AND FRACTURE RISK

CKD–mineral bone disease (MBD) leads to a high risk of bone fractures because of bone mineral density (BMD) changes and poor bone quality. Chronically high or low levels of PTH can negatively impact bone metabolism, and both have been linked to increased fracture rates. Meta-analyses and cohort studies confirm that DM is associated with a higher fracture risk.[188] DM and osteoporotic fractures are two of the most important causes of morbidity and mortality. Both T1DM and T2DM increase the risk of skeletal fracture, particularly at the hip.[189-191] DM in the aging population is associated with reduced muscle strength, poor muscle quality, and accelerated loss of muscle mass, which may result in sarcopenia and osteopenia.[126]

BMD measurement, which is a noninvasive method for identifying individuals with osteoporosis and possibly those at high risk of fractures, calculates bone density and is a core indicator of bone strength. A single BMD combined with a fracture history assessment can predict fracture risk over 20 to 25 years.[192] This measurement is compared to the reference population of a group of healthy young adults. If the BMD is 2.5 standard deviations or more below the average reference-group BMD, there is presence of osteoporosis. BMD scores are reduced in patients with T1DM but normal or increased in patients with T2DM.[189-191] This paradox may be due to the fact that DM may affect bone metabolism by multiple pathways.

One explanation for a reduced BMD in patients with T1DM is a deficiency of insulin which may cause bone fragility.[193] The disease burden and increased risk of falling may further explain the higher fracture incidence in patients with DM with respect to the general population. Poor vision and reduced peripheral nerve function can predispose patients to increased fracture risk, not necessarily solely dependent of BMD. Other risk factors include the presence of DKD and DN, lack of physical activity, and autonomic and other neuropathic changes that could promote a loss of bone mineral composition. Therefore, an increased risk of falling in persons with DM could account for the elevated hip fracture risk in the face of normal or elevated BMD.[194]

Bone cells and the integrity of the matrix can be influenced in several ways. Increased blood glucose levels can have a negative impact.[195] In vitro studies suggest that hyperglycemia has a deleterious effect on osteoblasts, impeding bone formation, but this has not been confirmed in clinical studies.[196] A meta-analysis reported no effect of glycemic control on BMD.[197] However, diabetic ketoacidosis, severe hyperglycemia, or metabolic acidosis could cause hyperphosphatemia due to massive cellular shifts of phosphate out of the cells. Another possible explanation for increased bone fragil-

ity in DM is the accumulation of AGEs within bone collagen, leading to increased stiffness of the collagen network.[198] An excessive formation of AGE cross-links changes bone integrity and increases fracture risk.[199]

The role of antidiabetic agents on bone health varies with some being protective and others increasing the risk of MBD. Metformin has a direct effect on bone tissue and can reverse the adverse impact of AGE accumulation.[200] Incretin therapies inhibit bone resorption and may protect the skeleton.[201,202] Thiazolidinediones are associated with bone loss.[203] Some SGLT2i have shown an increased incidence of bone fractures in clinical trials.[27,34]

Individuals with DM and CKD should be evaluated thoroughly for evidence of CKD–MBD (see Chapter 10 for more information). Further studies are needed to understand the mechanisms of bone loss in patients with DKD to develop more effective treatments to reduce bone loss and improve bone density. It is reasonable to expect that close metabolic control of DM may improve bone status, although its effect on reduction of fracture risk has not yet been demonstrated in clinical studies.

ORAL HEALTH AND DENTAL DISEASE

Periodontal disease has been referred to as the overlooked DM complication, being more severe and probably more prevalent in patients with DM than those without DM; and there is a bidirectional relationship between the two.[145,204,205] Periodontal inflammation causes poor glycemic control and is a major source of inflammation in PD.[205] Patients with CKD suffer from numerous systemic complications that contribute to poor oral health as a consequence of uremic metabolic, endocrinological, and immunological imbalances.[206] Diabetic oral health complications include xerostomia, dental caries, tooth loss, gingivitis, periodontitis, odontogenic abscesses, candidiasis, burning mouth syndrome, halitosis, and soft-tissue lesions of tongue and mucosa.[1,205,206] CKD has been reported to affect the teeth, oral mucosa, bone, periodontium, salivary glands, tongue, mouth cavity, and temporomandibular joint.[206] A study of oral and dental manifestations in patients on dialysis showed that patients with DM had a higher prevalence of caries and more severe dry mouth, taste changes, and mucosal pain.[207] DM and a longer dialysis vintage are independently associated with the severity of periodontitis, which involves bone loss around the teeth as a result of subgingival bacterial infection; and there are also correlations with malnutrition, inflammation, and systemic infection, with possible association with cardiovascular mortality in the population with ESKD.[1,206] Salivary dysfunction can adversely affect oral and nutritional health as well as immune response and inflammation; and hyposalivation in DM has been associated with hyperglycemia, neuropathy, and xerogenic medications.[1,208] Periodontal gum disease, an infectious disease process that occurs in the presence of bacteria, may be due to prolonged exposure to hyperglycemia, while the immune response to infection also is altered by hyperglycemia.[1,208] Proactive, preventive dental care and assessment are important management strategies, and periodontal therapy may improve glycemic control.[1,144] Periodontal care and treatment are useful for ameliorating a variety of the inflammatory manifestations in those with diabetic nephropathy.[205] The importance of dental disease related to DM cannot be dismissed, as it could ultimately influence a patient's ability to consume an adequate diet and help deter malnutrition.

HIV

Patients on dialysis with HIV may be prone to DM. The ADA recommends screening for DM and prediabetes in those with HIV, although the HbA1c value should not be used as a screening factor because it underestimates glycemia in this population.[144] There is an increased risk for abnormal carbohydrate metabolism, IR, T2DM, and poor CVD outcomes with HIV due to the metabolic effects of individual or combination therapies for HIV infection.[209-211] People with both HIV and DM are at a significantly increased risk of CKD compared to those with either disease alone, even after adjusting for traditional CKD risk factors.[212]

MALNUTRITION

Related complications and presence of comorbidities with DM contribute to malnutrition. Multiple microvascular and macrovascular complications affect daily activities, access to food supply, preparation of food, food's appeal, and taste. GAN has a major influence with its side effects. Oral health problems contribute to difficulty chewing and local infections. Foot problems and associated surgery may alter the protein requirements due to infection and wound healing needs. Inadequate nutritional intake, especially protein intake, increases the risk of sarcopenia and frailty in the aging population with DM.[126]

However, IR and DM play major roles. Insulin is both an anabolic and anticatabolic hormone. Insulin therapy affects parameters of protein kinetics, enhances amino acid uptake, and stimulates protein synthesis. Protein metabolism is more sensitive to the DM control status than is generally appreciated "clinically."[8,199,213,214] DM is the most significant predictor of lean body mass loss in patients on dialysis. This loss is independent of inadequate dialysis dose, metabolic acidosis, and an insufficient protein intake.[215] In addition to insulin deficiency, which increases muscle protein breakdown, the data appears to point to the potential protein catabolic effects of IR for a combined effect.[216] Patients with acidemia and CKD need higher-than-normal levels of insulin to inhibit proteolysis.[217] Alteration of protein metabolism by insulin may lead to changes in body tissue composition, which may become clinically evident in conditions characterized by low insulinemia, such as fasting and low energy intakes, that could overlap with alterations in insulin sensitivity occurring in normal aging.[217] Attention to modifiable factors of IR may help improve the situation.

OBESITY AND BARIATRIC SURGERY

Obesity is a predisposing factor in both DM and CKD. The AACE/ACE have designated adiposity-based chronic disease as the medical diagnostic term for overweight/obesity and view this as needing a long-term management commitment.[34] The ADA and AACE/ACE have similar recommendations regarding weight loss, involving a combination of a healthy lower-calorie diet, physical activity, and behavioral therapy for all overweight persons or individuals with obesity and T2DM or at risk for DM.[34,218] Dietary interventions may differ by macronutrient goals and food choices as long as they create the necessary energy deficit to promote weight loss while also considering the determination of food availability and other cultural circumstances that could affect dietary patterns.[218] A medication's effect on weight gain needs to be considered when prescribed.[218]

The ADA recommendations for obesity include the use of nonjudgmental patient-centered communication, and accommodations should be made to provide privacy during weighing. Many patients may perceive their weight as sensitive information and may have been stigmatized by previous experiences.[218] This may now be compounded by the frequency of being weighed with dialysis treatments and an ongoing focus on volume status. Those who are obese and have DM may have a more pressing need to understand and differentiate the concept of fluid weight gains and losses and how these relate to actual body mass and target weight. This area may need further exploration, if we are to be successful in achieving both body weight goals and fluid control in this population. It also warrants concern, as those on dialysis may need to lose weight to achieve a BMI deemed as acceptable for a transplant program acceptance.

The appropriate weight management of patients with CKD remains a controversial topic. The 2007 Clinical Practice Guidelines for DM and CKD recommend a BMI within the normal range (18.5–24.9) which is based on extrapolation from other populations.[42] A number of studies have indicated that higher values of BMI reflecting both overweight and obesity seemed to be associated with better survival rates in patients with ESKD, but there is limited data regarding this pattern of reverse epidemiology in patients with CKD.[219,220]

It is unknown whether weight management may lower the risk for developing DKD and progressing to ESKD, as there are no specific weight loss interventions tailored to patients with DKD. A systematic review of 13 studies on patients with CKD failed to demonstrate

a change in GFR with nonsurgical weight loss interventions, but a statistically significant improvement in proteinuria was observed during a short follow-up period.[221] Surgical intervention with bariatric surgery normalized glomerular hyperfiltration. There is a lack of long-term studies to address weight loss interventions on the progression of CKD.

Individuals with T2DM are at risk for obesity-related comorbidities; however, persons with T1DM have traditionally had a lower BMI, but current research has demonstrated otherwise.[222,223] The prevalence of obesity in patients with T1DM has increased at a faster rate compared to the general population. Individuals with T1DM can have both obesity and IR commonly observed in patients with T2DM. Little is known about effective weight management interventions in this population. Multiple approaches could be targeted, such as dietary modifications, increased physical activity, adjustment of insulin, and other pharmacotherapies that impact weight loss. Often, increased physical activity is identified as a barrier to weight management due to the fear of hypoglycemia which can occur up to 24 hours after exercising.[224] To prevent the occurrence of hypoglycemia, the insulin dose can be reduced prior to activity, but typically patients prefer to consume carbohydrates before and during activity, which can result in subsequent weight gain.

While lifestyle modification is recommended as a primary treatment approach for patients with T2DM, there is limited evidence on the development and progression of DKD. The Action for Health in Diabetes Trial did not demonstrate that intensive management could reduce cardiovascular events in patients with overweight or obesity issues and T2DM.[224,225] Long-term weight loss was achieved with a mean weight loss of 4.7% at 8 years with 27% of the study participants maintaining a 10% weight loss. The intensive managed lifestyle group had a 31% lower incidence of developing CKD, which could suggest a role for lifestyle management in the development and progression of DKD.

The FDA has approved medications for both short- and long-term weight management. All weight loss medications need to be used with the appropriate cautions in CKD stages 3 through 5.[226] GI interventions have been suggested as treatments for T2DM, and in that context, they are termed *metabolic surgery*; but the role in T1DM will require more study despite seeing metabolic profile improvement.[218] Bariatric surgery is by far the most effective and has even been shown in some patients to be renoprotective, primarily reflected by a reduction in proteinuria and remission of DM.[227] The nutritional interventions in DM and CKD should incorporate a multifaceted approach to reduce risk factors as well as promote healthy behaviors. Studies are needed to determine safe approaches for effective and sustained weight loss in adults with CKD and DM.

PHYSICAL CONDITIONING AND EXERCISE

Physical activity enhances insulin sensitivity and endothelial function and lowers inflammatory markers, which are associated with an improvement in CVD and all-cause mortality in the general population and those with CKD. However, most people with CKD do not meet the physical activity levels that are recommended by the AHA and the American College of Sports Medicine.[30,228] Exercise potential in those on dialysis may be limited due to the physical problems caused by CKD–MBD, secondary hyperparathyroidism and metastatic calcification, metabolic acidosis, and malnutrition.

Having DM further complicates the patient's ability to achieve or maintain a level of physical activity. Although physical activity can acutely increase albumin excretion, no evidence indicates that vigorous exercise will accelerate the rate of progression of DKD.[148] Each person with T1DM has a variable glycemic response to exercise that needs to be considered when recommending the type and duration of exercise.[148] Certain types of exercise may be unadvisable or predispose the person with DM to injury. During a preexercise evaluation for exercise, patients need to be assessed for conditions such as uncontrolled HTN, untreated proliferative retinopathy, AN, peripheral neuropathy, and a history of foot ulcers or Charcot foot.[148] Peripheral neuropathy can lead to muscle atrophy. There is also low-activity

tolerance due to decreased maximal oxygen consumption, the presence of CAN, and/or anemia. Additional instruction may be needed regarding when it is safe to exercise depending on blood sugar levels and presence of ketosis, possible need to alter antidiabetic medications prior to exercising, adjustment of intake to prevent hypoglycemia, treatment of hypoglycemia should it occur, and use of proper footwear. Physical therapists can develop appropriate exercise programs to increase the patient's functional capacity, and occupational therapists can help the patient develop strategies for activities of daily living.

The KDIGO recommendations and consideration for patients with DM and CKD include the following[30]:

- Patients should be advised to undertake moderate-intensity physical activity for a cumulative duration of at least 150 minutes per week (spread throughout the week when possible) or to a level compatible with their cardiovascular and physical tolerance.
- Physical activity recommendations should consider age, ethnic background, presence of other comorbidities, and access to resources.
- Patients should be advised to avoid sedentary behavior.
- For patients at higher risk of falls, health care providers should advise on the intensity of physical activity and the type of exercises.
- Many short bouts of exercise with less intensity can still offer health benefits.
- Patients should engage in multicomponent physical activities, which include aerobic and muscle-strengthening activities along with balance-training activities as tolerated.

PSYCHOLOGICAL AND MENTAL HEALTH ISSUES

The prevalence of clinically significant psychopathology diagnoses are considerably more common in people with DM, and accompanying symptoms can interfere with the person's ability to carry out daily DM self-management.[144] Anxiety disorders, depression, eating disorders, and serious mental illness are addressed in the ADA Standards of Medical Care, and there could also be an impact on issues relating to dialysis care management.[144,148] The association between DM and depression or depressive symptoms is a major public health problem. Several studies suggest that there may be a mutually reinforcing relationship between depressive symptoms and poorer adherence to self-care behaviors.[225]

DM distress refers to significant negative psychological reactions related to emotional burdens and worries specific to a person's experience in having to manage a severe, complicated, and demanding chronic disease.[148] This concept could be applicable to those needing dialysis. DM distress can lead to worse adherence and outcomes, while there may also be shared biological and behavioral mechanisms that merit consideration to understand the link between depression and DM.[1,148,229] Mindful self-compassion training may be beneficial to deal with DM distress.[148]

Lower health-related quality of life scores with DM were associated with dialysis, blindness, symptomatic neuropathy, foot ulcers, amputations, debilitating stroke, and CHF.[230] A study with a small sample size raised interesting points as to how individuals with DM perceive kidney failure, and a clear distinction was made between losses due to DM vs intrusion into lifestyle, including diet, fluid control, and emphasis on time factors with dialysis.[231] Conditions for coverage for ESKD require a qualified social worker to assess the psychosocial needs of patients via use of a standardized mental and physical tool and inclusion of this assessment's results in the patient's plan of care.[232] The Kidney Disease Quality of Life tool is one such standardized tool and includes questions related to appetite and perceived burden of diet and fluid restrictions.[233] Collaborative decision-making is viewed as important for positive interactions with health care providers and the creation of individualized treatment plans for more effective self-management.[231,234] More attention and psychosocial support may be warranted when these dual diagnoses are present in patients with CKD.

Summary

Living with either DM or CKD can be challenging. Managing DM in the presence of CKD requires additional effort on the part of the patient, caregivers, and health care team to improve outcomes and decrease the morbidity and mortality in this population. The nutrition needs of patients with DM and CKD change as the progression and the management of the diseases evolve. Understanding the treatment goals of each stage is crucial to maximize the nutritional status of patients throughout this process and individualize their MNT accordingly while endeavoring to enhance their quality of life. As new advances occur regarding CKD and DM, it is important to stay abreast of new guidelines (eg, the KDOQI, the KDIGO, and the ADA Medical Standards of Care in Diabetes) and integrate them into practice and patient care.

References

1. Schatz SR, Pagenkemper J. Nutrition management of diabetes in chronic kidney disease. In: Byham-Gray L, Stover J, Wiesen K, eds. *A Clinical Guide to Nutrition Care in Kidney Disease*. 2nd ed. Academy of Nutrition and Dietetics; 2013:111-139.

2. Tuttle KR, Bakris GL, Bilous R, et al. Diabetic kidney disease: a report from an ADA consensus conference. *Diabetes Care*. 2014;37(10):2864-2883. doi:10.2337/dc14-1296

3. United States Renal Data System. Executive Summary 2019: Overview of Kidney Disease in United States. USRDS website. January 2019. Accessed January 9, 2020. https://usrds.org/media/2371/2019-executive-summary.pdf

4. United States Renal Data System. 2017 USRDS Annual Data Report. January 2017. Accessed September 2, 2018. https://usrds.org/media/1652/v1_00_execsummary_17.pdf

5. Centers for Disease Control and Prevention. Chronic Kidney Disease in the United States, 2019. CDC website. March 2019. Accessed January 9, 2020. www.cdc.gov/kidneydisease/pdf/2019_National-Chronic-Kidney-Disease-Fact-Sheet.pdf

6. United States Renal Data System. US Renal Data System 2019 Annual Data Report: Epidemiology of Kidney Disease in the United States. National Institute of Health, National Institute of Diabetes and Digestive and Kidney Diseases website. January 2019. Accessed February 11, 2020. www.usrds.org/annual-data-report/previous-adrs

7. McFarlane P, Cherney D, Gilbert R, Senior P. Diabetes Canada Clinical Practice Guidelines Expert Committee. 2018 Clinical Practice Guidelines Chronic Kidney Disease in Diabetes. *Can J Diabetes*. 2018;42:S201-S209. doi:10.1016/j.jcjd.2017.11:004

8. American Diabetes Association. 11. Microvascular complications and foot care: standards of medical care in diabetes—2021. *Diabetes Care*. 2021;44(suppl 1):S151-S167. doi:10.2337/dc21-S011

9. Senior PA. Diabetes and chronic kidney disease: concern, confusion, clarity? *Can J Diabetes*. 2014;38(5):287-289. doi:10.1016/j.jcjd.2014.08.001

10. American Diabetes Association. 2. Classification and diagnosis of diabetes: standards of medical care in diabetes—2021. *Diabetes Care*. 2021;44(suppl 1):S15-S331. doi:10.2337/dc21-S002

11. Narasimhan S, Weinstock RS. Youth-onset type 2 diabetes mellitus: lessons learned from the TODAY study. *Mayo Clin Proc*. 2014;89(6):806-816. doi:10.1016/j.mayocp.2014.01.009

12. Afkarian M. Diabetic kidney disease in children and adolescents. *Pediatr Nephrol*. 2015;30(1):65-74. doi:10.1007/s00467-014-2796-5

13. Jellinger PS, Handelsman Y, Rosenblit P, et al. American Association of Clinical Endocrinologists and American College of Endocrinology guidelines for management of dyslipidemia and prevention of cardiovascular disease. *Endocr Pract*. 2017;23(suppl 2):1-87. doi:10.4158/EP171764.APPGL

14. Prasad GV. Metabolic syndrome and chronic kidney disease: current status and future directions. *World J Nephrol*. 2014;3(4):210-219. doi:10.5527/wjn.v3.i4.210

15. Comini LO, de Oliveira LC, Borges LD, et al. Individual and combined components of metabolic syndrome with chronic kidney disease in individuals with hypertension and/or diabetes mellitus accompanied by primary health care. *Diabetes Metab Syndr Obes*. 2020;13:71-80. doi:10.2147/DMSO.S223929

16. Zammit AR, Katz MJ, Derby C, Bitzer M, Lipton R. Chronic kidney disease in non-diabetic older adults: associated roles of the metabolic syndrome, inflammation, and insulin resistance. *PLoS One*. 2015;10(10):e0139369. doi:10.1371/journal.pone.0139369

17. Shinohara K, Shoji T, Emoto M, et al. Insulin resistance as an independent predictor of cardiovascular mortality in patients with end-stage renal disease. *J Am Soc Nephrol*. 2002;13(7):1894-1900. doi:10.1097/01.asn.0000019900.87535.43

18. Liu J, Rosner MH. Lipid abnormalities associated with end-stage renal disease. *Semin Dial*. 2006;19(1):32-40. doi:10.1111/j.1525-139X.2006.00117.x

19. Abe M, Kalantar-Zadeh K. Haemodialysis-induced hypoglycaemia and glycaemic disarrays. *Nat Rev Nephrol*. 2015;11(5):302-313. doi:10.1038/nrneph.2015.38

20. Bailey JL. Insulin resistance and muscle metabolism in chronic kidney disease. *ISRN Endocrinol*. 2013;329606. doi:10.1155/2013/329606

21. Koppe L, Pelletier CC, Alix C, et al. Insulin resistance in chronic kidney disease: new lessons from experimental models. *Nephrol Dial Transplant*. 2014;29(9):1666-1674. doi:10.1093/ndt/gft435

22. Palmer BF. Carbohydrate and insulin metabolism in chronic kidney disease. Uptodate.com website. March 2019. Accessed January 9, 2020. www.uptodate.com/contents/carbohydrate-and-insulin-metabolism-in-chronic-kidney-disease

23. Lin-Tan DT, Lin J-L, Wang LH, et al. Fasting glucose levels in predicting 1-year all-cause mortality in patients who do not have diabetes and are on maintenance hemodialysis. *J Am Soc Nephrol*. 2007;18(8):2385-2391. doi:10.1681/ASN.2006121409

24. American Diabetes Association. 3. Prevention or delay of type 2 diabetes: standards of medical care in diabetes—2021. *Diabetes Care*. 2021;44(suppl 1):S34-S39. doi:10.2337/dc21-S003

25. Chu YW, Wu WS, Hsu CF, Wang JJ, Weng SF, Chien CC. Bidirectional association between ESRD dialysis and diabetes: national cohort study. *PLoS One*. 2017;12(3):e0173785. doi:10.1371/journal.pone.0173785

26. Centers for Disease Control and Prevention. National Chronic Kidney Disease Fact Sheet, 2017. January 2017. Accessed September 2, 2018. www.cdc.gov/diabetes/pubs/pdf/kidney_factsheet.pdf

27. American Diabetes Association. 9. Pharmacologic approaches to glycemic treatment: standards of medical care in diabetes—2021. *Diabetes Care*. 2020;44(suppl 1):S111-S124. doi:10.2337/dc21-S009

28. Inzucchi SE, Bergenstal RM, Buse JB, et al. Management of hyperglycemia in type 2 diabetes, 2015: a patient-centered approach: update to a position statement of the American Diabetes Association and the European Association for the Study of Diabetes. *Diabetes Care.* 2015;38(1):140-149. doi:10.2337/dc14-2441

29. Davies MJ, D'Alessio DA, Fradkin J, et al. Management of hyperglycemia in type 2 diabetes, 2018. A consensus report by the American Diabetes Association (ADA) and the European Association for the Study of Diabetes (EASD). *Diabetologia.* 2018;61:2461-2498. doi:10.1007/s00125-018-4729-5

30. Kidney Disease: Improving Global Outcomes (KDIGO) Diabetes Work Group. KDIGO 2020 Clinical practice guideline for diabetes management in chronic kidney disease. *Kidney Int.* 2020;98(4S):S1-S115. doi:10.1016/j.kint.2020.06.019

31. Sanchez-Rangel E, Inzucchi SE. Metformin: clinical use in type 2 diabetes. *Diabetologia.* 2017;60(9):1586-1593. doi:10.1007/s00125-017-4336-x

32. Davidson JA. SGLT2 inhibitors in patients with type 2 diabetes and renal disease: overview of current evidence. *Postgrad Med.* 2019;131(4):251-260. doi:10.1080/00325481.2019.1601404

33. Greco EV, Russo G, Giandalia A, Viazzi F, Pontremoli R, De Cosmo S. GLP-1 receptor agonists and kidney protection. *Medicina (Kaunas).* 2019;55(6):223. doi:10.3390/medicina55060233

34. Garber AJ, Handelsman YH, Grunberger G, et al. Consensus Statement by the American Association of Clinical Endocrinologists and American College of Endocrinology on the Comprehensive Type 2 Diabetes Management Algorithm—2020 Executive Summary. *Endocr Pract.* 2020;26(1):107-139. doi:10.4158/CS-2019-0472

35. Beck J, Greenwood D, Blanton L, et al. 2017 National Standards for Diabetes Self-Management Education and Support. *Diabetes Care.* 2017;40(10):1409-14619. doi:10.2337/dci17-0025

36. American Association of Diabetes Educators. An effective model of diabetes care and education: revising the AADE7 self-care behaviors. *Diabetes Educ.* 2020;46(2)139-160. doi:10.1177/0145721719894903

37. Gheith O, Farouk N, Nampoory N, Halim M, Al-Otaibi T. Diabetic kidney disease: world wide difference of prevalence and risk factors. *J Nephropharmacol.* 2016;5(1):49-56. doi:10.4103/1110-9165.197379

38. Alicic RZ, Rooney MT, Tuttle KR. Diabetic kidney disease: challenges, progress, and possibilities. *Clin J Am Soc Nephrol.* 2017;12(12):2032-2045. doi:10.2215/CJN.11491116

39. Pugliese G, Penno G, Natali A, et al. Diabetic kidney disease: new clinical and therapeutic issues. Joint position statement of the Italian Diabetes Society and the Italian Society of Nephrology on "The natural history of diabetic kidney disease and treatment of hyperglycemia in patients with type 2 diabetes and impaired renal function." *J Nephrol.* 2020;33(1):9-35. doi:10.1007/s40620-019-00650-x

40. Mogensen CE. Microalbuminuria predicts clinical proteinuria and early mortality in maturity-onset diabetes. *N Engl J Med.* 1984;310(6):356-360. doi:10.1056/NEJM198402093100605

41. Kidney Disease: Improving Global Outcomes. KDIGO 2012 Clinical practice guideline for the evaluation and management of chronic kidney disease. *Kidney Int Suppl.* 2013;3(1):1-150.

42. National Kidney Foundation. KDOQI Clinical practice guidelines and clinical practice recommendations for diabetes and chronic kidney disease. *Am J Kidney Dis.* 2007;49(2 suppl 2):S12-S154. doi:10.1053/j.ajkd.2006.12.005

43. The Diabetes Control and Complications (DCCT) Research Group. Effect of intensive therapy on the development and progression of diabetic nephropathy in the Diabetes Control and Complications Trial. *Kidney Int.* 1995;47(6):1703-1720. doi:10.1038/ki.1995/236

44. Orchard TJ, Dorman JS, Maser RE, et al. Prevalence of complications in IDDM by sex and duration. Pittsburgh Epidemiology of Diabetes Complications Study II. *Diabetes.*1990;39(9):1116-1124. doi:10.2337/diab.39.9.1116

45. Patel A, MacMahon S, Chalmers J, et al. ADVANCE Collaborative Group. Intensive blood glucose control and vascular outcomes in patients with type 2 diabetes. *N Engl J Med.* 2008;358(24):2560-2572. doi:10.1056/NEJMoa0802987

46. Ismail-Beigi F, Craven T, Banerji MA, et al. Effect of intensive treatment of hyperglycaemia on microvascular outcomes in type 2 diabetes: an analysis of the ACCORD randomised trial. *Lancet.* 2010;376(9739):419-430. doi:10.1016/S0140-6736(10)60576-4

47. Duckworth W, Abraira C, Moritz T, et al. Glucose control and vascular complications in veterans with type 2 diabetes. *N Engl J Med.* 2009;360(2):129-139. doi:10.1056/NEJMoa0808431

48. de Boer IH, Afkarian M, Rue TC, et al. Renal outcomes in patients with type I diabetes and macroalbuminuria. *J Am Soc Nephrol*. 2014;25(10):2342-2350. doi:10.1681/ASN .2013091004

49. Hovind P, Tarnow L, Rossing P, et al. Predictors for the development of microalbuminuria and macroalbuminuria in patients with type 1 diabetes: inception cohort study. *BMJ*. 2004;328(7448):1105. doi:10.1136/bmj.38070.450891.FE

50. Bakris GL, Williams M, Dworkin L, et al. Preserving renal function in adults with hypertension and diabetes: a consensus approach. *Am J Kidney Dis*. 2000;36(3):646-661. doi:10.1053/ajkd.2000.16225

51. Levey AS, Beto JA, Coronado BE, et al. Controlling the epidemic of cardiovascular disease in chronic renal disease: what do we know? What do we need to learn? Where do we go from here? National Kidney Foundation Task Force on Cardiovascular Disease. *Am J Kidney Dis*. 1998;32(5):853-906. doi:10.1016/s0272-6386(98)70145-3

52. Moen MF, Zhan M, Hsu VD, et al. Frequency of hypoglycemia and its significance in chronic kidney disease. *Clin J Am Soc Nephrol*. 2009;4(6):1121-1127. doi:10.2215/CJN.00800209

53. Biesenbach G, Raml A, Schmekal B, Eichbauer-Strum G. Decreased insulin requirement in relation to GFR in nephropathic type 1 and insulin-treated type 2 diabetic patients. *Diabet Med*. 2003;20(8):642-645. doi:10.1046/j.1464-5491.2003 .01025.x

54. Snyder RW, Berns JS. Use of insulin and oral hypoglycemic medications in patients with diabetes mellitus and advanced kidney disease. *Semin Dial*. 2004;17(5):365-370. doi:10.1111/j.0894-0959.2004 .17346.x

55. Horton ES, Johnson C, Lebovitz HE. Carbohydrate metabolism in uremia. *Ann Intern Med*. 1968;68(1):63-74. doi:10.7326/0003-4819-68-1-63

56. Dieter BP, Alicic RZ, Tuttle KR. GLP-1 receptor agonists in diabetic kidney disease: from the patient-side to the bench-side. *Am J Physiol Renal Physiol*. 2018; 315(6):F1519-F1525. doi:10.1152 /ajprenal.00211.2018

57. Klahr S, Levey AS, Beck GJ, et al. The effects of dietary protein restriction and blood-pressure control on the progression of chronic renal disease. Modification of Diet in Renal Disease Study Group. *N Engl J Med*. 1994;330(13):877-884. doi:10.1056 /NEJM199403313301301

58. Hunsicker LG, Adler S, Caggiula A, et al. Predictors of the progression of renal disease in the modification of diet in renal disease study. *Kidney Int*. 1997;51(6):1908-1919. doi:10.1038/ki.1997.260

59. Pedrini MT, Levey AS, Lau J, Chalmers TC, Wang PH. The effect of dietary protein restriction on the progression of diabetic and nondiabetic renal disease: a meta-analysis. *Ann Intern Med*. 1996;124(7):627-632. doi:10.7326/0003-4819-124 -7-199604010-00002

60. Kovesdy CP, Kopple JD, Kalantar-Zadeh K. Management of protein-energy wasting in non-dialysis-dependent chronic kidney disease: reconciling low protein intake with nutritional therapy. *Am J Clin Nutr*. 2013;97(6):1163-1177. doi:10.3945/ajcn.112.036418

61. Academy of Nutrition and Dietetics Evidence Analysis Library. EAL-KDOQI (CKD) Guideline. Eatright website. August 2020. Accessed October 23, 2020. www.andeal.org/topic.cfm?menu=5303 &cat=5557

62. Ikizler TA, Burrowes JD, Byham-Gray LD, et al. KDOQI Clinical Practice Guidelines for nutrition in CKD: 2020 update. *Am J Kidney Dis*. 2020;76(3 suppl 1):S1-S107. doi:10.1053/j.ajkd.2020.05.006

63. Kalantar-Zadeh K, Moore LW, Tortorici AR, et al. North American experience with low protein diet for non-dialysis-dependent chronic kidney disease. *BMC Nephrol*. 2016;17(1):90. doi:10.1186/s12882 -016-0304-9

64. Ko GJ, Obi Y, Tortorici AR, Kalantar-Zadeh K. Dietary protein intake and chronic kidney disease. *Curr Opin Clin Nutr Metab Care*. 2017;20(1):77-85. doi:10 .1097/MCO.0000000000000342

65. Kasiske BL, Lakatua JD, Ma JZ, Louis TA. A meta-analysis of the effects of dietary protein restriction on the rate of decline in renal function. *Am J Kidney Dis*. 1998;31(6):954-961. doi:10.1053/ajkd.1998 .v31.pm9631839

66. Muntner P, Whelton PK, Woodward M, Carey R. A comparison of the 2017 American College of Cardiology/American Heart Association Blood Pressure Guideline and the 2017 American Diabetes Association Diabetes and Hypertension Position Statement for U.S. Adults with Diabetes. *Diabetes Care*. 2018;41(11):2322-2329. doi:10 .2337/dc18-1307

67. Fryar CD, Ostchega Y, Hales C, Zhang GZ, Kruszon-Moran, D. Hypertension prevalence and control among adults: United States, 2015–2016. US Department of Health and Human Services: Centers for Disease Control and Prevention website. October 2017. Accessed February 3, 2020. www.cdc.gov/nchs/data/databriefs/db289.pdf

68. Norgaard K, Feldt-Rasmussen B, Borch-Johnsen K, Saelan H, Deckert T. Prevalence of hypertension in type 1 (insulin-dependent) diabetes mellitus. *Diabetologia*. 1990;30(7):407-410. doi:10.1007/BF00404089

69. Van Buren PN, Toto R. Hypertension on diabetic nephropathy: epidemiology, mechanisms, and management. *Adv Chronic Kidney Dis*. 2011;18(1):28-41. doi:10.1053/j.ackd.2010.10.003

70. American Diabetes Association. 10. Cardiovascular disease and risk management: standards of medical care in diabetes—2021. *Diabetes Care*. 2021;44(suppl 1):S125-S150. doi:10.2337/dc21-S010

71. Wright J, Cavanaugh K. Dietary sodium in chronic kidney disease: a comprehensive approach. *Semin Dial*. 2010;23(4):415-421. doi:10.1111/j.1525-139X.2010.00752.x

72. Dietary Guidelines for Americans 2015–2020. 8th ed. Home of the Office of Disease Prevention and Health Promotion. December 2015. Accessed October 28, 2018. https://health.gov/dietaryguidelines/2015/resources/2015-2020DietaryGuidelines.pdf

73. James PA, Oparil S, Carter BL, et al. 2014 evidence-based guideline for the management of high blood pressure in adults: report from panel members appointed to the Eighth Joint National Committee (JNC 8). *JAMA*. 2014;311(5):507-520. doi:10.1001/jama.2013.284427

74. National Kidney Foundation. K/DOQI Clinical practice guidelines on hypertension and antihypertensive agents in chronic kidney disease. *Am J Kidney Dis*. 2004;43(5 suppl 1):S1-S290. doi:10.1053/j.ajkd.2004.03.003

75. Matchar DB, McCrory DC, Orlando LA, et al. Systematic review: comparative effectiveness of angiotensin-converting enzyme inhibitors and angiotensin II receptor blockers for treating essential hypertension. *Ann Intern Med*. 2008;148(1):16-29. doi:10.7326/0003-4819-148-1-200801010-00189

76. Kunz R, Friedrich C, Wolbers M, Mann JFE. Meta-analysis: effect of monotherapy and combination therapy with inhibitors of the renin angiotensin system on proteinuria in renal disease. *Ann Intern Med*. 2008;148(1):30-48. doi:10.7326/0003-4819-148-1-200801010-00190

77. Bakris GL, Ruilope L, Locatelli F, et al. Treatment of microalbuminuria in hypertensive subjects with elevated cardiovascular risk: results of the IMPROVE trial. *Kidney Int*. 2007;72(7):879-885. doi:10.1038/sj.ki.5002455

78. Bilo H, Coentrao L, Couchoud C, et al. Clinical practice guideline on management of patients with diabetes and chronic kidney disease stage 3b or higher (eGFR <45 ml/min). *Nephrol Dial Transplant*. 2015;30(suppl 2):ii1–ii142. doi:10.1093/ndt/gfv100

79. Heaf J, Petersons A, Vernere B, et al. Why do physicians prescribe dialysis? A prospective questionnaire study. *PLoS One*. 2017;12(12):e0188309. doi:10.1371/journal.pone.0188309

80. Rivara MB, Chen CH, Nair A, Cobb D, Himmelfarb J, Mehrotra R. Indication for dialysis initiation and mortality in patients with chronic kidney failure: a retrospective cohort study. *Am J Kidney Dis*. 2016;69(1):41-50. doi:10.1053/j.ajkd.2016.06.024

81. Rhee CM, Kovesdy CP, Ravel V, et al. Association of glycemic status during progression of chronic kidney disease with early dialysis mortality in patients with diabetes. *Diabetes Care*. 2017;40(8):1050-1057. doi:10.2337/dc17-0110

82. Sattar A, Argyropoulos C, Weissfeld L, et al. All-cause and cause-specific mortality associated with diabetes in prevalent hemodialysis patients. *BMC Nephrology*. 2012;13:130. doi:10.1186/1471-2369-13-130

83. Sun CY, Lee CC, Wu MS. Hypoglycemia in diabetic patients undergoing hemodialysis. *Ther Apher Dial*. 2009;13(2):95-102. doi:10.1111/j.1744-9987.2009.00662.x

84. Kazempour-Ardebili S, Lecamwasam VL, Dassanyake T, et al. Assessing glycemic control in maintenance hemodialysis patients with type 2 diabetes. *Diabetes Care*. 2009;32(7):1137-1142. doi:10.2337/dc08-1688

85. Rodbard HW, Jellinger PS, Davidson JA, et al. Statement by an American Association of Clinical Endocrinologists/American College of Endocrinology consensus panel on type 2 diabetes mellitus: an algorithm for glycemic control. *Endocr Pract*. 2009;15(6):540-549. doi:10.4158/EP.15.6.540

86. Tzamaloukas AH, Ing TS, Elisaf M, et al. Abnormalities of serum potassium concentration in dialysis-associated hyperglycemia and their correction with insulin: review of published reports. *Int Urol Nephrol*. 2011;43(2):451-459. doi:10.1007/s11255-010-9830-8

87. Tzamaloukas A, Ing T, Siamopoulos K, et al. Body fluid abnormalities in severe hyperglycemia in patients on chronic dialysis: theoretical analysis. *J Diabetes Complications*. 2007;21(6):374-380. doi:10.1016/j.jdiacomp.2007.05.007

88. Kim YL. Can we overcome the predestined poor survival of diabetic patients? Perspectives from pre- and post-dialysis. *Perit Dial Int*. 2007;27(suppl 2):S171-S175.

89. Cotovio P, Rocha A, Rodrigues A. Peritoneal dialysis in diabetics: there is room for more. *Int J Nephrol*. 2011;914849. doi:10.4061/2011/91489

90. National Kidney Foundation. KDOQI Clinical Practice Guideline for Diabetes and CKD: 2012 update. *Am J Kidney Dis*. 2012;60(5):850-886. doi:10.1053/j.ajkd.2012.07.005

91. Kuriyama S. Peritoneal dialysis in patients with diabetes: are the benefits greater than the disadvantages? *Perit Dial Int*. 2007;27(suppl 2):S190-S195.

92. Bastos KA, Villar KR, Andrade MP Jr, Barbosa LM, Lôbo JV, Lima FL. Predictors of peritoneal dialysis-related peritonitis. *Perit Dial Int*. 2007;27(3):S25.

93. Ueda R, Nakao M, Maruyama Y, et al. Effect of diabetes on incidence of peritoneal dialysis-associated peritonitis. *PLoS One*. 2019;14(12):e0225316. doi:10.1371/journal.pone.0225316

94. Rodríguez-Carmona A, Pérez-Fontán M, Lopez-Muniz A, Ferreiro-Hermida T, Garcia-Falcon T. Correlation between glycemic control and the incidence of peritoneal and catheter tunnel and exit-site infections in diabetic patients undergoing peritoneal dialysis. *Perit Dial Int*. 2014;34(6):618-626. doi:10.3747/pdi.2012.00185

95. Berns JS, Glickman JD. Management of hyperglycemia in patients with type 2 diabetes and pre-dialysis chronic kidney disease of end-stage renal disease. UptoDate website. November 2018. Accessed November 15, 2020. www.uptodate.com/contents/management-of-hyperglycemia-in-patients-with-type--diabetes-and-pre-dialysis-chronic-kidney-disease-or-end-stage-renal-disease

96. Gokal R, Moberly J, Lindholm B, Mujais S. Metabolic and laboratory effects of icodextrin. *Kidney Int*. 2002;62(suppl 81):S62-S71. doi:10.1046/j.1523-1755.62.s81.9.x

97. Baxter Corporation. Peritoneal Dialysis Solution Product Monograph Extraneal. September 27, 2016. Accessed February 10, 2020. www.baxter.ca/sites/g/files/ebysai1431/files/2018-11/Extraneal_EN.pdf

98. Wong T, Szeto CC, Chow KM, Leung CB, Lam C, Li P. Rosiglitazone reduces insulin requirement and c-reactive protein levels in type 2 diabetes patients receiving peritoneal dialysis. *Am J Kidney Dis*. 2005;46(4):713-719. doi:10.1053/j.ajkd.2005.06.020

99. Quellhorst E. Insulin therapy during peritoneal dialysis: pros and cons of various forms of administration. *J Am Soc Nephrol*. 2002;13(suppl 1):S92-S96.

100. Huang CC. Treatment targets for diabetic patients on peritoneal dialysis: any evidence? *Perit Dial Int*. 2007;27(suppl 2):S176-S179.

101. National Kidney Foundation. KDOQI Clinical Practice Guidelines for nutrition in chronic renal failure. *Am J Kidney Dis*. 2000;35(6 suppl 2):S40-S61.

102. Strid H, Simrén M, Johansson AC, Svedlund J, Samuelsson O, Björnsson ES. The prevalence of gastrointestinal symptoms in patients with chronic renal failure is increased and associated with impaired psychological well-being. *Nephrol Dial Transplant*. 2002;17(8):1434-1439. doi:10.1093/ndt/17.8.1434

103. Van V, Schoonjans RS, Struijk DG, et al. Influence of dialysate on gastric emptying time in peritoneal dialysis patients. *Perit Dial Int*. 2002;22(1):32-38.

104. Yao Q, Lindholm B, Heimbürger O. Peritoneal dialysis prescription for diabetic patients. *Perit Dial Int*. 2005;25(suppl 3):S76-S79.

105. Hecking M, Haidinger M, Döller D, et al. Early basal insulin therapy decreases new-onset diabetes after renal transplantation. *J Am Soc Nephrol*. 2012;23(4):739-749. doi:10.1681/ASN.2011080835

106. Chakkera HA, Weil EJ, Castro J, et al. Hyperglycemia during the immediate period after kidney transplantation. *Clin J Am Soc Nephrol*. 2009;4(4):853-859. doi:10.2215/CJN.05471008

107. Sharif A, Hecking M, de Vries AP, et al. Proceedings from an International Consensus Meeting on posttransplantation diabetes mellitus: recommendations and future directions. *Am J Transplant*. 2014;14(9):1992-2000. doi:10.1111/ajt.12850

108. Yates CJ, Fourlanos S, Hjelmesaeth J, Colman PG, Cohney SJ. New-onset diabetes after kidney transplantation—changes and challenges. *Am J Transplant*. 2012;12(4):820-828. doi:10.1111/j.1600-6143.2011.03855.x

109. Hornum M, Jørgensen KA, Hansen JM, et al. New-onset diabetes mellitus after kidney transplantation in Denmark. *Clin J Am Soc Nephrol*. 2010;5(4):709-716. doi:10.2215/CJN.05360709

110. Santos AH Jr, Chen C, Casey M, Worner K, Wen X. New-onset diabetes after kidney transplantation: can the risk be modified by choosing immunosuppression regimen based on pretransplant viral serology? *Nephrol Dial Transplant.* 2018;33(1):177-184. doi:10.1093/ndt/gfx281

111. Valderhaug TG, Jenssen T, Hartmann A, et al. Fasting plasma glucose and glycosylated hemoglobin in the screening for diabetes mellitus after renal transplantation. *Transplantation.* 2009;88(1):429-434. doi:10.1097/TP.0b013e3181af1f53

112. Sharif A, Baboolal K. Risk factors for new-onset diabetes after transplantation. *Nat Rev Nephrol.* 2010;6(7):415-423. doi:10.1038/nrneph.2010.66

113. Sharif A, Moore R, Baboolal K. Influence of lifestyle modification in renal transplant recipients with postprandial hyperglycemia. *Transplantation.* 2008;85(3):353-358. doi:10.1097/TP.0b013e3181605ebf

114. American Diabetes Association. 6. Glycemic targets: standards of medical care in diabetes-2021. *Diabetes Care.* 2021;44(suppl 1):S73-S84. doi:10.2337/dc21-S006

115. Hoshino J, Larkina M, Karaboyas A, et al. Unique hemoglobin A1c level distribution and its relationship with mortality in diabetic hemodialysis patients. *Kidney Int.* 2017;92(2):497-503. doi:10.1016/j.kint.2017.02.008

116. Hahr AJ, Molitch ME. Management of diabetes mellitus in patients with chronic kidney disease. *Clin Diabetes Endocrinol.* 2015;1:2. doi:10.1186/s40842-015-0001-9

117. Tuttle KR, Bakris GL, Bilous RW, et al. Diabetic kidney disease: a report from an ADA consensus conference. *Diabetes Care.* 2014;37(10):2864-2883. doi:10.2337/dc14-1296

118. Oomichi T, Emoto M, Tabata T, et al. Impact of glycemic control on survival of diabetic patients on chronic regular hemodialysis: a 7-year observational study. *Diabetes Care.* 2006;29(7):1496-1500. doi:10.2337/dc05-1887

119. Kalantar-Zadeh K, Kopple JD, Regidor DL, et al. A1c and survival in maintenance hemodialysis patients. *Diabetes Care.* 2007;30(5):1049-1055. doi:10.2337/dc06-2127

120. Ishimura E, Okuno S, Kono K, et al. Glycemic control and survival of diabetic hemodialysis patients—importance of lower hemoglobin A1c levels. *Diabetes Res Clin Pract.* 2009;83(3):320-326. doi:10.1016/j.diabres.2008.11.038

121. Molitch ME, Adler AI, Flyvbjerg A, et al. Diabetic kidney disease: a clinical update from kidney disease: improving global outcomes. *Kidney Int.* 2015;87(1):20-30. doi:10.1038/ki.2014.128

122. National Kidney Foundation. KDOQI Clinical practice guideline for diabetes and CKD: 2012 update. *Am J Kidney Dis.* 2012;60(5):850-886. doi:10.1053/j.ajkd.2012.07.005

123. Navaneethan SD, Schold JD, Jolly SE, Arrigan S, Winkelmayer WC, Nally J Jr. Diabetes control and the risks of ESRD and mortality in patients with CKD. *Am J Kidney Dis.* 2017;70(2):191-198. doi:10.1053/j.ajkd.2016.11.018

124. Kalantar-Zadeh K. A critical evaluation of glycated protein parameters in advanced nephropathy: a matter of life or death. *Diabetes Care.* 2012;35(7):1625-1628. doi:10.2337/dc12-0483

125. Alsahli M, Gerich JE. Hypoglycemia in patients with diabetes and renal disease. *J Clin Med.* 2015;4(5):948-964. doi:10.3390/jcm4050948

126. American Diabetes Association. 12. Older adults: standards of medical care in diabetes - 2021. *Diabetes Care.* 2021;44(suppl 1):S168-S179. doi:10.2337/dc21-S012

127. Molitch ME. Glycemic control assessment in the dialysis patient: is glycated albumin the answer? *Am J Nephrol.* 2018;47(1):18-20. doi:10.1159/000485844

128. Schatz SR. Report from the American Diabetes Association (ADA) 77th Scientific Sessions. *Renal Nutrition Forum.* 2017;36(4):26-27.

129. Raghav A, Ahmad J. Glycated albumin in chronic kidney disease: pathophysiologic connections. *Diabetes Metab Syndr.* 2018;12(3):463-468. doi:10.1016/j.dsx.2018.01.002

130. Selvin E, Sacks DB. Monitoring glycemic control in end-stage renal disease: what should be measured? *Clin Chem.* 2017;63(2):447-449. doi:10.1373/clinchem.2016.265744

131. Imran SA, Agarwal G, Bajaj HS, et al. 2018 Clinical practice guidelines: targets for glycemic control. *Can J Diabetes.* 2018;40:S42-S46. doi:10.1016/j.jcjd.2017.10.030

132. Frankel A, Kazempour-Ardebili S, Bedi R, et al. Management of adults with diabetes on the hemodialysis unit: summary of new guidance from the Joint British Diabetes Societies and the Renal Association. *Diabet Med.* 2018;35(8):1018-1026. doi:10.1111/dme.13676

133. Gan T, Liu X, Gaosi X. Glycated albumin versus HbA1c in the evaluation of glycemic control in patients with diabetes and CKD. *Kidney Int Rep.* 2017;3(3):542-554. doi:10.1016/j.ekir.2017.11.009

134. Freitas P, Ehlert L, Camargo J. Glycated albumin: a potential biomarker in diabetes. *Arch Endocrinol Metab*. 2017;61(3):296-304. doi:10.1590/2359 -3997000000272

135. Dozio E, Corradi V, Proglio M, et al. Usefulness of glycated albumin as a biomarker for glucose control and prognostic factor in chronic kidney disease patients on dialysis (CKD-G5D). *Diabetes Res Clin Pract*. 2018;140:9-17. doi:10.1016/j .diabres.2018.03.017

136. Chen CW, Drechsler C, Suntharalingam P, et al. High glycated albumin and mortality in persons with diabetes mellitus on hemodialysis. *Clin Chem*. 2017;63(2):477-485. doi:10.1373/clinchem.2016 .258319

137. American Diabetes Association. 7. Diabetes Technology: Standards of Medical Care in Diabetes-2021. *Diabetes Care*. 2021;44(suppl 1):S85-S99. doi:10.2337/dc21-S007

138. American Diabetes Association. Hypoglycemia (Low Blood Sugar). American Diabetes Association website. January 2020. Accessed February 14, 2020. www.diabetes.org/diabetes/medication -management/blood-glucose-testing-and-control /hypoglycemia

139. Klonoff DC. Continuous glucose monitoring: roadmap for 21st century diabetes therapy. *Diabetes Care*. 2005;28(5):1231-1239. doi:10.2337 /diacare.28.5.1231

140. Graham C. Continuous glucose monitoring and global reimbursement: an update. *Diabetes Technol Ther*. 2017;19(S3):S60-S66. doi:10.1089 /dia.2017.0096

141. Williams ME. The role of glycemic control in diabetic ESRD patients. Renal and Urology News website. March 11, 2010. Accessed February 14, 2020. www.renalandurologynews.com/home /departments/commentary/expert-reviews/the-role -of-glycemic-control-in-diabetic-esrd-patients/2/

142. Williams ME. Diabetic kidney disease in elderly individuals. *Med Clin N Am*. 2013;97(1):75-89. doi:10 .1016/j.mcna.2012.10.011

143. Panduru NM, Nistor I, Groop P-H, Van Biesen W, Farrington K, Covic A. Considerations on glycaemic control in older and/or frail individuals with diabetes and advanced kidney disease. *Nephrol Dial Transplant*. 2017;32(4):591-597. doi:10.1093/ndt /gfx021

144. American Diabetes Association. 4. Comprehensive medical evaluation and assessment of comorbidities: standards of medical care in diabetes—2021. *Diabetes Care*. 2021;44(suppl 1):S40-S52. doi:10.2337/dc21-S004

145. Shi C, Liu S, Yu H-F, Han B. Glycemic variability and all-cause mortality in patients with diabetes receiving hemodialysis: a prospective cohort study. *J Diabetes Complications*. 2020;34(4):107549. doi:10.1016/j.jdiacomp.2020.107549

146. National Kidney Foundation. *Diabetes and Chronic Kidney Disease: Clinical Handbook*. National Kidney Foundation; 2007.

147. Tzamaloukas AH, Leehey DJ, Friedman EA. Diabetes. In: Daugirdas JT, Blake PG, Ing TS, eds. *Handbook of Dialysis*. 4th ed. Wolters Kluwer Health/Lippincott Williams & Wilkins; 2007:490-507.

148. American Diabetes Association. 5. Facilitating behavior change and well-being to improve health outcomes: standards of medical care in diabetes—2021. *Diabetes Care*. 2021;44(suppl 1):S53-S72. doi:10.2337/dc21-S005

149. Evert A, Dennison M, Gardner C, et al. Nutrition therapy for adults with diabetes or prediabetes: a consensus report. *Diabetes Care*. 2019;42:731-754. doi:10.2337/dci19-0014

150. MacLeod J, Franz MJ, Handu D, et al. Academy of Nutrition and Dietetics Nutrition practice guideline for type 1 and type 2 diabetes in adults: nutrition intervention evidence reviews and recommendations. *J Acad Nutr Diet*. 2017;117(10):1637-1658. doi:10.1016/j.jand.2017 .03.023

151. Franz D, Zheng Y, Leeper N, Chandra V, Montez-Ruth M, Chang T. Trends in rates of lower extremity amputation among patients with end-stage renal disease who receive dialysis. *JAMA Intern Med*. 2018;178(8):1025-1032. doi:10.1001 /jamainternmed.2018.2436

152. Schatz SR. Glycemic index and glycemic load: a new look at an old topic. *The Cutting Edge*. 2014;35.

153. Campbell AP, Rains TM. Dietary protein is important in the practical management of prediabetes and type 2 diabetes. *J Nutr*. 2015;145(1):164S-169S. doi:10.3945/jn.114.194878

154. Chumlea WC, Cockram DB, Dwyer JT, Han H, Kelly MP. Nutrition assessment in chronic kidney disease. In: Byham-Gray LD, Burrowes JD, Chertow GM, eds. *Nutrition in Kidney Disease*. Humana Press; 2008:60-61.

155. Kalantar-Zadeh K, Regidor DL, Kovesdy C, et al. Fluid retention is associated with cardiovascular mortality in patients undergoing long-term hemodialysis. *Circulation*. 2009;119(5):671-679. doi:10.1161/CIRCULATIONAHA.108.807362

156. Sung J-M, Kuo S-C, Guo H-R, Chuang S-F, Lee S-Y, Huang J-J. The role of oral dryness in interdialytic weight gain by diabetic and non-diabetic haemodialysis patients. *Nephrol Dial Transplant*. 2006;21(9):2521-2528. doi:10.1093/ndt/gfl236

157. Schatz SR. Chronic diseases: diabetes, cardiovascular disease, and human immunodeficiency virus infection. In: Byham-Gray LD, Burrowes JD, Chertow GM, eds. *Nutrition in Kidney Disease*. Humana Press; 2008:387-418.

158. Tzamaloukas AH, Avasthi PS. Serum potassium concentration in hyperglycemia of diabetes mellitus with long-term dialysis. *West J Med*. 1987;146(5):571-575.

159. Wu J, Geng J, Liu L, Teng W, Liu L, Chen L. The relationship between estimated glomerular filtration rate and diabetic retinopathy. *J Ophthalmol*. 2015;10:326209. doi:10.1155/2015/326209

160. Man R, Sasongko MB, Wang JJ, et al. The association of estimated glomerular filtration rate with diabetic retinopathy and macular edema. *Invest Opthalmol Vis Sci*. 2015;56(8):4810-4816. doi:10.1167/iovs.15-16987

161. Rodríguez-Poncelas A, Mundet-Tudurí X, Miravet-Jiminez, et al. Chronic kidney disease and diabetic retinopathy in patients with type 2 diabetes. *PLoS One*. 2016;11(2):e0149448. doi:10.1371/journal.pone.0149448

162. Deli G, Bosnyak E, Pusch G, Komoly S, Feher G. Diabetic neuropathies: diagnosis and management. *Neuroendocrinology*. 2013;98(4):267-280. doi:10.1159/000358728

163. Pasnoor M, Dimachkie MM, Kluding P, Barohn R. Diabetic neuropathy part 1: overview and symmetric phenotypes. *Neurol Clin*. 2013;31(2):425-445. doi:10.1016/j.ncl.2013.02.004

164. Vinik AI, Nevoret M-L, Casellini C, Parson H. Diabetic neuropathy. *Endocrinol Metab Clin North Am*. 2013;42(4):747-787. doi:10.1016/j.ecl.2013.06.001

165. Juster-Switlyk K, Smith AG. Updates in diabetic peripheral neuropathy. Version 1 *F1000Res*. 2016;5:F1000 Faculty Rev-738. doi:10.12688/f1000research.7898.1

166. Pop-Busui R, Boulton A, Feldman E, et al. Diabetic neuropathy: a position statement by the American Diabetes Association. *Diabetes Care*. 2017;40(1):136-154. doi:10.2337/dc16-2042

167. Duby JJ, Campbell RK, Setter SM, White JR, Rasmussen KA. Diabetic neuropathy: an intensive review. *Am J Health Syst Pharm*. 2004;61(2):160-173. doi:10.1093/ajhp/61.2.160

168. Vinik A, Casellini C, Nevoret M-L. Diabetic neuropathies. In: Feingold KR, Anawalt B, Boyce, et al, eds. Endotext. February 5, 2018. Accessed February 16, 2020. www.ncbi.nlm.nih.gov/books/NBK279175/

169. Valabhji J. Foot problems in patients with diabetes and chronic kidney disease. *J Ren Care*. 2012;38(suppl 1):99-108. doi:10.1111/j.1755-6686.2012.00284.x

170. Boulton A, Armstrong DG, Albert SF, et al. Comprehensive foot examination and risk assessment. *Diabetes Care*. 2008;31(8):1679-1685. doi:10.2337/dc08-9021

171. Saha H, Leskinen Y, Salenius J, Lahtela J. Peripheral vascular disease in diabetic peritoneal dialysis patients. *Perit Dial Int*. 2007;27(suppl 2):S210-S214.

172. National Kidney Foundation. K/DOQI clinical practice guidelines for cardiovascular disease in dialysis patients. *Am J Kidney Dis*. 2005;45(suppl 3):S1-S154. doi:10.1053/j.ajkd.2005.01.019

173. Meaney B. Diabetic foot care: prevention is better than cure. *J Ren Care*. 2012;38(suppl 1):90-98. doi:10.1111/j.1755-6686.2012.00276.x

174. Herzog RI, Chyun D, Young LH. Cardiac autonomic neuropathy. *Practical Diabet*. 2006;25:34-38.

175. Maisey A. A practical approach to gastrointestinal complications of diabetes. *Diabetes Ther*. 2016;7(3):379-386. doi:10.1007/s13300-016-0182-y

176. Gatopoulou A, Papanas N, Maltezos E. Diabetic gastrointestinal autonomic neuropathy: current status and new achievement for everyday clinical practice. *Eur J Intern Med*. 2012;23(6):499-505. doi:10.1016/j.ejim.2012.03.001

177. Krishnasamy S, Abell TL. Diabetic gastroparesis: principles and current trends in management. *Diabetes Ther*. 2018;9(suppl 1):S1-S42. doi:10.1007/s13300-018-0454-9

178. Avalos DJ, Sarosiek I, Loganathan P, McCallum W. Diabetic gastroparesis: current challenges and future prospects. *Clin Exp Gastroenterol*. 2018;11:347-363. doi:10.2147/CEG.S131650

179. Rayner CK, Samsom M, Jones KL, Horowitz M. Relationships of upper gastrointestinal motor and sensory function with glycemic control. *Diabetes Care*. 2001;24(2):371-381. doi:10.2337/diacare.24.2.371

180. National Institute of Diabetes and Digestive and Kidney Diseases. Treatment for Gastroparesis. January 2018. Accessed October 15, 2018. www.niddk.nih.gov/health-information/digestive-diseases/gastroparesis/treatment

181. Törnblom H. Treatment of gastrointestinal autonomic neuropathy. *Diabetologia*. 2016;59(3):409-413. doi:10.1007/s00125-015-3828-9

182. Lok CE, Oliver MJ, Rothwell DM, Hux JE. The growing volume of diabetes-related dialysis: a population based study. *Nephrol Dial Transplant*. 2004;19(12):3098-3103. doi:10.1093/ndt/gfh540

183. Komici K, Femminella GD, de Lucia C, et al. Predisposing factors to heart failure in diabetic nephropathy: a look at the sympathetic nervous system hyperactivity. *Aging Clin Exp Res*. 2019;31(3):321-330. doi:10.1007/s40520-018-0973-2

184. Banerjee D, Ma JZ, Collins A, Herzog CA. Long-term survival of incident hemodialysis patients who are hospitalized for congestive heart failure, pulmonary edema, or fluid overload. *Clin J Am Soc Nephrol*. 2007;2(6):1186-1190. doi:10.2215/CJN.01110307

185. Drechsler C, Krane V, Ritz E, Marz W, Wanner C. Glycemic control and cardiovascular events in diabetic hemodialysis patients. *Circulation*. 2009;120(24):2421-2428. doi:10.1161/CIRCULATIONAHA.109.857268

186. Ishimura E, Okuno S, Kitatani K, et al. Different risk factors for peripheral vascular calcification between diabetic and non-diabetic haemodialysis patients—importance of glycaemic control. *Diabetologia*. 2002;45(10):1446-1448. doi:10.1007/s00125-002-0920-8

187. Cooper M. Importance of advanced glycation end products in diabetes-associated cardiovascular and renal disease. *Am J Hypertens*. 2004;17(12 Pt 2):31S-38S. doi:10.1016/j.amjhyper.2004.08.021

188. Isidro ML, Ruano B. Bone disease in diabetes. *Curr Diabetes Rev*. 2010;6(3):144-145. doi:10.2174/157339910791162970

189. Chen Z, Kooperberg C, Pettinger MB, et al. Validity of self-report for fractures among a multiethnic cohort of postmenopausal women: results from the Women's Health Initiative observational study and clinical trials. *Menopause*. 2004;11(3):264-274. doi:10.1097/01.gme.0000094210.15096.fd

190. Nicodemus KK, Folsom AR; Iowa Women's Health Study. Type 1 and type 2 diabetes and incident hip fractures in postmenopausal women. *Diabetes Care*. 2001;24(7):1192-1197. doi:10.2337/diacare.24.7.1192

191. Janghorbani M, Feskanich D, Willett WC, Hu F. Prospective study of diabetes and risk of hip fracture: the Nurses' Health Study. *Diabetes Care*. 2006;29(7):1573-1578. doi:10.2337/dc06-0440

192. Black DM, Cauley JA, Wagman R, et al. The ability of a single BMD and fracture history assessment to predict fracture over 25 years in postmenopausal women: the study of osteoporotic fractures. *J Bone Miner Res*. 2018;33(3):389-395. doi:10.1002/jbmr.3194

193. McCabe LR. Understanding the pathology and mechanisms of type I diabetic bone loss. *J Cell Biochem*. 2007;102(6):1343-1357. doi:10.1002/jcb.21573

194. Schwartz AV, Sellmeyer DE. Women, type 2 diabetes, and fracture risk. *Curr Diab Rep*. 2004;4(5):364-369. doi:10.1007/s11892-004-0039-z

195. Saito M, Fujii K, Soshi S, Tanaka T. Reductions in degree of mineralization and enzymatic collagen cross-links and increases in glycation-induced pentosidine in the femoral neck cortex in cases of femoral neck fracture. *Osteoporosis Int*. 2006;17:986-995. doi:10.1007/s00198-006-0087-0

196. Schwartz AV, Sellmeyer MD. Diabetes, fracture and bone fragility. *Curr Osteoporos Rep*. 2007;5(3):105-111. doi:10.1007/s11914-007-0025-x

197. Vestergaard P. Discrepancies in bone mineral density and fracture risk in patients with type 1 and type 2 diabetes—a meta-analysis. *Osteoporosis Int*. 2007;18(4):427-444. doi:10.1007/s00198-006-0253-4

198. Saito M, Marumo K. Bone quality in diabetes. *Front Endocrinol*. 2013;14(4):72:1-9. doi:10.3389/fendo.2013.00072

199. Shiraki M, Kuroda T, Tanaka S, Saito M, Fukunaga M, Nakamura T. Nonenzymatic collagen cross-links induced by glycoxidation (pentosidine) predicts vertebral fractures. *J Bone Miner Metab*. 2008;26(1):93-100. doi:10.1007/s00774-007-0784-6

200. Antonopoulou M, Bahtiyar G, Banerji M, Sacerdote AS. Diabetes and bone health. *Maturitas*. 2013;76:253-259.

201. Ceccarelli E, Guarino EG, Merlotti D, et al. Beyond glycemic control in diabetes mellitus: effects of incretin-based therapies on bone metabolism. *Front Endocrinol*. 2013;4:73. doi:10.3389/fendo.2013.00073

202. Krieger NS, Frick KK, Bushinsky DA. Mechanism of acid-induced bone resorption. *Curr Opin Nephrol Hypertens*. 2004;13(4):423-436. doi:10.1097/01.mnh.0000133975.32559.6b

203. Rzonca SO, Suva LJ, Gaddy D, Montague DC, Lecka-Czernik B. Bone is a target for the antidiabetic compound rosiglitazone. *Endocrinology*. 2004;145(1):401-406. doi:10.1210/en.2003-0746

204. Dunning T. Periodontal disease—the overlooked diabetes complication. *Nephrol Nurs J.* 2009;36(5):489-495.

205. Nazir MA, AlGhamdi L, AlKadi M, AlBeajan N, AlRashoudi L, AlHussan M. The burden of diabetes, its oral complications and their prevention and management. *Open Access Maced J Med Sci.* 2018;6(8):1545-1553. doi:10.3889/oamjms.2018.294

206. Akar H, Akar GC, Carrero JJ, Stenvinkel P, Lindholm B. Systemic consequences of poor oral health in chronic kidney disease patients. *Clin J Am Soc Nephrol.* 2011;6(1):218-226. doi:10.2215/CJN.05470610

207. Chuang SF, Sung JM, Kuo SC, Huang JJ, Lee SY. Oral and dental manifestations in diabetic and nondiabetic uremic patients receiving hemodialysis. *Oral Surg Oral Med Oral Pathol Oral Radiol Endod.* 2005;99(6):689-695. doi:10.1016/j.tripleo.2004.06.078

208. Miyata Y, Obata Y, Mochizuki Y, et al. Periodontal disease in patients receiving dialysis. *Int J Mol Sci.* 2019;20(15):3805. doi:10.3390/ijms20153805

209. Ryan JG. Increased risk for type 2 diabetes mellitus with HIV-1 infection. *Insulin.* 2010;5(1):37-45. doi:10.1016/S1557-0843(10)80008-9

210. Sattler F. Body habitus changes related to lipodystrophy. *Clin Infect Dis.* 2003;36(suppl 2):S84-S90. doi:10.1086/367563

211. Gelato MC. Insulin and carbohydrate dysregulation. *Clin Infect Dis.* 2003;36(suppl 2):S91-S95. doi:10.1086/367564

212. Medapalli R, Parikh CR, Gordon K, et al. Comorbid diabetes and the risk of progressive chronic kidney disease in HIV-infected adults: data from the veterans aging cohort study. *J Acquir Immune Defic Syndr.* 2012;60(4):393-399. doi:10.1097/QAI.0b013e31825b70d9

213. Deger SM, Sundell MB, Siew ED, et al. Insulin resistance and protein metabolism in chronic hemodialysis patients. *J Ren Nutr.* 2013;23(3):e59-e66. doi:10.1053/j.jrn.2012.08.013

214. Gougeon R, Marliss EB, Jones PJ, Pencharz PB, Morais JA. Effect of exogenous insulin on protein metabolism with differing nonprotein energy intakes in type 2 diabetes mellitus. *Int J Obes Relat Metab Disord.* 1998;22(3):250-261. doi:10.1038/sj.ijo.0800577

215. Pupim LB, Heimbürger O, Qureshi AR, Ikizler TA, Stenvinkel P. Accelerated lean body mass loss in incident chronic dialysis patients with diabetes mellitus. *Kidney Int.* 2005;68(5):2368-2374. doi:10.1111/j.1523-1755.2005.00699.x

216. Ikizler TA. Effects of glucose homeostasis on protein metabolism in patients with advanced chronic kidney disease. *J Ren Nutr.* 2007;17(1):13-16. doi:10.1053/j.jrn.2006.10.004

217. Garibotto G, Sofia A, Russo R, et al. Insulin sensitivity of muscle protein metabolism is altered in patients with chronic kidney disease and metabolic acidosis. *Kidney Int.* 2015;88(6):1419-1426. doi:10.1038/ki.2015.247

218. American Diabetes Association. 8. Obesity management for the treatment of type 2 diabetes: standards of medical care in diabetes—2021. *Diabetes Care.* 2021;44(suppl 1):S100-S110. doi:10.2337/dc21-S008

219. Kalantar-Zadeh K, Block G, Humphreys M, Kopple J. Reverse epidemiology of cardiovascular risk factors in maintenance dialysis patients. *Kidney Int.* 2003;63(3):793-808. doi:10.1046/j.1523-1755.2003.00803.x

220. Kovesdy CP, Anderson JE. Reverse epidemiology in patients with chronic kidney disease who are not yet on dialysis. *Semin Dial.* 2007;20(6):566-569. doi:10.1111/j.1525-139X.2007.00335.x

221. Navaneethan SD, Yehnert H, Moustarah F, Schreiber MJ, Schauer PR, Beddhu S. Weight loss interventions in chronic kidney disease: a systematic review and meta-analysis. *Clin J Am Soc Nephrol.* 2009;4(10):1565-1574. doi:10.2215/CJN.02250409

222. Conway B, Miller RG, Costacou T, et al. Temporal patterns in overweight and obesity in type I diabetes. *Diabet Med.* 2010;27(4):398-404. doi:10.1111/j.1464-5491.2010.02956.x

223. Mottalib A, Kasetty M, Mar, JY, Elseaidy T, Ashrafzadeh, Hamdy O. Weight management in patients with type I diabetes and obesity. *Curr Diab Report.* 2017;17(10):92. doi:10.1007/s11892-017-0918-8

224. Look AHEAD Research Group. Severe hypoglycemia in the Look AHEAD Trial. *J Diabetes Complications.* 2016;30(5):935-943. doi:10.1016/j.jdiacomp.2016.03.016

225. Look AHEAD Research Group: Effect of a long-term behavioural weight loss intervention on nephropathy in overweight or obese adults with type 2 diabetes: a secondary analysis of the Look AHEAD randomised clinical trial. *Lancet Diabetes Endocrinol.* 2014;2(10):801-809. doi:10.1016/S2213-8587(14)70156-1

226. Garvey WT, Mechanick JI, Brett EM, et al. American Association of Clinical Endocrinologists and American College of Endocrinology Comprehensive Clinical Practice Guidelines for medical care of patients with obesity. *Endocr Pract.* 2016;22 (suppl 3):1-203. doi:10.4158/EP161365.GL

227. Friedman AN, Wolfe B. Is bariatric surgery an effective treatment for type II diabetic kidney disease? *Clin J Am Soc Nephrol.* 2016;11(3):528-535. doi:10.2215/CJN.07670715

228. Evans N, Forsyth E. End-stage renal disease in people with type 2 diabetes: systemic manifestations and exercise implications. *Phys Ther.* 2004;84(5):454-463.

229. Holt RIG, de Groot M, Lucki I, Hunter C, Sartorius N, Golden SH. NIDDK international conference report on diabetes and depression: current understanding and future directions. *Diabetes Care.* 2014;37(8):2067-2077. doi:10.2337/dc13-2134

230. Coffey JT, Brandle M, Zhou H, et al. Valuing health-related quality of life in diabetes. *Diabetes Care.* 2002;25(12):2238-2243. doi:10.2337/diacare.25.12.2238

231. Ravenscroft EF. Diabetes and kidney failure: how individuals with diabetes experience kidney failure. *Nephrol Nurs J.* 2005;32(5):6-13.

232. Department of Health and Human Services Centers for Medicare & Medicaid Services. 42 CFR Parts 405, 410, 413 et al. Medicare and Medicaid Programs; Conditions for Coverage for End-Stage Renal Disease Facilities; Final Rule. Federal Register. 2008;73(73):20379-20484. April 15,2008. Accessed February 18, 2018. www.cms.gov/Regulations-and-Guidance/Legislation/CFCsAndCoPs/downloads/esrdfinalrule0415.pdf

233. KDQOL Complete. January 2018. Accessed September 17, 2018. www.kdqol-complete.org

234. Rubin RR, Peyrot M. Patients' and providers' perspectives in diabetes care. *Pract Diabetes.* 2005;24:6-13.

CHAPTER 10

Mineral and Bone Disorders and Kidney Disease

Rachael R. Majorowicz, RDN, CSR, LDN, FNKF

Introduction

Chronic kidney disease (CKD) is associated with disruption to normal mineral homeostasis. The term "CKD–mineral and bone disorder" (CKD–MBD) refers to the systemic syndrome affecting mineral, bone, and cardiac calcification disorders in patients with kidney disease. It was coined by the Kidney Disease: Improving Global Outcomes (KDIGO) work group as either one or a combination of the following:

1. abnormalities of calcium, phosphorus, parathyroid hormone (PTH), or vitamin D metabolism;
2. abnormalities of bone physiology, high bone turnover, bone mineralization, bone volume, growth, and/or strength; or
3. vascular or other soft-tissue calcification.[1]

These disturbances are implicated as key risk factors in high cardiovascular morbidity and mortality, decreased quality of life, and extraskeletal calcification in patients with CKD.[2,3]

Normal Physiology

In normal kidney function, small reductions in extracellular ionized calcium concentrations stimulate PTH production, which is instrumental in the following:

- releasing calcium and phosphorus from the bone into the blood
- stimulating the kidneys to reabsorb calcium and reduce renal tubular reabsorption of phosphorus,

increasing serum calcium and removing more phosphorus in the urine

- stimulating the kidneys to convert 25-hydroxyvitamin D to the active form 1,25-dihydroxyvitamin D (or calcitriol), which then stimulates absorption of calcium and phosphorus from the intestine, as well as increases the expression of the vitamin D receptor (VDR) in the parathyroid gland, resulting in reduction of PTH synthesis and secretion through a decrease in PTH gene transcription[4]

These three functions result in normalizing serum calcium levels from bone resorption, increasing kidney reabsorption and increasing gut absorption, whereas serum phosphorus is maintained within range due to the increased kidney excretion to counteract the increases in bone resorption and gut absorption (Figure 10.1 on page 186).

Maintaining calcium homeostasis is the primary function of the parathyroid glands.[5] The parathyroid gland calcium-sensing receptors (CaSRs) detect ionized extracellular calcium levels.[6] In addition, fibroblast growth factor-23 (FGF-23) and klotho hormones have been identified as key players in phosphorus and vitamin D metabolism and may be the earliest identifiable disturbances in CKD–MBD and cardiovascular disease (CVD).[7] Notably, because these hormones are not typically measured or used within clinical practice, their inclusion here is solely to better understand the physiology of CKD–MBD.

185

FIGURE 10.1 | Mineral and bone metabolism in healthy kidneys

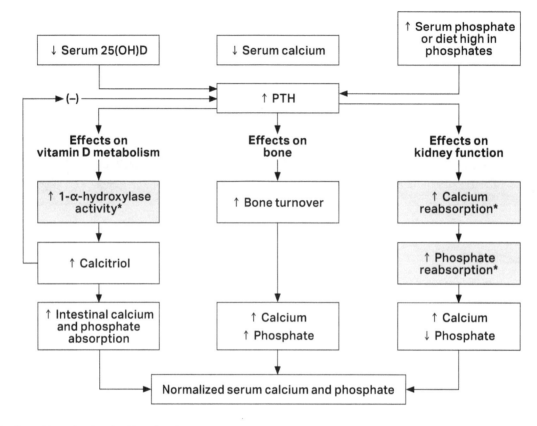

* Directly affected by reductions in kidney function.

FGF-23 is produced by osteoblasts in response to increases in serum phosphorus (although the sensing mechanism is not yet clear) and acts on the kidneys and parathyroid glands as the major sites of action.[5] These cumulatively maintain phosphorus homeostasis by increasing urinary phosphorus excretion and reducing phosphorus absorption in the gut by inhibiting the production and secretion of PTH in the parathyroid glands[7] and within the kidneys in FGF-23.[6-8] FGF-23 does the following:

- stimulates urinary phosphaturic effect (ie, excretion of phosphorus via urine) within the renal proximal tubules
- inhibits 1-α-hydroxylase activity, preventing conversion of 25-hydroxyvitamin D to 1,25-dihydroxyvitamin D and enhances the catabolism of both 25-hydroxyvitamin D and 1,25-dihydroxyvitamin D, theoretically reducing the intestinal phosphorus absorption

- increases calcium reabsorption within the distal tubules, also aided by the PTH

Klotho, a coreceptor for FGF-23, is necessary for FGF-23 to more readily bind to the FGF receptor in the kidney, thereby having an effect on calcium and phosphorus metabolism.[7] Expression of klotho is inhibited in CKD, resulting in resistance to FGF-23, reduced phosphorus excretion in the urine and reduced inhibition of PTH excretion.[7,8]

Disordered Physiology and Progression of Disease

FGF-23 is one of the earliest markers of CKD progression as it becomes elevated prior to PTH, phosphorus, or creatinine.[9] FGF-23 increases throughout the progression of kidney disease, resulting in lower 1,25-dihydroxyvitamin D, and in a compensatory manner, it aids in the prevention of hyperphosphatemia in early kidney disease. Lower 1,25-dihydroxyvitamin D levels lead to a rise in PTH with progression of CKD, not from changes in serum calcium or phosphorus as these are not typically abnormal until a later stage of kidney disease. By the time patients reach late CKD stage 2, 1,25-dihydroxyvitamin D levels have dropped to the lower limit of the reference range, and near the end of CKD stage 3, many patients have levels below normal, along with increasing PTH levels. Low levels of 25-hydroxyvitamin D have also been seen in many patients with CKD; although these levels do not correlate with 1,25-dihydroxyvitamin D levels, they likely limit the production of 1,25-dihydroxyvitamin D.[10] The PTH levels are above the normal reference range in approximately 40% of patients with CKD stage 3 and 70% of patients with CKD stage 4.[10]

Parathyroid hyperplasia develops from chronically low serum calcium and calcitriol levels or elevated serum phosphorus, causing an excess of PTH production and likely resistance to FGF-23.[5] Left untreated, the glands develop an irreversible decrease of VDRs and CaSRs, making medical therapy more difficult.[10] Secondary hyperparathyroidism (SHPT) develops as a result of this ongoing stimulation of the parathyroid gland, deficiency of 1,25-dihydroxyvitamin D, decreased expression of VDRs and CaSRs, hyperphosphatemia, hypocalcemia, and skeletal resistance to PTH.[11,12] SHPT develops fairly early in the course of CKD, progressing as the estimated glomerular filtration rate (eGFR) decreases.[13] Numerous abnormalities may result from SHPT and progression of CKD.

MINERAL AND HORMONAL ABNORMALITIES

Calcium

Serum calcium is the primary regulator of PTH; therefore, hypocalcemia is a powerful stimulant of PTH secretion. As kidney disease and SHPT progress, the reabsorption of calcium in the kidneys and the conversion of 25-hydroxyvitamin D to calcitriol are inhibited, resulting in less intestinal calcium absorption. As se-

rum calcium levels decline, PTH levels rise, resulting in increased bone turnover in order to release calcium and correct low serum calcium levels.

The increase in bone turnover also releases phosphorus, contributing to hyperphosphatemia and a rise in FGF-23. This, too, inhibits the conversion of 25-hydroxyvitamin D to calcitriol, furthering the calcium imbalance.

The stimulation of PTH secretion results in further phosphorus resorption from bone. The end result is hyperphosphatemia, hypocalcemia, and calcitriol deficiency. If severe SHPT ensues, the parathyroid gland becomes less sensitive to normalized serum calcium or vitamin D levels. This can lead to a transition from hypocalcemia to hypercalcemia with progression to end-stage kidney disease (ESKD).

Another reason for high PTH levels in SHPT may be the shift in the set point for calcium, and potentially fewer CaSRs, so that a higher serum calcium level is required to decrease PTH production.[12] A small study of 20 patients showed that patients with mildly elevated PTH levels or adynamic bone disease (ie, near absence of bone turnover) required a higher calcium level in the blood to decrease PTH production.[14]

Vitamin D

In the general population, most vitamin D is synthesized by the skin from 7-dehydrocholesterol after exposure to ultraviolet B rays from sunlight, while some is obtained through the diet (cholecalciferol, vitamin D3). Ergocalciferol, vitamin D2, is available from enriched foods and vitamin D supplements. Ergocalciferol and cholecalciferol are converted primarily in the liver to 25-hydroxyvitamin D2 (ercalcidiol) or 25-hydroxyvitamin D3 (calcidiol), respectively, but can also be activated to a lesser degree in other tissues for biologic functions. 25-hydroxyvitamin D2 and 25-hydroxyvitamin D3 are then activated by the enzyme 1-α-hydroxylase in the kidneys (see Figure 10.2 on page 188 for calcitriol formation).

1,25-dihydroxyvitamin D3 (calcitriol), which is the most active vitamin D metabolite with endocrine function, has only an 8-hour half-life, whereas 25-

FIGURE 10.2 | Calcitriol production[15]

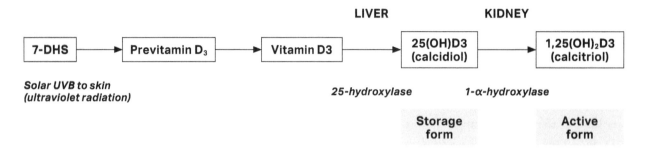

hydroxyvitamin D is the most accurate indicator of bodily vitamin D status and is, therefore, the routine serum measure.[5,12] 25-hydroxyvitamin D has a half-life of 2 to 3 weeks and in circulation is bound to vitamin D–binding protein (80%–90%), albumin (10%–15%), and less than 1% existing in a free form; free and albumin-bound 25-hydroxyvitamin D constitute the bioavailable 25-hydroxyvitamin D.[16]

Reasons for 25-hydroxyvitamin D deficiency in the general population include decreased exposure to the sun due to wide use of sunscreen or avoidance of the sun, decreased production in the skin of aging individuals, malabsorption or malnutrition, and dietary deficiency from avoiding high-phosphorus foods, such as milk and milk products, that are typically fortified with vitamin D.[12] Normal levels of 25-hydroxyvitamin D are generally suggested as greater than 30 ng/mL in the general population; no recommendations have been set for CKD.

Vitamin D deficiency is recognized as highly common in populations with CKD.[17] Low levels of 25-hydroxyvitamin D as a substrate for calcitriol are gaining recognition as a key factor for SHPT in patients with early kidney disease, despite most bodily organs having some ability to activate vitamin D, including the intestine, kidneys, bone, bone marrow, parathyroid glands, skin, liver, muscle, and lymphoid tissues.

Phosphorus

In early CKD, the kidneys respond to increased production of FGF-23 and secretion of PTH by increasing both excretion of phosphorus and the production of calcitriol. This is likely why serum phosphorus levels

usually remain in the normal range during CKD stages 2 and 3. By CKD stage 4, changes in phosphorus excretion and calcitriol production are not maintained by the reduced kidney function. FGF-23 resistance results in increased serum phosphorus levels, lower calcitriol levels, and increased PTH secretion.[18]

Because changes in serum values may be small and within the currently accepted ranges of serum phosphorus, these subtle changes in phosphorus levels may go unrecognized. The data from the Kidney Early Evaluation Program and the National Health and Nutrition Examination Survey (NHANES) showed only a small increase in mean phosphorus levels from 3.7 to 4.15 mg/dL as the eGFR dropped substantially from nearly 60 mL/min/1.73 m² to less than 30 mL/min/1.73 m².[19]

Phosphorus stimulates synthesis and secretion of PTH, independent of serum calcium or calcitriol.[20] Furthermore, a high-phosphorus diet appears to result in rapid parathyroid cell growth.[4] These cells have reduced levels of VDRs and CaSRs; thus, they are resistant to conventional therapy.[20]

Parathyroid Hormone

High levels of intact PTH result, in part, from increased secretion as well as from decreased catabolism secondary to the decreased number of nephrons. The kidneys are the only organs responsible for the removal of carboxy-terminal PTH fragments, so it is common that an accumulation of these fragments occurs in patients with kidney failure[21] (for further explanation, see the section Measurement of Parathyroid Hormone on page 194).

Skeletal resistance to PTH occurs early and in nearly every stage of CKD, including in some posttransplant patients and in patients with AKI. Due to this, supranormal levels of PTH may be required for achieving bone turnover.[12] Some evidence suggests that a deficiency of 1,25-dihydroxyvitamin D may be a factor or may be due, in part, to downregulation of PTH receptors.[4,21] A summary of these expected laboratory abnormalities in CKD–MBD is presented in Table 10.1.

TABLE 10.1 | Abnormal Laboratory Markers in Chronic Kidney Disease–Mineral and Bone Disorders

	Early	Late
Calcium	Low	High-normal or elevated
Phosphorus	Normal or elevated	Elevated
Parathyroid hormone	Normal, trending up within goal range or elevated	Normal to significantly elevated
25-hydroxyvitamin D	Trending down or low	Low
Alkaline phosphatase	Normal or trending up	Elevated

Adapted with permission from McCann L, ed. *Pocket Guide to Nutrition Assessment of the Patient With Kidney Disease*. 6th ed. National Kidney Foundation; 2021.[22]

Hyperparathyroidism has long been associated with pruritus.[12] But a recent analysis has found no association between PTH, phosphorus, calcium, calcium–phosphorus product, or Kt/V in patients receiving hemodialysis (HD).[23] Sukul and colleagues[24] had consistent findings, but they also determined that pruritus affects significantly more predialysis patients than providers are aware; one in four patients with CKD stages 3 through 5 suffer from pruritus, which directly impacts quality of life, sleep, and depression. Studies have shown that antihistamines are ineffective and are no longer recommended.[23] Because it may not be clear whether itching is a result of dry skin and the majority of patients tend to prefer a topical treatment, it may be worthwhile to try initially an emollient with few risks of side effects; in most cases, gabapentin in small doses has been associated with the greatest relief, but any side effects should be monitored.[23]

CARDIOVASCULAR DISEASE

The rates of CVD morbidity and mortality are higher in patients with CKD than in people with normal kidney function and are above the level expected with traditional risk factors. The risk of calcification rises directly with the progression of CKD, and vascular calcification (VC) is one of the strongest predictors for risk of heart disease and death in patients with CKD.[25,26] CVD accounts for 30% to 50% of all causes of death in patients with kidney disease.[27] Several traditional risk factors, including CKD, diabetes, and atherosclerosis, contribute to the development of VC.[26] Yet these factors cannot fully explain the unreasonably high CVD mortality in patients with CKD and is why nontraditional risk factors (eg, abnormal mineral metabolism) are suspected to play a role.[27] Total alkaline phosphatase is also associated with inflammation and mortality in all stages of CKD or transplant and diverse ethnicities.[28]

Abnormal mineral metabolism is known to be a critical component of the pathogenesis of VC, potentially stimulated by excess use of vitamin D or its analogs, hypercalcemia or calcium-based phosphate binders, calcium supplements, higher calcium dialysate, inflammation, and hyperphosphatemia.[6] Several observational studies have consistently shown increased risk of VC and mortality associated with increased serum calcium, phosphorus, PTH, and FGF-23.[6] Elevated FGF-23 and hyperphosphatemia are the most significant risk factors for CVD and mortality in patients with CKD, as well as risk of calciphylaxis.[5,8] In the Chronic Renal Insufficiency Cohort (CRIC) study of more than 3,000 patients with CKD, left ventricular mass and the risk of left ventricular hypertrophy were independently associated with FGF-23 levels.[25] Other studies have associated elevated FGF-23 with VC, left ventricular hypertrophy, inflammation, and mortality in patients on dialysis although the role of FGF-23 in CKD–MBD needs to be better understood and studied.[29] Furthermore, FGF-23 has been found to inhibit angiotensin production, enhancing the production of aldosterone which allows greater transport of phosphorus into vascular smooth muscle cells; aldosterone enhances inflammation via tumor necrosis factor α.[30]

Calcium and phosphorus balance are crucial for life, and positive balances are associated with VC, cardiac events, and higher morbidity and mortality.[26] Calcium–phosphorus product has historically been used as a marker of MBD, but it does not entirely represent true calcium or phosphorus balance nor deposition in soft tissues.[26] Calcium phosphate crystals have demonstrated toxic cellular effects, contributing to inflammation and VC.[27] The relationship between high calcium intake, serum calcium concentrations, and mortality has long been a topic of study. A study of 40,538 patients receiving HD found a 20% increased risk of death with each incremental increase of serum calcium by 0.25 mmol/L.[3] There are currently no treatments to reverse VC, so studies continue to explore its relationship with abnormal mineral metabolism for potential prevention options.[27]

Even in predialysis patients, a relationship exists between high phosphorus and all-cause mortality risk. A recent meta-analysis demonstrated a 20% mortality risk for every 1 mg/dL increase in phosphorus in patients with CKD, as well as identified phosphorus as an independent risk factor for progression of kidney disease.[31] A study evaluating predialysis patients found a significant association between the progression of coronary artery calcification (CAC) and serum phosphorus in patients with CKD, although the majority of the patients had serum phosphorus levels in the normal range according to the stage of CKD. This suggests that CAC progression could be enhanced by phosphorus at levels that are currently thought to be normal.[32]

The results of another large study of patients with CKD also showed an association between elevated serum phosphorus levels and the risk for mortality and myocardial infarction (MI). There was again an association between higher phosphorus levels and mortality risk in patients with phosphorus levels in the high-to-normal range.[33] Similar increases of 0.5 and 1 mg/dL in serum phosphorus levels were associated with increased mortality in another study.[34]

Hyperphosphatemia represents an independent risk factor for death, mainly from CVD causes, in patients on HD.[35] For a variety of reasons, the CVD mortality rate is 20 to 40 times higher for adults on HD than for the general population.[36] The original large studies using data from the United States Renal Data System (USRDS) found that for patients on dialysis for at least 1 year, the relative risk from cardiac mortality was 41% higher in those with serum phosphorus levels greater than 6.5 mg/dL.[37]

Numerous factors contribute to VC, including an imbalance of calcification inhibitors (eg, pyrophosphate, adenosine, and others) and calcification inducers (eg, hypercalcemia, inflammation, hyperphosphatemia, elevated PTH, and others). The reduction of VC inhibitors and elevated VC inducers may explain the abnormally high rates of VC in patients with CKD.[27] This may be due to in vitro data suggesting that the transformation of aortic smooth muscle cells into osteoblast-like cells that are thought to be involved in the soft-tissue and CV calcification related to phosphorus occurs at a phosphorus concentration of approximately 6 mg/dL and above.[38] Several studies of patients receiving dialysis also showed a significant risk of CVD mortality with high phosphorus and can be increased by as much as 27% for every increase of 1 mg/dL phosphorus.[39]

Vitamin D deficiency is also well documented to show an association with CVD events or mortality in observational literature. This may be due, in part, to the association of vitamin D deficiency with hypertension in observational studies; these data indicate that high levels of vitamin D inhibit the renin angiotensin system, improving blood pressure.[8] Treatment with 1, 25-dihydroxyvitamin D in patients with earlier CKD has had mixed results, with only some studies finding that supplementation of cholecalciferol may prevent VC.[8,30] Conversely, treatment with calcitriol or vitamin D analogs in patients with ESKD has been associated with improved mortality risk.

The roles of these nutrients, as well as vitamin K, continue to be examined in ongoing studies. Numerous studies have consistently associated low vitamin K levels and increased risk of VC and heart disease.[26] This may be due, in part, to the association of vitamin K–dependent proteins in vascular smooth muscle cells as anti-inflammatory agents, calcification inhibitors, and inhibitors of calcium phosphate crystal formation. Low vitamin K levels can be the result of restrictive diet, high demand in VC management, the use of vitamin K antagonist anticoagulants, and the potential for binding by phosphate binders.[26] A review by Floege[40] demonstrated that not all binders interact with vitamin K2; one study showed that sucroferric oxyhydroxide and sevelamer carbonate did not interfere with vitamin K in vitro, yet other reports indicate that sevelamer aggravates vitamin K deficiency. Warfarin is strongly correlated with calciphylaxis, and some studies have found that vitamin K2 treatments improve bone markers in adynamic bone disease.[41] This continues to be an area of interest, and additional clinical trials are currently under way to study vitamin K and VC.

Magnesium also plays a role with calcium in cardiac conduction and bone formation; dialysates with low magnesium levels have been associated with increased risk of death.[8] Recent studies have found an inverse association between CAC density and serum magnesium levels in patients with CKD and higher phosphorus levels, as well as a higher CVD mortality risk in patients undergoing HD with increased serum phosphorus levels, except in those with higher magnesium levels.[41]

Yet initial attempts at reducing FGF-23, phosphorus-lowering therapies, vitamin D supplementation, or use of calcimimetics to lower PTH have resulted in mixed results or increased risks, indicating that these associations may not be causal but simply may be confounding factors.[8] Lipid control has also failed to improve cardiac outcomes in patients with ESKD.[26]

CALCIPHYLAXIS

According to Vedvyas and colleagues,[42] calciphylaxis (also known as calcific uremic arteriolopathy) is an "ischemic small-vessel vasculopathy seen in 1% to 4%" of patients on HD that is associated with profound pain and mortality rates. Although the cause of calciphylaxis remains unclear, risk factors include elevated calcium or phosphorus, use of calcium-containing phosphate binders, vitamin D therapy, and SHPT; in addition, increased risks have been observed in females; White individuals; and persons with obesity, diabetes, warfarin use, low albumin, and trauma. Proposed preventive measures include use of lower calcium dialysate, limited use of vitamin D and calcium supplements, and improvement of the nutritional status in hypoalbuminemia. Medical treatment currently includes pain control measures, provision of sodium thiosulfate during or after dialysis, use of calcimimetics instead of vitamin D, substitution of non–calcium-based binders for calcium-based options, and hyperbaric oxygen treatments; parathyroidectomy, bisphosphonates, or corticosteroids have also been reported in some cases to result in improvement.

Causes and Types of Renal Bone Disease

Renal osteodystrophy (ie, renal bone disease) is the bone disorders aspect of CKD–MBD, which includes several types of bone diseases as described in this section.[1,43] Abnormal bone quality, mass, and strength result from numerous hormonal and metabolic disorders common in kidney disease (eg, hypocalcemia, hyperphosphatemia, SHPT, 25-hydroxyvitamin D deficiency, decreased synthesis of calcitriol, metabolic acidosis, and inflammation).[44]

Metabolic acidosis is progressively present in patients with CKD stage 3 through initiation of dialysis. It is generally indicated when serum carbon dioxide is less than 22 mmol/L. Chronic metabolic acidosis alters bone composition and alters the homeostatic relationships between blood ionized calcium, PTH, and 1, 25-dihydroxyvitamin D such that bone dissolution is exaggerated and bone fractures are a relatively common result. Furthermore, metabolic acidosis causes a shift of intracellular phosphate to extracellular phosphate and reduces renal calcium reabsorption.[5,6] Evidence is limited as to whether a correction of metabolic acidosis alone leads to an improvement or correction of osteodystrophy.[45] Metabolic acidosis also impacts osteodystrophy in that vitamin D analog therapy seems to be more effective in the absence of acidosis.[45]

In patients with CKD not on dialysis, recent studies have found predominantly low-turnover bone disease throughout CKD stages 2 through 5, although Barreto's study found high incidence of high-turnover bone disease as CKD progressed through stages 4 and 5.[43,46] Studies have demonstrated that the incidence of age-adjusted hip fracture in patients with CKD has actually increased in recent decades despite an intensive focus on treatments for renal osteodystrophy, such as PTH and phosphorus-lowering therapies.[47]

In the dialysis population, there has been a change in the prevalence of the different types of bone turnover in recent decades, with more adynamic bone and less high-turnover bone disease. This is likely due to changes in the therapy of renal osteodystrophy, age of patients, increased incidence of diabetes, and dialysis techniques.[21,43] Recent studies have shown a definitive shift toward primarily low-turnover bone disease in White patients on HD, whereas Black patients have demonstrated high-turnover bone disease via biopsy.[48] Similar findings were reported years later by an international study of patients undergoing dialysis, in which low-turnover bone disease was prominent, as well as the realization that PTH was quite limited in predicting bone turnover.[49]

Patients with CKD stages 3 through 5D have increased hip fracture rates compared to the general population, with escalated risk as CKD advances.[44] This risk extends even for kidney transplant recipients, especially in the first year and up to 5 years following transplant.[44,50] Furthermore, patients with HD and fracture have a fourfold increased risk of rehospitalization and death, especially within the first month of fracture.[51] For those requiring hospitalization, the risk of mortality doubles.

Patients often have no symptoms of bone disease, or symptoms appear late in the process. Most symptoms are nonspecific, such as pain and stiffness in joints, higher risk of fracture, spontaneous tendon rupture, or proximal muscle weakness. Similar symptoms are seen with both low- and high-turnover types of disease.

There is no approved or standardized terminology for the various types of renal bone diseases. The most commonly referenced will be described.

HIGH-TURNOVER BONE DISEASE

High-turnover bone disease, also known as osteitis fibrosa, results from persistent SHPT.[4,52] It is characterized by increased bone turnover and increased number and activity of osteoblasts and osteoclasts, escalating bone formation and resorption rates so that newly formed bone is not adequately mineralized or properly structured.[51,52] The disease severity seems proportional to the amount and the duration of hyperparathyroidism.[52]

While high-turnover bone disease was once the most prominent form, the occurrence has declined in recent decades with the rise of adynamic bone disease. This disorder is seen more often in patients on HD than in patients undergoing peritoneal dialysis (PD). Bone is prone to fracture and common symptoms include joint and bone pain.[12,52]

LOW-TURNOVER BONE DISEASE

Low-turnover bone disease is subdivided into adynamic bone disease and osteomalacia.

Adynamic Bone Disease

With adynamic bone, almost all bone formation is absent. Bone formation and resorption are decreased due to the reduced number of osteoblasts and osteoclasts. Adynamic bone is associated with oversuppression of PTH by the use of calcium, active vitamin D, vitamin D analogs, and calcimimetics.[51] PTH levels are typically less than 150 pg/mL but can be up to 300 pg/mL in patients receiving dialysis.[12] It is seen more often in the elderly, female patients, White patients, or in patients on PD with high dialysate calcium concentrations, diabetes mellitus, and total parathyroidectomy.[4,12,52] Low bone turnover caused by aluminum deposition due to use of aluminum-based phosphate binders is no longer common. Since bone turnover is minimal, serum calcium and phosphorus levels may be elevated due to the bones' inability to buffer calcium and phosphorus loads.[12]

Other tissues are susceptible to the accumulation of calcium when bone will not buffer available calcium. Patients with adynamic bone are reported to have increased VC and increased risk of calciphylaxis.[6] Higher fracture rates, more bone pain, delayed healing, and higher morbidity and mortality may be associated with adynamic bone as well.[50]

Osteomalacia

Osteomalacia is characterized by low rates of bone turnover and low bone mineralization, perceived as prolonged mineralization time and increased thickness, surface area, and osteoid.[51,52] Historically, the most common cause of osteomalacia was related to the accumulation of aluminum, but now it may be more related to metabolic acidosis by inhibiting osteoblasts and osteoclasts.[51] In recent years, there has been a low prevalence of osteomalacia, mainly due to the avoidance of aluminum-based phosphate binders and aluminum-free dialysate.[52]

MIXED-UREMIC BONE DISEASE

Historically, mixed-uremic bone disease, or mixed renal osteodystrophy, was defined as having a combination of high- and low-turnover bone disease (ie, impaired bone formation and mineralization).[12,52] Areas of bone can show high- or low-remodeling activities, as well as defective mineralization with or without increased bone formation. Currently, it is differentiated between type 1 or type 2 mixed-uremic bone disease.[51] Factors influencing the formation of mixed bone include increased PTH activity, metabolic acidosis, calcium and calcitriol deficiency, aluminum toxicity, skeletal resistance to active vitamin D and PTH, and hyperphosphatemia.

OSTEOPOROSIS

Many medical conditions can lead to osteoporosis. The World Health Organization (WHO) defines osteoporosis based on bone mineral density (BMD) determined by dual-energy x-ray absorptiometry (DXA). According to the National Institutes of Health, osteoporosis is defined with an emphasis on bone strength based on bone density and bone quality. Therefore, patients with CKD with low BMD or poor bone quality may technically have osteoporosis.[47]

Osteoporosis in the general population and renal osteodystrophy develop by different mechanisms.[53] Postmenopausal women or patients with age-related osteoporosis unknowingly may have CKD stage 1 up to early stage 3.[53] It is no surprise then that fractures in CKD stages 1 through 3 are more likely to be caused by some form of osteoporosis, rather than renal bone disease, and many patients initiate dialysis at an advanced age and may have preexisting osteoporosis.[30,52,54]

Uremic osteoporosis is a recent term coined to explain the effect of uremic toxins on bone quality and quantity, which explains the association of patients with uremia having higher rates of bone disease than the general population.[30]

Classifying Renal Osteodystrophy

A bone biopsy is considered the "gold standard" for diagnosis in order to fully characterize bone quality and type of renal bone disease via its ability to determine bone volume, turnover, mineralization, and collagen structure.[12,44] But because this procedure is invasive, expensive, and limited to that point in time and biopsy location, other less invasive tests have been used for identifying and monitoring bone turnover. The 2017 KDIGO update suggests BMD testing to assess fracture risk or bone biopsy to determine type of renal bone disease, if the results of either will affect treatment decisions.[55] This change in recommendations reflects recent studies that revealed reliable DXA prediction of bone fractures throughout the spectrum of CKD (stages 3 through 5D), as well as elevated bone-specific alkaline phosphatase.[56,57] Although DXA does not distinguish types of renal bone disease and its accuracy may be affected by hydration status, it may be a useful tool in combination with total alkaline phosphatase trends to predict bone turnover, and consideration of bone biopsy when results are inconsistent, or in other complex cases.[55,58] Yet bone biopsy or BMD testing may not be practical in clinical practice due to patient resistance, cost, and limited experience reading the results.

Bone-specific alkaline phosphatase best distinguishes between low-to-normal-turnover and high-turnover bone disease in patients on dialysis and is the most specific for bone disease, but it is expensive and is, therefore, rarely drawn.[52] Bone-specific alkaline phosphatase is a component of total alkaline phosphatase and thereby total alkaline phosphatase still offers indication of osteoblast activity or bone turnover as long as there is no liver disease.[28] Osteoblast markers can include alkaline phosphatase and osteocalcin, among others, as well as tests to determine osteoclast function and number.[44] Although fluid overload may increase total alkaline phosphatase, it is not affected by decline in kidney function, unlike PTH.[28] Due to limitations of each test, serial measurements of both PTH and alkaline phosphatase should be used to monitor fracture risk or bone turnover activity.[12]

Bone abnormalities of renal osteodystrophy are classified by turnover, mineralization, and volume.[58] Turnover theoretically includes both resorption rate and formation rate. Mineralization is abnormal in osteomalacia and in mixed disease. Bone volume is important because it is directly related to bone strength. But volume is not yet used to define types of renal osteodystrophy and future research may show how turnover and mineralization relate to bone volume.

There could be high, low, or normal bone volume with each of the forms of renal osteodystrophy.[58] A low blood level of PTH (<100 pg/mL) and occasionally hypercalcemia typically suggest adynamic bone; however, a high PTH does not exclude adynamic bone, as PTH levels greater than 400 pg/mL have been found in patients with adynamic bone.[45,52] Bover and colleages[28] state that as "PTH is only indirectly associated with bone formation," inaccurate detection of PTH fragments, and resistance to PTH in patients with CKD are indications of why achieving PTH within normal goal range is not recommended in patients with early CKD. There is agreement that PTH less than twice the upper normal limit is associated with adynamic bone disease; yet the ideal PTH ranges for normal bone formation or survival in patients with CKD remain unknown.

MEASUREMENT OF PARATHYROID HORMONE

The PTH molecule consists of 84 amino acids and is referred to as 1–84 PTH. Various amino-terminal and carboxy-terminal fragments (ie, non-1–84 PTH) result from the metabolism of PTH in the liver and kidneys. The carboxy-terminal fragments are mainly inactive. These are excreted by the kidneys, so the circulating levels of these inactive fragments tend to increase with kidney disease progression.[59]

Initially, PTH levels were measured by first-generation competitive radioimmunoassay. Second-generation "intact" PTH immunoassays were thought to provide a more accurate assessment. These assays rely on two detection antibodies to avoid measurement of intact PTH fragments. Newer third-generation "whole" PTH assays measure only the biologically active 1–84 PTH molecule, but their clinical usefulness has yet to be determined.[12] At this time, the third-generation assays have not proven to be superior to the second-generation assays in clinical practice, so there is no current recommendation to switch from the second-generation to the third-generation assays.[60]

Prevention and Management

Prevention of renal osteodystrophy is a primary goal. Choosing the best prevention or management regimen requires evaluating clinical, biochemical, and financial factors specific to the individual patient. Parameters to evaluate include PTH, calcium, phosphorus, alkaline phosphatase, 25-hydroxyvitamin D, dialysate calcium, medications, symptoms, and current bone disease (if known by bone biopsy). Despite emphasis on dietary or medical management of individual markers, the literature, in fact, shows that the coregulation of PTH, calcium, and phosphorus reduces mortality risk.[26]

The risks of treatment options must be evaluated since new, avoidable problems can develop if careful decisions are not made. The KDIGO Clinical Practice Guideline for the Diagnosis, Evaluation, Prevention, and Treatment of CKD–MBD was updated in 2017 to provide guidance in making treatment decisions. See Box 10.1 for a comparison of the 2009 and 2017 KDIGO CKD–MBD and the Kidney Disease Outcomes Quality Initiative (KDOQI) Clinical Practice Guidelines for Nutrition in CKD: 2020 Update.

CALCIUM

The majority of calcium in the diet is absorbed throughout the small intestine and is predominantly passive between intestinal cells, especially when intestinal concentrations of calcium are high. This route is indirectly influenced by calcitriol by allowing the junctions to be more permeable to calcium, but calcitriol is more

BOX 10.1 | Comparison of the 2009 and 2017 KDIGO Clinical Practice Guidelines for Adults With CKD–MBD Related to Nutrition Practice and the 2020 KDOQI Nutrition Guidelines[53,55,61]

GUIDELINE	Kidney Disease Outcomes Quality Initiative (KDOQI) 2020	KDIGO 2017	KDIGO 2009
CALCIUM GOAL AND MANAGEMENT	**Chronic kidney disease (CKD) 3 through 4:** Suggest striving for 800 to 1,000 mg calcium per day, if not also taking vitamin D analogs. **CKD 5D^a:** Consider adjusting calcium intake (all sources included) with concurrent use of vitamin D or analogs and calcimimetics to avoid hypercalcemia.	**CKD 3 through 5D:** Avoid hypercalcemia. Use dialysate calcium 2.5 to 3.0 mEq/L (1.25–1.5 mmol/L). **Transplant:** See Box 10.2 for laboratory frequency.	**CKD 3a through 5D:** Maintain within the normal range and use dialysate calcium 2.5 to 3.0 mEq/L.
PHOSPHORUS GOAL AND MANAGEMENT	**CKD 3 through 5D:** Adjust phosphorus intake to maintain serum levels within goal range. **CKD 1 through 5D and transplant:** Consider bioavailability of phosphate sources (eg, plant vs animal-based or additives) to decide plan for phosphorus restriction. **Transplant:** In hypophosphatemia, consider high phosphorus intake (all sources) to replete serum levels.	**CKD 3a through 5D:** Lower elevated phosphorus toward the normal range and base phosphate-lowering treatment on chronically elevated levels. Limit calcium-based phosphate binders. Limit phosphorus intake to treat hyperphosphatemia or in combination with other treatments. Consider phosphorus sources (eg, additive, animal, and vegetable) in recommendations. **CKD 5D:** Increase dialytic phosphorus removal with persistent elevation (nocturnal or daily dialysis). **Transplant:** See Box 10.2 for laboratory frequency.	**CKD 3a through 5:** Maintain in the normal range. **CKD 5D:** Lower elevated levels toward the normal range and increase dialytic phosphorus removal with persistent elevation. **CKD 3a through 5D:** Limit phosphorus intake to treat hyperphosphatemia or in combination with other treatments. Use phosphate-binding agents in the treatment of high levels but limit calcium-based binders and vitamin D or analog with recurrent high calcium, presence of arterial calcification, adynamic bone disease, or ongoing low PTH levels. **CKD 5D:** Increase dialytic phosphorus removal with persistent elevation (nocturnal or daily dialysis).

Continued on next page

Continued from previous page

GUIDELINE	Kidney Disease Outcomes Quality Initiative (KDOQI) 2020	KDIGO 2017	KDIGO 2009
VITAMIN D MANAGEMENT	**CKD 1 through 5D and transplant:** Suggest cholecalciferol or ergocalciferol supplementation to correct 25-hydroxyvitamin D deficiency or insufficiency.	**All stages and transplant:** Treat deficiency and insufficiency using recommendations for the general population.	**All stages and transplant:** Treat deficiency and insufficiency using recommendations for the general population.
PARATHYROID HORMONE (PTH) GOAL AND MANAGEMENT	N/A	**CKD 3a through 5:** Ideal value is not known. If PTH level is increasing over time or is chronically elevated, monitor for high phosphorus levels or high intake, low calcium, and low vitamin D. Do not routinely use calcitriol or vitamin D analogs. Reserve these for CKD 4 through 5 with progressively or severely elevated PTH. **CKD 5D:** Maintain levels within two to nine times the upper normal limit for the assay. Profound shifts in either direction within this range prompt an initiation or change in therapy to prevent levels outside this range. For PTH-lowering therapy, use calcimimetics, calcitriol, vitamin D analogs, or a combination of these. **Transplant** No recommendations.	**CKD 3a through 5:** Ideal value is not known. Evaluate and treat patients for hyperphosphatemia, low calcium, and vitamin D deficiency when PTH level is above the upper normal limit of the assay. Correct abnormalities with lower phosphorus diet, phosphate binders, calcium supplements, and vitamin D. If PTH level is increasing despite corrections, treat with calcitriol or vitamin D analogs. **CKD 5D:** Maintain PTH level in the range of approximately two to nine times the upper normal limit for the assay. For PTH-lowering therapy, use calcimimetics, calcitriol, vitamin D analogs, or a combination of these.
MINERAL BONE DISEASE TREATMENT	See calcium, phosphorus, and vitamin D information above.	**CKD 3a through 5D:** Based on trends of phosphorus, calcium, and PTH levels considered together, rather than calcium–phosphorus product calculation. Within 12 months of transplant, eGFR greater than 30 and low bone density: consider use of vitamin D or analogs and antiresorptive agents.	**CKD 3a through 5D:** Based on trends of phosphorus, calcium, and PTH levels considered together, rather than calcium–phosphorus product calculation.

[a] 5D is dialysis

directly involved in the active absorption of calcium transcellularly.[5] As the concentration gradient of calcium declines, calcitriol stimulates the VDRs in intestinal cells to synthesize absorption mechanisms (such as calbindin and others), which bind calcium and move it across intestinal cells.[5]

Total serum calcium includes three components: ionized (48%), protein bound (46%), and complexed fractions (7%) bound to other molecules such as citrate and phosphate.[5] Approximately 98% to 99% of calcium filtered by the kidneys is reabsorbed throughout the tubules, but the majority is passively reabsorbed in the proximal convoluted tubule (60%–70%). The terminal nephron is responsible for regulation of calcium excretion.[5] The 10% to 15% of calcium reabsorbed via active transport in the proximal tubule is regulated by calcitriol and PTH.[5] Numerous factors influence calcium reabsorption in the kidneys, including PTH, calcitriol, calcium concentration, fluid shifts, metabolic acidosis or alkalosis, and diuretics.[5] Increases in extracellular fluid, metabolic acidosis, and loop diuretics result in enhanced calcium excretion, whereas thiazide diuretics increase calcium absorption.[5]

Serum calcium does not reflect total body calcium and bone status. Serum calcium levels may remain within normal ranges until CKD stage 4, when they tend to decline due to low PTH and lower vitamin D.[5,12] Low calcium levels stimulate production of PTH and synthesis of 1,25-dihydroxyvitamin D. Treatment of hypocalcemia helps prevent exacerbation of this disorder in earlier stages of CKD. Vitamin D supplementation to correct deficiency will increase gut calcium absorption, or calcium supplementation may be considered; however, caution is advised to stay within the recommended ranges. If a patient is on a calcium-based phosphate binder, this may also help correct serum calcium levels. See Box 10.1 for the 2020 KDOQI and 2017 KDIGO guidelines regarding calcium.

In patients with ESKD, serum calcium levels tend to normalize or trend in the upper range of normal due to the progression of SHPT and the removal of calcium from bone. Limitation of dairy products due to potassium and phosphorus content leads to an inherently low-calcium diet. If hypercalcemia or upward trend in serum calcium arises, it is prudent to verify limitation of dairy products and no recent intake or initiation of calcium-fortified foods, calcium supplements, or antacids.

Excess calcium is unlikely to be stored in bone, especially in the presence of adynamic bone disease.[62] Hypocalcemia may still be present in a smaller subset of patients with ESKD on dialysis. Calcium supplementation is generally contraindicated in patients with ESKD because numerous studies have demonstrated an increased risk of calcification or mortality with high calcium intake (dietary or medication sources). The 2017 KDIGO CKD–MBD guidelines indicate that higher serum calcium levels are increasingly associated with CVD events and increased mortality in adults with use of higher calcium concentrations. Furthermore, a lack of adverse outcomes in patients with mild or moderate hypocalcemia has led to a change to individualize hypocalcemia management, no longer treating hypocalcemia for all patients.[55] Hypocalcemia may be acceptable when the patient is taking calcimimetic medication because mild or asymptomatic hypocalcemia may be harmless; treatment should be individualized and addressed in pronounced or symptomatic hypocalcemia.[55] See Box 10.2 on page 198 for frequency of laboratory monitoring recommended by the KDIGO 2017 guidelines.

MAGNESIUM

Daily magnesium intake approximates 300 mg with intestinal absorption of 25% in high-magnesium diets and up to 75% in lower-magnesium diets.[5] Absorption occurs primarily in the small intestine and, to a smaller degree, within the colon via passive and active pathways. The majority of magnesium is stored intracellularly in bone (at least 50%), muscle, and soft tissues; of the 1% within the extracellular space, 30% is albumin-bound, 60% is free in its active form for physiologic functions, and the remainder is bound to serum anions. Long-term use of proton pump inhibitor medications are associated with low magnesium. Numerous other factors impair magnesium absorption,

BOX 10.2 | Frequency of Laboratory Monitoring[55]

1 THROUGH 3BT

Calcium	Every 6 to 12 months
Phosphorus	Every 6 to 12 months
Parathyroid hormone	Baseline with rechecks as needed
Alkaline phosphatase	No recommendation in chronic kidney disease (CKD)
25-hydroxyvitamin D	Baseline with rechecks as needed for all stages of CKD

CKD 3A THROUGH 5D AND TRANSPLANT MAINTENANCE (AS NEEDED BASED ON ABNORMALITIES AND CKD PROGRESSION)

3a through 3b

Calcium	Every 6 to 12 months
Phosphorus	Every 6 to 12 months
Parathyroid hormone	Baseline with rechecks as needed
Alkaline phosphatase	Same as 4 through 5T
25-hydroxyvitamin D	Baseline with rechecks as needed for all stages of CKD

4 and 4T

Calcium	Every 3 to 6 months
Phosphorus	Every 3 to 6 months
Parathyroid hormone	Every 6 to 12 months
Alkaline phosphatase	Annually, or more often, if parathyroid hormone (PTH) level is elevated
25-hydroxyvitamin D	Baseline with rechecks as needed for all stages of CKD

5, 5D, and 5T

Calcium	Every 1 to 3 months
Phosphorus	Every 1 to 3 months
Parathyroid hormone	Every 3 to 6 months
Alkaline phosphatase	Annually, or more often, if PTH level is elevated
25-hydroxyvitamin D	Baseline with rechecks as needed for all stages of CKD

TRANSPLANT–IMMEDIATE ACUTE

Calcium	Weekly until stable
Phosphorus	Weekly until stable
Parathyroid hormone	No recommendation
Alkaline phosphatase	No recommendation
25-hydroxyvitamin D	No recommendation

[a] T = transplant

including chronic diarrhea, metabolic acidosis, hypercalcemia, low phosphorus or potassium, diuretics, immunosuppressants, and other medications.[5] Low magnesium levels are associated with hypocalcemia and low PTH levels; symptoms may include weakness, cramps, numbness, arrhythmia, or seizures.[5]

Magnesium may promote vitamin D deficiency and hypocalcemia, resulting in disordered homeostasis.[8] Magnesium is a growing topic of study to better understand its role in CKD–MBD.

PHOSPHORUS

Phosphorus control is a primary therapy in the treatment and prevention of hyperphosphatemia, secondary hyperparathyroidism, renal osteodystrophy, and soft-tissue calcification. Hyperphosphatemia results in decreased 1,25-dihydroxyvitamin D levels and increased PTH levels; therefore, management of phosphorus is crucial in the prevention of furthering SHPT.

Phosphorus typically does not become elevated until GFR declines below 45 mL/min/1.73 m² and becomes increasingly prevalent with progression toward ESKD.[61] Furthermore, serum phosphorus levels are reported to fluctuate (being lowest in the morning and increasing 16% by midday) and also seasonally, with serum levels potentially being higher in summer months.[6] With these variables and complex physiology, management of serum phosphorus is a challenge requiring multiple facets; interventions include modifications to diet, use of phosphate binders, and dialysis, in patients with ESKD.

Diet

The majority of phosphorus is absorbed in the small intestine, specifically the jejunum and ileum, via paracellular passive absorption and the rate-limiting sodium-dependent phosphate cotransporters, such as sodium phosphate cotransporter and others.[6,8] Approximately 60% of phosphorus is absorbed via these mechanisms; 40% remains unabsorbed and excreted via feces.[6] There is also a component of individuality in the absorption rates of phosphorus among patients, where some patients have lower urinary or fecal excretion of phosphorus.[63] Others may potentially be superabsorbers. A low-phosphorus diet and calcitriol stimulate kidney and intestinal sodium phosphate transporters to increase phosphorus absorption in the gut and reabsorption within the proximal tubules, reportedly up to 80% of phosphorus absorption with calcitriol.[5,6,8] Thereby these mechanisms may, in theory, negate the goal of a lower phosphorus diet, but this has not been demonstrated.

Several randomized, controlled trials of predialysis patients and those undergoing in-center HD demonstrated that serum phosphorus levels can be improved via dietary modification. In predialysis patients with CKD, recent randomized control trials reported near-significant or significant reduction in serum phosphorus levels on a low-protein diet or very low-protein diet supplemented with keto-analogs.[64] According to the KDOQI Clinical Practice Guidelines for Nutrition in CKD: 2020 Update work group, phosphorus restriction may be valid independently in predialysis patients, but "the serum phosphate reductions achieved solely by limiting dietary intake are modest (especially for dialysis patients) and recommend this strategy as only one" of several options to control serum phosphorus.[61]

Studies on phosphorus restriction and mortality are conflicting in patients on dialysis. Two randomized, control trials demonstrated that dietary counseling on limiting phosphorus or education on identifying phosphate additives can reduce serum phosphorus levels.[65,66] One study found an association between higher mortality and higher phosphorus intake based on 3-day food recalls.[67] Another study assessed the association between dietary phosphorus restriction and mortality via post hoc analysis of the Hemodialysis (HEMO) study.[68] An association was found between markers of poorer nutritional status with greater need for nutrition supplements with more restrictive dietary phosphorus recommendations; greater survival was found with more liberal phosphorus guidelines.

Since the clinical consequences of dietary phosphorus restriction are not well documented, less emphasis on restriction was recommended in the 2017 KDIGO CKD–MBD guideline update which stated the following: "there is an absence of data showing that phosphorus restriction improves clinical outcomes."[55] In addition, greater phosphorus restriction in the diet has been correlated with worse nutritional status and increased need for nutrition support and higher mortality.[61] The KDOQI Clinical Practice Guidelines for Nutrition in CKD: 2020 Update mirrored this change and no longer recommend a defined phosphorus allowance. Rather, emphasis should be placed on individualizing recommendations to each patient's needs with the goal of maintaining serum phosphorus levels within the goal range based on laboratory trends (rather than a single value), and in consideration of serum calcium and PTH trends. The guidelines also suggest that the bioavailability of phosphorus sources (eg, plant, animal, and additive) be considered.[61]

Historically, it was difficult to recommend adequate protein for patients undergoing dialysis because higher protein foods were considered high in phosphorus, making it difficult to achieve simultaneously protein and phosphorus goals. Now, if phosphorus levels become elevated, the clinician can emphasize reducing sources of added phosphates in processed and convenience foods and adjusting phosphate binders to better ensure a well-balanced diet. In earlier stages of CKD, phosphorus restriction likely is not necessary and more balanced dietary approaches, such as the Dietary Approaches to Stop Hypertension (DASH) or Mediterranean diets, may offer protective benefits and healthful antioxidants.[26] It is advisable to monitor serum phosphorus trends and adjust intake to maintain levels within goal ranges.

Natural vs added phosphorus Phosphates exist in organic and inorganic forms, both of which are found in foods and of which the bioavailability varies considerably. Natural foods contain organic phosphorus, while phosphorus added to foods as a preservative during processing is often referred to as inorganic phosphorus. Estimated organic phosphorus absorption in the gut is 40% to 60% for animal food sources and less than 20% to 50% for plant-based foods due to being in the form of indigestible phytate in the outer coating of grains and seeds, whereas the inorganic phosphate additives in processed foods are estimated to be absorbed up to 100%, but this has not been demonstrated.[69]

There are currently dozens of phosphate additives used in food manufacturing and listed by the Food and Drug Administration as "generally regarded as safe." Phosphorus additives serve many functions, including emulsifiers, anticaking agents, antimicrobials, and leavening agents. These additives can improve texture, taste, acidity, moisture binding, color stability, iron binding, reduction of cooking time, buffering,

maintenance of firmness in freezing and canning, and nutrient fortification.[70] These phosphate food additives are even more widely used in the preparation of fast foods and convenience foods, which are generally more highly processed. Convenience foods that are partially or fully premade or instant have added phosphate salts, enabling them to cook faster or require little or no cooking. More working families and single adults are becoming reliant on these foods due to lack of ability or time for food preparation from scratch.[71]

Studies have shown that the content of phosphate additives in foods has more than doubled since 1990.[72] One study by Carrigan and colleagues[73] found that diets including foods with phosphate additives were 30% to 40% (483–790 mg) higher in phosphorus than those without. Leon and colleagues[70] demonstrated that up to 72% of processed foods contain phosphate additives. Food categories found to have the highest phosphorus content, comparatively with foods without additives, were processed cheeses, cereals, and enhanced meats, whereas bread, soups, and canned vegetables with added phosphates had minimally more phosphorus than their counterparts without these additives. The authors calculated that diets with multiple daily servings of foods with phosphate additives may have 736 mg more phosphorus per day.[70]

Enhanced meats, fish, and seafood—seemingly "fresh" foods that have been treated with sodium phosphates to increase shelf life and improve appearance—should also be limited or avoided. Sherman and Mehta[74] found that processed meats or seafood containing added phosphates had a 62% higher phosphorus:protein ratio than those without phosphates. Additionally, they found that phosphorus was not listed universally on ingredient lists; several foods with added phosphates listed these as broths or flavorings. Benini and colleagues[75] found that chicken, turkey, or ham with phosphate additives contained nearly 70% more phosphorus than options without additives. Unfortunately, organic foods are not necessarily better options, even if conducive to budgets, as they may still contain additives. One strategy can be to recommend "natural" or "all natural" poultry, fish, or seafood as these typically do not contain added phosphorus, are not typically more expensive, and are found in a variety of brands.

Commercial beverages, such as canned or bottled teas, colas, flavored waters, and many others, may contain phosphoric acid or other phosphate additives. A 2015 study of popular beverages found that 78% of beverages contained more phosphorus than indicated in nutrient databases and that many beverages contain significantly more phosphorus than colas.[76] Since phosphorus is not listed on most nutrition labels, there is no way for consumers to know the phosphorus content of these beverages. The only way to identify added phosphates is by reading the ingredient list for "phos" ingredients. Even then, there is no indication if there is 2 mg vs 200 mg within any product, so it is considered best that patients should limit or avoid beverages with these ingredients and that alternatives for better choices be provided.[77]

Other foods shown to be high in added phosphates include fast food, processed cheeses, processed meats, beer, packaged/convenience foods, chocolate, and wine. A recent study showed that wines can be higher in phosphorus than many beers, so these can no longer be assumed as safe alternatives.[78] Furthermore, food insecurity, food deserts, or limited access to healthful foods affect the ability to manage phosphorus intake. A cross-sectional analysis of 2,879 participants found higher serum phosphorus values associated with low socioeconomic status, regardless of race, gender, or other variables. All patients living within the lowest income category had a twofold incidence of hyperphosphatemia than those in the highest income level, indicating poverty may be a novel risk factor for hyperphosphatemia.[79]

Since phosphorus content is not required to be published on food labels, it can be difficult for patients to identify safe food choices. Therefore, it is crucial to educate patients with hyperphosphatemia on strategies to choose foods without added phosphates, identify foods with phosphate additives, moderate intake of foods with higher natural phosphate bioavailability, and provide

lists of safer alternatives. As opposed to recommendations of the past, whole grains no longer have to be routinely discouraged and may again be included in a healthful, balanced diet. Considering the lower bioavailability of whole grains, comparison of the phosphorus content of white rice vs brown or wild rice, as well as other whole grains compared with their refined counterparts, showed minimal or no phosphorus benefit.[80]

Monitoring laboratory results for the need to moderate some of these foods or modifying preparation techniques may be necessary. A recent study has shown that boiling or pressure cooking sliced or cubed beef for 10 to 30 minutes and discarding the water after can reduce phosphorus content approximately 50% without detriment to the protein content.[81] A previous study had similar findings—up to 50% phosphorus reduction in boiled beef and chicken when the water was discarded.[82] Notably, neither of these studies specified whether the protein sources contained phosphate additives, and since phosphates are commonly added to poultry products, this leads us to question whether natural vs added phosphates were removed with boiling. In addition, boiling meats may, of course, change the palatability of some protein foods and may be better tolerated in some dishes than in others.

Allowing more varied and healthful food choices may be more amenable to patients with CKD with plant-based eating habits. A study of nine patients with CKD comparing a meat diet vs a vegetarian diet with similar protein and phosphorus content demonstrated lower serum phosphorus with the vegetarian diet.[83] For vegetarian patients with ESKD, diet modification to control phosphorus while providing adequate protein may be a challenge but is possible. Again, flexibility may be needed to include some dairy products, legumes, or appropriate protein supplements with close monitoring of laboratory values. It can be useful to calculate estimated phosphorus:protein ratios of plant-based foods with animal-based foods in order to best guide patient education, particularly when these are adjusted for potential phosphate bioavailability. As there is reported to be an average of 15 to 17 mg phosphorus per gram of animal proteins (without phosphate additives), plant-based options can be compared with animal-based counterparts.[71]

The diet should be individualized to maintain nutritional quality while limiting phosphorus, if indicated by elevated laboratory results. A detailed diet history is useful in assessing the patient's diet and revealing foods ingested on a regular basis. Both traditional and unique cultural foods should be evaluated and considered for benefit to nutrition content and phosphorus control.

Phosphates in Medications and Supplements

Phosphorus is widely used in medications as an inert ingredient or as a main ingredient in over-the-counter nutrition supplements. Calvo and Uribarri[71] noted that phosphorus was commonly listed as an inactive ingredient in medications or supplements. They found that commonly used multivitamin or multimineral supplements contributed 31 to 130 mg phosphorus per day (108 mg average).

Sherman and colleagues[84] found that of the 200 most commonly prescribed dialysis medications, 11.5% listed phosphorus in the ingredients but in unreported amounts. Of these, phosphorus content ranged from 1.4 to 111.5 mg per tablet with varying phosphorus content with differing manufacturers of the same drug. This also held true for the two dialysis renal vitamins where one contained 1.7 mg phosphorus and the other contained 37.7 mg phosphorus. Megestrol acetate (Megace) was also reported to contain significant phosphorus content.[84] Significant phosphorus content was found in common medications for blood pressure, cholesterol, and depression, among others. Furthermore, they found that branded medications that did not contain phosphorus were also very likely not to contain phosphorus in the generic as well.[84]

PHOSPHATE BINDERS

Phosphate binders are medications that bind to dietary phosphorus in the gastrointestinal tract, creating insoluble compounds, preventing absorption, and subsequently eliminating it via the gut.[6] Numerous studies have been published on phosphate-binding potential (ie, potential effectiveness at binding phosphate) and phosphate binder equivalent doses.[85] See Table 10.2 for comparing common phosphate-binding medications and details.

Drugs containing aluminum, such as aluminum hydroxide (Alucaps) and later aluminum carbonate, were commonly used as phosphate binders in the 1970s.[86] These were very effective as phosphorus binders but are now used sparingly due to the association with osteomalacia, aluminum toxicity, anemia, and encephalopathy. The KDIGO guidelines recommend avoidance of long-term use of aluminum-containing binders at all CKD stages.[55]

Soon after, calcium-based binders were found to be effective in binding phosphorus and continue to be used widely. Examples include calcium carbonate (TUMS) and calcium acetate (Eliphos, Calphron, PhosLo, PhosLyra), whereas the use of calcium citrate is discouraged due to enhancing the absorption of aluminum that is found in various medications, leading to increased aluminum absorption and potential for side effects. Calcium carbonate has considerably higher calcium content than calcium acetate. For example, calcium carbonate is 40% elemental calcium; so 1,000 mg contributes 400 mg elemental calcium, whereas 667 mg calcium acetate contains only 168 mg calcium and is 10,000 times more dissolvable than calcium carbonate.[87] Notably, calcium carbonate has demonstrated reduced phosphate binding when used in combination with proton pump inhibitors or H_2 blockers, which are often prescribed in this population.[40] In patients with CKD and hypocalcemia who are not receiving dialysis, calcium carbonate is often used as a calcium supplement at night or, if hyperphosphatemia is also present, it can be taken during meals to improve both calcium and phosphorus levels. Since numerous studies have shown the potential increased calcification and mortality risk with higher calcium intakes in persons with ESKD, choosing binders with lower or no calcium burden are prudent in this population.

TABLE 10.2 | Comparison of Common Phosphate Binders[104]

Product and cost (availability)	Form	Starting dose	Usual dose	Medication interactions	Estimated equivalent dose[a] (1 tablet)	Advantages	Adverse effects and warnings
Calcium acetate (Rx: PhosLo, Eliphos, Calphron)	667 mg capsule/tablet	667 mg/meal	667-1,334 mg/meal (1-3 per meal)	Antibiotics, Synthroid	0.67	25% elemental calcium	Contributes to hypercalcemia, calcification, and PTH suppression
(Rx: Phoslyra)	667 mg/5 mL liquid					Liquid	Not as affordable as previously
(OTC: Generic calcium acetate)	668 mg tablet						
Calcium carbonate (OTC: TUMS)	500, 750, 1,000 mg liquid, tablet, gum, capsule, chewable	Possibly 1 per meal	In end-stage kidney disease: keep minimal	Antibiotics, Synthroid	0.5, 0.75, 1.0, respectively	Easily acquired, chewable, and inexpensive	40% elemental calcium; Contributes to hypercalcemia, calcification, and PTH suppression
Ferric citrate (Rx: Auryxia)	1 g coated tablets (210 mg ferric iron)	2 g per meal (2 tablets)	8-9 tablets daily, max: 12	Antibiotics, Synthroid	0.6; Manufacturer claims equivalent to calcium acetate or sevelamer	Noncalcium, absorbable iron	Contraindicated with iron overload, may overload iron stores; Gastrointestinal issues: diarrhea, discolored stool, constipation, nausea, vomiting
Lanthanum carbonate (Rx: Fosrenol)	500 mg, 750 mg, and 1,000 mg chewable wafers; 750 or 1,000 mg powder	500 mg per meal	750-1,000 mg per meal; Max: 4,500 mg/d	Antibiotics, Synthroid, antacids, and some heart medications, blood thinners, or blood pressure medications	1.0, 1.5, 2.0, respectively	Noncalcium; Chewable or powdered form	Contraindicated with bowel obstruction, severe constipation, and history of gastrointestinal surgery; Gastrointestinal issues: abdominal pain, bowel obstruction, nausea, vomiting
Sevelamer carbonate (Rx: Renvela or generic)	800 mg capsules; 0.8 or 2.4 g powder packets	800 mg or 0.8 g per meal	6.4-7.2 g per day	Antibiotics, immunosuppressants, Synthroid	0.6	Noncalcium; Improves lipids; Renvela available in powdered form and does not worsen acidosis	Large capsules and cannot be cut; Bowel obstruction or perforation, abdominal pain, constipation, diarrhea, nausea, vomiting
Sevelamer HCl (Rx: Renagel or generic)	800 mg capsules	800 mg per meal	6.4-7.2 g capsules per day	Antibiotics, immunosuppressants, Synthroid	0.6		Renagel may worsen acidosis
Sucroferric oxyhydroxide (Rx: Velphoro)	500 mg chewable tablets (2,500 mg sucroferric oxyhydroxide or 500 mg elemental iron)	500 mg per meal (1 tablet)	3-4 tablets per day; Max: 6 tablets per day	Antibiotics, Synthroid	1.6; Manufacturer claims need for half as many tablets as sevelamer	Noncalcium; Chewable, less absorbable iron; Lower pill burden	Monitor iron stores; Caution with history of gastrointestinal surgery; Gastrointestinal issues: diarrhea, discolored stool, nausea

OTC = over-the-counter | PTH = parathyroid hormone | RX= requires a prescription

[a] Estimated equivalent dose provides a comparison of phosphate binders based on phosphate-binding potential, using 1 g calcium carbonate as the baseline (ie, 1.0). For example, one 500 mg lanthanum carbonate is potentially equivalent to two 500-mg calcium carbonate or two 800-mg sevelamer carbonate since these medications have approximately half the equivalent dose of the lanthanum carbonate.

Unbound calcium is absorbed in the gut, leading to hypercalcemia in approximately 50% of patients undergoing dialysis, especially when patients are receiving active forms of vitamin D.[62] Hypercalcemia or high calcium intake suppresses PTH, leading to adynamic bone disease.[88] Calcium-based binders are associated statistically with soft tissue and VC, often thought to be due to calcium loading.[89] If serum calcium or corrected calcium becomes elevated, avoid other dietary sources of calcium (eg, use of antacids, calcium-fortified foods, or calcium supplements) and consider reducing the dosage of calcium-based binders, adjusting calcitriol or vitamin D analogs, and adding non–calcium-based binders as needed to control phosphorus.

Whether the use of calcium-based binders is safe remains a matter of opinion. The 2003 KDOQI guidelines recommended limiting total elemental calcium from binders to 1,500 mg/d, and the total calcium, including dietary calcium, should not exceed 2,000 mg/d.[45] The KDIGO recommendations have not included these criteria and continue to offer no recommendations for patients on dialysis or with a kidney transplant. See Box 10.1 for current KDOQI and KDIGO calcium recommendations.

A variety of non–calcium-based phosphate binders have been developed with growing evidence that higher calcium loads increase mortality risk in patients with ESKD. Sevelamer hydrochloride (Renagel) and sevelamer carbonate (Renvela) are phosphate binders without aluminum, calcium, or magnesium. Sevelamer is an ion-exchange polymer that interacts with phosphorus in the gastrointestinal tract.[6] Sevelamer carbonate has the same polymeric structure as sevelamer hydrochloride but in which the carbonate replaces chloride as the anion. This replacement may buffer some of the acid load that accumulates in patients with kidney disease, as well as reduce some gastrointestinal side effects from sevelamer hydrochloride.

A previous meta-analysis and a Cochrane meta-analysis and systematic review suggested insufficient data to determine if non–calcium-based binders were superior to calcium-based options.[90,91] A more recent meta-analysis of randomized controlled trials by Patel and colleagues[92] found significantly lower all-cause mortality with sevelamer as opposed to calcium-based binders, although evidence was lacking to show benefit of use in predialysis patients. Urinary excretion studies have reported reduced phosphate binding with higher doses of sevelamer.[93]

Aside from being a noncalcium binder, sevelamer acts as a bile acid sequestrant and may provide a cardioprotective benefit by reducing low-density lipoprotein cholesterol and total cholesterol levels; it may also bind bile acids or interfere with absorption of fat-soluble vitamins.[94]

Adverse effects of sevelamer hydrochloride include GI disturbances, cost, difficulty swallowing large tablets, and potential metabolic acidosis; sevelamer carbonate carries the same price tag but may improve metabolic acidosis and reduce GI symptoms.[95] There are also reports of sevelamer crystals causing GI mucosal injury, erosion, or perforation, so it is not recommended in patients with a recent history of GI surgery.[40] Sevelamer carbonate powder is available for patients with difficulty swallowing the large pills or seeking to reduce pill burden.

Magnesium-based binders, such as magnesium carbonate (MagnaBind), have been used with caution in some practices due to the potential risk of magnesium accumulation. Conversely, studies cited by Hamano[41] report increased cardiovascular risk in hyperphosphatemic patients with low magnesium levels, indicating that a magnesium-based binder may offer potential cardioprotective benefit. Patients appeared to tolerate magnesium carbonate well, although there was risk for diarrhea. There are no studies to evaluate the long-term effects of magnesium-based binders on VC, bone histology, and mortality.

Lanthanum carbonate (Fosrenol) is a chewable wafer or powdered phosphate binder that does not contain aluminum, calcium, or magnesium. Maximal phosphate binding is reported at lower pH levels (3–5) and, similar to other binders, phosphate binding has been reported to decline with higher lanthanum doses.[85,93] A post hoc analysis of a 2-year randomized control trial of lanthanum carbonate found a reduced mortality rate in patients aged greater than 65 years, but not in younger patients.[96] A recent systematic review and meta-analysis by Jamal and colleagues[97] found a 22% reduced all-cause mortality rate with use of non–calcium-based binders (sevelamer or lanthanum), as opposed to calcium-based, in every stage of CKD, although the majority of studies were in the population undergoing HD.[97] The risk of lanthanum accumulation or benefit in earlier CKD has not been adequately studied, whereas a 5-year observational study showed no evidence of accumulation in bone, toxicity, or liver damage.[6,40]

Another new class of noncalcium binders is iron-based. Both medications improved serum phosphorus approximately 30% from baseline and FGF-23 levels by two-thirds, which has not been observed with calcium-based binders.[29] There are no comparative studies between iron-based and calcium-based binders.[86] Most common side effects in iron-based binders include discolored bowel movements, diarrhea, nausea, and constipation.[86,98] Larger trials exploring mortality outcomes are still needed.[41] Options include sucroferric oxyhdroxide and ferric citrate.

Sucroferric oxyhydroxide (Velphoro) are berry-flavored chewable tablets that should be taken during meals and can also be crushed. Each chewable tablet contains 500 mg elemental iron (equivalent to 2,500 mg sucroferric oxyhydroxide), claiming to bind up to 130 mg phosphorus per tablet and requiring half as many tablets per day as sevelamer.[98] The starting dose is one tablet per meal with a titration increase of one tablet per day.[98] In a 52-week study of patients receiving HD and PD comparing sucroferric oxyhydroxide and sevelamer carbonate, similar reductions in FGF-23 and phosphate-lowering potential were found, but potentially with a much lower pill burden with sucroferric oxyhydroxide.[29] These results were confirmed in other studies of Black patients and patients on PD.[40] Sucroferric oxyhydroxide is unique as it touts low iron absorption.[12]

Ferric citrate (Auryxia) comes in tablet form and binds with phosphorus to form ferric phosphate, which is excreted. It is a more absorbable form of iron and, thus, requires monitoring of iron stores.[12] It has been found to reduce cardiac-related hospitalizations by 45%, potentially due to lower use of erythropoiesis-stimulating agents and possibly reduction of VC.[41] In

a review of recent studies, Floege[40] reported effective phosphate binding in patients pre dialysis and on dialysis; reduction in FGF-23 levels compared to lanthanum; fewer hospitalizations; and increases in hemoglobin, ferritin, and transferrin saturation. Another study demonstrated comparable effectiveness at reducing serum phosphorus as calcium acetate, no significant increase in aluminum levels, and improvement in PTH.[99]

Observational studies have shown improved survival rate in patients on phosphate binders and receiving HD.[100,101] It is unclear whether this is due to improved phosphorus control or better nutritional status in these patients resulting from better intake. A review of phosphate binders by Ruospo et al[86] found predominantly studies of small sample size, short duration, and no placebo-controlled studies examining all-cause mortality. The HiLo study is currently underway to fill this void.[102]

Much uncertainty regarding the benefit or harm of phosphate binders continues to exist as studies remain inconsistent.[26,40] A study of patients with moderate CKD found only modest improvement in phosphorus despite relatively high binder doses and improved BMD,[103] whereas more recent meta-analysis in patients with CKD and ESKD found no evidence of any phosphate binder improving CVD outcomes (ie, cardiovascular events or mortality).[26] Due to the limited reduction of serum phosphorus despite significant reduction in urinary phosphate, the authors surmised that serum phosphorus may be a poor marker of binder adherence as CKD progresses.[103] Daugirdas and colleagues[93] reported only 26 mg of phosphorus bound by each tablet of sevelamer, whereas each calcium acetate bound up to 33 mg phosphorus. Furthermore, some findings report lower levels of phosphorus bound with higher doses of sevelamer.

There may be individual patient variability on the effectiveness of phosphate binders, where phosphorus absorption has been reportedly reduced by 15% to 54% between the study participants.[63] Variability may also be due to the effect pH has on the absorption of phosphorus within the gut, phosphate binders acting as antacids and altering the pH (excluding sevelamer), and the common use of acid-suppressing medications (eg, proton pump inhibitors, antacids, and H2-blockers) in patients with kidney disease.[6] Some phosphate binders are also theoretically less effective in the lower pH environments of the stomach or upper duodenum where phosphate additives are likely absorbed.[63] The newer classes of noncalcium phosphate binders may be less dependent on pH and, therefore, may provide more benefit in diets high in phosphate additives.[87]

The 2017 KDIGO CKD–MBD guidelines add the following suggestions on binder usage[55]:

- Safety of phosphate-binding medication in CKD stages 3 through 4 is unproven. Phosphorus-lowering therapies (ie, diet or medications) should be considered only in "progressive or persistent hyperphosphatemia," not for the sake of prevention.
- Different phosphate-binding medications are no longer considered interchangeable as new evidence demonstrates the benefit of limiting calcium-based binders. Excess calcium from all sources (eg, diet, dialysate, and medications) may cause harm at any stage of CKD, regardless of previously identified risk markers (eg, hypercalcemia, calcification, etc).
- The work group was unable to make recommendations regarding the safe maximal dose of calcium-containing phosphate-binding medications. This is left to the discretion of clinicians, while recognizing that a safe upper calcium limit may exist.

PHOSPHATE TRANSPORT INHIBITORS

Inhibitors of intestinal phosphate transporters are being studied as novel approaches to improving hyperphosphatemia. In rodents, the majority of active phosphorus absorption occurs through the sodium phosphate-2b cotransporter, whereas phosphate transporter-1 and -2 may play more minor roles.[105] The mechanism is not yet clear in humans and remains under study.

Sodium Phosphate-2b Inhibitors

Thus far, nicotinamide (niacinamide) has been the only sodium phosphate-2b inhibitor to reduce serum phos-

phorus levels in humans.[105] Oral nicotinamide also demonstrated a beneficial increase in serum high-density lipoprotein and a decrease in low-density lipoprotein.[62] More recent trials of niacin in patients with CKD stage 3 have shown significant reductions in serum phosphorus.[106] However, side effects (eg, diarrhea, flushing, nausea, vomiting and hyperglycemia) may be barriers.[11]

In a small study of 19 patients with ESKD, a sodium phosphate-2b inhibitor that demonstrated substantial improvement in serum phosphorus in rat studies failed to show any improvements in urinary or fecal excretion of phosphorus or improved serum phosphorus levels in human beings.[107]

Sodium Phosphate-2b, Phosphate Transporter-1, and Phosphate Transporter-2 Inhibitors

A study in healthy and hyperphosphatemic rats found that an inhibitor of sodium-dependent phosphate transporters sodium phosphate-2b, phosphate transporter-1, and phosphate transporter-2 successfully and dose-dependently increased fecal phosphorus levels and reduced urinary phosphate excretion, indicating reduced phosphorus absorption.[108]

A small phase 1b study in patients receiving HD found promising results on reducing intestinal phosphate absorption with EOS789, a novel pan-inhibitor of these phosphate transporters. Fractional phosphate absorption declined incrementally at a higher dose, with or without sevelamer use, and was well tolerated.[109] Further study is needed.

Tenapanor

Tenapanor (Ibsrela) is a tablet taken twice daily to inhibit intestinal sodium-hydrogen exchanger (NHE3) activity. NHE3 exchanges sodium from outside the cell with protons from inside the cell. Inhibition of NHE3 increases protons inside the cell which selectively tightens junctions between cells, thereby reducing paracellular phosphate absorption. A recent study by Block and colleagues[110] found that tenapanor significantly improved serum phosphorus in patients on HD. Since sodium absorption is also impaired, the primary side effect is diarrhea, although this study demonstrated a weekly increase of only 2.8 bowel movements and an increase of less than 1 point (ie, slightly less firm) on the Bristol Stool Form Scale. It is not yet clear what dose provides ideal responses or the percentage of patients who will be successfully treated with this therapy. Additional study is warranted.

ADHERENCE

Medication and diet nonadherence are common problems in patients receiving dialysis. Following a kidney diet is challenging for many patients due to the complexity of the recommendations and difficulties determining which foods are acceptable. Potential barriers to following the dialysis diet were examined in a study by St-Jules and colleagues[111] in structured patient interviews, in which they found lower dietary adherence due to limitations in time, difficulty finding the right foods when grocery shopping, inability or lack of time to cook fresh foods, fatigue, poor appetite, and frustration with the limited acceptable options.

Another study identified barriers to be infrequent interaction with the health care team, older age, financial limitations, low education level, and balancing employment, dialysis, and managing their health. Adhering even only to the phosphorus restriction has been reported by patients undergoing dialysis to be the most complicated and challenging part of the entire diet. Individualized diet counseling, focusing on only one to two key education points at a time, providing lists of foods patients can enjoy (specific to their culture), involving family or caregiver support, and including the patient in goal setting can be useful in overcoming these barriers. A systematic review and meta-analysis of educational interventions in patients on HD identified several strategies to achieve desired behavior change: self-evaluation, easy-to-apply skills that fit within their current lifestyle, individualized counseling by a dietitian who specializes in renal nutrition, ongoing education, and providing education prior to dialysis, rather than during dialysis (found in one study).[112]

Compliance with phosphate binders can be a particular challenge. One study showed 61% of patients with unintentional nonadherence for those who take binders, and 48% have some intentional nonadherence; those with intentional nonadherence reported doing so because of making them feel worse, having no symptoms, or taking phosphate binders was inconvenient. Furthermore, phosphorus-related knowledge and medication refill rates at the pharmacy were not associated with improved phosphorus control.[113] Fissell and colleagues[114] found that up to 57% of patients missed at least one phosphate binder dose in a month, with increasing rates of nonadherence with the higher amount of binders prescribed and higher resulting serum phosphorus and PTH levels. Factors that influence medication adherence include increased dosage frequency and number of pills, complexity of the regimen, adverse gastrointestinal reactions, length of treatment, low education level, and lower socioeconomic status.[115] Patients who skipped phosphate binders more frequently were also reported to be younger, single, more likely to skip or shorten dialysis treatments, or have a greater likelihood of a psychiatric disorder.[114] The limited fluid allotment is also a disincentive to taking multiple binders.

Improved medication and dialysis attendance adherence may be related to a good patient–physician relationship and whether the staff were perceived as caring in these predominantly Black patients.[116] Other possible factors are simplification of regimen, visual reminders, using medication boxes, written instructions, education, and incentives, rather than negative feedback. Positive encouragement and reinforcement by the dietitian and other team members are needed to help patients succeed. Patients should also be counseled regarding the proper timing of binders (ie, during meals and snacks). Dosage should be customized to the patient's phosphorus consumption throughout the day, as patients rarely eat three meals of equal size.

The choice of phosphate binder is complicated and may go beyond the opinions of the practitioner regarding the best choice. Patients' ability to pay, comorbid illnesses, swallowing ability, and gastrointestinal side effects are often considerations when deciding on a binder. Including patients on these decisions and including dose adjustments may improve the likelihood of buy-in and adherence.

DIALYSIS

Serum phosphorus levels fluctuate (being lowest in the morning and rising through mid-afternoon) in patients on continuous ambulatory peritoneal dialysis (CAPD) and HD, although the fluctuations are less pronounced in those on CAPD (being more similar to the healthy population).[117]

Phosphorus removal during dialysis is dependent on several factors, including frequency and duration of dialysis, dialyzer type, PTH, ultrafiltration volume, and predialysis serum phosphorus level (ie, higher serum phosphorus levels result in greater phosphorus removal during dialysis).[118,119] Bertocchio and colleagues[120] also reported that excess bicarbonate (ie, alkalosis) during dialysis may impair phosphorus mobilization and, thereby, removal.

Increasing dialytic blood flow rate removes higher amounts of urea and electrolytes but fails to improve phosphorus removal.[121] Several studies in the literature indicate that the first 1 to 2 hours of dialysis allow for rapid removal of phosphorus, after which removal is markedly reduced due to the slow transfer of phosphorus extracellularly as the concentration gradient difference falls; this may also explain the rebound in serum phosphorus levels commonly seen post dialysis.[6,118] More recently, Elias and colleagues[119] found that phosphorus removal during HD sessions is fairly consistent throughout the treatment, despite serum phosphorus normalizing within the first hour.

Phosphorus removal is generally not adequate via typical HD or PD techniques.[118] Yet Svara and colleagues[122] showed that newer high-flux membranes and hemodiafiltration were significantly more effective at phosphorus removal than lower-flux HD. Experts previously considered that PD was superior at removing phosphorus since these patients typically had better controlled phosphorus levels; yet Evenepoel and colleagues[123] showed that total phosphorus clearance is lower in patients on PD compared to those on HD, even when kidney clearance is incorporated. This indicates that the improved phosphorus control of PD is due primarily to kidney phosphorus clearance; hence,

the risk of hyperphosphatemia is likely to rise as residual kidney function (RKF) declines. When Evenepoel and colleague compared PD modalities, CAPD demonstrated significantly more dialytic clearance of phosphorus than automated PD, potentially related to differences in treatment time. Wang and colleagues[124] also demonstrated the challenge of maintaining serum phosphorus levels within goal ranges in patients on CAPD; those with RKF experienced hyperphosphatemia nearly half as often as those with anuria.

The transfer of phosphorus is a rate-limiting process in traditional 3- to 4-hour dialysis treatments; therefore, conventional dialysis falls short of removing the amount of phosphorus consumed by diet.[118] Historically, it was estimated that HD removed an average of 2,500 mg phosphorus per week, but more recent studies have shown considerable variability ranging from 250 to 1,400 mg per dialysis session (750–4,200 mg/wk).[63] PD removes approximately 250 to 360 mg/d of phosphorus (1,750–2,520 mg/wk).[6] More gradual dialysis treatment options may allow for a slower equilibration of phosphorus between body compartments, such as longer dialysis times (eg, nocturnal dialysis), or more frequent dialysis (eg, short daily HD), and may allow for more efficient phosphorus removal.[6] Zupančič and colleagues[125] demonstrated greater phosphorus removal with nocturnal dialysis as compared to traditional HD, with total phosphorus removal of 5,195.7 ± 1,898 mg/d.

Patients with considerable RKF or on more frequent HD (eg, six times per week) have somewhat improved phosphorus control and an increased percentage may have acceptable phosphorus control without binders, with the exception of patients on PD. The data from the Frequent Hemodialysis Network Daily and Nocturnal Trials found that patients on dialysis six times per week (12 hours per week on average) had serum phosphorus levels improve by nearly 0.5 mg/dL and reduced quantity of phosphate binders; patients on frequent nocturnal dialysis 6 to 8 hours six times per week improved serum phosphorus levels by nearly 1.25 mg/dL; all of the patients were able to discontinue phosphate binders, and 42% of patients required phosphorus to be added to the dialysate to prevent hypophosphatemia.[126] In another report, patients on HD for more than 30 hours per week were able to discontinue phosphate binders.[118]

OVERVIEW OF PHOSPHORUS CONTROL

To improve rising or persistently elevated phosphorus:

- Assess trends in phosphorus in combination with calcium and PTH. Maximize SHPT therapy to prevent release of phosphorus from the bone into the blood.
- Review dietary recall for highly absorbable phosphorus foods or hidden sources of phosphorus (ie, processed meats, processed cheeses, baked goods, and others).
  - Identify one to two problematic foods to limit and offer alternatives.
  - Ensure no overconsumption of natural phosphorus foods (eg, dairy products).
  - Provide education on choosing fresh foods, label reading and choosing foods without phosphate additives, when possible. Recommend "natural" or "all natural" poultry, fish, or seafood, as these typically do not contain added phosphorus.
- Binders may be advised at CKD stage 5 if dietary control has been unsuccessful and with monitoring laboratory trends, rather than a single value. Educate patients that binders only help reduce a small portion of phosphorus; hence, making good food choices is so important.
  - Recommend the binder type most suitable to each patient's economic and physical needs (ie, affordability, swallowing ability, dentition, patient preference, and tolerance). Consider concentrated forms to reduce pill burden.
  - Match the number of binders to the phosphorus content of the meals and snacks. Binders should be taken during meals for optimal effect. If patients experience gastrointestinal upset with binders, ensure they are not taken on an empty stomach before transitioning to a new binder type.
    - Consider increasing binder dosage if phosphorus level is greater than 5.5 mg/dL or is trending toward elevation, the patient is compliant with diet and binders, and the maximum recommended binder dosage has not been reached.
    - Reduce binder dosage if phosphorus level drops to less than 3.0 mg/dL. Evaluate oral intake for nutritional adequacy.
- Assess for risk of food insecurity and needed resources to maximize outcomes.
- Recognize that many causes of elevated phosphorus are out of the patient's control (eg, phosphate additives in foods and medications, the amount removed by dialysis, the little phosphorus eliminated by binders), so you can help prioritize what is actually achievable or will make the most impact with each patient.

VITAMIN D

Ergocalciferol and cholecalciferol comprise "nutritional" vitamin D.[16] Cholecalciferol is more potent than ergocalciferol in the human body, yet ergocalciferol (50,000 IU) is the only high-dose commercial version in the United States. Cholecalciferol is found in drugstores at doses such as 400 IU, 1,000 IU, 2,000 IU, and 5,000 IU per capsule or tablet.

Use of vitamin D has variable success in treating CKD–MBD, depending on the stage of kidney disease. Ergocalciferol, cholecalciferol, and calcitriol are used regularly in the predialysis population for treatment of vitamin D deficiency and hypocalcemia in order to prevent overproduction of PTH. Nutritional vitamin D treatment can be quite effective in the earlier stages, but becomes less so in the later stages due to reduced VDRs in hyperplastic parathyroid glands.[12] A study of 52 predialysis patients with vitamin D deficiency and elevated PTH levels received treatment with ergocalciferol. The 25-hydroxyvitamin D levels normalized in patients with CKD stages 3 and 4. PTH decreased in stage 3 but did not significantly decrease in patients with CKD stage 4.[127] Another study demonstrated reduction of PTH in patients with CKD and vitamin D deficiency treated with high-dose cholecalciferol.[8]

In patients on dialysis, there is concern that the use of active vitamin D may result in hypercalcemia or hyperphosphatemia due to increased absorption in the gut. Vitamin D analogs used in these populations are considered to have a lesser calcemic effect yet are equally effective in suppressing PTH, so they are used more commonly.[12,128] However, more recent literature indicates that their calcemic effect may be more equal than previously thought.[16]

As many as 80% of patients on HD have 25-hydroxyvitamin D levels equal to or less than 31 ng/mL (mean baseline of 18.4 ng/mL); after ergocalciferol supplementation dosed at 50,000 IU/wk for 24 weeks, total 25-hydroxyvitamin D levels rose significantly to a mean of 42 ng/mL.[17] In another study, greater SHPT improvement was demonstrated with a combination of cholecalciferol and vitamin D analog, than via vitamin D analog alone in patients on HD; therefore, it should be considered that these are provided concurrently.[30]

Calcium-based phosphate binders have been reported to hinder the effect of vitamin D in SHPT management, potentially by raising serum calcium levels.[30] It has also been reported that high doses of active vitamin D may contribute to 25-hydroxyvitamin D deficiency and increased catabolism, resulting in a shortage in other organs or tissues that also rely on or activate 25-hydroxyvitamin D.[30]

The 2020 KDOQI Clinical Practice Guidelines on Nutrition suggest cholecalciferol or ergocalciferol supplementation to correct 25-hydroxyvitamin D deficiency or insufficiency in CKD stages 1 through 5D and posttransplant patients.[61] Additional research is needed to determine the optimal levels for 25-hydroxyvitamin D. No randomized control trials have shown reduced cardiac events or mortality with vitamin D therapies.[8]

PARATHYROID HORMONE

The majority of patients with kidney disease develop SHPT. This typically worsens with the longer duration of advanced kidney disease or duration on dialysis. The associated vitamin D deficiency, reduced sensitivity of parathyroid CaSR, and other factors of severe SHPT result in greater difficulty achieving desirable serum laboratory results.

Historically, the therapy for renal bone disease has centered on the use of active vitamin D and its analogs. These medications are given orally or intravenously depending on the type of dialysis therapy, stage of kidney disease, or desired effect. Oral therapy is often used intermittently, two to three times per week, or daily. Because intravenous (IV) medications are given at the time of dialysis, adherence is better than with oral calcitriol. IV calcitriol has also been shown to improve bone remodeling after 6 months of therapy when compared with oral pulse or oral intermittent calcitriol therapy, despite similar changes in PTH levels.[15] When comparing oral to pulse intraperitoneal calcitriol, a study in patients on PD showed that pulse intraperitoneal calcitriol is more effective than pulse oral calcitriol at lowering PTH and resolving renal osteodystrophy. There was also a lower incidence of hyperphosphatemia.[129]

While calcitriol therapy is effective in lowering PTH, it brings with it the risk of increased gastrointestinal absorption of both calcium and phosphorus. Increased levels of calcium and phosphorus are associated with increased mortality in patients receiving dialysis.[130] These disturbances are associated with progression of VC and coronary artery disease. Therapies should focus on PTH suppression without initiating or worsening hypercalcemia and overt hyperphosphatemia.

Vitamin D analogs are synthetic forms of active vitamin D. Paricalcitol (Zemplar) is indicated for the prevention and the treatment of SHPT in patients with CKD, HD, and PD. It is used intravenously for patients with CKD stage 5D or orally in capsule form for patients at CKD stages 3, 4, or 5 and for those receiving PD.

Doxercalciferol (Hectorol) is another vitamin D analog that is indicated in the treatment of SHPT in patients with CKD stages 3 and 4 (capsules) and in patients on dialysis (capsules or injection). In the oral vs IV doxercalciferol study in patients on HD, IV doxercalciferol appeared to have less of an effect on serum calcium and phosphorus levels than oral treatment.[131]

Calcifediol (Rayaldee) is the newest in this class and is indicated for use in patients with CKD stages 3 and 4 and low vitamin D levels; it is not for patients with CKD stage 5 or ESKD. It comes as extended-release capsules to be taken at bedtime and swallowed whole (not chewed).[132]

The target range for PTH is two to nine times the upper limit of normal for the assay.[53] With vitamin D therapy, serum calcium and phosphorus should be monitored when initiating or titrating the dose of vitamin D. Successful treatment of SHPT depends on appropriate timing for initial therapy, adequate dosing, and careful monitoring for side effects, such as hypercalcemia, hyperphosphatemia, or over-suppressed PTH. Discontinuation of vitamin D or vitamin D analogs should be considered in cases of severe hyperphosphatemia, hypercalcemia, low PTH (not related to parathyroidectomy), low-turnover bone disease, or calciphylaxis.[12]

CALCIMIMETICS

Calcimimetics are medications that mimic the action of calcium in activating CaSRs on bodily tissues (eg, the parathyroid gland) in treating SHPT. These are used in established SHPT where there is a decrease in the expression of the CaSR. The CaSR regulates PTH release; these medications shift the set point for PTH secretion so that a 50% decrease in PTH occurs at a lower ionized calcium concentration, allowing a lower serum calcium level to suppress PTH.[133] Cinacalcet (Sensipar) and etelcalcitide (Parsabiv) are the calcimimetics approved for use in patients with ESKD. They are not recommended for use in predialysis patients.

Cinacalcet is an oral tablet indicated for the treatment of SHPT in patients with CKD on dialysis. Cinacalcet binds to the CaSR on the parathyroid gland to increase the sensitivity to calcium and thereby reduces PTH secretion.[6] It is particularly helpful in cases when hyperparathyroidism occurs in conjunction with marginal or overt hypercalcemia, as the medication results in serum calcium reduction.[12] Although it is well tolerated by many patients, the most commonly reported adverse effects are nausea, vomiting, and diarrhea.

During cinacalcet therapy, there is a concomitant decrease in serum calcium levels, although there rarely are hypocalcemic symptoms.[134] Potential harm from positive calcium balance and the lack of negative effects of hypocalcemia with calcimimetic use in the Evaluation of Cinacalcet Hydrochloride Therapy to Lower Cardiovascular Events trial (EVOLVE) led the KDIGO work group to modify the previous recommendation.[55] Therefore, the KDIGO guidelines now discourage the unnecessary use of calcium supplementation in patients with mild or asymptomatic hypocalcemia.[55]

The manufacturer recommends starting cinacalcet at 30 mg once daily, typically taken during the evening or largest meal, and at least 12 hours prior to PTH laboratory work. Cinacalcet should be titrated no more than every 2 to 4 weeks using sequential doses of 60 mg, 90 mg, 120 mg, and 180 mg once daily, until PTH targets are met. Serum calcium value of less than 8.4 mg/dL is a contraindication for initiating cinacalcet. Tablets should be taken with food and should never be cut or divided. Serum calcium levels should be monitored weekly at initiation or with dose changes, where PTH would be rechecked within 4 weeks.[135]

Studies exploring the use of cinacalcet to improve CVD or mortality outcomes in patients with kidney disease have had conflicting findings. The ADVANCE study found that patients on HD with moderate or severe SHPT had reduced progression of CAC with cinacalcet combined with vitamin D therapy, compared to active vitamin D therapy alone.[136] The EVOLVE trial found that cinacalcet demonstrated improvement in FGF-23, PTH, and phosphorus, as well as reduced rates of parathyroidectomies and calciphylaxis; yet a reduction in cardiac events or survival advantage was not seen in patients with ESKD randomized on cinacalcet compared with a placebo due to study limitations.[8,25] However, a recent post hoc analysis of the EVOLVE trial showed that higher baseline FGF-23 levels were likely the cause of the increased risk of mortality and CVD events; patients receiving cinacalcet HCl had greatly reduced FGF-23 levels; a 30% or more reduction was associated with a lower incidence of CVD risk, independent of phosphorus, PTH, calcium, and vitamin D levels.[25] Patients with ESKD on dialysis receiving combined vitamin D analogs and cinacalcet are reported to have the most favorable outcomes.[8]

Etelcalcetide, which is an IV calcimimetic developed for patients with ESKD, is provided during dialysis rinse back up to three times per week. It forms conjugates with serum albumin and acts to activate the CaSR, which is a longer-acting mechanism than cinacalcet. The starting dose is 5 mg and can be increased to 7.5 mg, 10 mg, 12.5 mg, or 15 mg. Severe hypocalcemia may result if patients take cinacalcet concurrently with etelcalcetide. Therefore, the manufacturer recommends discontinuing cinacalcet use at least 7 days prior to initiating etelcalcetide. As with cinacalcet, etelcalcetide has demonstrated a calcium-lowering effect; therefore, therapy should only be initiated if serum calcium is equal to or greater than 8.3 mg/dL, the dose reduced if 7.5 mg/dL to 8.3 mg/dL, and held for 1 month if less than 7.5 mg/dL.[137] Side effects can include hypocalcemia, muscle spasms, nausea, diarrhea, and paresthesia (abnormal skin tingling or numbness) but the gastrointestinal symptoms seem to occur less frequently than with oral cinacalcet.

Patients on calcimimetics are at risk of hypocalcemia, which can result in QT interval prolongation and ventricular arrhythmia. Serum calcium should be checked weekly and PTH should be checked monthly after initiating either therapy, until the results are stabilized within goal ranges. These are recommended for use alone or in combination with calcium, calcium-based binders, or vitamin D analogs.

PARATHYROIDECTOMY

Therapy for SHPT may not be successful in all patients. The KDIGO guideline recommends consideration of a parathyroidectomy in patients with CKD stages 3a through 5D and severe SHPT who fail to respond adequately to PTH-lowering therapies or medical interventions.[55]

Normal parathyroid glands weigh 30 to 40 mg; by comparison, hyperplastic glands may weigh 2 to 3 g. Most people have four glands, but more or fewer glands may be present.

There are no randomized control trials, demonstrating improved outcomes with parathyroidectomy or benefit over medical therapies. A few retrospective analyses have shown that parathyroidectomy may improve fracture risk and mortality risk.[138,139] Conversely, a more recent cohort study found that parathyroidectomy resulted in a higher mortality risk, 39% increased hospitalizations, increased days in the hospital, 20-fold increase in emergency department visits due to hypocalcemia, and a 69% increase in intensive care unit admissions within the subsequent year.[140]

Following parathyroidectomy, alkaline phosphatase levels are likely to remain elevated initially and normalize within 6 months, and bone density has been reported to improve by up to 332% within a year, whereas some patients with ESKD may develop osteomalacia after a year.[140] Performing a parathyroidectomy prior to transplant is controversial and a total parathyroidectomy is not recommended because control of calcium levels may be difficult to manage post transplant.[45]

Parathyroidectomy Procedures

The following procedures are available to reduce parathyroid tissue[141]:

- Subtotal parathyroidectomy: This procedure involves the removal of all parathyroid tissue except for a portion of the least hyperplastic gland. This may have a lower risk of adynamic bone disease.
- Total parathyroidectomy with reimplantation: This procedure involves the removal of all of the parathyroid glands that are evident during surgery with a small amount of tissue transplanted typically into the forearm. This allows easier removal from the arm if a repeat surgery is needed, but reexploration of the neck may still be necessary.
- Total parathyroidectomy: This procedure involves removal of all of the parathyroid tissue. Although it is less commonly performed, it can be appropriate for patients requiring dialysis.[12] This procedure reduces the risk of recurrent disease. The disadvantages of total parathyroid removal include development of hypocalcemia, adynam-

ic bone disease, permanent hypoparathyroidism, and need for long-term calcium and vitamin D therapy.

Following subtotal or parathyroidectomy with reimplantation, the rate of recurrence is similar and hyperparathyroidism can recur in roughly 10% of patients.[12] Expert opinions remain divided on the ideal method between these two procedures.[141]

Postparathyroidectomy Therapy

A short-term decline in serum calcium levels is common following parathyroidectomy, whereas hungry bone syndrome often refers to serum calcium values less than 8.4 mg/dL for 2 to 4 days following surgery. The sudden drop in PTH abruptly stops osteoclastic bone resorption and osteoblastic activity rises in conjunction with alkaline phosphatase levels. Therefore, the bone dramatically increases uptake of calcium, phosphorus, and magnesium as new bone is formed. Severe hypocalcemia and hypophosphatemia often result.

The risks for bone hunger occurrence in SHPT include the following preoperative scenarios[140]:

- PTH more than 1,000 pg/mL,
- alkaline phosphatase greater than three times the upper limit,
- age greater than 60 years, or
- elevated osteoclast counts in bone biopsy or radiologic findings.

Serum calcium and phosphorus levels should be monitored regularly until stabilized. Careful monitoring is paramount as the severity of bone hunger tends to be directly related to the severity of SHPT prior to parathyroidectomy. Severe hypocalcemia can occur, resulting in tingling, muscle spasms, or seizures, potentially persisting for several months and in some cases over a year.[140]

There are no guidelines outlining the ideal treatment for bone hunger, and there are no known studies evaluating the long-term consequences of parathyroidectomy or the use of aggressive supplementation commonly applied in the treatment of hungry bone. Current suggestions include the following[140]:

- Administer 4 to 12 g calcium daily, preferably spread among numerous doses for optimal ab-

sorption. Calcium dialysate can be increased to 3 mEq/L.
- Use 2 to 4 mcg oral calcitriol daily for increased gut absorption of calcium and phosphorus.
- Supplement magnesium, depending on serum values.
- Discontinue phosphate binders and consider phosphorus supplementation if serum levels are less than 1 mg/dL.

IV calcitriol can be given with dialysis treatments if practitioners are unsure whether the patient will be adherent with the oral therapy. Phosphorus levels tend to rebound more quickly than calcium levels, especially in diets high in phosphate additives, and often these patients do not require supplementation. As serum calcium and phosphorus levels begin to stabilize within the normal range, supplements should be tapered and eventually discontinued.

Many patients do not receive complete parathyroidectomies, so recurrence of SHPT is possible, especially if hypocalcemia, hyperphosphatemia, or diets high in phosphorus additives are not corrected.

Kidney Transplant

The incidence of MBD in the posttransplant population is increasing and is affected by both the pretransplant MBD and the cumulative effects of posttransplant MBD, medications, and rising rates of transplantation. Adynamic bone disease is most commonly seen post transplant, affecting up to 50% of patients; conversely, high-turnover bone disease has been reported in as many as 25% to 50% of patients. Osteoporosis rates are estimated to be as high as 30%, and there is approximately a 22% fracture risk within 5 years of transplant. The risk of hip fracture is 34% higher in the immediate posttransplantation period than in patients with ESKD; this risk then declines after 6 months post transplant. The risk of death following hip fracture in this population is approximately 60% higher than that in the general population.[142]

PARATHYROID HORMONE

Following a transplant, PTH is increased in about two-thirds of patients immediately after transplant, which then decreases within the first several weeks with increased conversion of 25-hydroxyvitamin D3 to calcitriol to increase gut calcium absorption, both resulting in a gradual inhibition of PTH and increased serum calcium over the next 6 months.[142] However, in patients with severe SHPT, elevated PTH levels may persist for several years and result in significant bone loss and reduced graft survival.[142] A study by Wolf and colleagues[143] found that patients with PTH greater than 600 pg/mL improved to 203 pg/mL within 3 months and then continued to decline gradually throughout the remainder of the year. Patients with more controlled PTH levels demonstrated a more gradual decline in PTH levels; notably, 15% or less of patients achieved improvement up to less than 65 pg/mL within the year.

CALCIUM

Previous research has shown a transient decrease in calcium levels immediately after a transplant with an increase to normal or elevated levels by around week 2.[144] More recently, Wolf and colleagues[143] demonstrated progressively rising calcium levels through week 4, regardless of whether PTH was controlled or elevated, although those with elevated PTH levels also had persistently elevated calcium levels through 12 months. In patients with lower PTH levels, hypercalcemia can occur in up to 29% of patients within the first 2 weeks, which then near steadily declined throughout the year.[143] In patients with severe SHPT, elevated calcium levels can persist for years and leads to increased bone resorption.[142]

PHOSPHORUS

Phosphorus levels decrease rapidly in the first post-transplant months to normal or below normal, possibly due to increased kidney excretion of phosphorus related to elevated FGF-23 and PTH levels, glucocorticoids,

and suboptimal vitamin D levels.[61] Wolf and colleagues[143] found that serum phosphorus levels, regardless of whether PTH levels were controlled or elevated, improved within 4 weeks of transplant and remained nearly stable within normal limits throughout the year.

Hypophosphatemia was found to be as prevalent (up to 40%) in patients 6 months after transplantation and may peak by week 2 and progressively improve throughout the year, although it was unknown if supplementation was provided.[142,143] Per the KDOQI 2020 work group opinion, phosphorus supplementation or a high-phosphorus diet can be considered to remedy hypophosphatemia.[61] No replacement dose or target serum level to initiate supplementation was provided; the level should be based on clinical judgment. Phosphorus levels typically normalize within a year as FGF-23 levels stabilize.[142]

The benefits or harm of phosphate binder use in this population are being assessed in a review that is currently being updated.[86]

VITAMIN D

Wolf and colleagues[143] found an increase in 1,25-dihydroxyvitamin D3 and a slight reduction of 25-hydroxyvitamin D throughout the year, regardless of PTH control and without treatment. Vitamin D supplements or analogs are commonly used post transplant in reducing PTH levels and potentially improving bone density. Calcitriol and paricalcitol have been shown to improve PTH levels and bone density post transplant, although paricalcitol exhibits a possible association with adynamic bone disease and hypercalcemia.[142]

PREVENTION AND MANAGEMENT

As in other stages of kidney disease, bone biopsy is considered the gold standard for diagnosing MBD after transplant, but it is rarely performed due to the procedure invasiveness, cost, and limited analysis.[142] The use of the WHO's fracture risk assessment tool is suggested as a potentially validated tool for predicting the probability of fractures; DXA and computed tomography may provide additional useful information, although there have been no prospective studies have been studied specifically in the transplant population.[142]

See Table 10.1 for updated KDIGO guidelines in managing MBD and updated KDOQI nutrition guidelines. Furthermore, experts recommend measuring serum calcium and phosphorus weekly immediately post transplant until these values stabilize; vitamin D measurements and correction should match those for the general population.[55]

Vitamin D, vitamin D analogs, and calcimimetics are routinely used post transplant for PTH suppression. Calcimimetics have been shown to be effective in reducing persistent SHPT and hypercalcemia in patients with transplant, but not necessarily with improving bone density and may have an association with adynamic bone disease.[142]

There are numerous medications that can affect MBD post transplant, whether as side effects of immunosuppressants or used for the prevention of bone disease progression. Common immunosuppressants (eg, glucocorticoids such as prednisone and methylprednisolone) impair gut calcium absorption by reducing activation of vitamin D and increasing renal calcium excretion, as well as stimulating osteoclast activity and inhibiting osteoblasts. Calcineurin inhibitors (eg, cyclosporine and tacrolimus) can create high-bone turnover osteoporosis by raising PTH levels, lowering magnesium levels, and stimulating osteoclast activity at a higher degree than osteoblasts. Conversely, bisphosphonates decrease bone resorption and reduce osteoclastic activity, but may not reduce the incidence of fractures. Denosumab (Prolia & Xgeva) inhibits osteoclastic activity, but its use has been very limited in patients with CKD or transplant.

In a study of bone alterations post transplant, the degree of osteocyte cell death was related to total glucocorticoid use.[142] Experts speculate that rates of fracture and bone density abnormalities may improve as steroid-limiting protocols are enacted. Although this is not consistently seen in studies yet, a 45% reduction in hip fractures has been reported comparing data from 1997 to data from 2010.[142] Upcoming studies indicate that

mTOR inhibitors (eg, rapamycin and everolimus) may have a protective effect on bone by inhibiting bone resorption. Yet a previous study showed significant risk of osteoporosis with their use.[142]

Parathyroidectomy remains an option for treatment of SHPT and hypercalcemia that do not respond to medical management. Both total or subtotal parathyroidectomy has been demonstrated to be effective in improving SHPT in patients post transplant.[142] Long-term benefits and outcomes remain unknown. See Chapter 8 for further information regarding nutrition management for transplant patients.

Summary

CKD–MBD is a wide complex of disorders that includes SHPT, renal osteodystrophy, disorders of vitamin D metabolism, hyperphosphatemia, hypocalcemia and hypercalcemia, and VC. Together, these problems have a major impact on the morbidity and the mortality of patients with kidney disease. Many of these disorders can be modified through changes in concurrent monitoring of serum calcium, phosphorus, and PTH, the use of phosphorus binders, vitamin D and analogs, and calcimimetic therapy. The registered dietitian nutritionist plays a major role in implementing these therapies and improving the lives of patients with kidney disease.

References

1. Moe S, Drueke T, Cunningham J, et al. Definition, evaluation, and classification of renal osteodystrophy: a position statement from Kidney Disease: Improving Global Outcomes (KDIGO). *Kidney Int.* 2006;69(11):1945-1953. doi:10.1038/sj.ki.5000414

2. Kalantar-Zadeh K, Kuwae N, Regidor DL, et al. Survival predictability of time-varying indicators of bone disease in maintenance hemodialysis patients. *Kidney Int.* 2006;70(4):771-780. doi:10.1038/sj.ki.5001514

3. Block GA, Klassen PS, Lazarus JM, et al. Mineral metabolism, mortality, and morbidity in maintenance hemodialysis. *J Am Soc Nephrol.* 2004;15(8):2208-2218. doi:10.1097/01.ASN .0000133041.27682.A2

4. Martin KJ, Gonzalez EA. Metabolic bone disease in chronic kidney disease. *J Am Soc Nephrol.* 2007;18(3):875-885. doi:10.1681/ASN.2006070771

5. Blaine J, Chonchol M, Levi M. Renal control of calcium, phosphate, and magnesium homeostasis. *Clin J Am Soc Nephrol.* 2015;10(7):1257-1272. doi:10.2215/CJN.09750913

6. Shaman AM, Kowalski SR. Hyperphosphatemia management in patients with chronic kidney disease. *Saudi Pharm J.* 2016;24(4):494-505. doi:10 .1016/j.jsps.2015.01.009

7. Gutierrez OM. Fibroblast growth factor 23, Klotho, and disordered mineral metabolism in chronic kidney disease: unraveling the intricate tapestry of events and implications for therapy. *J Ren Nutr.* 2013;23(3):250-254. doi:10.1053/j.jrn.2013.01.024

8. Lunyera J, Scialla JJ. Update on chronic kidney disease mineral and bone disorder in cardiovascular disease. *Semin Nephrol.* 2018;38(6):542-558. doi:10 .1016/j.semnephrol.2018.08.001

9. Isakova T, Wahl P, Vargas GS, et al. Fibroblast growth factor 23 is elevated before parathyroid hormone and phosphate in chronic kidney disease. *Kidney Int.* 2011;79(12):1370-1378. doi:10.1038/ki.2011.47

10. Andress DL, Coyne DW, Kalantar-Zadeh K, et al. Management of secondary hyperparathyroidism in stages 3 and 4 chronic kidney disease. *Endocr Pract.* 2008;14(1):18-27. doi:10.4158/EP.14.1.18

11. Kovesdy CP, Kalantar-Zadeh K. Bone and mineral disorders in pre-dialysis CKD. *Int Urol Nephrol.* 2008;40(2):427-440. doi:10.1007/s11255-008 -9346-7

12. Feehally J, Floege J, Tonelli M, et al. Bone and mineral disorders in chronic kidney disease. In: *Comprehensive Clinical Nephrology.* Elsevier; 2019:979-995.

13. De Boer IH, Gorodetskaya I, Young B, et al. The severity of secondary hyperparathyroidism in chronic renal insufficiency is GFR-dependent, race-dependent, and associated with cardiovascular disease. *J Am Soc Nephrol.* 2002;13(11):2762-2769. doi:10.1097/01.asn.0000034202.91413.eb

14. Olaizola I, Aznarez A, Jorgetti V, et al. Are there any differences in the parathyroid response in the different types of renal osteodystrophy? *Nephrol Dial Transplant.* 1998;13 (suppl 3):15-18. doi:10 .1093/ndt/13.suppl_3.15

15. Turk S, Akbulut M, Yildiz A, et al. Comparative effect of oral pulse and intravenous calcitriol treatment in hemodialysis patients: the effect on serum IL-1 and IL-6 levels and bone mineral density. *Nephron.* 2002;90(2):188-194. doi:10.1159/000049041

16. Parikh C, Gutgarts V, Eisenberg E, et al. Vitamin D and clinical outcomes in dialysis. *Semin Dial.* 2015;28(6):604-609. doi:10.1111/sdi.12446

17. Blair D, Byham-Gray L, Lewis E, McCaffrey S. Prevalence of vitamin D [25(OH)D] deficiency and effects of supplementation wtih ergocalciferol (vitamin D2) in stage 5 chronic kidney disease patients. *J Ren Nutr.* 2008;18(4):375-382. doi:10 .1053/j.jrn.200804.008

18. Al-Badr W, Martin KJ. Vitamin D and kidney disease. *Clin J Am Soc Nephrol.* 2008;3(5):1555-1560. doi:10 .2215/CJN.01150308

19. Vassalotti JA, Uribarri J, Chen SC, et al. Trends in mineral metabolism: Kidney Early Evaluation Program (KEEP) and the National Health and Nutrition Examination Survey (NHANES) 1999-2004. *Am J Kidney Dis.* 2008;51(4 suppl 2):S56-S68. doi:10.1053/j.ajkd.2007.12.018

20. Slatopolsky E, Dusso A, Brown AJ. The role of phosphorus in the development of secondary hyperparathyroidism and parathyroid cell proliferation in chronic renal failure. *Am J Med Sci.* 1999;317(6):370-376. doi:10.1097/00000441 -199906000-00004

21. Elder G. Pathophysiology and recent advances in the management of renal osteodystrophy. *J Bone Miner Res.* 2002;17(12):2094-2105. doi:10.1359 /jbmr.2002.17.12.2094

22. McCann L, ed. *Pocket Guide to Nutrition Assessment of the Patient with Kidney Disease.* 6th ed. National Kidney Foundation; 2021.

23. Rayner HC, Larkina M, Wang M, et al. International comparisons of prevalence, awareness, and treatment of pruritus in people on hemodialysis. *Clin J Am Soc Nephrol.* 2017;12(12):2000-2007. doi:10.2215/CJN.03280317

24. Sukul N, Speyer E, Tu C, et al. Pruritus and patient reported outcomes in non-dialysis CKD. *Clin J Am Soc Nephrol.* 2019;14(5):673-681. doi:10.2215/CJN .09600818

25. Cianciolo G, Galassi A, Capelli I, et al. Klotho–FGF23, cardiovascular disease, and vascular calcification: black or white? *Curr Vasc Pharmacol.* 2018;16(2):143-156. doi:10.2174 /1570161115666170310092202

26. Viegas C, Araujo N, Marreiros C, et al. The interplay between mineral metabolism, vascular calcification and inflammation in chronic kidney disease (CKD): challenging old concepts with new facts. *Aging (Albany NY)*. 2019;11(12):4274-4299. doi:10.18632/aging.102046

27. Yamada S, Giachelli CM. Vascular calcification in CKD–MBD: roles for phosphate, FGF23, and klotho. *Bone*. 2017;100:87-93. doi:10.1016/j.bone.2016.11.012

28. Bover J, Urena P, Aguilar A, et al. Alkaline phosphatases in the complex chronic kidney disease-mineral and bone disorders. *Calcif Tissue Int*. 2018;103(2):111-124. doi:10.1007/s00223-018-0399-z

29. Ketteler M, Sprague SM, Covic AC, et al. Effects of sucroferric oxyhydroxide and sevelamer carbonate on chronic kidney disease–mineral bone disorder parameters in dialysis patients. *Nephrol Dial Transplant*. 2019;34(7):1163-1170. doi:10.1093/ndt/gfy127

30. Hou YC, Lu CL, Lu KC. Mineral bone disorders in chronic kidney disease. *Nephrology*. 2018;23(suppl 4):88-94. doi:10.1111/nep.13457

31. Da J, Xie X, Wolf M, et al. Serum phosphorus and progression of CKD and mortality: a meta-analysis of cohort studies. *Am J Kidney Dis*. 2015;66(2):258-265. doi:10.1053/j.ajkd.2015.01.009

32. Covic A, Kothawala P, Bernal M, et al. Systematic review of the evidence underlying the association between mineral metabolism disturbances and risk of all-cause mortality, cardiovascular mortality and cardiovascular events in chronic kidney disease. *Nephrol Dial Transplant*. 2009;24(5):1506-1523. doi:10.1093/ndt/gfn613

33. Kestenbaum B, Sampson JN, Rudser KD, et al. Serum phosphate levels and mortality risk among people with chronic kidney disease. *J Am Soc Nephrol*. 2005;16(2):520-528. doi:10.1681/Asn.2004070602

34. Schwarz S, Trivedi BK, Kalantar-Zadeh K, et al. Association of disorders in mineral metabolism with progression of chronic kidney disease. *Clin J Am Soc Nephrol*. 2006;1(4):825-831. doi:10.2215/CJN.02101205

35. Goodman WG, London G, Amann K, et al. Vascular calcification in chronic kidney disease. *Am J Kidney Dis*. 2004;43(3):572-579. doi:10.1053/j.ajkd.2003.12.005

36. Fatica RA, Dennis VW. Cardiovascular mortality in chronic renal failure: hyperphosphatemia, coronary calcification, and the role of phosphate binders. *Cleve Clin J Med*. 2002;69(suppl 3):S21-S27. doi:10.3949/ccjm.69.suppl_3.s21

37. Ganesh SK, Stack AG, Levin NW, et al. Association of elevated serum PO4, Ca × PO4 product, and parathyroid hormone with cardiac mortality risk in chronic hemodialysis patients. *J Am Soc Nephrol*. 2001;12(10):2131-2138.

38. Jono S, McKee MD, Murry CE, et al. Phosphate regulation of vascular smooth muscle cell calcification. *Circ Res*. 2000;87(7):E10-E17. doi:10.1161/01.res.87.7.e10

39. Tonelli M, Sacks F, Pfeffer M, et al. Relation between serum phosphate level and cardiovascular event rate in people with coronary disease. *Circulation*. 2005;112(17):2627-2633. doi:10.1161/Circulationaha.105.553198

40. Floege J. Phosphate binders in chronic kidney disease: an updated narrative review of recent data. *J Nephrol*. 2020;33(3):497-508. doi:10.1007/s40620-019-00689-w

41. Hamano T. Mineral and bone disorders in conventional hemodialysis: challenges and solutions. *Semin Dial*. 2018;31(6):592-598. doi:10.1111/sdi.12729

42. Vedvyas C, Winterfield LS, Vleugels RA. Calciphylaxis: a systematic review of existing and emerging therapies. *J Am Acad Dermatol*. 2012;67(6):e253-e260. doi:10.1016/j.jaad.2011.06.009

43. Massy Z, Drueke T. Adynamic bone disease is a predominant bone pattern in early stages of chronic kidney disease. *J Nephrol*. 2017;30(5):629-634. doi:10.1007/s40620-017-0397-7

44. McNerny EMB, Nickolas TL. Bone quality in chronic kidney disease: definitions and diagnostics. *Curr Osteoporos Rep*. 2017;15(3):207-213. doi:10.1007/s11914-017-0366-z

45. Eknoyan G, Levin A, Levin NW. KDOQI Clinical Practice Guidelines: bone metabolism and disease in chronic kidney disease. *Am J Kidney Dis*. 2003;42(suppl 3):1-201. doi:10.1016/S0272-6386(03)00905-3

46. Barreto FC, Barreto DV, Canziani ME, et al. Association between indoxyl sulfate and bone histomorphometry in pre-dialysis chronic kidney disease patients. *J Bras Nefrol*. 2014;36(3):289-296. doi:10.5935/0101-2800.20140042

47. Moe SM. Renal osteodystrophy or kidney-induced osteoporosis? *Curr Osteoporos Rep*. 2017;15(3):194-197. doi:10.1007/s11914-017-0364-1

48. Malluche HH, Mawad HW, Monier-Faugere MC. Renal osteodystrophy in the first decade of the new millennium: analysis of 630 bone biopsies in black and white patients. *J Bone Miner Res.* 2011;26(6):1368-1376. doi:10.1002/jbmr.309

49. Sprague SM, Bellorin-Font E, Jorgetti V, et al. Diagnostic accuracy of bone turnover markers and bone histology in patients with CKD treated by dialysis. *Am J Kidney Dis.* 2016;67(4):559-566. doi:10.1053/j.ajkd.2015.06.023

50. Evenepoel P, Behets GJS, Laurent MR, et al. Update on the role of bone biopsy in the management of patients with CKD–MBD. *J Nephrol.* 2017;30(5):645-652. doi:10.1007/s40620-017-0424-8

51. Tentori F, McCullough K, Kilpatrick RD, et al. High rates of death and hospitalization follow bone fracture among hemodialysis patients. *Kidney Int.* 2014;85(1):166-173. doi:10.1038/ki.2013.279

52. Daugirdas JT, Blake PG, Ing TS. *Handbook of Dialysis.* 5th ed. Wolters Kluwer Health, Inc; 2014.

53. Kidney Disease: Improving Global Outcomes (KDIGO) CKD–MBD Workgroup. KDIGO clinical practice guideline for the diagnosis, evaluation, prevention, and treatment of Chronic Kidney Disease–Mineral and Bone Disorder (CKD–MBD). *Kidney Int Suppl.* 2009;113:S1-S130. doi:10.1038/ki.2009.188

54. Miller PD. Diagnosis and treatment of osteoporosis in chronic renal disease. *Semin Nephrol.* 2009;29(2):144-155. doi:10.1016/j.semnephrol.2009.01.007

55. Kidney Disease: Improving Global Outcomes (KDIGO) CKD-MBD Workgroup. KDIGO 2017 clinical practice guideline update for the diagnosis, evaluation, prevention, and treatment of Chronic Kidney Disease–Mineral and Bone Disorder (CKD–MBD). *Kidney Int.* 2017;7(1):1-60.

56. Naylor KL, Garg AX, Zou G, et al. Comparison of fracture risk prediction among individuals with reduced and normal kidney function. *Clin J Am Soc Nephrol.* 2015;10(4):646-653. doi:10.2215/CJN.06040614

57. West SL, Lok CE, Langsetmo L, et al. Bone mineral density predicts fractures in chronic kidney disease. *J Bone Miner Res.* 2015;30(5):913-919. doi:10.1002/jbmr.2406

58. Ott SM. Renal osteodystrophy-time for common nomenclature. *Curr Osteoporos Rep.* 2017;15(3):187-193. doi:10.1007/s11914-017-0367-y

59. Reichel H, Esser A, Roth HJ, et al. Influence of PTH assay methodology on differential diagnosis of renal bone disease. *Nephrol Dial Transplant.* 2003;18(4):759-768. doi:10.1093/ndt/gfg144

60. Souberbielle JC, Boutten A, Carlier MC, et al. Inter-method variability in PTH measurement: implication for the care of CKD patients. *Kidney Int.* 2006;70(2):345-350. doi:10.1038/sj.ki.5001606

61. Ikizler TA, Burrowes JD, Byham-Gray LD, et al. KDOQI Nutrition in CKD Guideline Workgoup. KDOQI Clinical Practice Guidelines for nutrition in CKD: 2020. *Am J Kidney Dis.* 2020;76(3 suppl 1):S1-S107.

62. Hutchison AJ. Oral phosphate binders. *Kidney Int.* 2009;75(9):906-914. doi:10.1038/ki.2009.60

63. Sherman RA. Hyperphosphatemia in dialysis patients: beyond nonadherence to diet and binders. *Am J Kidney Dis.* 2016;67(2):182-186. doi:10.1053/j.ajkd.2015.07.035

64. Garneata L, Stancu A, Dragomir D, et al. Ketoanalogue-supplemented vegetarian very low-protein diet and CKD progression. *J Am Soc Nephrol.* 2016;27(7):2164-2176. doi:10.1681/ASN.2015040369

65. Lou LM, Caverni A, Gimeno JA, et al. Dietary intervention focused on phosphate intake in hemodialysis patients with hyperphosphatemia. *Clin Nephrol.* 2012;77(6):476-483.

66. Sullivan C, Sayre SS, Leon JB, et al. Effect of food additives on hyperphosphatemia among patients with end-stage renal disease a randomized controlled trial. *JAMA.* 2009;301(6):629-635. doi:10.1001/jama.2009.96

67. Noori N, Kalantar-Zadeh K, Kovesdy CP, et al. Association of dietary phosphorus intake and phosphorus to protein ratio with mortality in hemodialysis patients. *Clin J Am Soc Nephrol.* 2010;5(4):683-692. doi:10.2215/CJN.08601209

68. Lynch KE, Lynch R, Curhan GC, et al. Prescribed dietary phosphate restriction and survival among hemodialysis patients. *Clin J Am Soc Nephrol.* 2011;6(3):620-629. doi:10.2215/CJN.04620510

69. Kalantar-Zadeh K, Gutekunst L, Mehrotra R, et al. Understanding sources of dietary phosphorus in the treatment of patients with chronic kidney disease. *Clin J Am Soc Nephrol.* 2010;5(3):519-530. doi:10.2215/CJN.06080809

70. Leon JB, Sullivan CM, Sehgal AR. The prevalence of phosphorus-containing food additives in top-selling foods in grocery stores. *J Ren Nutr.* 2013;23(4):265-270. doi:10.1053/j.jrn.2012.12.003

71. Calvo MS, Uribarri J. Contributions to total phosphorus intake: all sources considered. *Semin Dial.* 2013;26(1):54-61. doi:10.1111/sdi.12042

72. Uribarri J, Calvo MS. Hidden sources of phosphorus in the typical american diet: does it matter in nephrology? *Semin Dial.* 2003;16(3):186-188. doi:10.1046/j.1525-139x2003.16037.x

73. Carrigan A, Klinger A, Choquette SS, et al. Contribution of food additives to sodium and phosphorus content of diets rich in processed foods. *J Ren Nutr.* 2014;24(1):13-19, 19e1. doi:10.1053/j.jrn.2013.09.003

74. Sherman RA, Mehta O. Dietary phosphorus restriction in dialysis patients: potential impact of processed meat, poultry, and fish products as protein sources. *Am J Kidney Dis.* 2009;54(1):18-23. doi:10.1053/j.ajkd.2009.01.269

75. Benini O, D'Alessandro C, Gianfaldoni D, et al. Extra-phosphate load from food additives in commonly eaten foods: a real and insidious danger for renal patients. *J Ren Nutr.* 2011;21(4):303-308. doi:10.1053/j.jrn.2010.06.021

76. Moser M, White K, Henry B, et al. Phosphorus content of popular beverages. *Am J Kidney Dis.* 2015;65(6):969-971. doi:10.1053/j.ajkd.2015.02.330

77. Karalis M, Murphy-Gutekunst L. Enhanced foods: hidden phosphorus and sodium in foods commonly eaten. *J Ren Nutr.* 2006;16(1):79-81. doi:10.1053/j.jrn.2005.11.001

78. Lindley E, Costelloe S, Bosomworth M, et al. Use of a standard urine assay for measuring the phosphate content of beverages. *J Ren Nutr.* 2014;24(6):353-356. doi:10.1053/j.jrn.2014.07.002

79. Gutierrez OM, Anderson C, Isakova T, et al. Low socioeconomic status associates with higher serum phosphate irrespective of race. *J Am Soc Nephrol.* 2010;21(11):1953-1960. doi:10.1681/ASN.2010020221

80. Sparks B. Is there room for more than white rice in the renal diet? A new look at ancient grains. *J Ren Nutr.* 2018;28(3):e15-e18. doi:10.1053/j.jrn.2018.02.002

81. Ando S, Sakuma M, Morimoto Y, et al. The effect of various boiling conditions on reduction of phosphorus and protein in meat. *J Ren Nutr.* 2015;25(6):504-509. doi:10.1053/j.jrn.2015.05.005

82. Cupisti A, Comar F, Benini O, et al. Effect of boiling on dietary phosphate and nitrogen intake. *J Ren Nutr.* 2006;16(1):36-40. doi:10.1053/j.jrn.2005.10.005

83. Moe S, Zidehsarai M, Chambers M, et al. Vegetarian compared with meat dietary protein source and phosphorus homeostasis in chronic kidney disease. *Clin J Am Soc Nephrol.* 2011;6(2):257-264. doi:10.2215/CJN.05040610

84. Sherman RA, Ravella S, Kapoian T. A dearth of data: the problem of phosphorus in prescription medications. *Kidney Int.* 2015;87(6):1097-1099. doi:10.1038/ki.2015.67

85. Gutekunst L. An update on phosphate binders: a dietitian's perspective. *J Ren Nutr.* 2016;26(4):209-218. doi:10.1053/j.jrn.2016.01.009

86. Ruospo M, Palmer SC, Natale P, et al. Phosphate binders for preventing and treating chronic kidney disease-mineral and bone disorder (CKD–MBD). *Cochrane Database Syst Rev.* 2018;8:CD006023. doi:10.1002/14651858.CD006023.pub3

87. Emmett M. A comparison of clinically useful phosphorus binders for patients with chronic kidney failure. *Kidney Int Suppl.* 2004;66(90):S25-S32. doi:10.1111/j.1523-1755.2004.09005.x

88. Goldsmith DJ, Covic A. Calcium and the saga of the binders: accumulating controversy, or building consensus? *Int Urol Nephrol.* 2008;40(4):1009-1014. doi:10.1007/s11255-008-9477-x

89. London GM, Marchais SJ, Guerin AP, et al. Association of bone activity, calcium load, aortic stiffness, and calcifications in ESRD. *J Am Soc Nephrol.* 2008;19(9):1827-1835. doi:10.1681/ASN.2007050622

90. Zhang Q, Li M, Lu Y, et al. Meta-analysis comparing sevelamer and calcium-based phosphate binders on cardiovascular calcification in hemodialysis patients. *Nephron Clin Pract.* 2010;115(4):c259-c267. doi:10.1159/000313484

91. Navaneethan SD, Palmer SC, Vecchio M, et al. Phosphate binders for preventing and treating bone disease in chronic kidney disease patients. *Cochrane Database Syst Rev.* 2011;2:CD006023. doi:10.1002/14651858.CD006023.pub2

92. Patel L, Bernard LM, Eler GJ. Sevelamer versus calcium-based binders for treatment of hyperphosphatemia in CKD: a meta-analysis of randomized controlled trials. *Clin J Am Soc Nephrol.* 2016;11(2):232-244. doi:10.2215/CJN.0680061

93. Daugirdas JT, Finn WF, Emmett M, et al. The phosphate binder equivalent dose. *Semin Dial.* 2011;24(1):41-49. doi:10.1111/j.1525-139X.2011.00849.x

94. Autissier V, Damment SJ, Henderson RA. Relative in vitro efficacy of the phosphate binders lanthanum carbonate and sevelamer hydrochloride. *J Pharm Sci.* 2007;96(10):2818-2827. doi:10.1002/jps.20956

95. Delmez J, Block G, Robertson J, et al. A randomized, double-blind, crossover design study of sevelamer hydrochloride and sevelamer carbonate in patients on hemodialysis. *Clin Nephrol.* 2007;68(6):386-391. doi:10.5414/cnp68386

96. Wilson R, Zhang P, Smyth M, et al. Assessment of survival in a 2-year comparative study of lanthanum carbonate versus standard therapy. *Curr Med Res Opin.* 2009;25(12):3021-3028. doi:10.1185/03007990903399398

97. Jamal SA, Vandermeer B, Raggi P, et al. Effect of calcium-based versus non-calcium-based phosphate binders on mortality in patients with chronic kidney disease: an updated systematic review and meta-analysis. *Lancet.* 2013;382(9900):1268-1277. doi:10.1016/S0140-6736(13)60897-1

98. Fresenius Medical Care. Velphoro prescribing information. Velphoro website. 2019. Accessed February 24, 2020. www.velphorohcp.com

99. Van Buren PN, Lewis JB, Dwyer JP, et al. The phosphate binder ferric citrate and mineral metabolism and inflammatory markers in maintenance dialysis patients: results from prespecified analyses of a randomized clinical trial. *Am J Kidney Dis.* 2015;66(3):479-488. doi:10.1053/j.ajkd.2015.03.013

100. Isakova T, Gutierrez OM, Chang Y, et al. Phosphorus binders and survival on hemodialysis. *J Am Soc Nephrol.* 2009;20(2):388-396. doi:10.1681/ASN.2008060609

101. Lopes AA, Tong L, Thumma J, et al. Phosphate binder use and mortality among hemodialysis patients in the dialysis outcomes and practice patterns study (DOPPS): evaluation of possible confounding by nutritional status. *Am J Kidney Dis.* 2012;60(1):90-101. doi:10.1053/j.ajkd.2011.12.025

102. Wolf M. HiLo Study. Accessed September 16, 2020. https://hilostudy.org

103. Block GA, Wheeler DC, Persky MS, et al. Effects of phosphate binders in moderate CKD. *J Am Soc Nephrol.* 2012;23(8):1407-1415. doi:10.1681/ASN.2012030223

104. Micromedex Solutions. Phosphate-binding agents comparative tables. December 2019. Accessed April 1, 2020. www.micromedexsolutions.com/micromedex2/librarian

105. Wagner CA. Coming out of the PiTs-novel strategies for controlling intestinal phosphate absorption in patients with CKD. *Kidney Int.* 2020;98(2):273-275. doi:10.1016/j.kint.2020.04.010

106. Ix JH, Ganjoo P, Tipping D, et al. Sustained hypophosphatemic effect of once-daily niacin/laropiprant in dyslipidemic CKD stage 3 patients. *Am J Kidney Dis.* 2011;57(6):963-965. doi:10.1053/j.ajkd.2011.03.010

107. Larsson TE, Kameoka C, Nakajo I, et al. NPT-IIb inhibition does not improve hyperphosphatemia in CKD. *Kidney Int Rep.* 2018;3(1):73-80. doi:10.1016/j.ekir.2017.08.003

108. Tsuboi Y, Ohtomo S, Ichida Y, et al. EOS789, a novel pan-phosphate transporter inhibitor, is effective for the treatment of chronic kidney disease–mineral bone disorder. *Kidney Int.* 2020;98(2):343-354. doi:10.1016/j.kint.2020.02.040

109. Hill Gallant KM, Stremke ER, Trevino L, et al. EOS789, a broad-spectrum inhibitor of phosphate transport, is safe with an indication of efficacy in a phase 1b randomized crossover trial in hemodialysis patients. *Kidney Int.* 2021;99(5):1225-1233. doi:10.1016/j.kint.2020.09.035

110. Block GA, Rosenbaum DP, Yan A, et al. Efficacy and safety of tenapanor in patients with hyperphosphatemia receiving maintenance hemodialysis: a randomized phase 3 trial. *J Am Soc Nephrol.* 2019;30(4):641-652. doi:10.1681/ASN.2018080832

111. St-Jules DE, Woolf K, Pompeii ML, et al. Exploring problems in following the hemodialysis diet and their relation to energy and nutrient intakes: the Balancewise Study. *J Ren Nutr.* 2016;26(2):118-124. doi:10.1053/j.jrn.2015.10.002

112. Karavetian M, de Vries N, Rizk R, et al. Dietary educational interventions for management of hyperphosphatemia in hemodialysis patients: a systematic review and meta-analysis. *Nutr Rev.* 2014;72(7):471-482. doi:10.1111/nure.12115

113. Joson CG, Henry SL, Kim S, et al. Patient-reported factors associated with poor phosphorus control in a maintenance hemodialysis population. *J Ren Nutr.* 2016;26(3):141-148. doi:10.1053/j.jrn.2015.09.004

114. Fissell RB, Karaboyas A, Bieber BA, et al. Phosphate binder pill burden, patient-reported non-adherence, and mineral bone disorder markers: findings from the DOPPS. *Hemodial Int.* 2016;20(1):38-49. doi:10.1111/hdi.12315

115. Loghman-Adham M. Medication noncompliance in patients with chronic disease: issues in dialysis and renal transplant. *Am J Manag Care.* 2003;9(2):155-171.

116. Kovac JA, Patel SS, Peterson RA, et al. Patient satisfaction with care and behavioral compliance in end-stage renal disease patients treated with hemodialysis. *Am J Kidney Dis.* 2002;39(6):1236-1244. doi:10.1053/ajkd.2002.33397

117. Viaene L, Meijers B, Vanrenterghem Y, et al. Daytime rhythm and treatment-related fluctuations of serum phosphorus concentration in dialysis patients. *Am J Nephrol.* 2012;35(3):242-248. doi:10.1159/000336308

118. Daugirdas JT. Removal of phosphorus by hemodialysis. *Semin Dial.* 2015;28(6):620-623. doi:10.1111/sdi.12439

119. Elias RM, Alvares VRC, Moyses RMA. Phosphate removal during conventional hemodialysis: a decades-old misconception. *Kidney Blood Press Res.* 2018;43(1):110-114. doi:10.1159/000487108

120. Bertocchio JP, Mohajer M, Gaha K, et al. Modifications to bicarbonate conductivity: a way to increase phosphate removal during hemodialysis? Proof of concept. *Hemodial Int.* 2016;20(4):601-609. doi:10.1111/hdi.12423

121. Gutzwiller JP, Schneditz D, Huber AR, et al. Increasing blood flow increases kt/V(urea) and potassium removal but fails to improve phosphate removal. *Clin Nephrol.* 2003;59(2):130-136. doi:10.5414/cnp59130

122. Svara F, Lopot F, Valkovsky I, et al. Phosphorus removal in low-flux hemodialysis, high-flux hemodialysis, and hemodiafiltration. *ASAIO J.* 2016;62(2):176-181. doi:10.1097/MAT.0000000000000313

123. Evenepoel P, Meijers BK, Bammens B, et al. Phosphorus metabolism in peritoneal dialysis- and haemodialysis-treated patients. *Nephrol Dial Transplant.* 2016;31(9):1508-1514. doi:10.1093/ndt/gfv414

124. Wang AY-M, Woo J, Sea MM-M, et al. Hyperphosphatemia in Chinese peritoneal dialysis patients with and without residual kidney function: what are the implications? *Am J Kidney Dis.* 2004;43(4):712-720. doi:10.1053/j.ajkd.2003.12.032

125. Zupančič T, Ponikvar R, Gubenšek J, et al. Phosphate removal during long nocturnal hemodialysis/hemodiafiltration: a study with total dialysate collection. *Ther Apher Dial.* 2016;20(3):267-271. doi:10.1111/1744-9987.12435

126. Daugirdas JT, Chertow GM, Larive B, et al. Effects of frequent hemodialysis on measures of CKD mineral and bone disorder. *J Am Soc Nephrol.* 2012;23(4):727-738. doi:10.1681/ASN.2011070688

127. Zisman AL, Hristova M, Ho LT, et al. Impact of ergocalciferol treatment of vitamin D deficiency on serum parathyroid hormone concentrations in chronic kidney disease. *Am J Nephrol.* 2007;27(1):36-43. doi:10.1159/000098561

128. Kumar R. New clinical trials with vitamin D and analogs in renal disease. *Kidney Int.* 2011;80(8):793-796. doi:10.1038/ki.2011.260

129. Gadallah MF, Arora N, Torres C, et al. Pulse oral versus pulse intraperitoneal calcitriol: a comparison of efficacy in the treatment of hyperparathyroidism and renal osteodystrophy in peritoneal dialysis patients. *Adv Perit Dial.* 2000;16:303-307.

130. Malluche HH, Mawad H, Koszewski NJ. Update on vitamin D and its newer analogues: actions and rationale for treatment in chronic renal failure. *Kidney Int.* 2002;62(2):367-374. doi:10.1046/j.1523-1755.2002.00450.x

131. Coburn JW, Maung HM, Elangovan L, et al. Doxercalciferol safely suppresses PTH levels in patients with secondary hyperparathyroidism associated with chronic kidney disease stages 3 and 4. *Am J Kidney Dis.* 2004;43(5):877-890. doi:10.1053/j.ajkd.2004.01.012

132. OPKO Renal. Rayaldee prescribing information. 2020. Rayaldee website. Accessed May 5, 2020. https://rayaldee.com

133. Nemeth EF, Heaton WH, Miller M, et al. Pharmacodynamics of the type II calcimimetic compound cinacalcet HCl. *J Pharmacol Exp Ther.* 2004;308(2):627-635. doi:10.1124/jpet.103.057273

134. Chonchol M, Locatelli F, Abboud HE, et al. A randomized, double-blind, placebo-controlled study to assess the efficacy and safety of cinacalcet HCl in participants with CKD not receiving dialysis. *Am J Kidney Dis.* 2009;53(2):197-207. doi:10.1053/j.ajkd.2008.09.021

135. Amgen. 2018. Sensipar website. Accessed January 20, 2020. www.sensipar.com

136. Raggi P, Chertow GM, Torres PU, et al. The ADVANCE study: a randomized study to evaluate the effects of cinacalcet plus low-dose vitamin D on vascular calcification in patients on hemodialysis. *Nephrol Dial Transplant.* 2011;26(4):1327-1339. doi:10.1093/ndt/gfq725

137. Amgen. Parsabiv prescribing information. Parsabiv website. 2018–2019. Accessed February 21, 2020. www.parsabiv.com

138. Rudser KD, de Boer IH, Dooley A, et al. Fracture risk after parathyroidectomy among chronic hemodialysis patients. *J Am Soc Nephrol.* 2007;18(8):2401-2407. doi:10.1681/Asn.2007010022

139. Dussol B, Morand P, Martinat C, et al. Influence of parathyroidectomy on mortality in hemodialysis patients: a prospective observational study. *Ren Fail.* 2007;29(5):579-586. doi:10.1080/08860220701392447

140. Ishani A, Liu J, Wetmore JB, et al. Clinical outcomes after parathyroidectomy in a nationwide cohort of patients on hemodialysis. *Clin J Am Soc Nephrol.* 2015;10(1):90-97. doi:10.2215/CJN.03520414

141. Chen J, Jia X, Kong X, et al. Total parathyroidectomy with autotransplantation versus subtotal parathyroidectomy for renal hyperparathyroidism: a systematic review and meta-analysis. *Nephrology (Carlton)*. 2017;22(5):388-396. doi:10.1111/nep.12801

142. Altman AM, Sprague SM. Mineral and bone disease in kidney transplant recipients. *Curr Osteoporos Rep*. 2018;16(6):703-711. doi:10.1007/s11914-018-0490-4

143. Wolf M, Weir MR, Kopyt N, et al. A prospective cohort study of mineral metabolism after kidney transplantation. *Transplantation*. 2016;100(1):184-193. doi:10.1097/TP.0000000000000823

144. Agrawal N, Josephson MA. Posttransplant bone disease. *Transplant Rev*. 2007;21(3):143-154.

CHAPTER 11

Cardiovascular Disease and Kidney Disease

D. Jodi Goldstein-Fuchs, DSc, CNN-NP, NP-C, RD, and Judith Beto, PhD, RDN, FAND

Introduction

Cardiovascular disease (CVD) is a major cause of morbidity and mortality in the population with chronic kidney disease (CKD). The prevalence of CVD in patients aged 66 years and older was reported to be 64.5% vs 32.4% for those individuals without CKD. CKD is recognized to be an independent risk factor for CVD; and death from CVD is greater than the occurrence of progression to end-stage kidney disease (ESKD) in this patient group. In the patient population with ESKD on kidney replacement therapy (KRT), CVD accounts for approximately 39% of all deaths.[1] Experts hypothesize that the factors responsible for this statistic are related to a panel of risk factors associated specifically with CKD that are in addition to the traditional and nontraditional factors for CVD. Traditional risk factors refer to the specific factors the Framingham Heart Study identified as resulting in an increased risk of CVD in the general population.[2,3] Nontraditional risk factors are additional risk parameters that continue to be identified since the Framingham Heart Study. Nonmodifiable risk factors are constitutional in nature and cannot be altered. These include race, age, gender, genetics, and ethnicity. Modifiable risk factors are those that can be influenced by lifestyle and management of disease. Box 11.1 on page 224 distinguishes between these four groups of risk factors for CVD.

Risk factors associated with both CKD and CVD are thought to account, in part, for similar traditional risk factors including diabetes mellitus (DM), dyslipidemia, family history, hypertension (HTN), left ventricular hypertrophy (LVH), physical inactivity, smoking, low serum high-density lipoprotein cholesterol (HDL-C), and advanced age.[1-5] In 2005, of 373,539 patients undergoing dialysis in the United States, 40% had both HTN and DM, increasing the risk of heart disease by fivefold to sixfold compared to patients without these conditions.[6] In addition to comorbidities, derangements in lipoprotein metabolism, anemia, vascular calcification (VC), and disorders of calcium and phosphate metabolism are thought to have a synergistic effect and contribute to the high prevalence of CVD in this patient population. Other nontraditional risk factors important in the pathophysiology of CVD for this patient population are inflammation and homocysteinemia (see Box 11.1).

Congestive heart failure (CHF) is an important cause of mortality risk in the patient population with CKD. In older patients receiving Medicare, adjusted survival probability was 77.8% vs 90.2% for Medicare patients without CKD.[1] Almost half of these patients had a diagnosis of atrial fibrillation (AF). Angiotensin-converting enzyme inhibitors and angiotensin receptor blockers are first-line therapy for heart failure, and the use of anticoagulants for AF is increasing in the patient population with CKD and CVD.[1] Management of hypervolemia in these patients is recognized as a critical factor and impacts medical nutrition therapy through therapeutic prescriptions for sodium and water.

BOX 11.1 | Categories of Risk Factors for Cardiovascular Disease

Traditional risk factors	Advanced age
	Diabetes mellitus
	Family history
	Hypercholesterolemia
	Low high-density lipoprotein
	High low-density lipoprotein
	Left ventricular hypertrophy
	Male gender
	Menopause
	Obesity
	Physical inactivity
	Smoking
Nontraditional risk factors	Abnormal mineral metabolism
	Albuminuria
	Anemia
	Autonomic imbalance
	Calcium–phosphorus imbalances
	Endothelial dysfunction
	Homocysteinemia
	Inflammation
	Malnutrition
	Oxidative stress
	Secondary hyperparathyroidism
	Vascular medial hyperplasia, sclerosis, and calcification
	Volume overload
Modifiable risk factors	Diabetes
	Diet
	Excessive alcohol
	High cholesterol
	Hypertension
	Obesity
	Sedentary lifestyle
	Smoking
Nonmodifiable risk factors	Family history
	Increasing age
	Male gender
	Menopause
	Race

The prevalence of CVD in the patient population with CKD is so significant that experts propose that CKD be regarded as a coronary disease risk.[1,7] In the general population, individuals with an estimated glomerular filtration rate (eGFR) of greater than 60 mL/min/1.73 m^2 have 21 cardiovascular events per 1,000 person-years. For individuals with CKD stages 1 through 3, the risk of cardiovascular events increases from 37 to 113 per 1,000 patient-years. This risk rate dramatically increases to 218 to 366 cardiovascular events per 1,000 person-years in CKD stages 4 and 5.[2,7,8] The predominant manifestations of cardiac disease in these patients are arrhythmia, cardiac ischemia, and heart failure. LVH is also highly prevalent and usually develops prior to CKD stage 5 as a result of multiple factors which often include HTN and volume overload.[2,9]

This chapter reviews the risk factors of CVD in persons with CKD that are recognized to have the potential to respond to nutrition and lifestyle interventions. Some of these interventions are often presented in the literature as therapeutic lifestyle changes (TLC). These components include maintaining a healthy body weight, exercising, avoiding smoking, and eating a healthy diet. Other kidney disease–specific components include the following: management of metabolic bone disease, anemia, and volume status. Therefore, nutrition intervention is aimed toward diet recommendations that facilitate the accomplishment of target range laboratory parameters. These parameters reflect each of these kidney disease components in addition to other recommendations for protein, carbohydrate, fat, electrolytes, and fluid (see Chapters 3, 5, 6, and 7).

Cardiac Pathology

Cardiac disease pathology and changes that occur in CKD are often described as those affecting the arteries (ie, blood vessels): arterial stiffness, endothelial dysfunction, increased wall thickness, and arterial calcification; and those affecting the heart: left ventricular dysfunction, valvular disease, dysrhythmia, myocardial fibrosis, and altered cardiac geometry.[9] Arteriosclerosis consists of three types of lesions: atherosclerosis, arteriosclerosis, and Mönckeberg medial calcific sclerosis. Arteriosclerosis is characterized by lipid-laden plaques within the intimal layer of the artery. Calcification, as a feature of arteriosclerosis, may or may not be present. Medial calcific sclerosis is defined by medial thickening, no atheroma, and heavy calcification.[9]

Arterial stiffening is a result of calcification and artery wall thickening. Carotid and aortic stiffness independently predict death in patients with CKD on hemodialysis (HD). The vascular endothelium maintains arterial tone mainly by production of nitric oxide. Nitric oxide protects blood vessels from developing arterial disease predominantly by inhibiting smooth muscle proliferation, monocyte adhesion, and platelet aggregation—all potential proinflammatory mechanisms of disease injury.

Endothelial dysfunction has been demonstrated in patients with CKD stages 4 and 5. Arterial calcification is a feature of both atherosclerosis and Mönckeberg sclerosis. The specific patterns of intima calcification found in these diseases are associated with alterations in bone metabolism resulting from abnormalities in phosphorus and calcium balance that are linked to this pathology. Calcification may also contribute to arterial stiffness.[2,9]

Cardiac muscle pathology includes an increase in LVH and/or left ventricular remodeling. These changes in cardiac muscle can lead to functional impairment that could include both diastolic and systolic dysfunction. Myocardial fibrosis and calcification as well as valvular calcification can be found in patients with CKD. Valvular disease is four times more common in patients on dialysis therapy than in matched controls and involves calcification of the aortic and/or mitral valves. This valvular calcification can accelerate aortic sclerosis and lead to an incompetent mitral valve. In terms of dysrhythmia, the majority of studies in CKD have been completed in patients on HD. Fluid and electrolyte shifts predispose these patients to dysrhythmias as do the autonomic neuropathy and reduced heart rate variability often found in this patient population. AF is very common in patients with CKD and can impair cardiac output in the presence of LVH. In the presence of CKD and AF, there is a higher risk of thromboembolic problems associated with this dysrhythmia.[9,10]

Dyslipidemia

Guidelines for the identification and the treatment of hyperlipidemia have been revised most recently by a Kidney Disease Improving Global Outcomes (KDIGO) work group.[11] Important changes pertain to the measurement of lipids and implementation of treatment. Experts now think that the main determinants of hyperlipidemia in the population with CKD are as follows: DM, degree of proteinuria, use of immunosuppressive agents, modality of KRT, eGFR, comorbidities, and nutritional status. This insight has altered the approach to the evaluation and management of hyperlipidemia. This shift has resulted in less emphasis on guiding therapy based on low-density lipoprotein cholesterol (LDL-C) levels to assessing the overall risk for CVD. Measurement of the lipid profile is recommended for the primary purpose of determining if the patient is presenting with hypercholesterolemia or hypertriglyceridemia and then ruling out secondary causes. Referral to a specialist is recommended if triglyceride levels are higher than 1,000 mg/dL (11.3 mmol/L) or if LDL-C levels exceed 190 mg/dL (4.9 mmol/L). The LDL-C is no longer recognized as a sole parameter for prescribing or modifying pharmacological treatment. Another new component of the KDIGO hyperlipidemia guidelines is that patients with CKD, including patients with ESKD receiving KRT, only require follow-up lipid profile measurements to assess cardiovascular risk in individuals who are aged 50 years or less and to evaluate adherence to statin therapy, changes in KRT, or suspicion of the development of secondary factors for dyslipidemia.[11] These KDIGO recommendations coincide with those of the 2018 Cholesterol Clinical Practice Guidelines published by the American College of Cardiology and American Heart Association Task Force (ACC/AHA).[12]

Traditionally, nutrition intervention for CVD has focused on the quantity of fat and avoidance of foods high in cholesterol and sources of saturated fatty acids.

While experts have maintained that it is important to limit fat to less than 25% to 30% of total energy intake and minimize cholesterol intake to less than 200 mg/d to 300 mg/d, the *type* of fatty acids ingested has been identified to have an important clinical effect on cardiovascular health.[12] The literature suggests a potential beneficial effect of omega-9 (olive oil) and particularly omega-3 (fish oil) fatty acids to reduce the risk of CVD.[3] Evidence-based recommendations to include omega-3 fatty acids in the diets of individuals with hypertriglyceridemia are still pertinent, as described by the Kidney Disease Outcomes Quality Initiative (KDOQI) and ACC/AHA guidelines.[3,12] Other than in hypertriglyceridemia, nutrition recommendations for cardiovascular risk reduction have now shifted to focus not just on one nutrient or substrate (eg, fat or carbohydrate) but to the dietary pattern of eating as a whole. While this philosophy is not new, evidence-based data with positive associations on risk reduction for CVD as well as CKD progression are a growing component of the CKD literature.[13] What many studies are demonstrating is that within each food component and food group, thoughtful food selection can potentially impact risk factors that contribute to the development of CVD. This approach is currently recommended by both the KDOQI and the ACC/AHA Guidelines.[3,12]

The 2013 KDIGO dyslipidemia guidelines include nutrition therapy for the treatment of hypertriglyceridemia with omega-3 fatty acids. The TLC of increasing physical activity, weight reduction, reducing alcohol intake, treating hyperglycemia when present, and dietary recommendations are specifically mentioned. The latter category specifies reducing total fat intake to less than 15% of total daily calories, reducing total carbohydrate, including reducing intake of monosaccharide and disaccharides, and in similarity to the KDOQI guidelines, recommends the use of fish oils (in individuals not malnourished).[11] These more recent recommendations by the KDIGO guidelines mirror those of the 2018 Guideline on the Management of Blood Cholesterol published by the ACC/AHA Task Force for severe hypertriglyceridemia defined as a triglyceride level 500 mg/dL or higher (≥5.7 mmol/L).[12]

The ACC and AHA have continued to include lifestyle therapies in their 2018 guidelines for management of hyperlipidemia. They are unchanged from the 2013 document and recommend a diet pattern that is rich in fruits, vegetables, and whole grains; allows lower fat versions of animal protein, specifically skinless chicken and fish/seafood; and includes nuts, legumes, and low-fat dairy products. Limiting red meat intake is recommended. In regard to fatty acids, nontropical vegetable oils are recommended, limiting both saturated and *trans* fats. Carbohydrate selection should steer away from refined sugars and sweets, including sweetened beverage products (ie, juices and sodas). Total calories are recommended to be individually adjusted for weight goals—be it weight loss, maintenance, or gain. At least 40 minutes of aerobic physical exercise is recommended three to four times per week at a moderate to intense level.[12] No specific guidelines for patients with CKD are found in these guidelines. However, risk factors for CKD are addressed within the nutrition guideline for metabolic syndrome, which is directed toward individuals with any three of the following five risk factors for atherosclerotic CVD[12]:

- elevated waist circumference
- elevated serum triglycerides
- elevated blood pressure
- elevated fasting glucose
- reduced HDL-C

Elevated blood pressure is a risk factor for patients with CKD. This section of the ACC/AHA guidelines emphasizes the importance of TLC for individuals with metabolic syndrome.[12]

Abnormal Mineral Metabolism

Abnormal mineral metabolism is characterized in the population with CKD by secondary hyperparathyroidism and resulting dysmetabolism of calcium and phosphorus, causing alterations in serum intact parathyroid hormone (iPTH), 1,25-dihydroxyvitamin D, 25-hydroxyvitamin D, phosphorus, and calcium levels.

This mineral bone disorder (MBD), in the population with CKD, is associated with LVH, CVD, death, VC, and bone disease.[14,15] Despite these associations, interventions for MBD to normalize vitamin D, calcium, phosphorus, and iPTH levels with 1,25-dehydroxy vitamin D analogs, calcimimetics, 25-hydroxyvitamin D supplements, phosphate binders, calcium supplements when indicated, and dietary modification of phosphorus and calcium intake have not been proven. This is due to a lack of prospective cohort and randomized clinical trials that demonstrate an impact on cardiovascular mortality or events.[14] This may also be due to newer evidence emerging pertaining to the variability of mineral metabolism markers by ancestry, gender, individual variation in phosphorus absorption, as well as genetic variants affecting all of these components. Genetic variants that influence gene activity for vitamin D metabolism, as well as calcium and phosphorus transport, are now being recognized as having a role in response to interventions and may further explain what clinicians currently label as noncompliance to phosphate binders. Approaches to management that are personalized based on these factors is an exciting newer area of CKD–MBD that has the potential to modify both the approach to and the outcomes of MBD and ascertain the impact on CVD outcomes.[16]

Altered mineral metabolism in CKD is a main risk factor for VC.[14] VC is the process of calcium deposition into the intimal layers and the medial of the vasculature. It is unclear whether there is an association between the location of calcium deposition and the resulting cardiovascular pathology.[17,18]

Calcium intake and control of serum phosphorus are critical elements influencing VC. Oral intake of large amounts (>1,000 mg/d) of calcium supplements for the purpose of dietary phosphate binding can contribute to the progression of vascular damage, particularly once calcium intake exceeds skeletal buffering capability. Control of serum phosphorus levels within the goal of 3.5 to 5.5 mg/dL is important. High serum phosphorus, in a climate of hypercalcemia from oral calcium intake and active vitamin D therapy, can exacerbate the accumulation of calcium in blood vessels and increase the risk

of morbidity and mortality.[17-19] Genetic polymorphisms have also been identified to have a role in impacting both the severity and the outcomes of cardiovascular calcification. Identification of these genetic polymorphisms has not been widely studied as of this date, but research is in progress. For example, a novel functional assay (ie, T50) measures the propensity of human blood toward calcification risk. Studies on T50 in patients receiving HD have been reported, but more research is needed to determine specificity and reliability.[14]

CHRONIC KIDNEY DISEASE–MINERAL BONE DISORDER, CARDIOVASCULAR RISK, AND MANAGEMENT

Block and colleauges [20] further confirmed the relationship between mineral imbalances and relative risk of cardiovascular mortality. Serum phosphorus concentrations from 5.0 mg/dL to 5.5 mg/dL and 5.5 mg/dL to 6.0 mg/dL were associated with significant increases in the relative risk of death: 1.10 mg/dL and 1.25 mg/dL, respectively. Strong relationships exist between elevated serum phosphorus, calcium phosphate product, parathyroid hormone (PTH), and cardiac causes of death in patients undergoing HD.[17-18,21]

Some data demonstrate that in varying doses, active vitamin D can promote atherosclerosis from plaque calcification in patients with kidney disease.[17,18,21] Hypercalcemia can contribute to soft-tissue calcification. Adynamic bone disease resulting from oversuppression of the parathyroid gland is another potential contributing factor for VC. A calcimimetic, which lowers PTH by binding to calcium-sensing receptors, is a viable adjunct therapy for managing secondary hyperparathyroidism. It is particularly advantageous for patients who exhibit hypercalcemia with active vitamin D therapy. Low-dose active vitamin D with calcimimetics (ie, dual therapy) is a viable option to consider in patients on KRT.[16,22]

Since these parameters have been found to be independently associated with increased morbidity and mortality, the National Kidney Foundation (NKF) KDOQI Bone Disease work group has established target goals for these parameters along with the KDIGO update in

2017 (see Chapter 10).[15] Additional commentaries discuss applications to clinical practice.[23,24] An important point raised in all of these CKD–MBD national and international publications is that the registered dietitian nutritionist (RDN) plays a key role in the successful management and outcomes of CKD–MBD.[15,16]

Hypertension

Reduction of blood pressure in individuals without CKD has been shown to reduce the risk for cardiovascular events. In patients with CKD, there is evidence in early stages of CKD (stages 1 through 3 and with serum creatinine in the 1.4 mg/dL range) that lowering blood pressure reduces the risk for stroke, cardiovascular death, and MI. In patients with CKD and later stages of disease, including those on HD, analyses of larger trials reported that lowering blood pressure reduced the incidence of cardiovascular deaths and events. Meta analyses of several large trials evaluating the effect of blood pressure reduction and specific antihypertensive agents on cardiovascular outcomes in patients with CKD found that blood pressure reduction lessened the prevalence of cardiovascular events and deaths in patients receiving HD compared to controls. A reduction of 4 to 5 mm Hg in mean systolic blood pressure values and 2 to 3 mm Hg in mean diastolic blood pressure values resulted in a 29% reduction in cardiovascular events and mortality in comparison with a control group.[9] This is similar to what has been observed in the general population. The optimal blood pressure goal is not known, and the most effective and safe agents to lower blood pressure and improve cardiovascular outcomes have also not yet been identified.

A previous blood pressure target was defined as accomplishing a blood pressure of less than 130/80 mm Hg for patients with CKD. The 2012 KDIGO Clinical Practice Guideline for Management of Blood Pressure in CKD identified a blood pressure target of less than 140/90 mm Hg for patients without proteinuria, and less than 130/80 mm Hg if proteinuria is greater than 3 mg/mmol.[25] These guidelines continue to be debated and modified to best accomplish cardiovascular health in the patient population with CKD.[26] Blood pressure lowering to ranges as described above are critical to the risk reduction of cardiovascular morbidities, and mortality including stroke, MI, and CHF in patients with CKD.

Nutrition recommendations to support these goals include the following: achievement and maintenance of a healthy body weight; lowering of sodium intake to less than 90 mmol (<2 g) per day or 5 g sodium chloride; unless contraindicated, participating in a regular exercise program focused on cardiac health, at least 30 minutes, 5 days per week; and limiting alcohol intake to one drink per day for women and up to two drinks per day for men (see Chapter 3).[27]

Homocysteinemia

Patients with ESKD have higher homocysteine (Hcy) levels compared with the general population.[27] Hyperhomocysteinemia has been linked to CVD in the general population as well as in the population on dialysis. Several studies have suggested that hyperhomocysteinemia is an independent risk factor for CVD; however, a causal relationship between the two factors has not been established. As kidney failure progresses, there is decreased metabolism of Hcy by the renal parenchyma. Furthermore, the cofactors involved in Hcy metabolism, such as folic acid, vitamins B6 (ie, pyridoxine), and B12 (ie, cobalamin), are low due to dialysis loss and overall decreased intake with dietary restrictions.[27]

Supplementation of folic acid, riboflavin, vitamin B12, and vitamin B6 has demonstrated a decrease in serum Hcy levels by as much as 30% to 50% and may also have cardioprotective effects.[27] Research has shown that folic acid supplementation of 5 to 10 mg/d may help decrease serum Hcy levels. However, there is no strong evidence to demonstrate that supplementing patients who have CKD with folic acid has any beneficial effect on lowering Hcy levels or impacting cardiovascular outcomes. This was the conclusion of the NKF KDOQI Clinical Practice Guidelines for Cardiovascular Disease in Dialysis Patients panel with no new evidence to support otherwise at this time.[3]

Inflammation

It is unclear whether inflammation is a maladaptive response to or a causative factor in the pathogenesis of CKD. Nonetheless, CKD is now characterized as a disease that is associated with the presence of a low-grade, chronic inflammatory mileu.[28,29] Increased markers of inflammation in patients with CKD were first reported in the 1990s when the inflammatory cytokine interleukin-1 was hypothesized to be the initiator of the major comorbid conditions in patients with CKD and a significant contributor to the high mortality rate of this patient group.[28] Multiple other markers of inflammation have since been identified, including C-reactive protein (CRP), interleukin-6, and tumor necrosis factor-α. The prevalence of inflammation has been reported to be in the range of 30% to 75%. This large range is due to multiple factors that can affect inflammation, such as dialysis therapy, residual kidney function, genetics, and criteria by which CRP identifies inflammation.[29] Malnutrition, muscle wasting, VC, CVD—all common comorbid conditions in patients with ESKD and contributors to mortality risk—are recognized to be associated with chronic inflammation. Systemic inflammation has been reported to worsen in patients with CKD when they start dialysis.[28-30] Hemodialysis itself confers a systemic inflammatory state through biomaterial activation of the complement system, resulting in thromboinflammatory changes during the HD process. Development of specific complement inhibitors and other specific site inflammatory mediators is an active area of research.[30] Malnutrition –inflammation scores have been developed to evaluate and monitor the presence of inflammation in association with malnutrition.[31] However, intervention, including diet therapy, for amelioration of this proinflammatory, aggressive systemic state has not yet been identified.

Kidney Transplantation and Cardiovascular Disease

A recent review by Rao and Coates[32] of CVD risk post–kidney transplant is highlighted in this section. The high risk of CVD is also present for individuals who receive a kidney transplant and continues to be a major cause for mortality. There is a higher incidence of CHF and a twofold higher risk of death.[1] The overall incidence is three to five times higher in the kidney transplant recipient than in the general population. Factors that contribute to this high incidence are CVD risk factors at baseline and comorbidities (eg, anemia, sodium and fluid retention, HTN, aortic stenosis, and arteriosclerosis). Immunosuppression therapy, infection, and systemic inflammation also play a role. Other risk factors for the development of CVD post transplant are DM, HTN, dyslipidemia, and presence of a functioning arteriovenous fistula. The latter factor is a risk for CVD due to the diversion by the fistula of a significant proportion of cardiac output required by the fistula to function. This results in increased cardiac stroke volume to maintain the increased cardiac output. This increased cardiac output may be contributing to the increased incidence of cardiovascular events characterizing the population with ESKD. Rao and Coates[32] demonstrated that fistula closure may be beneficial.

With regard to HTN and CVD risk post transplant, a study by Opelz and colleagues[33] found that kidney transplant recipients whose systolic blood pressure was greater than 140 mm Hg post transplant at 1 year—but reduced to less than or equal to 140 mm Hg by 3 years—had improved graft outcomes in the long term, compared with transplant recipients with blood pressures that continued to be in the greater or equal to 140 mm Hg systolic range. Dyslipidemia is common post transplant and is reported to be present in 71.3% of patients. Dyslipidemia has been reported to increase the risk of MI. Kidney transplant recipients are recommended to receive long-term management to control dyslipidemia with statin therapy.[11]

Immunosuppression therapy also has a role in the risk of CVD post–kidney transplant. It is challenging to change immunosuppressive agents post transplant due to the risk of developing donor-specific antibodies and subsequent graft rejection. Some transplant centers do make efforts to implement steroid withdrawal. One transplant group in Albany, NY, reported a significant CVD risk reduction over a 10-year period with this approach.[34]

Posttransplant DM, obesity, and the metabolic syndrome all contribute significant risks to the development of CVD. Posttransplant DM has been reported in up to 50% of cases in the United States post transplant. Some data suggests that patients who maintained normoglycemia during the immediate first 3 months post–kidney transplant were reported to be unlikely to develop DM. TLC are recommended to avoid and intervene for DM, obesity, and the metabolic syndrome.[34]

Treatment strategies for the prevention and management of posttransplant CVD include six lifestyle modifications:

- achieve a healthy body weight;
- increase exercise;
- encourage smoking cessation;
- highlight greater use of preemptive transplant (ie, living donors);
- achieve control of HTN and dyslipidemia, consideration for arteriovenous fistula closure, modification of immunosuppression therapy when able; and
- minimize use of steroids.

ANTICOAGULATION

There is a significant risk of stroke in the patient population with CKD, more than threefold higher in patients with CKD stage 5D, when compared to the general population. In addition, AF, which is a strong risk factor for stroke and mortality, is the most common arrhythmia in patients with CKD, and affects more than 7% of this patient population with nonvalvular AF. The use of anticoagulation therapy in CKD is a subject of debate since there is a significant risk of bleeding that is specific to CKD pathology.[9,10] Even aspirin has been reported to increase the risk of intracranial and extracranial bleeds.[9] While warfarin is the gold standard anticoagulant for nonvalvular AF, new oral agents

have emerged onto the CKD platform. More clinical trials are needed to best ascertain the risk:benefit ratio of implementing anticoagulation therapy in all stages of CKD.

The Registered Dietitian Nutritionist's Role in Managing Cardiovascular Disease

RDNs play a key role in preventing and treating cardiovascular risk factors for individuals with all stages of CKD. Nutrition-focused interventions with evidence-based data to support implementation include maintaining adequate energy and protein intake; management of calcium, phosphorus, and PTH; and evaluation/modification of lipid, sodium, and fluid intake. All interventions need to be individualized within these treatment strategies. RDNs can also play a role in anemia management, blood pressure control, glucose control for people with DM, and promotion of exercise and weight management. They may assist with encouraging patients to pursue smoking cessation. Patient education, when individualized appropriately, can be applied to this particular patient population to motivate healthier eating patterns in order to reduce CVD risk, regardless of the patient's CKD stage.

MAINTAINING ADEQUATE PROTEIN AND ENERGY INTAKE IN PATIENTS AT RISK FOR MALNUTRITION

The recommendations discussed in this section are reserved for patients with CKD who are well nourished, report a stable appetite, and are able to maintain an adequate nutritional status. Modification of cholesterol and fatty acid intake is not indicated for patients who are not nutritionally stable. Weight loss, albumin depletion, and reporting of poor appetite accompanied by abnormal laboratory values, such as a low phosphorus and potassium, are examples of several indicators that a patient is at risk for malnutrition. For these patients, the priority for the RDN is to guide and educate individuals on how to reverse this trend by maximizing oral dietary intake as best as possible. Utilization of oral supplements that provide complete nutrition and/or modular types are recommended as needed and within dietary modifications for electrolytes and fluid (see Chapter 18).

NUTRITION INTERVENTIONS FOR CALCIUM, PHOSPHORUS, AND PARATHYROID HORMONE

The RDN plays a large role in the management of helping patients with CKD to achieve and maintain target levels of calcium, phosphorus, and PTH to reduce cardiovascular risk, prevent VC, and lessen the development of bone disease (see Chapter 10).

NUTRITION INTERVENTIONS TO MODIFY DIETARY FAT INTAKE

The RDN can evaluate lipid intake by quantifying total fat intake in grams per day and percentage of calories. In addition, the patient's dietary intake should be evaluated for sources of saturated and polyunsaturated fats (ie, omega-3, omega-6, and omega-9 fatty acids). The RDN may advise patients of food products enriched in omega-3 and omega-6 fatty acids to facilitate the incorporation of these fats in their diet. Canola oil is an excellent source of both omega-3 and omega-9 fatty acids, and, as mentioned previously, olive oil is rich in omega-9 fatty acids. Either of these can be used in lieu of other vegetable oils. While studies have not shown the addition of fibric acid derivatives and nicotinic acid options to be overly effective, increasing dietary fiber and incorporating plant-based options can both play a role in modification to fat reduction.[11,12]

ANEMIA MANAGEMENT

Anemia in the patient population with CKD is due to functional iron deficiency, erythropoietin deficiency, and inflammation, among other factors.[9] It typically occurs in the later stages of CKD when GFR is significantly reduced. Anemia in this patient population is associated with LVH. Whether anemia is a cause of structural cardiac abnormalities is unclear as total or partial correction of anemia has not been shown to correct cardiovascular mass index with certainty. Large randomized trials have been completed to attempt to correct and identify anemia targets that are associated with improved cardiovascular outcomes.[35] These trials identified that higher levels of hemoglobin (≥13 g/dL) did not confer any advantage with regard to cardiovascular outcomes. These higher levels of hemoglobin resulted in excess risk for vascular access thrombosis and nonfatal MI; death, MI hospitalization for heart failure, and more cardiovascular end points were observed in subjects with CKD stage 3 or 4 participating in the Cardiovascular risk Reduction by Early Anemia Treatment with Epoetin Beta (CREATE) trial, by targeting a normal range hemoglobin of 13 to 15 g/dL vs 10.5 to 11.5 g/dL.[36] Current anemia targets include a hemoglobin of 10 to 12 g/dL.[35] Rapid changes in hemoglobin levels with erythropoietin-stimulating agents (ESA) can increase blood viscosity and HTN, both risk factors for CVD, and should be avoided. Based on these and other trials, ESAs have not been shown to reduce cardiovascular risk by correcting anemia.

The RDN can help patients achieve the hemoglobin goal by confirming adequacy of protein intake in patients and evaluating total iron intake. The RDN can also monitor the patient's response to ESAs as well as serum iron saturation and ferritin levels and communicate the results to team members responsible for dose adjustments (see Chapter 2).[27]

DIETARY ASPECTS OF HYPERTENSION MANAGEMENT

Sodium restriction is a mainstay of HTN management.[37] Recommendations depending on the stage of CKD and individual variation can range from less than 2,300 mg/d to a broader range of 2,000 to 3,000 mg/d.[37,38] The Dietary Approaches to Stop Hypertension (DASH) diet can be considered for patients in all stages of CKD with modification to the quantity of protein, potassium, and phosphorus content in the more advanced stages (see Chapters 3, 5, 6, and 7).[38,39] Other approaches include the traditional 2,000 mg/d sodium restriction, which focuses on minimizing foods with added sodium.

For the patient with CKD requiring fluid restriction due to cardiovascular, kidney, or other related comorbid conditions, the RDN needs to calculate urine output, adding 500 mL for insensible losses or more, as individually determined. Fluid management, when needed, and sodium restriction work together to maximize obtaining and maintaining goal blood pressure ranges.[40]

DIABETES MANAGEMENT

There have been many studies evaluating the risk of cardiovascular events with intensive glycemic control with conflicting results. Currently, experts recommended that to reduce the incidence of microvascular and macrovascular disease in individuals with DM, the hemoglobin A1c (HbA1c) goal should remain less than 7% to 8% and should be checked regularly.[41] Individuals who have been diagnosed with diabetes for less than 10 years may benefit from setting a goal of less than 6.5%, if severe hypoglycemia can be avoided.[41] The HbA1c target that is associated with the best clinical outcomes in CKD stage 5 is not known.[19] Multifactorial risk reduction includes smoking cessation, blood pressure control, regular intake of aspirin, reduction in serum lipids, and exercise. Nutrition intervention includes dietary patterns of eating similar to the lifestyle modifications discussed earlier in this chapter. Specific examples of how to maximize a healthier pattern of eating was recently published as part of a joint American Diabetes Association/American Society of Nephrology Expert Panel on DM and CKD.[42] In high-risk patients, such as those with CKD, an angiotensin-converting enzyme inhibitor is recommended for all patients with type 2 diabetes.[43] The RDN can educate patients with CKD on how to merge all these seemingly separate diet recommendations into one diet that incorporates CKD specifics, including electrolyte, mineral, fluid, carbohydrate, and protein recommendations (see Chapter 9).

WEIGHT MANAGEMENT

Unlike the general population without kidney disease, a survival advantage exists in patients with obesity requiring dialysis.[44] In the general population with normal kidney function, obesity is associated with increased CVD risk, and weight reduction is recommended. In the past, weight reduction was not recommended for patients undergoing dialysis unless they met the guidelines for obesity with a body mass index (BMI) of 30 or higher.[45] However, a recent study shows that waist-to-hip ratio (WHR), not BMI, is associated with cardiac events in the population with CKD. The study concluded that abdominal obesity is a high risk for all-cause and cardiovascular mortality in the population with ESKD.[44] Experts recommend that individuals with CKD stages 2 to 4 who are overweight and demonstrate a high WHR lose weight and maintain a healthy BMI. The RDN can individually develop a diet for weight loss incorporating the kidney diet–specific elements for patients with CKD stages 2 to 4. At a minimum, the overweight patient with CKD stage 5 receiving KRT should be encouraged to follow healthy eating guidelines and focus on avoiding further weight gain.

SMOKING CESSATION

Smoking contributes to CVD risk, but smoking cessation has not been shown to benefit cardiovascular outcomes in patients with CKD stage 5.[11] However, because the data regarding the hazards of smoking are so compelling, smoking cessation is recommended in all patients with CKD.[4,9] The RDN has an important role in assisting the patient to obtain and maintain healthy dietary habits while undergoing smoking cessation. Adherence to CKD dietary guidelines will continue to be needed. Appropriate snack foods and any new diet cravings or challenges that may present themselves while a patient is undergoing smoking cessation are best addressed by the experienced RDN.

EXERCISE

Decreased mortality has been associated with exercise for patients on dialysis and for patients in the general population. The exercise program should be approved by a physician to identify the limits beyond which exercise could impart stress to the patient. The current ACC/AHA guidelines recommend aerobic, moderate-to-vigorous intensity exercise in 40-minute sessions, three to four times per week.[12,46] The RDN can encourage and support patient involvement in an approved exercise regimen and evaluate diet intake for adequacy, particularly with regard to protein and energy intake. The RDN can also monitor musculature development by completing body composition measurements and monitoring waist circumference.

Summary

CVD prevention and risk reduction in relation to diet for the patient with CKD involves addressing an array of dietary- and kidney disease–specific factors (see Box 11.1). Dietary intake with regard to lipid, protein, energy, phosphorus, calcium, and sodium are all important. In addition, the patient's overall dietary intake pattern needs to be considered. Experts recommend that the pattern shift toward increased servings of fresh fruits and vegetables, low-fat dairy, limited red meat and lower fat proteins, inclusion of plant-based foods, and complex carbohydrates in lieu of simple sugars. This pattern of intake, when individualized appropriately, can be accomplished even with the later stages of CKD. Nutritional status needs to be defined and maintained in optimal condition. TLC, including exercise and smoking cessation, work together to help decrease risk. Intervention for secondary hyperparathyroidism, altered calcium and phosphorus metabolism, and anemia control also impact CVD outcomes. All of these interventions require continuous monitoring, reevaluation, education, and patient input. Experienced RDNs have the knowledge and consistent patient involvement to be able to recognize changes in patients and possible need for revision to the plan of care. The RDN can provide leadership with regard to communication of these concerns to the nephrology care team, modification of diet therapy, and the assurance of timely interventions by the clinical team.

References

1. United States Renal Data System. 2018 USRDS Annual Data Report: epidemiology of kidney disease in the United States. National Institutes of Health, National Institute of Diabetes and Digestive and Kidney Diseases website. 2018. Accessed April 20, 2020. http://usrds.org

2. Weiner D, Sarnak M. Cardiac function and cardiovascular disease in chronic kidney disease. In: Greenburg A, ed. *Primer on Kidney Diseases*. Elsevier; 2009:499-509.

3. National Kidney Foundation. K/DOQI clinical practice guidelines for cardiovascular disease in dialysis patients. *Am J Kidney Dis*. 2005;45(4 suppl 3):S1-S153. doi:10.1053/j.ajkd.2005.01.019

4. Longenecker JC, Coresh J, Powe NR, et al. Traditional cardiovascular disease risk factors in dialysis patients compared with the general population: the CHOICE study. *J Am Soc Nephrol*. 2002;13(7):1918-1927. doi:10.1097/01.asn.0000019641.41496.1e

5. Landray MJ, Thambyrajah J, McGlynn FJ, et al. Epidemiological evaluation of known and suspected cardiovascular risk factors in chronic renal impairment. *Am J Kidney Dis*. 2001;38(3):537-546. doi:10.1053/ajkd.2001.26850

6. Xue JL, Frazier ET, Herzog CA, Collins AJ. Association of heart disease with diabetes and hypertension in patients with ESRD. *Am J Kidney Dis*. 2005;45(2):316-323. doi:10.1053/j.ajkd.2004.10.013

7. Weiner DE, Krassilnikova M, Tighiouart H, Salem DN, Levey AS, Sarnak MJ. CKD classification based on estimated GFR over three years and subsequent cardiac and mortality outcomes: a cohort study. *BMC Nephrol*. 2009;10:26. doi:10.1186/1471-2369-10-26

8. Levey AS, Coresh J, Balk E, et al. National Kidney Foundation practice guidelines for chronic kidney disease: evaluation, classification, and stratification. *Ann Intern Med*. 2003;139(2):137-147. doi:10.7326/0003-4819-139-2-200307150-00013

9. Haynes R, Wheeler D, Landray M, Baigent C. Cardiovascular aspects of kidney disease. In: Skorecki K, Chertow G, Marsden P, Yu A, Taal M, eds. *The Kidney*. 10th ed. Elsevier; 2016:1854-1874.

10. Bansal VK, Herzog CA, Sarnak MJ, et al. Oral anticoagulants to prevent strokes in nonvalvular atrial fibrillation in patients with CKD stage 5D: an NKF–KDOQI controversies report. *Am J Kidney Dis.* 2017;70(6):859-868. doi:10.1053/j.ajkd.2017.08.003

11. Kidney Disease: Improving Global Outcomes (KDIGO) Lipid Work Group. KDIGO clinical practice guideline for lipid management in chronic kidney disease. *Kidney Int Suppl.* 2013;3:259-305.

12. Grundy S, Stone J, Bailey A, et al. 2018 AHA/ACC/ AACVPR/AAPA/ABC/ACPM/ADA/AGS/APhA/ASPC/ NLA/PCNA guideline on the management of blood cholesterol: a report of the American College of Cardiology/American Heart Association Task Force on Clinical Practice Guidelines. *J Am Coll Cardiol.* 2019;73(24):e285-e350. doi:10.1016/j.jacc.2018 .11.003

13. Goldstein-Fuchs DJ. What common practices in dialysis units can be altered to improve patient care? *Semin Dial.* 2004;17(1):19-21. doi:10.1111/j .1525-139X.2004.17109.x

14. Jovanovich A, Kendrick J. Personalized management of bone and mineral disorders and precision medicine in end-stage kidney disease. *Semin Nephrol.* 2018;38(4):397-409. doi:10.1016/j .semnephrol.2018.05.009

15. Kidney Disease: Improving Global Outcomes (KDIGO) CKD-MBD Update Work Group. KDIGO 2017 clinical practice guideline update for the diagnosis, evaluation, prevention and treatment of chronic kidney disease–mineral and bone disorder (CKD–MBD). *Kidney Int Suppl.* 2017;7(1):14. doi:10 .1016/j.kisu.2017.04.001

16. Beto J, Bhatt N, Gerbeling T, Patel C, Drayer D. Overview of the 2017 KDIGO CKD-MBD update: practice implications for adult hemodialysis patients. *J Ren Nutr.* 2019;29(1):2-15. doi:10.1053/j .jrn.2018.05.006

17. McCullough PA, Agarwal M, Agrawal V. Risks of coronary artery calcification in chronic kidney disease: do the same rules apply? *Nephrology.* 2009;14(4):428-436. doi:10.1111/j.1440-1797 .2009.01138.x

18. London GM, Guerin AP, Marchais SJ, Métivier F, Pannier B, Adda H. Arterial media calcification in end-stage renal disease: impact on all-cause and cardiovascular mortality. *Nephrol Dial Transplant.* 2003;18(9):1731-1740. doi:10.1093/ndt/gfg414

19. Chmielewski M, Carrero JJ, Nordfors L, Lindholm B, Stenvinkel P. Lipid disorders in chronic kidney disease: reverse epidemiology and therapeutic approach. *J Nephrol.* 2008;21(5):635-644.

20. Block GA, Klassen PS, Lazarus JM, Ofsthun N, Lowrie EG, Chertow GM. Mineral metabolism, mortality, and morbidity in maintenance hemodialysis. *J Am Soc Nephrol.* 2004;15(8):2208-2218. doi:10.1097/01.ASN.0000133041.27682.A2

21. McCullough PA, Sandberg KR, Dumler F, Yanez JE. Determinants of coronary vascular calcification in patients with chronic kidney disease and end-stage renal disease: a systematic review. *J Nephrol.* 2004;17(2):205-215.

22. Ketteler M, Martin KJ, Wolf M, et al. Paricalcitol versus cinacalcet plus low-dose vitamin D therapy for the treatment of secondary hyperparathyroidism in patients receiving haemodialysis: results of the IMPACT SHPT study. *Nephrol Dial Transplant.* 2012;27(8): 3270-3278. doi:10.1093/ndt/gfs018

23. Tanenbaum N, Quarles D. Bone disorders in chronic kidney disease. In: Greenburg A, ed. *Primer on Kidney Diseases.* Elsevier; 2009:487-497.

24. Isakova T, Nickolas TL, Denburg M, et al. KDOQI US Commentary on the 2017 KDIGO Clinical Guideline Update for the Diagnosis, Evaluation, Prevention and Treatment of Chronic Kidney Disease–Mineral and Bone Disorder (CKD–MBD). *Am J Kidney Dis.* 2017;70(6):737-751. doi:10.1053/j.akjd.2017.07.019

25. Kidney Disease: Improving Global Outcomes (KDIGO) blood pressure work group. KDIGO clinical practice guideline for the management of blood pressure in chronic kidney disease. *Kidney Int Suppl.* 2012;5(2):337-414. doi:10.1038/kisup.2012.46

26. Taler S, Agarwal R, Bakris G, et al. KDOQI US Commentary on the 2012 KDIGO Clinical Practice Guideline for Management of Blood Pressure in CKD. *Am J Kidney Dis.* 2013;62(2):201-213. doi:10 .1053/j.ajkd.2013.03.018

27. Perna A, De Santo N. Homocysteine. In: Kopple J, Massry S, eds. *Nutritional Management of Renal Disease.* 2nd ed. Lippincott Williams &Wilkins; 2004:117-124.

28. Mihai S, Codrici E, Popescu I, et al. Inflammation-related mechanisms in chronic kidney disease prediction, progression, and outcome. *J Immunol Res.* 2018;2018:1-16. doi:10.1155/2018/2180373

29. Avesani CM, Carrero JJ, Axelsson J, Qureshi AR, Lindholm B, Stenvinkel P. Inflammation and wasting in chronic kidney disease: partners in crime. *Kidney Int.* 2006;70(104):s8-s13. doi:10.1038/sj/ki.5001969

30. Kalantar-Zadeh K, Kopple JD, Block G, Humphreys MH. A malnutrition-inflammation score is correlated with morbidity and mortality in maintenance hemodialysis patients. *Am J Kidney Dis.* 2001;38(6):1251-1263. doi:10.1053/ajkd.2001 .29222

31. Mastellos D, Reis E, Biglarnia A, et al. Taming hemodialysis-induced inflammation: are complement C3 inhibitors a viable option? *Clin Immunol.* 2019;198:102-105. doi:10.1016/j.clim.2018.11.010

32. Rao N, Coates P. Cardiovascular disease after kidney transplant. *Semin Nephrol.* 2018;38(3):291-297. doi:10.1016/j.semnephrol.2018.02.008

33. Opelz G, Dohler B, Collaborative Transplant Study. Improved long-term outcomes after kidney transplantation associated with blood pressure control. *Am J Transplant.* 2005;5(11):2725-2731. doi:10.1111/j.1600-6143.2005.01093.x

34. Lopez-Soler RI, Chan R, Martinolich J, et al. Early steroid withdrawal results in improved patient and graft survival and lower risk of post-transplant cardiovascular risk profiles: a single-center 10-year experience. *Clin Transplant.* 2017;31(2):e12878. doi:10.1111/ctr.12878

35. Kidney Disease Improving Global Outcomes (KDIGO) Anemia Work Group. KDIGO clinical practice guidelines for anemia for chronic kidney disease. *Kidney Int Suppl.* 2012;2:279-335.

36. Drueke TB, Locatelli F, Clyne N, et al. Normalization of hemoglobin level in patients with chronic kidney disease and anemia. *N Engl J Med.* 2006;355(20):2071-2084. doi:10.1056/NEJMoa062276

37. Vennegoor M. Salt restriction and practical aspects to improve compliance. *J Ren Nutr.* 2009;19(1):63-68. doi:10.1053/j.jrn.2008.10.019

38. Appel LJ, Moore TJ, Obarzanek E, et al. A clinical trial of the effects of dietary patterns on blood pressure. *N Engl J Med.* 1997;336(16):1117-1124. doi:10.1056/NEJM199704173361601

39. Sacks FM, Obarzanek E, Windhauser MM, et al. Rationale and design of the Dietary Approaches to Stop Hypertension trial (DASH). A multicenter controlled-feeding study of dietary patterns to lower blood pressure. *Ann Epidemiol.* 1995;5(2):108-118. doi:10.1016/1047-2797(94)00055-x

40. Smith K, Coston M, Glock K, et al. Patient perspectives on fluid management in chronic hemodialysis. *J Ren Nutr.* 2010;20(5):334-341. doi:10.1053/j.jrn.2009.09.001

41. National Kidney Foundation. KDOQI Clinical Practice Guidelines and clinical recommendations for diabetes and chronic kidney disease. *Am J Kidney Dis.* 2007;49(2 suppl 2):S62-S73. doi:10.1053/j.ajkd.2006.12.005

42. Tuttle KR, Bakris GL, Bilous RW, et al. Diabetic kidney disease: a report from an ADA consensus conference. *Diabetes Care.* 2014;37(10):2864-2883. doi:10.2337/dc14-1296

43. Brown A, Reynolds LR, Bruemmer D. Intensive glycemic control and cardiovascular disease: an update. *Nat Rev Cardiol.* 2010;7(7):369-375. doi:10.1038/nrcardio.2010.35

44. Postorino M, Marino C, Tripepi G, Zoccali C, CREDIT Working Group. Abdominal obesity and all-cause and cardiovascular mortality in end-stage renal disease. *J Am Coll Cardiol.* 2009;53(15):1265-1272. doi:10.1016/j.jacc.2008.12.040

45. Elsayed EF, Tighiouart H, Weiner D, et al. Waist-hip-ratio and body mass index as risk factors for cardiovascular events in CKD. *Am J Kidney Dis.* 2008;52(1):49-57. doi:10.1053/j.ajkd.2008.04.002

46. Lobelo F, Young DR, Sallis R, et al. Routine assessment and promotion of physical activity in healthcare settings: a scientific statement from the American Heart Association. *Circulation.* 2018;137(18):e495-e522. doi:10.1161/CIR.0000000000000559

CHAPTER 12

Pregnancy and Chronic Kidney Disease

Jean Stover, RD, LDN

Many reports exist which describe pregnancy and kidney outcomes in women with chronic kidney disease (CKD), but the comparison of these outcomes is limited by small sample size, restricted clinical data, and a variety of other limiting factors. Pregnancy in women with known CKD, those receiving dialysis, or even those with a functional kidney transplant pose a challenging clinical approach relative to higher maternal–fetal morbidity.[1] Two large retrospective studies reporting pregnancy outcomes for 778 American women with CKD have shown that compared to low-risk healthy controls, these women have greater maternal risk for preeclampsia, cesarean section, and an increased fetal risk for preterm birth, poor growth, low birth weight, and neonatal intensive care admission.[1,2] With improvements in the care of women with CKD who become pregnant, there is now cautious optimism for this population.[1] Informed decisions between the patient and her clinicians is extremely important. A multidisciplinary approach must be present, including all specialists in patient comorbidities, such as diabetes, hypertension (HTN), and immunologic diseases.[1,3]

Compared to women with normal kidney function, the rate of women undergoing dialysis who will complete a full-term pregnancy and give birth is still about 1:100.[3] Fertility usually returns for women with well-functioning kidney transplants, but immunosuppressive drug therapy, especially cyclosporine, has been known to result in babies who are small for gestational age. These medications have not been associated with an increase in congenital anomalies, except for mycophenolate mofetil, which is now thought to be teratogenic.[4] All women with CKD, even after transplantation, are at risk for premature births.[4]

Given the circumstances and risk, care for a woman with CKD who becomes pregnant presents many challenges to the health care team, as substantive research regarding the specialized medical and nutrition needs for this unique patient population is lacking. Thus, the nephrology and high-risk obstetrics health care teams in addition to the previously mentioned specialists dependent on comorbidities must work together to monitor closely the patient's clinical parameters to increase the likelihood of successful maternal and fetal outcomes. Adequate nutrition, including vitamin and mineral therapy, is particularly important during pregnancy to promote a positive outcome for the mother and baby. Also, for patients receiving dialysis, the amount of treatment time must be increased during pregnancy to more closely assimilate the function of normal kidneys during fetal development. Since the 1990s, successful birth rates have increased to 70% to 90% with more intense dialysis.[1]

Medical Considerations

Individuals in the later stages of CKD and those undergoing dialysis usually require a pelvic ultrasound, in addition to the serum measurement of the β subunit of human chorionic gonadotropin (hCG) that is commonly done to confirm pregnancy. This is due to the healthy kidney normally excreting small amounts of hCG produced by somatic cells; thus, in kidney failure, this test can appear positive by normal standards.[1]

Once pregnancy is confirmed, medications prescribed for these women may need modification. Control of HTN before and during pregnancy even in patients without CKD is of significant importance. One meta-analysis of nearly 800,000 hypertensive pregnant women without CKD has shown marked increases in preeclampsia, preterm birth, cesarean section, intensive care admissions, and perinatal death. Although research is lacking on a common consensus for blood pressure (BP) targets and treatment-related modification for those with CKD who are hypertensive during pregnancy, the National Institute for Health and Care Excellence guidelines do recommend maintaining BP measurements of less than 140/90 mm Hg in women with CKD.[1] Some antihypertensive medications which are still considered acceptable for this population include α-methyldopa, labetalol, and nifedipine. The groups of antihypertensives that are contraindicated during pregnancy include both angiotensin-converting enzyme (ACE) inhibitors and angiotensin receptor blockers (ARBs). These types of medications have been associated with oligohydraminos, dysplastic kidneys, restricted intrauterine growth, and even fetal death. Recent studies suggest that these anomalies may be related to HTN and other comorbidities, and not specifically to ACE inhibitors. Since there is a benefit of ARBs reducing proteinuria, continuing these medications until pregnancy is confirmed may be acceptable in women with proteinuria.[1]

Anemia becomes worse during pregnancy due to increased plasma volume without an increase in red blood cell (RBC) mass. Erythropoiesis usually increases in the first trimester for women without kidney disease to provide the needed increase in RBC mass, but this process is limited or absent for individuals with CKD.[5] Generally, goals have been set to keep the hemoglobin levels in the range defined for nonpregnant individuals with CKD. Erythropoietin-stimulating agents (ESAs) are generally required and doses are increased, as needed, to achieve or maintain hemoglobin levels within the goal range. Epoetin α has commonly been given to pregnant women on dialysis, and this medication has not been associated with congenital anomalies in infants.[6] Studies have reported that darbepoetin α has been given successfully to pregnant women with CKD prior to dialysis, while undergoing dialysis, and after kidney transplantation.[7,8]

Although parathyroid hormone (PTH) may be elevated for the pregnant patient receiving dialysis, cinacalcet is not recommended due to the lack of information regarding its use during pregnancy and is labeled a category C drug accordingly. This medication should only be used during pregnancy if its benefits outweigh its risks. Etelcalcetide is also not generally given for the same reason but has not been assigned a category for pregnancy.[9] Vitamin D analogs, however, have been given to pregnant patients without documented adverse effects (see Box 12.1 on page 238).

Dialysis Regimen

Studies have shown that the best outcomes of pregnancy for women undergoing hemodialysis (HD) occur with dialysis times of 24 hours or more per week, with residual kidney function taken into account.[1,10] Women undergoing this therapy must understand that an increased time commitment to dialysis is recommended during pregnancy. In small retrospective observations from Canada, nocturnal home hemodialysis (HHD) seems to promote fertility and allows a greater gestation period with much better fetal outcomes. These patients increased dialysis times from an average of 36 hours per week to 48 hours per week during pregnancy.[10] This seems to be an ideal dialysis therapy for women contemplating pregnancy.

There are some case reports of pregnancy in individuals with CKD undergoing peritoneal dialysis (PD) and continuing this mode of therapy until delivery. Conception seems to occur less frequently in women

BOX 12.1 | Suggested Management Guidelines for Pregnancy and Chronic Kidney Disease[6,10,12-20]

MEDICAL NUTRITION THERAPY

Energy[a]	Approximately 25 to 35 kcal/kg + 300 kcal/d (2nd and 3rd trimesters)	
Protein[a]	Chronic kidney disease stages 3 through 5:	(0.55 to 0.6 g/kg) + (10 to 25 g/d)
	Hemodialysis/peritoneal dialysis:	(1.0 to 1.2 g/kg) + (10 to 25 g/d)
Sodium, potassium, phosphorus, and fluid	Chronic kidney disease:	Sodium restriction 2 to 3 g/d, as needed, based on blood pressure/fluid status; potassium/phosphorus restrictions, as needed, based on serum levels
	Hemodialysis/peritoneal dialysis:	Potentially liberalize intake of potassium, phosphorus, sodium, and fluid with more intensive dialysis
Multivitamin supplements	Chronic kidney disease stages 1 through 3:	Prenatal
	Chronic kidney disease stages 4 and 5:	Renal vitamin or prenatal
	Hemodialysis/peritoneal dialysis:	Renal vitamin and total daily intake of 2 to 4 mg folic acid
Vitamin D	Chronic kidney disease:	Vitamin D2 or vitamin D3, if deficient
	Hemodialysis/peritoneal dialysis:	Vitamin D analogs have been given intravenously to some pregnant patients on dialysis; no documented adverse effects on fetal outcomes have been reported

Other nutrients

Zinc	Chronic kidney disease:	11 mg/d
	Hemodialysis/peritoneal dialysis:	15 mg/d
Calcium	Chronic kidney disease stages 3 and 4:	Approximately 800 to 1,000 mg/d
	Hemodialysis/peritoneal dialysis:	Supplement as needed to keep serum calcium/phosphorus levels within normal limits
Iron	Chronic kidney disease:	30 mg/d
	Hemodialysis/peritoneal dialysis:	Intravenous iron may be given as iron sucrose without noted complications to maintain serum ferritin and transferrin saturation within goals for patients on dialysis; some physicians prefer oral iron alone or included in vitamin preparations

MEDICATIONS

Epoetin α may be given to maintain hemoglobin within normal limits for nonpregnant patients with chronic kidney disease; monitor hemoglobin weekly. Darbopoetin α has also been given.

Antihypertensives: Needed if patient is euvolemic but blood pressure is at or above 140/90 mm Hg; α-methyldopa, labetalol, and calcium channel blockers are acceptable. Avoid angiotensin-converting enzyme (ACE) inhibitors and angiotensin receptor blockers (ARBs).

DIALYSIS REGIMEN

Dialysis 24 h/wk or more seems to provide the best outcomes. Frequent dialysis is also recommended to avoid hypertension or hypotension with less fluid weight gain and more gentle fluid removal.

A 2.5-mEq/L calcium dialysate should be adequate, especially if providing frequent dialysis and oral calcium preparations; monitor calcium and phosphorus levels.

May need a 3-mEq/L potassium dialysate due to increased frequency of dialysis.

May need a lower bicarbonate dialysate due to frequency of dialysis; monitor serum bicarbonate levels.

Suggest that calcium, phosphorus, potassium, and bicarbonate levels be monitored weekly.

[a] Weight based on pregravida weight.

undergoing PD than in those receiving HD.[1,10] It is also quite difficult to manipulate PD exchanges to achieve adequate dialysis and also prevent extreme abdominal discomfort as the pregnancy progresses. Chang and colleagues[11] reported in 2002 that using tidal PD with a cycling machine could improve both dialysis clearance and abdominal symptoms during pregnancy in patients with CKD. Some patients may be encouraged to change to in-center HD during pregnancy if PD becomes too uncomfortable.

Although the fetus requires adequate calcium for proper skeletal development, especially in the third trimester of pregnancy, it is usually unnecessary to increase the dialysate calcium content when calcium-containing medications are taken and more frequent dialysis is given. Generally, a dialysate containing 2.5 mEq/L is acceptable (in the United States). There is also some production of calcitriol by the placenta, which makes it important to frequently monitor serum calcium levels to avoid hypercalcemia.[12,13]

Also, due to increased dialysis time and frequency, a dialysate with a higher potassium concentration (3 mEq/L in the United States) may be required to prevent hypokalemia despite liberalization of the dietary potassium content.[12,13] The bicarbonate concentration of the dialysate may also need to be decreased. With more frequent dialysis, nausea, and vomiting during pregnancy, the possibility of developing metabolic alkalosis exists.[12] Serum bicarbonate levels should be monitored accordingly. See Box 12.1 for a summary of dialysis regimen recommendations.

Nutritional Management

PROTEIN AND ENERGY

In addition to the literature on calorie and protein requirements for pregnant women with CKD, it is helpful to use the National Kidney Foundation Kidney Disease Outcomes Quality Initiative (KDOQI) guidelines combined with the Dietary Reference Intakes for the general population during pregnancy. Generally,

25 to 35 kcal/kg pregravida body weight per day are prescribed in the first trimester, and an average of at least 300 kcal/d is added to this value for the second and third trimesters during all stages of CKD and after kidney transplantation. Protein needs of approximately 0.8 g/kg/d for CKD stages 1 and 2 are thought to be reasonable (although data are inconclusive), and this value plus 10 to 25 g/d for pregnancy seems feasible.[15] For CKD stages 3 through 5 without dialysis, a lower protein intake of 0.55 to 0.6 g/kg plus 10 to 25 g/d may be advised, but it would be difficult to meet energy needs with this restriction.[16] Most likely a woman who becomes pregnant in these stages would need dialysis at some point during the pregnancy.

Protein needs for pregnant women undergoing HD and PD are generally at least 1.0 to 1.2 g/kg/d, plus at least 10 to 25 g/d, with the higher end of this range with more frequent dialysis prescribed during pregnancy.[15-18] It may be easier to meet these needs for the pregnant patient undergoing dialysis, as the diet can frequently be liberalized for sodium, potassium, and phosphorus content due to increased solute removal with more intensive dialysis. The mother may require protein or calorie/protein supplements to attain her estimated energy and protein requirements. Medical experts and practitioners know that the expected decrease in serum albumin during the course of pregnancy, however, is at least 1 g/dL, even in women without CKD.[18]

VITAMINS

A standard prenatal vitamin is generally given to women in the early stages of CKD and after kidney transplantation.[14] Historically, standard renal multivitamin doses have been doubled for women undergoing dialysis because of increased requirements for water-soluble vitamins during pregnancy, as well as increased losses anticipated with more intensive dialysis. Because folate deficiency has been linked to neural tube defects in infants born to women without CKD, ensuring at least 2 mg of folic acid per day for pregnant women undergoing dialysis has been encouraged.[17] Even 3 to 4 mg folic acid daily has been recommended due to more intensive dialysis.[13] Some of the renal vitamins with greater than 1 mg folate may be appropriate for this population.

Vitamin D analogs have been given intravenously during dialysis to pregnant women needing suppression of PTH and to maintain normal serum levels of calcium. No definitive information is available about whether these forms of vitamin D cross the placental barrier and, if so, whether they are safe relative to fetal development.[19-21]

However, the potential impact of vitamin D deficiency during pregnancy, combined with the inability of the diseased kidney to activate vitamin D, may be reason enough to use small doses of vitamin D analogs for pregnant patients receiving dialysis.[22,23] The use of supplemental 25 hydroxyvitamin D is also a consideration, as it does cross the placental barrier and may be utilized by the fetus.[22,23]

MINERALS

For CKD stages 3 to 4, it has been recommended that a daily intake of at least 800 to 1,000 mg calcium be provided.[15] For patients undergoing dialysis, calcium-containing phosphate binders are generally used, but a binder may not be required due to increased phosphate removal with more frequent dialysis. Sometimes, the phosphorus is less than goal range, and then calcium supplements in the form of calcium carbonate are given between meals, and phosphate supplements are prescribed, if needed. Calcium levels should be kept within normal range for nonpregnant patients undergoing dialysis. This is usually achieved easily for patients undergoing frequent HD with a 2.5 mEq/L dialysate content (see dialysis recommendations).

Also, zinc supplementation is prescribed in an effort to prevent increased risks of fetal malformation, preterm delivery, low birth weight, and pregnancy-induced HTN. The latter three factors are known to be risks for pregnant women with CKD. The recommended zinc supplementation for women with kidney disease during pregnancy is at least 11 mg/d for CKD not on dialysis and 15 mg/d for women undergoing dialysis.[13,18]

At least 30 mg/d of iron is recommended during pregnancy, so women with CKD who are not receiving dialysis could receive this as an oral preparation.[18] Intravenous (IV) iron sucrose has been administered effectively to pregnant women undergoing dialysis without noted adverse effects.[20] Ferric gluconate has been labeled category B in pregnancy, which means that experimental studies have not shown harm with this drug during pregnancy and no adequate human studies have been performed.[13,18] As anemia worsens during pregnancy, IV iron is usually required in addition to ESAs to stimulate RBC production. IV iron is given to maintain iron levels within normal ranges for nonpregnant patients undergoing dialysis, and either oral or IV iron is given to those with CKD not yet on dialysis.

See Box 12.1 for a summary of nutritional management recommendations.

WEIGHT GAIN

One of the most difficult evaluations during pregnancy for women with CKD, especially those undergoing dialysis, is solid weight gain. This is because fluid retention is a factor in the later stages of CKD. Only approximately 1.6 kg weight gain normally occurs in the first trimester, and the literature suggests that in the second and third trimesters, the recommended weight gain is 0.3 to 0.5 kg/wk.[12] This is naturally dependent on energy and protein intake and volume status, and it must be evaluated based on a team approach. Ongoing consultations with dialysis technicians, nurses, the registered dietitian nutritionist (RDN), and physicians are helpful when making target weight determinations.

Breastfeeding

This issue is frequently questioned, especially for women undergoing dialysis. There is not much in the literature regarding the safety or efficacy of breastfeeding an infant born to a mother with CKD. Most women who plan to breastfeed decide not to after the infant is born because the pregnancy has been so difficult. The theoretical question is always whether the content of the breast milk will be high in urea for those in later stages of CKD and those back on their regular schedule of dialysis. High urea concentration could cause diuresis in the infant that must be supplemented with extra water.

Also, patients with transplant have generally been advised against breastfeeding due to the antirejection medications they are taking. However, the benefits of breastfeeding preterm infants in this population may be greater than the theoretical risks of adverse effects. Therefore, options should be discussed with the mother prior to delivery.

Data is limited for the safety of many immunosuppressants, while glucocorticoids and azathioprine are considered relatively safe. Data also now suggest that there is minimal fetal exposure via breast milk to tacrolimus and cyclosporine.[1] There are databases available as references for safe medications during breastfeeding; one recommended resource is Lactmed (from the National Institutes of Health).[24] Counseling practices do differ among transplant centers, however.

Antihypertensive medications believed to be safe for women with CKD during pregnancy are still appropriate during breastfeeding, in addition to some ACE inhibitors.[1]

Summary

Although kidney transplantation seems to be the best treatment modality for women with CKD who want to have children, there are still increased risks of maternal and fetal morbidity during pregnancy.[13,25] The collaboration between the kidney transplant and high-risk obstetrics health care teams in prenatal management continues to be very important to promote successful outcomes. Women with well-functioning kidney transplants (acceptable creatinine level and other criteria are determined by the transplant center) should follow the same nutrition recommendations as for women without CKD.[18]

In summary, women with CKD who become pregnant are considered high risk whether they are in the early stages of the disease, undergoing dialysis, or post–kidney transplant. Close monitoring by nephrology, high-risk obstetric, and other medical specialty teams, if needed, is very important to achieve positive outcomes, especially in the later stages of CKD and for women undergoing dialysis.

Case Study

The following case study is a general overview of the course of a patient who became pregnant while undergoing HHD. The information is from reviewing summarized notes and data provided by a colleague who followed this patient, access to electronic data, as well as the patient herself. The patient has given consent for this information to be presented in this publication, although fictitious first and last initials are used.

In July of 2015, E.M., a 35-year-old female who had been undergoing HHD, reported that she was pregnant. This was confirmed by pelvic ultrasound that showed she was 9 weeks gestation in the middle of August 2015.

Her height is 67 inches and her target weight (TW) was stated as 74.5 kg in July 2015. Her medical history includes CKD due to focal segmental glomerulosclerosis and HTN. She underwent in-center HD for 6 weeks prior to receiving a living related kidney transplant in 2004. In December 2010, she needed to return to in-center HD when the kidney transplant failed.

In July 2012, E.M. began training for HHD and remained on this modality until 2015. She did undergo a partial parathyroidectomy in June 2014 (PTH 2,316 pg/mL in May 2014). When reported to be pregnant in July 2015, she expressed to the dialysis team that she really wanted to attempt to carry her pregnancy to term. She then began training for nocturnal HHD with a dialysis prescription of 8-hour treatments 6 nights per week. Unfortunately, there was not a PTH accessible at this time.

At her HHD clinic visit on July 29, 2015, E.M.'s weight was 80.7 kg and her physician established TW as 81 kg. She was educated on the need to increase this weight gradually during pregnancy. During a visit with her primary care physician, she had reported a high serum potassium level (6.3 mEq/L) after her serum potassium level of 5.2 mEq/L on July 22, 2015; this was prior to more frequent dialysis being prescribed. Dietary potassium restriction was continued until a repeat serum potassium level would be checked with the new dialysis prescription. Also, of note, on July 22, 2015, the serum calcium level was 5.2 mg/dL, and her albumin was 4.1 g/dL. She had reported tingling in her fingers. In June 2015, her serum calcium level was high (12.2 mg/dL); thus, active vitamin D medication (calcitriol) and calcium carbonate were decreased. Repeat serum calcium in June 2015 was 10.2 mg/dL. Based on her newest very low calcium level, these medications were again increased and the calcium content of the HD bath was changed to 3.0 mEq/L.

At E.M.'s HHD clinic visit on August 14, 2015, her calcium acetate was decreased from three thrice daily to one capsule thrice daily and her diet was liberalized in phosphorus content by the RDN due to a recent low phosphorus level of 2.4 mg/dL. Also, 15 mg/d of zinc was added due to general recommendations for pregnancy and due to increased needs for those individuals undergoing HD. At this visit, she reported difficulty adhering to the increased HHD regimen due to many distractions. She was then transferred to another facility where she would undergo intense in-center dialysis. Her dialysis schedule was 4 hours per treatment on Monday, Wednesday, Friday, and Saturday. She was also prescribed 8 hours on nocturnal HD three times per week. This new dialysis prescription provided the patient with dialysis 40 h/wk. Her epoetin α dose was increased to 60,000 units per week due to recent hemoglobin levels of 8.2 to 8.5 g/dL and the known decrease in hemoglobin during pregnancy even in the individual without CKD. Recommendations, as previously mentioned, are to keep the hemoglobin goals within acceptable range for nonpregnant individuals undergoing HD.

On August 24, 2015, E.M. reported to the RDN that she had decreased appetite and was unable to eat very much. She had been prescribed 2,500 calories and 85 g protein, with pregnancy nutritional needs in addition to those for a patient undergoing dialysis. At this time, she was encouraged to eat more, including bringing meals/snacks to eat during dialysis. Donated Boost Plus was also provided to the patient to aid her in reaching protein and calorie goals. Her most recent serum potassium level was now 3.6 mEq/L. E.M.'s diet was liberalized and the potassium content of the HD bath was increased from 2 mEq/L to 3 mEq/L. Her serum calcium was 10.4 mg/dL; thus, the calcium content of the HD bath was changed from 3 mEq/L to 2.5 mEq/L. A decrease in calcium carbonate dose was prescribed as well. Of note was her PTH level of less than 6.3 pg/mL on August 17, 2015. She had a parathyroidectomy in June 2014; so this may have been accurate. Decreases in the calcium content of the HD bath and oral calcium supplements were also prescribed to increase the PTH level.

On September 1, 2015, her nephrologist summarized her August 24, 2015 visit. At the time of his writing, E.M. was 12 weeks pregnant. He stated that her BP had been high with systolic levels frequently more than 160 mm Hg. He felt that possibly the very high dose of epoetin α may have contributed to the increased BP levels. After her hemoglobin reached a low level of 7.5 g/dL, this blood level was now increasing so the epoetin α dose was decreased to 15,000 units three times per week given subcutaneously (as opposed to the IV route) because it was thought to be less likely to cause HTN. Given the patient's high BP levels, the plan was to obtain a hemoglobin goal of 8 to 9 g/dL. Labetelol was also started to help decrease BP. Serum calcium was now reasonable (in a 10 mg/dL range) with decreasing oral calcium supplements and the change in HD bath from 3.0 to 2.5 mEq/L. Calcitriol dose was unchanged due to the need for absorbing more phosphorus (despite low PTH level). The most recent serum phosphorus level was 1.5 mg/dL. Her diet had already been liberalized and calcium acetate discontinued; thus, K-Phos Neutral was started at one tablet two times per day (250 mg phosphorus, 298 mg sodium, and 45 mg potassium per tablet).

On September 21, 2015, the RDN reported that E.M. was 14 weeks pregnant. Her TW was still at

81 kg, but had most likely been overestimated initially; a liberal potassium and phosphorus diet was continued. BP was improved and most recent albumin calculation was still within the goal range at 4.2 g/dL. E.M. was then undergoing 36 hours HD per week, as 40 hours per week had just been too much for her due to other medical appointments and family commitments.

Again on October 13, 2015, the RDN indicated that E.M.'s TW was still at 81 kg. The physician still felt that her TW was overestimated early on and that she was now catching up, as shown by an improved BP, now without antihypertensive medication. Her diet then was completely liberal and a protein/energy supplement was encouraged if she was not able to improve intake. The albumin level was still within the goal range at 4.0 g/dL (according to laboratory results from October 7, 2015). The patient still had not started the zinc supplement, but was encouraged to do so. Laboratory results were continued to be monitored weekly.

E.M.'s serum potassium was very high at 6.5 mEq/L on October 19, 2015. Her HD bath had just been changed to 2K due to a serum potassium value of 5.7 mEq/L prior to this level. Per her physician, the RDN encouraged her to decrease her intake of high-potassium foods as well, but she had also missed some dialysis time on a few occasions.

On November 23, 2015, the RDN reported that E.M. was 24 weeks pregnant. She was concerned that E.M. still had not gained much actual weight. Her albumin was reported to be 4.0 g/dL (as of November 5, 2015), but again, she was encouraged to supplement her intakes with a protein/energy nutritional supplement due to lack of solid weight gain. Serum potassium was now acceptable at 4.0 on a dialysate potassium content of 2 mEq/L. Serum samples drawn that day (November 23, 2015) revealed potassium 4.8 and phosphorus 3.7.

On January 13, 2016, the RDN reported that E.M. was now 31 weeks pregnant and continued with 36 hours HD per week. TW was now 84 kg (3 kg increase in the last month). The patient was, however, recently hospitalized for high BP. Close monitoring of E.M.'s weight and BP continued accordingly. In the hospital, the last hemoglobin value was 10.1 g/dL. Her

albumin levels had decreased to 3.8 on December 9, 2015 and then to 3.4 in January 2016; thus, the RDN reinforced adequate intake of protein and calories. E.M. was willing again to take Boost Plus nutritional supplements. She had apparently had another low serum potassium level recently, and the HD bath was changed back to a potassium content of 3 mEq/L. The serum potassium level improved on this HD bath, and the bicarbonate level was acceptable as well.

On January 20, 2016, the RDN reported that E.M. was now 32 weeks pregnant. Per her physician, her TW was now increased to 85 kg. She did complain of an upper respiratory infection and some diarrhea, however. Protein/energy rich food sources were again encouraged and she was advised to use Boost Plus nutritional supplements, if tolerated. Serum potassium and phosphorus levels continued to be checked weekly, and E.M. was now taking K-Phos Neutral, two tablets thrice daily.

Because E.M. was absent from her scheduled dialysis treatment on January 28, 2016, the dialysis nurse learned that she had been admitted to the hospital on approximately January 27, 2016 for possible volume overload. He was later informed that she had delivered her baby boy at 33 weeks, 3 days gestation on January 29, 2016. The baby weighed 4 lb 7 oz and spent 10 days in the neonatal intensive care unit before being discharged.

This patient has since received a second kidney transplant in November 2016. Despite her struggles post transplant, she and her son are doing well. At the time of this writing, the infant is now approximately 2.5 years old and in the 83rd percentile for height and 94th percentile for weight for his age.

References

1. Fitzpatrick A, Mohammedi F, Jesudason S. Managing pregnancy in chronic kidney disease: improving outcomes for mother and baby. *Int J Womens Health.* 2016;8:273-285. doi:10.2147/IJWH.S76819
2. Li Y, Wang W, Wang Y, Chen Q. Fetal risks and maternal renal complications in pregnancy with preexisting chronic glomerulonephritis. *Med Sci Monit.* 2018;24:1008-1016. doi:10.12659/msm.905494

3. Piccoli GB, Attini R, Cabiddu G. Kidney diseases and pregnancy: a multidisciplinary approach for improving care by involving nephrology, obstetrics, neonatology, urology, diabetology, bioethics, and internal medicine. *J Clin Med*. 2018;7(6):E135. doi:10.3390/jcm7060135

4. Cabiddu G, Spotti D, Genone G, Maroni G, Gregorini G, Santoro D. A best-practice position statement on pregnancy after kidney transplantation: focusing on the unsolved questions. The Kidney and Pregnancy Study Group of the Italian Society of Nephrology. *J Nephrol*. 2018;31(5):665-681. doi:10.1007/s40620-018-0499-x

5. Chang JY, Jang H, Chung BH, et al. The successful clinical outcomes of pregnant women with advanced chronic kidney disease. *Kidney Res Clin Pract*. 2016;35(2):84-89. doi:10.1016/j.krcp.2015.12.005

6. Reddy SS, Holley J. Management of the pregnant dialysis patient. *Adv Chron Kidney Dis*. 2007;14(2):146-155. doi:10.1016/s1073-4449(98)70011-1

7. Sobiło-Jarek L, Popowska-Drojecka J, Muszytowski M, Wanic-Kossowska M, Kobelski M, Czekalski S. Anemia treatment with darbepoetin alpha in pregnant female with chronic renal failure: report of two cases. *Adv Med Sci*. 2006;51:309-311.

8. Goshorn J, Youell TD. Darbepoetin alfa treatment for post-renal transplantation anemia during pregnancy. *Am J Kidney Dis*. 2005;46(5):e81-e86. doi:10.1053/j.ajkd.2005.07.047

9. Etelcalcetide. Drugs.com website. Accessed July 19, 2020. www.drugs.com/mtm/etelcalcetide.html

10. Hou S. Pregnancy in women treated with dialysis: lessons from a large series over 20 years. *Am J Kidney Dis*. 2010;56(1):5-6. doi:10.1053/j.ajkd.2010.05.002

11. Chang H, Miller MA, Bruns FJ. Tidal peritoneal dialysis during pregnancy improves clearance and abdominal symptoms. *Perit Dial Int*. 2002;22(2):272-274.

12. Manisco G, Poti M, Maggiulli G, Di Tullio M, Losappio V, Vernaglione L. Pregnancy in end-stage renal disease patients on dialysis: how to achieve a successful delivery. *Clin Kidney J*. 2015;8(3):293-299. doi:10.1093/ckj/sfv016

13. Hou S. Pregnancy and renal disease. In: *Educational Review Manual in Nephrology*. 2nd ed. Castle Connolly Graduate Medical Publishing; 2008:251-278.

14. Grossman S, Hou S. Obstetrics and gynecology. In: Daugirdas JT, Blake PG, Ing TS, eds. *Handbook of Dialysis*. 4th ed. Lippincott Williams & Wilkins; 2006:672-684.

15. Ikizler TA, Burrowes JD, Byham-Gray LD, et al; KDOQI Nutrition in CKD Guideline Work Group. KDOQI Clinical Practice Guidelines for nutrition in CKD: 2020 update. *Am J Kidney Dis*. 2020;76(3) (suppl 1):S1-S107. doi:10.1053/j.ajkd.2020.05.006

16. Institute of Medicine. Dietary Reference Intake tables. U.S. National Library of Medicine website. Accessed September 9, 2020. www.ncbi.nlm.nih.gov/books/NBK222881

17. Stover J. Nutritional management of pregnancy in chronic kidney disease. *Adv Chronic Kidney Dis*. 2007;14(2):212-214. doi:10.1053/j.ackd.2007.01.011

18. Wiggins KL. Nutrition care of adult pregnant ESRD patients. In: *Guidelines for Nutrition Care of Renal Patients*. 3rd ed. American Dietetic Association; 2002:105-107.

19. Stover J. Pregnancy in chronic kidney disease (CKD). In: Byham-Gray L, Stover J, Wiesen K. *A Clinical Guide to Nutrition Care in Kidney Disease*. American Dietetic Association; 2013:151-156.

20. Fredericksen MC. Physiologic changes in pregnancy and their effect on drug disposition. *Sem Perinatol*. 2001;25(3):120-123. doi:10.1053/sper.2001.24565

21. Vidal LV, Ursu M, Martinez A, et al. Nutritional control of pregnant women on chronic hemodialysis. *J Ren Nutr*. 1998;8(3):150-156. doi:10.1016/S1051-2276(98)90007-3

22. Hollis BW, Wagner CL. Nutritional vitamin D status during pregnancy: reasons for concern. *CMAJ*. 2006;174(9):1287-1290. doi:10.1503/cmaj.060149

23. Schroth RJ, Lavelle CL, Moffatt ME. Review of vitamin D deficiency during pregnancy: who is affected? *Int J Circumpolar Health*. 2005;64(2):112-120. doi:10.3402/ijch.v64i2.17964

24. Lactmed. U.S. National Library of Medicine website. Accessed July 2020. www.ncbi.nlm.nih.gov/books/NBK501922

25. Tan PK, Tan ASA, Tan HK, Vathsala A, Tay SK. Pregnancy after renal transplantation: experience in Singapore General Hospital. *Ann Acad Med Singapore*. 2002;31(3):285-289.

CHAPTER 13

Kidney Disease in the Pediatric Patient

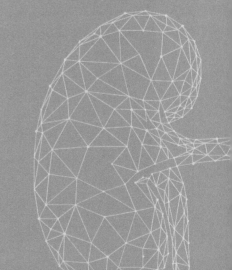

Christine Benedetti, MS, RDN, CSR, LD, FNKF, and Jenni Carvalho-Salemi, MPH, RDN, LD, CSP

Introduction

A common expression in pediatric medicine is "children are not simply little adults." In fact, the etiology and management of kidney disease are quite unique in pediatric patients. First, the principal causes of chronic kidney disease (CKD) in children—congenital abnormalities of the kidney and urinary tract, hereditary nephropathies, and pediatric glomerular diseases—are distinct from leading CKD etiologies in adults. Unlike age-related CKD caused primarily by hypertension (HTN) and diabetes (DM), pediatric kidney disease by its very nature presents during infancy or childhood, and therefore requires unique nutritional management.[1,2] Second, severe growth impairment and malnutrition are common in all ages of children with CKD. Infants and children are at increased risk for malnutrition because they have low nutrition stores and increased energy demands with rapid physical growth and brain development. Adolescents are also at risk due to the maturation demands of puberty.[3] Finally, impaired linear growth secondary to childhood CKD increases the risk of poor clinical outcomes, as well as obesity later in life. Extremes at both ends of body mass index (BMI) are associated with an increased risk for morbidity and mortality in children with kidney disease and worsened outcomes post transplant.[4-6] Aggressive management of malnutrition is vital as it impacts the long-term growth potential, neurocognitive development, and quality of life for pediatric patients.[3,7-10]

The overall goal of nutrition interventions for pediatric patients with CKD is to maximize nutrient intake in childhood and prevent growth decline exacerbated by reduced energy intake, gastrointestinal disturbances (eg, vomiting and diarrhea, chronic disease, uremic toxicity, and metabolic and electrolyte abnormalities). Pediatric nutrition management—especially for adolescent patients—involves consideration of long-term disease management, posttransplant quality of life, and transition to adulthood. Medical nutrition therapy (MNT) is an ongoing process that requires frequent monitoring and adjustments to the nutrition plan based on changes in age, development, anthropometrics, residual kidney function (RKF), biochemistries, medications, kidney replacement therapy (KRT), and psychosocial status. Input from the child and family/caregiver is important and is attained through frequent contact, regular communication, and development of strong rapport. The consistent promotion of the benefits of dietary modification and provision of practical information and emotional support to children and their families can positively influence treatment plan adherence and clinical outcomes and minimize stress related to nutrition issues. Full compliance with all dietary restrictions is not always realistic. Priorities should be identified on an individual basis, depending on the patient's dietary goals, physical and medical status, emotional needs, and social situation.

Assessment of Nutritional Status

Compared with adults, children with CKD have distinct nutritional requirements in terms of growth. Changes in their physical, social, emotional, and cognitive development require a nutritional needs assessment on an ongoing basis.[11] The recommended frequency for nutrition assessment of children with CKD stages 2 through 5 and those with CKD stage 5 on dialysis (5D) varies according to the child's age and stage of kidney disease.[11] Table 13.1 gives the minimum guidelines; more frequent assessment may be necessary. In particular, infants and children with polyuria, evidence of poor growth, decreasing or poor BMI, comorbid conditions influencing growth or nutrient intake, or recent acute changes in dietary intake or medical status may need closer follow-up.[11] In addition to diet and growth assessment, a thorough evaluation should consider medical and psychosocial history, quality of life, nutrition-related biochemical parameters, blood pressure, bowel habits, urine output, and fluid balance.

DIETARY EVALUATION

A thorough and accurate diet history will provide information for both quantitative and qualitative evaluation. A 3-day food record is preferred to the 24-hour dietary recall method and may be requested annually or as often as bimonthly, depending on the child's age, stage of CKD, and nutritional status and goals.[11] A short series of 24-hour recalls may be more feasible for adolescents. A variety of social and cultural factors influence food consumption and choices. A diet assessment should include the person responsible for food preparation and provision, location and timing of meals, frequency of eating out, and consumption of nonfood items (pica).

TABLE 13.1 | Recommended Frequency of Assessment for Children With Chronic Kidney Disease Stages 2 to 5 and Those With 5D[11]

Measure	Age 0 to <1 year CKD 2-3	CKD 4-5	CKD 5D	Age 1-3 years CKD 2-3	CKD 4-5	CKD 5D	Age >3 years CKD 2	CKD 3	CKD 4-5	CKD 5D
Dietary intake	0.5-3	0.5-3	0.5-2	1-3	1-3	1-3	6-12	6	3-4	3-4
Height or length-for-age percentile or SDS	0.5-1.5	0.5-1.5	0.5-1	1-3	1-2	1	3-6	3-6	1-3	1-3
Height or length velocity-for-age percentile or SDS	0.5-2	0.5-2	0.5-1	1-6	1-3	1-2	6	6	6	6
Estimated dry weight and weight-for-age percentile or SDS	0.5-1.5	0.5-1.5	0.25-1	1-3	1-2	0.5-1	3-6	3-6	1-3	1-3
BMI-for-height-age percentile or SDS	0.5-1.5	0.5-1.5	0.5-1	1-3	1-2	1	3-6	3-6	1-3	1-3
Head circumference-for-age percentile or SDS	0.5-1.5	0.5-1.5	0.5-1	1-3	1-2	1-2	N/A	N/A	N/A	N/A
nPCR	N/A	N/A	N/A	N/A	N/A	N/A	N/A	N/A	N/A	1[a]

BMI = body mass index | CKD = chronic kidney disease | N/A = not applicable | nPCR = normalized protein catabolic rate | SDS = standard deviation score

[a] Applies only to adolescents receiving hemodialysis

Reproduced with permission from National Kidney Foundation. KDOQI Clinical Practice Guidelines for nutrition in children with CKD: 2008 update. *Am J Kidney Dis*. 2009;53(suppl 2):S16.11.

FEEDING DIFFICULTIES

Feeding difficulties, reduced oral intake, emesis, and delay of oral motor skills are common in pediatric patients with CKD. Infants and toddlers with CKD often exhibit delayed or absence of progression through the normal stages of acquired feeding skills. A lack of interest in formula, breast milk, and solid foods is common, as is a rejection of varied food textures. Unless there is severe developmental delay or medical contraindication, the goal should be to introduce solids and advance textures at the same age as for healthy children. Signs of feeding difficulties should be investigated further, and the expertise of appropriate specialists (ie, child psychologist, speech or occupational therapist) should be utilized. Parents should be educated on initiating responsive feeding techniques and avoiding forced or pressured oral intake.[12]

Enteral nutrition is often required to meet nutrition goals as infants with CKD feed poorly, vomit easily, and have altered taste sensations. During the first 2 years of life, adequate nutrition is critical for growth; therefore, timely assessment and management are key.[10] Infants and children with polyuria are at risk for chronic hyponatremia and dehydration; they typically prefer water over breast milk/formula to satisfy their thirst.[13] Decreased appetite, early satiety, and a high incidence of gastroesophageal reflux (GER), delayed gastric emptying, nausea, and vomiting make it challenging for caregivers to meet the infant's nutrition needs orally.[14] Cytokines and hormones normally involved in the modulation of hunger and satiety are significantly altered, potentially contributing to anorexia and gastrointestinal dysfunction.[15-17] Guidelines for the treatment of infants with GER recommend reduced feeding volumes and permit the use of thickened feeds when there is regurgitation and emesis. In refractory cases, clinicians may recommend a 2- to 4-week trial of extensively hydrolyzed protein or amino acid-based formula.[18] Medications such as prokinetic agents and gastric acid-suppressing agents (eg, proton pump inhibitors and histamine-2 receptor antagonists) are commonly prescribed, although there is a critical need for additional research into their efficacy and safety in pediatric populations. Aluminum-containing antacids are not recommended for use in infants or in children with kidney impairment due to the risk of aluminum accumulation and toxicity.[18]

ANTHROPOMETRICS

Recumbent length (for children <2 years old) or standing height (for children ≥2 years old who are able to cooperatively stand straight and still), weight, and head circumference (for children ≤36 months old) are the basic measurements performed to evaluate growth. Weight-for-length (for children <2 years old) or BMI are calculated from these measures to evaluate weight relative to length or height. Measurement of growth parameters should be performed regularly by the same person, using standardized procedures and consistent, calibrated equipment.[11] A recumbent length board and a wall-mounted height stadiometer are essential for accurate results. These measurements are compared with measurements of a healthy reference population by plotting them on age- and gender-appropriate growth charts and the corresponding percentile is identified. Recommended growth charts include the World Health Organization (WHO) Child Growth Standards for birth to 2 years and the United States Centers for Disease Control and Prevention (CDC) growth charts for ages 2 years and older.[11,19,20] While use of percentiles is common in the clinical setting, use of standard deviation scores (SDS) or z scores (ZS) is now recommended.[21]

When evaluating anthropometrics of preterm infants outside of the neonatal intensive care setting, growth can be assessed with the WHO Child Growth Standards, using corrected age for prematurity until the age of 36 months, when appropriate.[21,22]

Length/Height and Linear Growth

Growth failure and short stature are common and visible features of CKD in children.[23-26] Short stature and poor growth velocity are associated with psychosocial and medical comorbidities, including an increased risk of mortality.[4,5,27-29] Patients whose linear growth is impaired due to malnutrition during early childhood are also at increased risk for being overweight and obese as adolescents and adults.[21]

The causes and degree of growth failure are multifactorial and are influenced by the age at the onset of CKD, the degree of kidney impairment, metabolic acidosis and electrolyte disturbances, mineral bone disorders, abnormalities in the growth hormone/insulin-like growth factor axis, and insufficient energy intake.[30] Linear growth is most sensitive to nutritional deprivation during infancy; hence, timely nutrition therapy and prevention and management of metabolic derangements are essential for optimizing growth.[11] Infants with salt-wasting and polyuria often need supplementary sodium and water in addition to a calorically dense diet.[9]

According to the WHO, impaired linear growth, or "stunting," is defined as having a height-for-age 2 standard deviations (SD) below the child growth standards median; likewise, the Kidney Disease Outcomes Quality Initiative (KDOQI) guidelines define "short stature" as falling below −1.88 SD.[11,21]

Clinical judgment should be applied to carefully assess a child's growth and potential benefits of treatment. Genetic potential based on parental heights should also be considered. Tanner's formula is traditionally used to estimate a child's "midparental" or target height for boys and girls (all measurements in centimeters)[31]:

Midparental Height (boy) =

$$\frac{\text{(Paternal Height + Maternal Height + 13 cm)}}{2}$$

Midparental Height (girl) =

$$\frac{\text{(Maternal Height + Paternal Height − 13 cm)}}{2}$$

When length-/height-for-age is monitored over time, the clinician can track growth velocity. This is considered a superior measure of pediatric growth, as it provides a more accurate picture of recent gains and declines in nutrition status. More importantly, it has the advantage of, ideally, cautioning the clinician to in-

tervene prior to the child's consequent growth failure.[32] Growth velocity is generally calculated over a period of 2 to 6 months in children under 2 years old and over a period of 1 year (measured in cm/year) for older children. Length or height velocity percentiles or ZS can be generated using data from the WHO Child Growth Standards for children under 2 years old and US data for older children.[19,20] The WHO length velocity ZS for children from birth to 24 months are available online. Online calculators and software programs, such as Child Metrics, can be useful in generating data for older children.[33]

Height velocity below the 25th percentile is considered growth stunting.[31] Per best practice, any decline in height-for-age greater than 1 ZS is considered an indicator of suboptimal growth velocity and necessitates an investigation into its etiology and appropriate interventions.[34]

Weight

Estimating true euvolemic weight or dry weight can be more challenging in children with CKD because, unlike adults, weight gain is expected in growing children. Weight and blood pressure fluctuations, laboratory markers of hydration (eg, serum sodium and albumin), dietary interviews, and physical examination for edema are all useful tools when estimating a child's dry weight.[11] For children on dialysis, tolerance of ultrafiltration should also be considered. For children on hemodialysis (HD), dry weight should be measured post dialysis; for children on peritoneal dialysis (PD), dry weight should be calculated as weight minus the weight of indwelling dialysate. Rapid weight gain without adequate energy intake should be viewed suspiciously and investigated before assuming it is true dry weight gain. Rate of weight gain, expressed as grams per day (g/d) can be assessed by a comparison with reported average rates of weight gain for healthy infants and children.[35,36] Rate of weight gain should be calculated as an average of the change in weight over a longer period of time (eg, change in weight in 1 week divided by 7 days for infants), rather than actual weight change over 1 or 2 days.

Dry weight should be frequently measured, and the ZS for age should be assessed using an appropriate growth chart. Weight-for-age provides an indicator that is not based on stature and is, therefore, critical to documenting acute changes in nutrition status in growth-stunted children.[21]

Weight-for-Length

Weight-for-length is an index used in the early years of life (<2 years) to consider a child's weight relative to height. The WHO weight-for-length growth standards are recommended for infants and toddlers until 24 months of age. Since the weight-for-height index does not consider age, it has limited applicability after 24 months, given the wide variability in the timing of growth spurts during childhood. For these reasons, BMI-for-age is now the recommended index of weight relative to height for children 2 years and older.[11]

Body Mass Index

In pediatrics, starting at the age of 2 years, BMI is calculated similarly for children and adults: weight (measured in kg) divided by height (measured in m²). However, unlike that of adults, a child's BMI will vary based on age and gender. BMI declines during the preschool years, typically reaching a low nadir around 4 to 6 years of age; gradually it increases thereafter, a phenomenon referred to as BMI rebound.

Age- and gender-specific growth charts are utilized to identify the child's BMI percentile and calculate his or her BMI ZS.[20] The CDC recommends the following BMI-for-age cutoffs for the screening of pediatric malnutrition and obesity: underweight equal to or less than 5th percentile, obesity equal to or greater than 95th percentile, overweight 85th through 95th percentile.[37] Both upper and lower extremes of BMI-for-age have been associated with mortality in children with CKD stage 5.[5] When a child's anthropometrics place them at percentile extremes, ZS are recommended as they facilitate quantification of degree in comparison to growth standard and monitoring progress over time.[38,39] The following has been recommended for the quantification of degree of pediatric malnutrition: mild

−1 to −1.9 ZS, moderate −2 to −2.9 ZS, severe −3 or greater ZS.[40] Because of the high prevalence of growth failure or stunting in children with CKD, research suggests that BMI-for-height age (ie, the age at which the child's height would be at the 50th percentile), rather than chronological age, be used when assessing weight relative to height for children with CKD.[41]

Finally, it is important to consider the patient's bone age and Tanner stage when using height-based anthropometrics like BMI. These considerations are essential for proper nutrition assessment as well as for establishing appropriate intervention strategies. For example, maintaining caloric intake despite "overweight" BMI status may be appropriate for a 2-year old girl with severe stunting but inappropriate for an 18-year-old female with a growth impairment following a history of malnutrition. In fact, the older adolescent patient will likely not benefit from hypercaloric intake goals once she has reached full adult height and her epiphyses are closed. On the contrary, such intake might increase her risk for obesity.

Mid-Upper Arm Circumference

The 2008 KDOQI pediatric guidelines do not recommend mid-upper arm circumference (MUAC) as part of the routine nutrition assessments.[11] Limitations of the MUAC include potential confounding due to the irregularities in fluid status, body composition, and lean body mass distribution of patients with CKD, as well as variance in the medical literature as to how to interpret the MUAC in the context of growth stunting. Moreover, the KDOQI publication noted that the lack of research available at that time was related to the use of MUAC in pediatric populations with CKD. Despite these limitations, however, the MUAC has since been used as a proxy for reduced muscle mass by researchers studying pediatric patients with CKD and was one of five indicators utilized to define protein–energy wasting (PEW) in children as part of the Chronic Kidney Disease in Children (CKiD) cohort study.[39]

The benefits of using the MUAC-for-age in clinical assessment are as follows: it has proven to be highly predictive of morbidity and mortality in high-risk populations; it allows for increased ease of measurement in children who are wheelchair bound or in whom accurate height measurements are difficult to obtain; it is considered a single data point indicator for pediatric malnutrition; and expanded age-based ZS for children 2 months to 18 years of age are now easily accessible online.[40,42,43] Of course, the MUAC, like any anthropometric indicator, has its own set of limitations. Clinical interpretation is necessary in the setting of growth stunting and changes in fluid status. Although studies have shown it to be less affected by fluid status than weight-dependent measurements, such as weight-for-age and BMI, the MUAC should be assessed during euvolemia when possible; otherwise, clinical judgment is needed to assess whether the child is affected by edema in the upper extremities.[21,44] Furthermore, while the MUAC may seem inherently less skewed than the BMI in the context of growth stunting, its interpretation in this context has not been thoroughly researched.

Other Measurements

Impaired functional outcomes, such as impaired immunity, learning and behavioral disorders, and muscle dysfunction, should be considered when determining and documenting both the cause and the effects of chronic malnutrition in pediatric patients.[34]

Muscle dysfunction is an established consequence of malnutrition and a predictor of functional status in hospitalized patients. Early CKD is associated with loss of muscle strength; this is especially true for those patients with concurrent growth retardation, low physical activity, or need for nutritional support. Handgrip strength is a validated tool to assess muscle strength and functional status. Its use is limited by both age and cognition, as the patient must be able to use the dynamometer of his or her own volition, and normative values are unavailable for children under the age of 3 years.[45,46]

Skinfold thickness measures using calipers, bioelectrical impedance analysis, and dual-energy x-ray absorptiometry (DXA) are methods for estimating body composition primarily in the pediatric research setting. The accuracy of each method is affected by abnormal

fluid status in the body, and their validity and clinical usefulness in children with CKD have not been well tested.[47] They are not recommended for routine nutrition assessment in children with CKD.[11]

Hypoalbuminemia occurs frequently in children with CKD and has been associated with increased risk of morbidity and mortality in this population.[48] Because it will decline with systemic inflammation and edema, in addition to malnutrition, it cannot be utilized as a stand-alone parameter for assessing nutritional status.[11,49-51] Yet despite its limitations, hypoalbuminemia is useful in overall clinical assessment and may be used with other nutrition indicators to establish and document PEW among pediatric patients with CKD.[39]

Nutrition Focused Physical Exam

A nutrition focused physical exam (NFPE) uses assessment findings to identify nutrient deficiencies or toxicities and their possible etiology. It can be a helpful tool in the pediatric population, especially in determining malnutrition status. Pediatric patients may become malnourished faster than adults, and malnutrition can negatively impact their growth and development. A focused or comprehensive NFPE can be utilized to help identify muscle wasting, subcutaneous fat loss, and edema. A focused NFPE is system specific based on the practitioner's medical record review or interview, and a comprehensive NFPE is a total review of systems in an organized sequence. Several techniques may be used for an effective NFPE, such as inspection, palpation, percussion, and auscultation. Potential etiologies of deficiencies or malnutrition are chronic disease, like CKD, long-term tube feedings, or long-term parenteral nutrition.[52,53]

The practitioner should begin with hand washing, asking the patient or family permission to begin the exam, explaining the process along the way, and ensuring the patient's privacy. Note the patient's positioning, for example, supine, and begin a general survey looking at overall appearance, level of consciousness or orientation, body movements, affect, and ability to communicate. When conducting a head-to-toe physical examination, useful exam areas include assessing subcutaneous fat, muscle losses, and edema (see Box 13.1 and Table 13.2 on page 253).[54] When conducting a micronutrient examination, hair, scalp, fontanel, eyes, face, mouth, skin, lips, teeth, tongue, gums, taste, neck, nails, and systems (eg, gastrointestinal, skeletal, muscular, and nervous) are all areas where signs of a nutrient deficiency can be identified. Vitamins and minerals play important roles in our body, and the implications of deficiency or accumulation may be detrimental in children with CKD, especially with respect to growth. Micronutrients of potential concern are aluminum, biotin, calcium, cobalamin, copper, folate, iron, magnesium, manganese, niacin, pantothenic acid, phosphorus, potassium, pyridoxine, riboflavin, selenium, sodium, thiamin, vitamins C, K, and D, and zinc. Other potential concerns are an essential fatty acid deficiency, protein–calorie malnutrition, malabsorption, hyperlipidemia, inadequate hydration, or vitamin A toxicity. A child's underlying diagnosis and requirement for KRT

BOX 13.1 | Physical Exam: Parameters Useful in the Assessment of Nutritional Status[54,58,59]

SUBCUTANEOUS FAT LOSS

Orbital region: surrounding the eye

Tips: View patient when standing directly in front of the practitioner, touch above cheekbone

Severe malnutrition	Hollow look, depressions, dark circles, loose skin
Mild-to-moderate malnutrition	Slightly dark circles, somewhat hollow look
Well nourished	Slightly bulged fat pads; fluid retention may mask loss

Upper arm region: triceps/biceps

Tips: Arm bent, roll skin between fingers, do not include muscle in pinch

Severe malnutrition	Very little space between folds, fingers touch
Mild-to-moderate malnutrition	Some depth in pinch, but not ample
Well nourished	Ample fat tissue obvious between folds of skin

Thoracic and lumbar region: ribs, lower back, midaxillary line

Tip: Have patient press hands hard against a solid object

Severe malnutrition	Depression between the ribs very apparent; iliac crest very prominent
Mild-to-moderate malnutrition	Ribs apparent, depressions between them less pronounced; iliac crest somewhat prominent
Well nourished	Chest is full, ribs do not show; slight to no protrusion of the iliac crest

MUSCLE LOSS

Temple region: temporalis muscle

Tips: View patient when standing directly in front of the practitioner; ask patient to turn head side to side

Severe malnutrition	Hollowing, scooping, depression
Mild-to-moderate malnutrition	Slight depression
Well nourished	Can see/feel well-defined muscle

Clavicle bone region: pectoralis major, deltoid, trapezius muscles

Tips: Look for prominent bone; make sure patient is not hunched forward

Severe malnutrition	Protruding, prominent bone
Mild-to-moderate malnutrition	Visible in male, some protrusion in female
Well nourished	Not visible in male, visible but not prominent in female

Continued on next page

Continued from previous page

Clavicle and acromion bone region: deltoid muscle

Tip: Patient arms at side, observe shape

Severe malnutrition	Shoulder to arm joint looks square; bones prominent; acromion protrusion very prominent
Mild-to-moderate malnutrition	Acromion process may slightly protrude
Well nourished	Rounded, curves at arm/shoulder/neck

Scapular bone region: trapezius, supraspinus, infraspinus muscles

Tips: Ask patient to extend hands straight out; push against solid object

Severe malnutrition	Prominent, visible bones, depressions between ribs/scapula or shoulder/spine
Mild-to-moderate malnutrition	Mild depression or bone may show slightly
Well nourished	Bones not prominent; no significant depressions

Dorsal hand: interosseous muscle

Tips: Look at thumb side of hand; look at pads of thumb when tip of forefinger touching tip of thumb

Severe malnutrition	Depressed area between thumb and forefinger
Mild-to-moderate malnutrition	Slightly depressed
Well nourished	Muscle bulges; could be flat in some well-nourished people

LOWER BODY (LESS SENSITIVE TO CHANGE)

Patellar region: quadricep muscle

Tip: Ask patient to sit with leg propped up, bent at knee

Severe malnutrition	Bones prominent, little sign of muscle around knee
Mild-to-moderate malnutrition	Kneecap less prominent, more rounded
Well nourished	Muscles protrude; bones not prominent

Anterior thigh region: quadricep muscles

Tips: Ask patient to sit; prop leg up on low furniture; grasp quads to differentiate amount of muscle tissue from fat tissue

Severe malnutrition	Depression/line on thigh, obviously thin
Mild-to-moderate malnutrition	Mild depression on inner thigh
Well nourished	Well-rounded, well-developed

Posterior calf region: gastrocnemius muscle

Tip: Grasp the calf muscle to determine amount of tissue

Severe malnutrition	Thin, minimal to no muscle definition
Mild-to-moderate malnutrition	Not well-developed
Well nourished	Well-developed bulb of muscle

EDEMA

Rule out other causes of edema (renal, liver, heart-related), patient at dry (target) weight

Tips: View sacrum in activity-restricted patient and ankles in mobile patient; press for 5 seconds.

Severe malnutrition	Deep to very deep pitting, depression that persists, extremity looks swollen (3–4+)
Mild-to-moderate malnutrition	Mild-to- moderate pitting, slight swelling of the extremity, indentation persists (1–2+)
Well nourished	No sign of fluid accumulation or barely perceptible

TABLE 13.2 | Edema Assessment[59]

Edema	Depth	Time for rebound	Degree
1+	≤2 mm indentation	Disappears rapidly	Mild pitting edema
2+	2-4 mm	15 seconds to rebound	Moderate pitting edema
3+	4-6 mm	30 seconds to rebound	Moderately severe pitting edema
4+	6-8 mm	>60 seconds to rebound	Severe pitting edema

may alter the likelihood of deficiency or accumulation. After determining a nutritional deficiency may be present based on the NFPE, the next step is to speak with the appropriate medical provider, request specific laboratory measures, and potentially recommend additional provider consultations.[52,55-59]

In infants and toddlers, muscle and fat stores should be assessed together as general wasting, as it is difficult to differentiate in the early years of life. If edema is known to be illness related, as in CKD, this should not be included as potential malnutrition; instead, assess weight change and edema together to ensure that tissue wasting is not masked by fluid status.[54]

Malnutrition and Protein–Energy Wasting

It is well established that nutritional status impacts clinical outcomes. Population-based studies in the United States have demonstrated that a clinical diagnosis of malnutrition among hospitalized children is associated with longer length of stay, increased vulnerability to infection and complications, and increased intensity of health care services.[60] In 2013, the American Society for Parenteral and Enteral Nutrition (ASPEN) expert work group proposed a comprehensive, etiology-based paradigm for defining pediatric malnutrition incorporating five domains of assessment, including anthropometrics, growth, chronicity, etiology, and functional status (see Box 13.2).[34] Reflected in this model is a recognition that disease-based malnutrition is multifactorial, and that anthropometric indicators of malnutrition often used in the general pediatric population may not, by themselves, be adequate for the complete assessment of nutritional status in children with chronic disease.

The International Society of Renal Nutrition and Metabolism has proposed the term *PEW* to describe malnutrition in the context of kidney disease.[61] The pathology of PEW is complex and multifactorial, and it is distinct from protein–energy malnutrition caused

BOX 13.2 | Recommended Domains for Defining Pediatric Malnutrition[a,34]

DOMAIN	HIGHLIGHTED EXEMPLIFICATIONS
Anthropometrics	Measure weight, height, body mass index, and mid-upper arm circumference; head circumference in children aged 2 years or less.
Growth	Record changes in weight and length velocity over time.
	Note that decline of more than 1 *z* score necessitates investigation into the etiology of growth failure and potential interventions.
Chronicity	Note that duration of malnutrition is acute if less than 3 months or chronic if 3 months or longer.
Etiology	Identify illness-related malnutrition.
	Identify predominant mechanisms of nutrient imbalance.
Impact of malnutrition on functional status	Include nutrition focused physical assessment whenever possible.
	Include validated objective measures of functional status (eg, handgrip).
	Document relevant developmental or neurocognitive findings, when applicable.

[a]This box is for illustrative purposes only. Clinical judgment is recommended prior to implementation. Refer to reference 34 for a comprehensive description of recommended domains.

by decreased nutrient intake alone.[62] Specifically, PEW refers to malnutrition secondary to CKD defined by disease-associated alterations in addition to low dietary intake; these include systemic inflammation, metabolic derangements, comorbidities, and hypercatabolism.[61]

To establish an operational definition of PEW specific to pediatric populations, the CKiD study, the largest multicenter study of children with CKD in North America, evaluated several adult and pediatric malnutrition indicators based on their relative ability to predict clinical outcomes (eg, incident hospitalization within 2 years).[39] The following set of criteria was adapted for this clinical guide. PEW may be defined as having both items 1 and 2:

1. Two or more of the nutrition-related clinical indicators listed as follows:
   a. Serum albumin less than 3.8 mg/dL
   b. Reduced body mass: BMI-for-height-age less than 5th percentile at entry *or* decline in BMI-for-height age and sex greater than 10% between first and second annual measurements
   c. Reduced muscle mass: MUAC less than 5th percentile *or* decline in MUAC percentile greater than 10% between first and second annual measurements
   d. Decreased appetite
2. Positive indication of poor growth, defined as follows:
   a. Height-for-age and sex percentile less than 3rd percentile, *or*
   b. Poor growth velocity: decline in height-for-age percentile greater than 10% between first and second annual measurements

While health care providers may find this proposed definition clinically useful for identifying patients at risk for poor clinical outcomes due to PEW, it is important to simultaneously adopt best practice guidelines with regard to malnutrition diagnosis. For instance, hepatic proteins (ie, albumin and prealbumin) are associated with poor outcomes and, therefore, may

be considered indicators for predicting risk for morbidity and mortality. However, it is essential for providers to understand that during illness, serum hepatic proteins change for multiple reasons unrelated to energy intake, including disease state, acute-phase response, hydration, severe zinc deficiency, altered distribution of albumin in intravascular and extravascular compartments, and kidney loss. It is, therefore, imperative that clinicians refer to current evidence-informed recommendations for the assessment and the diagnosis of pediatric malnutrition.[21,40] The Academy of Nutrition and Dietetics, ASPEN, and the Office of the Inspector General under the Department of Health and Human Services have clearly recommended that serum hepatic proteins not be used as defining indicators to either diagnose malnutrition or monitor changes in response to nutrient intake.[63-65] Furthermore, since appropriate and consistent documentation of malnutrition is fundamental to promoting continuity of care, payment for care, and adequate resources for treatment, the literature recommends that hospitals and clinics utilize evidence-informed indicators. Common best practice pediatric malnutrition diagnostic tools include the M-Tool: Michigan's Malnutrition Diagnostic Tool and the Texas Children's Hospital Pediatric Malnutrition Tool (see Table 13.3).[66] Another helpful resource for appropriate professional practice in this area is the Comprehensive Application of the Malnutrition Quality Improvement Initiative Toolkit to Pediatric Malnutrition.[67]

Furthermore, an expanded definition of PEW may be necessary for children with advanced CKD and patients receiving dialysis; such a definition may need to include additional biochemical parameters (eg, low cholesterol and low transferrin).[34]

Finally, it is important to note that the use of ZS in lieu of percentiles is now recommended for documenting nutrition assessment.[21] Clinicians can benefit from publicly available online assessment tools and ZS calculators, including those published by the WHO, CDC, and PediTools.

TABLE 13.3 | Texas Children's Hospital Pediatric Malnutrition Tool[a,b]

Primary indicators	Mild malnutrition	Moderate malnutrition	Severe malnutrition
Weight-for-length z score	−1 to −1.9	−2 to −2.9	−3 (wasting)[1]
BMI-for-age z score	−1 to −1.9	−2 to −2.9	−3
Length/height z score[10]	No data	−2 to −2.9[1]	−3 (stunting)[1]
Mid-upper arm circumference z score (6-60 mo[1,2]**; >60 mo**[3]**)**	−1 to −1.9	−2 to −2.9	−3

≥2 Data points and ≥2 indicators

		Mild malnutrition	Moderate malnutrition	Severe malnutrition
<2 y (pick one, if applies)	**Δ Weight-for-age**[1,4]	Decline in 1 z score	Decline in 2 z score	Decline in 3 z score
	WHO weight gain velocity[1]	−1 to −1.99 z score	−2 to −2.9 z score	−3 z score
	Weight gain velocity[2]	<75% of the norm for expected weight gain	<50% of the norm for expected weight gain	<25% of the norm for expected weight
2-20 y (pick one, if applies)	**Weight loss**[8,9]	5% usual body weight	7.5% usual body weight	10% usual body weight
	Δ Weight-for-age[8,9]	Decline in 0.66 z- score (~1 major percentile)	Decline in 0.67-1.33 z score (~2 major percentiles)	Decline in 1.34 z score (~3 major percentiles)
Deceleration in weight-for-length/ height z score[2]		Decline of 1 z score	Decline of 2 z score	Decline of 3 z score
Inadequate nutrient intake[2,8]		51%-75% estimated energy/protein needs	26%-50% estimated energy/protein needs	≤25% estimated energy/protein needs
Physical assessment (muscle or fat loss)[5,8]		No loss	Moderate loss	Severe loss
Functional capacity for age (physiologic changes related to weight loss, poor muscle or fat mass)[5-8]		No impairment, able to perform age-appropriate activity	Reduced ability to perform previous ADLs; less energy, tired more often	Significant reduced ability to perform ADLs; little/no play, confined to bed or chair >50% of waking time; no energy

Measurably reduced[6]

Postural change in heart rate >20 beats/min or fall in systolic blood pressure >20 mm Hg or >10 mm Hg diastolic[7] |

ADL = activities of daily living | BMI = body mass index | WHO = World Health Organization
[a] Consider Tanner staging and bone age in which individuals may be at final adult maturation but <18 years of age.
[b] Consider medical anomalies/chronic disease and use clinical judgment.
Exclusion: <44 weeks PMA, <45 cm length. Use of adult criteria may be an option.
Adapted with permission from *Texas Children's Hospital Pediatric Nutrition Reference Guide.* 12th ed. Texas Children's Hospital; 2019.[66]

Treating Growth Failure

Frequent monitoring of growth (see Table 13.3) is imperative for timely identification and treatment of pediatric patients with CKD growth failure. While its etiology is multifactorial, amenable contributing factors should be aggressively treated; these include, but are not limited to, protein–energy malnutrition, metabolic acidosis, CKD–mineral and bone disorder, steroid usage, and sodium wasting secondary to polyuria.[31]

Linear growth challenges are more likely if the child is younger at the time of initial CKD diagnosis, has a lower estimated glomerular filtration rate (eGFR), undergoes a longer disease duration, is diagnosed with a nonglomerular CKD, or receives enteral feeds. Disturbances of the insulin-like growth factor I and of the growth hormone axis are often seen.[68-70]

As previously described, short stature is defined as having a height-for-age less than –1.88 ZS or the 3rd percentile in children who have remaining linear growth potential (ie, epiphyses not fused).[11] If growth failure continues (height velocity below the 25th percentile), recombinant human growth hormone (rhGH) therapy should be considered in children over the age of 6 months with CKD stages 3 through 5/5D.[11, 31]

Despite its demonstrated efficacy and safety, experts estimate that less than 25% of those who qualify utilize rhGH therapy. The reasons are multifactorial but include caregiver/patient overestimation of risk vs perceived benefit, refusal, burden or fear of daily injections, early transplant referral, financial burden, or concern as to potential side effects.[68,70]

Long-term therapy has resulted in catch-up growth, with many children achieving a final adult height within the normal range.[30,31,71-73] Response to rhGH therapy is greatest in prepubertal children with earlier stages of CKD; however, improvements in linear growth are also observed in older children with growth potential and those on dialysis or post transplantation.[72,74,75] The most dramatic response to rhGH occurs in the first year of treatment with a growth velocity greater than the 75th percentile, indicating adequate catch-up growth.[31] Optimal nutrition, with special attention to the correction

of nutrient deficiencies and metabolic abnormalities, is recommended prior to initiating rhGH; specific recommendations for the use of the rhGH in children with CKD are available from consensus documents.[11,30,31]

Nutrition Intervention

Every child with CKD and their caregiver should receive intensive MNT based on an individualized plan of care and targeted at an appropriate education level.[11,76] The registered dietitian nutritionist (RDN) should quickly establish rapport with both the child and the primary caregiver to enhance commitment to the nutrition regimen. The child's age, development, and degree of independence determines who becomes the focus of the RDN's attention. With an infant, the parents or primary caregiver are responsible for food intake and should be instructed accordingly. With a child in grade school, the child, parents, and secondary caregivers (eg, grandparents, babysitters, teachers) should be involved in dietary management. The adolescent usually eats independently and needs to receive information directly; however, in most cases the parents provide and prepare the food and should also be informed of changes to the dietary prescription. The parents' desire to maintain control of the medical and nutrition regimen may conflict with the adolescent's growing independence.[77] Family members and primary caregivers should be involved to have appropriate foods available and to provide support for food and fluid limitations, as well as encouragement for nutrient consumption. Caregivers outside of the immediate family should be asked to be consistent in care to help the child follow his or her diet recommendations.

Messages from the health care team about the importance of nutrition can intensify attention to food intake and may add to parental stress or the risk for feeding problems (eg, food refusal, oral aversions, self-induced vomiting).[78,79] Infants are typically satisfied with small volumes of oral feedings, and many exhibit posttraumatic feeding disorders, gastrointestinal (GI) motility disorders, and GER.[14,16,80] Toddlers and young children often have poor or fussy appetites and a preference for salty foods if they have a salt-wasting condition and for commercial fast foods rather than homemade foods if they have been exposed to them through family, friends, or television. Parents frequently express frustration in feeding their infant or child, and they may pressure children to eat or give inappropriate attention to undesired behaviors and reward desired behaviors with minimal interaction. Families need guidance and constant support to establish and consistently enforce limits about food and unacceptable conduct at mealtimes, including instruction on rewarding desirable eating behaviors and ignoring undesirable actions.[78] Adolescents may have poor and irregular eating habits, skip meals, drink large quantities of high-phosphorus fluids, and patronize fast food restaurants with their friends. Nutrition education should focus on cafeteria foods, fast foods, snacks, and alternative drinks that can help an adolescent make safer selections when eating away from home.

The nutrition care plan requires ongoing modification based on changes in the child's age and development; appetite; GI function; rate of weight gain and linear growth; kidney function; biochemistries; medication regimen; compliance with diet, fluids, and medication; psychosocial situation; and treatment modality.[11]

Clinical exercise evaluation and regular physical activity are important components of the child's overall care plan.[81] Many physiological and lifestyle factors contribute to sedentary behavior and decreased physical fitness in children with CKD, more so than the general pediatric population.[82] Catabolism of lean body mass is a consequence of CKD and uremia, especially when there is inadequate intake of energy and protein. Regular physical activity can counteract these adverse effects and increase protein utilization and muscle mass.[83] Age and medically appropriate physical activity should be prescribed and encouraged often.

Medications should be reviewed concurrently with biochemistries because normal serum electrolytes or stable blood pressure may be the result of drug therapy and/or dietary restriction, and they can mask the risk for an altered biochemical state (eg, a low-phosphorus diet restriction would still be indicated for a child who is normophosphatemic but on phosphorus-binding medications). Medications should also be evaluated in terms of potential drug–nutrient interactions, which could adversely affect nutritional status or drug efficacy.[84,85]

Nutrient recommendations for children with CKD, on maintenance dialysis (MD), and post transplant should be used as a starting point. Recommendations may require modification during periods of acute illness or catabolic stress, for children significantly above or below their ideal body weight (IBW), or when a child's response to these recommendations is suboptimal. Restrictions are imposed only when clearly needed and should be individualized according to age, development, and food preferences. The use of chronological age is recommended for determining requirements and providing age-appropriate dietary recommendations.[11]

To increase energy intake for undernourished children and to improve adherence, the dietary modifications for children are typically less restrictive than for adults. Meeting energy demands for linear growth (and brain development in infancy) is unique to pediatrics and is a priority in the nutrition care plan. Pediatric dietary restrictions usually take the form of a "low–nutrient X diet" (eg, low-sodium diet), with education provided on which foods are high in that nutrient and guidance about acceptable alternatives and portion control of these foods. Depending on the response in the parameter relevant to that nutrient (eg, blood pressure, biochemical value, edema), the restriction can be liberalized or tightened. Children who are in early stages of CKD, who are polyuric, who have RKF, or who are undergoing PD or frequent HD usually require fewer diet restrictions.

CHRONIC KIDNEY DISEASE

The etiology of CKD in children can be congenital, hereditary, acquired, or metabolic; all causes can eventually lead to the need for KRT. For all etiologies, early referral to a pediatric nephrology team and active care helps limit or prevent growth failure, minimize biochemical and physiological consequences of uremia, enhance quality of life, and improve survival. Different etiologies of CKD may result in different nutritional needs. In general, consuming a normal diet, as indicated initially, with fewer processed food items may be recommended. Dietary modifications may be imposed when indicated by progression of kidney disease and abnormalities in blood pressure, anthropometric and biochemical parameters.[86]

NEPHROTIC SYNDROME

Acquired nephrotic syndrome is a cause of CKD in children and is characterized by the presence of severe proteinuria, hypoalbuminemia, hyperlipidemia, and edema. In children, nephrotic syndrome occurs most often between the ages of 18 months and 4 years, and more frequently in boys than girls. Nutrition management includes sodium and fluid restrictions during active periods of proteinuria and caloric control if undesirable weight gain occurs as a result of an increase in appetite from steroid use.[87] Protein supplementation to account for urinary losses is not recommended because animal studies have shown that the additional protein is catabolized to urea and excreted in the urine rather than being used to correct hypoalbuminemia.[88] Many children with nephrotic syndrome will not progress to end-stage kidney disease (ESKD), such as those diagnosed with minimal change disease. However, kidney biopsy may reveal a more severe disease, such as focal segmental glomerulosclerosis (FSGS). FSGS is the most common acquired cause of stage 5 kidney disease in children. It is characterized by sclerosis of the glomeruli and nonresponsiveness to steroid therapy. Only 20% to 30% with FSGS respond to steroid therapy, and one of every three children with FSGS progress to dialysis and/or transplant, often requiring more significant nutrition intervention.[89]

DIALYSIS

In contrast to the adult population requiring dialysis, the majority (56%) of pediatric patients are treated with PD rather than HD. Two types of PD are available: continuous ambulatory peritoneal dialysis (CAPD) and various forms of automated PD, including continuous

cyclic peritoneal dialysis (CCPD), intermittent peritoneal dialysis, tidal peritoneal dialysis (TPD), and nocturnal intermittent peritoneal dialysis (NIPD), which is sometimes called cyclic intermittent peritoneal dialysis. Approximately 70% to 75% of children on maintenance PD in North America are on a form of automated PD, with the use of CAPD being more common in developing countries.[1] See Chapter 7 for information on the different methods of PD.

HD treatments for children and adolescents are typically performed three to four times per week for 3 to 4 hours. Infants are usually unstable on HD and appropriately sized dialysis equipment may be difficult to obtain, leading to PD as a preferred therapy. Having the patient eat meals or snacks or drink an energy supplement during HD, or infusing an enteral feeding during HD can provide the additional nutrition needed for growth; however, agreement on the acceptance of these practices is not universal.[80] Several studies in adults have demonstrated an association between eating during dialysis and hemodynamic instability, hypotension, cramps, or other gastrointestinal symptoms, whereas other studies have not reflected this association.[90] In contrast to adults, children rarely have comorbidities like DM or significant cardiovascular issues that may lead to postprandial complications on dialysis. Children who consistently experience these symptoms during dialysis may experience fewer complications if food and fluids are not consumed before or during dialysis. Experience in using frequent (>5 sessions/wk) in-center or home HD in children is limited; however, preliminary data suggest that dietary and fluid restrictions are rarely required, and some children may need high-protein and high-phosphorus diets.[91-93] Children who switch dialysis modality or who have dialysis temporarily withheld for access problems need education on the required changes to their diet prescription.

TRANSPLANT

Kidney transplantation is the preferred treatment for children with CKD stage 5. It is not a cure but a continuum of CKD. A well-functioning graft eases dietary and fluid restrictions required during the dialysis period; however, children continue to need dietary modifications after transplantation to manage acute and long-term nutrition-related problems, many of which are associated with adverse effects of immunosuppressant medications (see Chapter 8). Ideally, a preemptive transplant is the treatment of choice and benefits children by maintaining their quality of life and improving growth potential. Compared with children established on dialysis at the time of transplant, children with preemptive transplants had significantly less growth retardation and improved survival benefits.[94]

In the first 6 to 12 months post transplant, rapid weight gain, increased BMI, as well as alterations in nutritionally related biochemical parameters are commonly observed. A hypercaloric intake may be the result of an improved appetite, reduced uremia and toxin buildup, fewer dietary restrictions, limited physical activity, and high doses of immunosuppressive medications.[95] Dietary intervention may be necessary to reduce the risk of obesity post transplant, along with the associated cardiovascular disease (CVD) risk. In general, dietary restrictions and mineral supplementation can be liberalized or discontinued based on changes in associated serum parameters. Immunosuppressive agents may cause nutrition-related side effects, such as nausea, vomiting, constipation, diarrhea, hyperlipidemia, hyperglycemia, anorexia, hypomagnesemia or hypophosphatemia, and these should be addressed symptomatically.[96,97]

A strong emphasis on growth and development continues after transplant. Normal adult height is the goal and is dependent on age and degree of height deficit at the time of transplant, steroid usage and dosages, and graft function.[98,99] Catch-up growth is seen primarily in the youngest ages (ie, those younger than 6 years).[1] The use of rhGH has successfully accelerated growth in the transplant population, without adverse effects on graft function. Typically, rhGH therapy is not started until at least 1 year after transplantation.[100] Children who are able to reach a normal stature post transplant are shown to maintain their graft function with an eGFR above 45 mL/min/1.73 m² for a longer duration compared to

those with continued short stature.[101] Nutrition management of children with suboptimally functioning grafts should be based on fluid status, blood pressure, relevant anthropometric and biochemical parameters, and treatment modality, in the same way as children with similar eGFRs pre transplant.

Nutrition Management

One of the most challenging aspects of living with kidney disease is modification of food and fluid intake. Necessary changes to the macronutrient and micronutrient content of a child's diet intrude on food preferences and have the potential to severely limit food choices when multiple restrictions are required or appetite is poor. Specific nutrients may be limited or encouraged, with changes occurring throughout the course of the disease. RDNs can ease the burden of successfully adopting diet alterations by providing practical suggestions for modifying or replacing favorite foods or fluids. RDNs are able to provide individualized care using their knowledge about infant and toddler feeding skills; infant formulas, pediatric and adult enteral supplements, tube feeding products, and pediatric parenteral nutrition solutions; eating habits of children and adolescents; behavior modification techniques; and the nutrient content of popular homemade and commercial foods, snacks, and drinks, including those of different cultures. RDNs will also utilize their skills in evaluating growth; body composition; and the physical, developmental, educational, and social needs of children. A trained pediatric renal RDN is best suited to care for children with CKD.[11]

ENERGY

Adequate intake of energy is important not only to promote weight gain and growth but also prevent protein from being used as an energy source through gluconeogenesis. Energy recommendations for children with CKD have traditionally been based on requirements for healthy children because there is a lack of evidence to suggest that children with CKD have greater require-

TABLE 13.4 | Energy and Protein Requirements for Infants, Children, and Adolescents With Chronic Kidney Disease Stages 2 Through 5D Aged 0 to 18 Years[a]

Month	SDI for infants[b] Energy[c] (kcal/kg/d)	Protein (g/kg/d)	Protein (g/d)
0	93-107	1.52-2.5	8-12
1	93-120	1.52-1.8	8-12
2	93-120	1.4-1.52	8-12
3	82-98	1.4-1.52	8-12
4	82-98	1.3-1.52	9-13
5	72-82	1.3-1.52	9-13
6-9	72-82	1.1-1.3	9-14
10-11	72-82	1.1-1.3	9-15
12	72-120	0.9-1.14	11-14

	SDI for children and adolescents			
Year	Energy (kcal/kg/d) Male	Female	Protein (g/kg/d)	Protein (g/d)
2	81-95[d]	79-92[d]	0.9-1.05	11-15
3	80-82	76-77	0.9-1.05	13-15
4-6	67-93	64-90	0.85-0.95	16-22
7-8	60-77	56-75	0.9-0.95	19-28
9-10	55-69	49-63	0.9-0.95	26-40
11-12	48-63	43-57	0.9-0.95	34-42
13-14	44-63	39-50	0.8-0.9	34-50
15-17	40-55	36-46	0.8-0.9	Male: 52-65 Female: 45-49

SDI = standard dietary intake

[a] For children with poor growth, reference to the standard dietary intake for height age may be appropriate. Height age is the age that corresponds to an individual's height when plotted on the 50th percentile on a growth chart.

[b] Gestation of 37 to 40 weeks. Premature infants have higher energy and protein requirements. The increased need for these and other particular nutrients (sodium, potassium, calcium, and phosphorus) must be balanced against the nutritional interventions to control the effects of CKD. This is outside the scope of this clinical practice recommendation.

[c] SDI is based on the Physical Activity Level (PAL) used by the international bodies: 1 through 3 year PAL 1.4: 4 through 9 year PAL 1.6; and 10 through 17 year PAL 1.8. Where guidelines have given a range of energy requirements for different levels of PAL, the lowest PAL has been taken for SDI energy in consideration that children with chronic kidney disease (CKD) are likely to have low activity levels.

[d] Scientific Advisory Committee on Nutrition reports energy requirements as kcal/d; male, 1,040 kcal/d; female, 932 kcal/d.

Adapted with permission from Shaw V, Polderman N, Renken-Terhaerdt J, et al. Energy and protein requirements for children with CKD stages 2–5 and on dialysis—clinical practice recommendations from the Pediatric Renal Nutrition Taskforce. *Pediatr Nephrol.* 2020;35(3):519-531.[105]

ments than healthy children or that the growth of children with CKD improves if their intake exceeds these amounts.[102,103] Therefore, the initial prescribed energy intake for infants, children, and adolescents with CKD or post transplant should be 100% of the estimated energy requirements for chronological age, adjusted individually for the child's physical activity level and body size (ie, BMI).[11,104] Stunted and underweight children are at risk for PEW and may require additional energy to catch up in growth. However, overfeeding promotes additional fat mass without promoting muscle regain. RDNs are able to determine adequate but not excessive feeding requirements to promote optimal growth.[80] Energy and protein requirements for infants, children, and adolescents with CKD stages 2 through 5D are summarized in Table 13.4.[105] Energy requirements for

BOX 13.3 | Estimated Energy Requirements for Overweight Children Aged 3 Through 18 Years[104,106]

GENDER	WEIGHT MAINTENANCE TOTAL ENERGY EXPENDITURE, KCAL/D
Boys	114 – (50.9 × Age in years) + Physical activity coefficient × (19.5 × Weight in kg + 1161.4 × Height in meters)
	Physical activity coefficient (PA)
	• PA = 1.00 if physical activity level (PAL) is estimated to be = 1.0 < 1.4 (sedentary)
	• PA = 1.12 if PAL is estimated to be = 1.4 < 1.6 (low active)
	• PA = 1.24 if PAL is estimated to be = 1.6 < 1.9 (active)
	• PA = 1.45 if PAL is estimated to be = 1.9 < 2.5 (very active)
Girls	389 – (41.2 × Age in years) + Physical activity coefficient × (15.0 × Weight in kg + 701.6 × Height in meters)
	PA
	• PA = 1.00 if PAL is estimated to be = 1.0 < 1.4 (sedentary)
	• PA = 1.18 if PAL is estimated to be = 1.4 < 1.6 (low active)
	• PA = 1.35 if PAL is estimated to be = 1.6 < 1.9 (active)
	• PA = 1.60 if PAL is estimated to be = 1.9 < 2.5 (very active)

overweight children (over the age of 3 years) are lower, and specific equations for weight management are recommended (see Box 13.3). Modifications can be made based on the rate of the child's response in terms of weight gain or loss, and adjusted for other changes, such as acute illness or disease progression.

Infants with anorexia, delayed gastric emptying, or GER frequently require supplementation with oral or tube feedings of fortified expressed breast milk or high-calorie formula. See Table 13.5 for examples of formulas. Depending on volumes and age, high-calorie breast milk or formulas containing 22 to 60 kcal/oz may be needed to meet the requirements. Gradual, stepwise increases in energy density of 2 to 4 kcal/oz theoretically improve tolerance.[107,108] As en-

ergy density increases, oral intake and gastrointestinal tolerance may decrease, and supplemental tube feeding may be needed. The timing and route of feedings may be adjusted to improve overall tolerance.[80] Infant formulas such as Good Start (Nestlé) and kidney-friendly Similac PM 60/40 (Abbott) contain less phosphorus than other cow's milk formulas and may be required by some infants to maintain normal serum levels. Good Start, as a regular infant formula, costs less than Similac PM 60/40, is readily available where infant formulas are sold, and is 100% whey based, which may or may not increase the rate of gastric emptying.[109-111] Similac PM 60/40 is 60% whey based and is advantageous for infants with hyperkalemia due to its lower potassium content. Many institutions utilize potassium-lowering

TABLE 13.5 | Nutrient Content of Select Infant Feedings[a]

Product	Energy (kcal/L)	Protein (g/L)	Fat (g/L)	Carbohydrate (g/L)	Osmolality (mOsm/kg H_2O)	Sodium (mg/L)	Potassium (mg/L)	Phosphorus (mg/L)
Breast milk (mean ± SD), term	680	10.5	39	72	290 ± 5	177	531	143
Cow's milk-based formula								
Enfamil Enfacare (Mead Johnson)	744	21	39	77	310	270	780	490
Enfamil Infant (Mead Johnson)	676	13.5	36	76	300	183	730	290
Good Start Gentle (Gerber)	676	14.7	34.2	75	250	181	724	255
Similac Advance (Abbott)	643	13.3	36	69	310	161	707	283
Similac Alimentum (Abbott)	676	18.6	37.5	69	370	298	798	507
Similac PM 60/40 (Abbott)[b]	676	15	37.9	69	280	162	541	189
Soy-based formula								
Good Start Soy (Gerber)	676	16.9	34.5	75.1	180	271	785	426
Similac Soy Isomil (Abbott)	643	15.76	35.11	66.9	200	296	707	508
Enfamil Prosobee (Mead Johnson)	676	16.9	36	72	178	240	810	470

SD = standard deviation
[a] For the most current nutrient content, refer to product labels or packaging.
[b] Designed for dietary management of individuals with kidney failure 1 year and older.

medications to pretreat formula; however, minerals and electrolytes should be monitored closely as other nutrients may be altered as well. Soy formulas are not typically recommended for children with reduced kidney function or preterm infants due to known aluminum content; however, they may be provided in cases of parent preference or specific medical needs.[112]

Renastart (Vitaflo USA), a pediatric renal formula, is for children with kidney failure 1 year and older; however, it may be mixed with infant formula to further lower electrolyte content if a pretreatment medication will not be used. Hypokalemia and other nutrient deficiency have been reported as a consequence of its very low kidney-specific nutrient content. It should, therefore, be used cautiously as a stand-alone formula and only with appropriate nutrient-intake monitoring.

Often, it is not possible to increase the energy density of a formula by concentration because of the resulting increase in sodium, potassium, phosphorus, and other nutrients for which serum levels are already elevated. The choice to add a carbohydrate modular, a fat modular, or a combination of both modulars should be based on serum glucose and lipid profiles, the presence or the absence of malabsorption or respiratory distress (carbohydrate metabolism increases carbon dioxide production), and the preparation burden and cost to the family or caregiver. In addition, when making a formula with more than two to three increases in energy density, an attempt should be made to preserve a similar distribution of energy from carbohydrate and fat as in the base formula. Unless malabsorption is present, a heart-healthy oil such as corn, canola, or safflower may be used. To prevent the oil from separating out during continuous tube feedings, an oil that contains emulsified fat (Microlipid by Nestlé) may be useful. Table 13.6 provides examples of modular products.

Minimizing the number of restrictions in the diet with identification and modification of favorite and appropriate foods are the first steps to achieving energy goals for older children. Foods commonly found in the home will most likely have better acceptance than oral nutrition supplements. Children with poor appetites

TABLE 13.6 | Nutrient Content of Selected Modular Products[a]

Modular product	Energy (kcal)	Protein (g)	Fat (g)	Carbohydrate (g)	Sodium (mg)	Potassium (mg)	Phosphorus (mg)
Carbohydrate products (per 100 g)							
Polycal (Nutricia)	384	0	0	96	2	0	0
SolCarb (Medica)	376	0	0	94.5	70	1	8
Fat products (per 100 mL)							
Corn, canola, or safflower oil	813	0	92	0	0	0	0
Medium-chain triglycerides oil (Nestlé)	773	0	93	0	0	0	0
Microlipid (Nestlé)	450	0	50	0	0	0	0
Liquigen (Nutricia)	450	0	50	0	5	0.1	nl
Carbohydrate and fat products (per 100 g)							
Duocal (Nutricia)	492	0	22	73	≤20	≤5	≤5
Protein products (per 100 g)							
Protifar (Nutricia)	373	89	1.6	<1.5	30	50	700
Beneprotein (Nestlé)	357	86	0	0	215	500	215
Liquid protein fortifier (per mL)	0.67	0.167	0	0	0	0	0

nl = not listed
[a] For the most current nutrient content, refer to product labels or packaging.

TABLE 13.7 | Nutrient Content of Pediatric Feedings[a]

Formula	Energy (kcal/L)	Protein (g/L)	Fat (g/L)	Carbohydrate (g/L)	Osmolality (mOsm/kg H_2O)	Sodium (mg/L)	Potassium (mg/L)	Phosphorus (mg/L)
Compleat Pediatric (6.8 g of fiber per L) (Nestlé)	1,000	38	38	136	400	760	1,700	1,080
Compleat Pediatric Organic Blends, Chicken (Nestlé)	1,200	43	53	137	710	833	2,000	1,167
Nutren Junior/Nutren Jr With Fiber (6 g of fiber per L) (Nestlé)	1,000	30	49.6	110	350	460	1,320	840
Pediasure Enteral (Abbott)	1,000	30	38	139	335	380	1,308	844
Pediasure Enteral With Fiber (13 g of fiber per L) (Abbott)	1,000	30	38	143	350	380	1,308	844
Renastart (Vitaflo)	1,000	15	48	124	230	420	190	166
Pediasure 1.5 Cal (Abbott)	1,500	59	67.5	160	370	380	1,646	1,055
Boost Kid Essentials 1.0 (Nestlé)	1,000	29.2	38	133	550-600	625	1,458	938
Boost Kid Essentials 1.5 (Nestlé)	1,500	42	75	163	390-405	750	1,958	1,333

[a] For the most current nutrient content, refer to product labels or packaging.

may respond to small, frequent meals and snacks. Energy can be added to foods using heart-healthy butter or oils, cream and other fats, cream cheese, syrups, or carbohydrate modulars. Milkshakes and desserts with an added high-calorie modular or foods (eg, peanut butter, whole-fat milk and cream, or low–phosphorus nondairy products when hyperphosphatemia is an issue) may be encouraged. Low-calorie or calorie-free drinks should typically be avoided.

Supplemental nutrition support should be considered when a child is not gaining weight or growing normally and fails to meet requirements for energy. If intake is adequate and there is no sign of malnutrition, supplementation may cause obesity without improving linear growth. Oral supplementation is preferred, followed by tube feeding.[80,113] Commercial supplements (eg, fruit-flavored beverages, milkshake-type drinks, puddings, and bars) may be used; however, their phos-

phorus and potassium content should be considered. Nonrenal pediatric feedings designed for children older than 1 year (Table 13.7) have fairly high calcium and phosphorus content, which may prove problematic.

Renastart, a pediatric renal formula, is used for children with kidney failure aged 1 year and older. Adult renal products designed to be energy dense, high or low in protein, and low in electrolytes and phosphorus (see Chapter 15) are recommended for children aged 4 years and older but have been used successfully at diluted strength in children as young as 1 year of age, with some limited experience in those patients younger than 1 year.[114] Serum magnesium levels should be monitored carefully in toddlers who use these adult products because the magnesium content is significantly higher than in breast milk or infant and pediatric formulas. If necessary, these products can be mixed to provide the appropriate protein content for an individual child. The cost of products and the lack of third-party reimbursement may deter use of supplements; the involvement of a social worker is invaluable.

Enteral tube feeding should be considered when a child is unable to meet nutritional goals orally.[113] Nasogastric (NG), gastrostomy (G), and gastrojejunostomy (GJ) tubes have all been used successfully to provide additional nutrition by intermittent bolus or continuous infusion and improve weight gain and growth.[10,115-117] Reported complications associated with NG and G feeding include emesis, exit-site erythema and infection, leakage, and, for children on PD, peritonitis.[118] To minimize the risk of peritonitis, a G-tube insertion should ideally occur prior to placement of a PD catheter, whenever possible.[11,80,113] The choice of formula and feeding route is guided by age, mineral and electrolyte imbalances, fluid allowance, presence of vomiting, consideration of financial costs to the family or caregiver, and potential length of need. In most cases, minimizing the volume of feeds is necessary to maintain fluid balance, optimize feeding tolerance, and keep the duration of feeding times manageable within the child's daily schedule. Continuous overnight and daytime bolus feeds are often used in an individualized manner to meet a child's nutritional needs. In children who have long-term feeding needs, a G-tube or GJ-tube may be more appropriate due to reduced nasal irritation and possible impairment to oral intake. Infants and toddlers who have been tube fed may experience a difficult transition to oral feeding.[119] Careful attention to oral stimulation and involvement of a multidisciplinary feeding program enable most children who are tube fed to meet their nutrition requirements orally without tube feeding within 1 year post transplant.[115,120-123]

The progressive decline in kidney function often causes anorexia and failure to achieve prescribed energy goals.[26] The timely initiation of KRT in children may prevent malnutrition. In adults, the initiation of dialysis increased dietary protein intake (DPI), lean body mass, and the subjective global assessment rating in patients started on PD, and increased DPI and serum albumin in patients undergoing HD.[123]

Peritoneal Dialysis

Children undergoing PD may experience early satiety or anorexia due to feelings of fullness from the indwelling dialysate exerting pressure on the stomach or the negative effect of absorption of the dialysate glucose on the brain's appetite control center. Supplemental tube feeding may be required for children who are unable to meet their nutritional requirements orally; wherever possible, placement of G- or GJ-tubes should occur before starting PD to decrease the risk of peritonitis.[80,113] Intraperitoneal dialysate glucose absorption in children on CAPD increased energy obtained by approximately 7 to 10 kcal/kg.[124] The absorption of glucose during the shorter dwell times of CCPD, TPD, and NIPD have not been studied in children. Energy absorbed from the dialysate glucose should not be included in the total energy intake unless the child is gaining weight at a rate quicker than desired, despite oral and enteral intakes that are lower than average.[11] Obesity is most often seen in infants on PD, and occasionally in adolescents requiring dialysate with high glucose concentrations for ultrafiltration. The use of dialysate-containing icodextrin, a nonabsorbable glucose polymer, in place of dextrose may improve fluid removal, prevent weight gain, and limit excessive glucose uptake, which may aid in the management of hyperglycemia and hyperlipidemia.[125,126]

Hemodialysis

HD is a catabolic procedure leading to negative protein balance; children with CKD on MD are at risk for protein–energy malnutrition exacerbated by uremia, postdialysis fatigue, and anorexia due to loss of appetite. Intradialytic parenteral nutrition (IDPN) is a noninvasive method of providing carbohydrate, protein, and lipids to undernourished patients via HD venous access during dialysis. The parenteral nutrition volume is concurrently removed via ultrafiltration. Existing evidence shows that IDPN is a safe and effective treatment for malnutrition.[127] IDPN is costly; furthermore, lack of complete insurance coverage and availability limits its use in many facilities.

Procedures for initiating IDPN vary based on the institution. An example protocol from Texas Children's Hospital Renal Dialysis Unit is presented here.[127]

> IDPN is indicated if 2 or more of the following criteria are met:
> - >10% loss of body weight in 3 months in a patient with <90% IBW
> - Unable to meet nutritional needs with enteral feeds
>   o Fluid restriction
>   o Trials to increase enteral feeds fail
>   o Gastrointestinal disease (required for Medicare reimbursement for IDPN without objective data of malnutrition)
> - Clinical signs of malnutrition
>   o Serum albumin <3.5 mg/dL
>   o Low [normalized protein catabolic rate] nPCR <1 g/kg/d

Hyperglycemia, electrolyte derangements secondary to refeeding syndrome, and hyperlipidemia are common adverse effects. Glucose, triglycerides, and electrolytes need to be checked prior to IDPN initiation and carefully monitored. IDPN is not a sole source of nutrition and its use should be limited to supplement intake in organically malnourished children who cannot meet the requisite needs via oral and enteral routes.[11]

Transplant

Children receiving a successful kidney transplant often experience an increase in appetite that makes weight control a challenge. A rapid increase in weight ZS occurs across all ages within the first 6 months post transplant. Children increase an average of 0.81 ZS in weight in the first year after transplant, with comparative consistency in average weight ZS over the next 5 years.[1] Weight gain may be greater in children who were obese pretransplant.[128] Children with obesity who undergo kidney transplantation have shown decreased short- and long-term kidney graft survival and increased risk of mortality.[128-130] Large steroid doses in the first 6 months after transplant increase insulin secretion, causing glucose uptake by fat cells, impaired glucose tolerance, glycosuria, and a relative resistance to insulin. Posttransplant

DM occurs in less than 3% of pediatric transplant recipients; the immunosuppressive agent tacrolimus is another significant risk factor.[131] For these and other long-term health reasons (eg, HTN and hyperlipidemia), the goal is to achieve and maintain BMI-for-age within the healthy range by controlling total energy intake through limiting use of total and saturated fats and avoidance of simple sugars, as well as participating in regular physical activity. Water and drinks low in simple sugars are the suggested beverages for normal weight or overweight children with high minimum total fluid intakes in the posttransplant period.[11]

PROTEIN

DPI in children with CKD is typically far in excess of average requirements for healthy children; however, protein malnutrition may occur in spite of adequate protein intake when energy intake is low.[132-134] Requirements are increased by catabolism, peritonitis, and steroid use. Protein breakdown and amino acid oxidation are also increased to buffer excess hydrogen ions during metabolic acidosis. While adequate protein intake is necessary for optimal growth and health (see Table 13.8 on page 266), KDOQI Clinical Practice Guidelines suggests that excess protein intake be avoided.[11] While there is no evidence that protein restriction has a nephroprotective effect, therapeutic goals in CKD should focus on avoiding excessive protein intake for the purposes of preventing uremia, reducing metabolic acidosis, and limiting dietary intake of phosphorus, which is commonly found in protein-rich foods.[134] Studies suggest that children with CKD stage 3 limit their protein intake to 100% to 140% of the Dietary Reference Intake (DRI) for IBW and that children with CKD stage 4 or 5 limit their DPI to 100% to 120% of the DRI for IBW (see Table 13.8 as well as Table 13.4).[105]

Protein intake is occasionally inadequate, potentially in association with anorexia, chewing problems, or strict dietary phosphorus control. Protein intake should be increased if clinical evaluation suggests protein malnutrition (eg, suboptimal dietary intake, low serum urea, and an undesirable decrease in nPCR for adolescents

TABLE 13.8 | Recommended Dietary Protein Intake in Children With Chronic Kidney Disease Stages 3 Through 5, 5D, and Transplant

Dietary protein intake recommendation, g/kg/d					
Age	**DRI**	**CKD stage 3, 3T[a]**	**CKD stages 4-5, 4T to 5T[b]**	**HD[c]**	**PD[d]**
0-6 mo	1.5	1.5-2.1	1.5-1.8	1.6	1.8
7-12 mo	1.2	1.2-1.7	1.2-1.5	1.3	1.5
1-3 y	1.05	1.05-1.5	1.05-1.25	1.15	1.3
4-13 y	0.95	0.95-1.35	0.95-1.15	1.05	1.1
14-18 y	0.85	0.85-1.2	0.85-1.05	0.95	1.0

CKD = chronic kidney disease | DRI = Dietary Reference Intake | HD = hemodialysis | PD = peritoneal dialysis | T = transplant
[a] 100%–140% DRI
[b] 100%–120% DRI
[c] DRI + 0.1 g/kg/d to compensate for dialytic losses
[d] DRI + 0.15 to 0.3 g/kg/d, depending on patient's age to compensate for peritoneal losses
Adapted with permission from the National Kidney Foundation. KDOQI Clinical Practice Guidelines for nutrition in children with CKD: 2008 update. *Am J Kidney Dis*. 2009;53(suppl 2):S1-S124.[11]

on HD). Minced or chopped meat, chicken, fish, egg, tofu, or unenriched fat-free milk powder can be added to soups, pasta, or casseroles. Milk and milk products can be substituted for meat per preference; however, phosphorus intake may increase. Egg whites and egg white powder are low phosphorus sources of protein that can be used to supplement the diet. Plant-based protein sources can also be considered as phosphorus from plant foods is less bioavailable, although one must still be mindful of potassium content.[135] Protein modulars (see Table 13.6) can be added to expressed breast milk or infant formula, strained foods, cereals, beverages, and moist foods. Protein-containing liquid or pudding supplements are other alternatives. Vegetarians, especially those following strict vegan diets, may need specific dietary recommendations to meet individual protein needs.[136]

Dialysis

The initial DPI for children on dialysis should be based on 100% of the DRI for their chronological age plus an additional increment based on anticipated dialysis losses of amino acids and protein. In addition to traditional

methods of dietary evaluation, DPI can be indirectly estimated from urea kinetics, provided the child is in nitrogen balance. In stable children, the protein nitrogen appearance equals the DPI. In undernourished children with poor appetites, urea kinetic modeling can suggest if inadequate dialysis may be a factor. Children with a low urea may seem to be well dialyzed but may actually have a low Kt/V, which is indicative of insufficient dialysis, and poor protein intake.[11]

Peritoneal dialysis Protein losses are similar for CAPD, CCPD, and TPD but vary widely among individuals; protein losses range from 0.35 mg/kg/d for infants to 0.15 g/kg/d for older children.[137] Requirements are higher for infants and toddlers based on g protein per kg body weight because protein losses are inversely related to body weight and peritoneal membrane surface area, and rapid growth rates can occur during this time. Children unable to maintain adequate oral or enteral protein intake may benefit from the use of amino acids as the osmotic agent in the dialysis solution to compensate for protein and amino acid losses and improve nitrogen balance.[138] Therapy using amino acid-containing dialysis solutions (intraperitoneal amino acid [IPAA] therapy or intraperitoneal nutrition [IPN]) permits provision of nitrogen carriers without any phosphate load and has the ultrafiltering capacity of lower-concentration (1.36%) glucose-containing solutions. To avoid using the amino acids for energy, the solution has usually been given during the day when meals or snacks provide a source of energy. Recent studies have explored the benefit of giving the amino acid solution overnight via a cycler, coupled with the usual glucose solutions as an energy source, and results suggest an anabolic effect.[139-141] The routine use of IPAA is impractical due to high costs, and long-term studies of its use are needed.[11] Use of IPN remains limited.

The use of normalized protein equivalent of nitrogen appearance (PNA) as a measure of protein intake in children on PD has received some study and is performed in some centers a few times per year.[11] Equations for estimating total nitrogen appearance that consider the child's age and body size have been proposed.[142,143] From these equations, PNA can be calculated as follows:

Protein equivalent of nitrogen appearance =
Total nitrogen appearance × 6.25 g protein/g nitrogen

Hemodialysis The protein losses in children on HD have not been measured, and recommendations are based on extrapolation from adult data. KDOQI Clinical Practice Guidelines suggests that children on HD should have their initial DPI based on the DRI for chronological age with an additional increment of 0.1 g/kg/d to replace dialysis amino acid and protein losses.[11] Higher than expected predialysis urea levels can occur for a variety of reasons, including excessive protein intake, adequate protein but insufficient energy intake, catabolism (eg, infection), inadequate dialysis, and recirculation of blood secondary to the condition of the vascular access. Persistently low urea levels may indicate overall inadequate protein and energy intake.

There is limited research on the use of nPCR to estimate DPI in children on HD.[144] In a single-center study, nPCR values of less than 1 g/kg/d predicted sustained weight loss of equal to or greater than 2% body weight for 3 consecutive months in adolescents.[50] In infants and younger children, nPCR did not predict outcomes (ie, weight loss), possibly due to differences between younger and older children in nutritional status and intake, urine urea clearance, protein catabolism, and growth rates. Current clinical practice guidelines recommend monthly assessment of nPCR on HD as trends for a particular patient can provide an objective measure of protein intake or changes. nPCR can be calculated in children as follows[11]:

$$G\ (mg/min) = \frac{[(C2 \times V2) - (C1 \times V1)]}{t}$$

$$nPCR = \frac{5.43 \times Est\ G}{V1 + 0.17}$$

where G= urea generation rate; C1= postdialysis blood urea nitrogen (BUN) (mg/dL); C2 = predialysis BUN (mg/dL); V1 = postdialysis total body water in dL (V1 = 5.8 dL/kg × postdialysis weight in kg); V2 = predialysis total body water in dL (V2 = 5.8 dL/kg × predialysis weight in kg); t = time in minutes from the end of the dialysis treatment to the start of the following treatment; and Est G= estimated urea generation rate determined from calculation 1

Transplant

Higher protein requirements in the immediate post-transplant period to compensate for adverse consequences of surgical stress and high-dose steroid therapy (ie, high nitrogen losses, catabolism, and decreased anabolism) may be appropriate.[145] Protein requirements for children with well-functioning kidney transplants following surgical healing are similar to those for healthy children (ie, 100% of DRI). Recommended requirements for children with transplants whose eGFR is less than 60 mL/min/1.73 m^2 (ie, CKD stages 3 through 5T) are comparable to children without transplants who have a similar eGFR. A successful kidney transplant improves appetite in association with feeling well and promotes an increase in the quantity of food consumed; achieving adequate protein intake is rarely a concern. Children with CKD stages 2 through 5 who have had transplants should also avoid excessive DPI, similar to their peers who have not had transplants.[11]

FAT

Fats are a crucial source of energy for growing children; inadequate intake over time can lead to negative energy balance, malnutrition, and essential fatty acid deficiency. The recommended acceptable macronutrient distribution ranges (AMDRs) for adults is 20% to 35% of total energy from fat, whereas in children, the recommended ranges are 30% to 40% between the ages of 1 and 3 years and 25% to 35% between the ages of 4 and 18 years.[103]

Conversely, excessive caloric intake from fat, specifically *trans* fat and most types of saturated fats, is associated with an increase in low-density lipoprotein (LDL) cholesterol and may be associated with a risk of chronic diseases, such as coronary heart disease, obesity, and DM.[104] Hyperlipidemia (seen most often as hypertriglyceridemia, high very low-density lipoprotein [VLDL] and intermediate-density lipoprotein cholesterol, and normal to moderately elevated levels of total and high-density lipoprotein [HDL] cholesterol) occurs in children with CKD stage 3 and increases in prevalence in the later stages of CKD.[146-149] The metabolic abnormalities associated with dyslipidemia in this population are complex; decreased lipoprotein catabolism and increased lipogenesis are thought to be potential mechanisms.[147] Children diagnosed with glomerular disease or nephrotic range proteinuria demonstrated increased risks for high total cholesterol and LDL cholesterol. Overweight or obesity, elevated proteinuria, hypocalcemia, and 1,25-dihydroxyvitamin D deficiency were associated with low HDL cholesterol.[150] Atherosclerosis and the progression of glomerular injury are potential risks of elevated plasma lipids.[151]

Children with CKD are a high-risk population for CVD, and CVD is the leading cause of morbidity and mortality in this population.[152,153] Therefore, dietary measures to control dyslipidemia by promoting heart-healthy oils, avoiding saturated and *trans* fats, keeping total fat intake within recommended AMDRs, and choosing complex carbohydrates over simple sugars, whenever possible, are perceived to be prudent.[11,104] There are no AMDRs for children younger than 1 year old; therefore, when increasing the caloric density of infant formulas, it is suggested that the distribution of calories from macronutrients be kept within standards set by the WHO for formula manufacturers (ie, protein: 7%–12%; fat: 40%–54%; carbohydrate: 36%–56%).[154] When children with CKD received enteral feeding with formulas that provided an appropriate energy intake with a balanced fat and carbohydrate profile, serum lipid levels were not adversely affected.[155]

Therapeutic lifestyle changes—dietary modification, healthy weight maintenance, increased physical activity, and avoidance of hyperglycemia, if present—may be considered appropriate for children, particularly adolescents, with CKD. However, the patient's age, along with clinical circumstances, and risks and benefits of dietary modification to disease risk should be considered. Specifically, modifications to reduce total fat and calories should be adopted judiciously and may not be appropriate for undernourished children.[156,157] Family and cultural preferences should also be considered.

Dialysis

Dyslipidemia is characteristic of children on MD, particularly elevated triglyceride levels (TG). The etiology is multifactorial and thought to involve diminished clearance of VLDL and chylomicrons, as well as impaired HDL antioxidant, anti-inflammatory, and reverse cholesterol transport activities and maturation.

Given that dyslipidemia is associated with atherosclerotic CVD events and mortality in the general population, therapeutic lifestyle modifications are generally recommended for children on dialysis in order to improve dyslipidemia and prevent future CVD complications. Notably, however, that hypercholesterolemia, LDL cholesterol, and elevated TG:HDL cholesterol ratios may not be appropriate indicators for CVD risk in this population. Paradoxically, elevated levels of some of these traditional risk factors have been associated with improved survival in populations with CKD—a phenomenon termed *reverse epidemiology*.[158] In fact, very low levels of total cholesterol and TG may increase the risk for all-cause and CVD mortality likely due to their association with PEW—which, as discussed previously in this chapter, is a common concern in children with CKD.[157-160] Modifications to enhance energy intake in undernourished children and electrolyte restrictions generally take precedence and make macronutrient manipulations more challenging in pediatric populations with CKD.[11,153,156,157]

Clinicians should also be cognizant of the fact that CKD-related dyslipidemia does not restrict itself to affecting children who are overweight. While obesity and insulin resistance may likely worsen the condition, in children with CKD, dyslipidemia is equally attributable, if not more, to impaired lipid metabolism rather than dietary excess. For the aforementioned reasons, the NKF KDOQI work group recommends reserving therapeutic lifestyle changes specifically directed to reduce cholesterol intake in children with non–HDL cholesterol greater than 145 mg/dL or LDL cholesterol greater than 130 mg/dL or those who are overweight.[159] Likewise, the Kidney Disease: Improving Global Outcomes Guidelines suggest healthy lifestyle changes for children with severe hypertriglyceridemia (fasting serum levels TG >500 mg/dL) with the caveat that clinical judgment is needed before recommending dietary modifications, if at all, in children who are malnourished.[157]

Many of the medications currently used to treat adult dyslipidemia have not been approved in the pediatric population, and clinical practice guidelines suggest that children aged 18 years and younger with CKD not be treated with statin medications.[153,159] Research demonstrates that omega-3 supplementation has a beneficial effect on the lipid profile and oxidative stress in children with CKD.[157,161,162] Finally, carnitine depletion has the potential to contribute to hypertriglyceridemia due to its role in the transportation of long-chain fatty acids across the mitochondria to be oxidized in the production of cellular energy. Secondary carnitine deficiency in kidney disease is multifactorial; causes include insufficient renal production, reduced caloric intake, loss via dialysis, and altered urinary excretion. Unfortunately, pediatric clinical trials of L-carnitine supplementation for dyslipidemia are limited.[163-165] Furthermore, additional pediatric research is needed as to the use of L-carnitine supplementation to improve outcomes in areas that have shown benefit in adult nephrology, such as cardiovascular dysfunction, erythropoietin-resistant anemia, impaired exercise and functional capacities, and intradialytic hypotension.[165]

Transplant

Dyslipidemia occurs frequently in children with CKD even after transplantation.[157] Etiology is multifactorial; factors include immunosuppressant medications, obesity, recurring disease, and proteinuria in graft nephropathy.[96] Rates of prevalence may be lower with more recent immunosuppressant protocols that are corticosteroid free. Dietary modification remains the first-line therapy for hyperlipidemia in children with transplants, although some patients may need pharmacotherapy to reach target levels. Lowering total energy intake and reducing the percentage of calories from fats and added sugars may benefit weight management in children who are overweight and obese.[11] Omega-3 supplementation may also have positive results on lipid profiles and CVD risk factors in pediatric kidney transplant recipients, although there is limited research in the area.[166]

VITAMINS AND MINERALS

CKD alters the status of many vitamins and minerals that are essential for growth and development.[84] The risk for deficiencies is increased by limited volume or variety of dietary intake, abnormal gastrointestinal absorption, abnormal renal metabolism, drug–nutrient interactions, and dialysis losses. Little is known about the vitamin requirements or status of children with CKD. Experts recommended that all children with CKD stages 2 through 5, 5D, and 5T receive 100% of the DRI for B vitamins; vitamins A, C, E, and K; folic acid; copper; and zinc.[11,167-170] Supplementation is suggested when dietary intake is less than 100% of the DRI or if there is clinical or laboratory evidence of deficiency or potential loss.[11]

Hyperhomocysteinemia, a risk factor for vascular disease, is a feature of CKD and is associated with low folate status when compared with rates in healthy children. Supplementation with folic acid increases serum red cell folate levels and reduces homocysteine levels in children with CKD; however, correction of hyperhomocysteinemia in adults with CKD has not resulted in risk reduction of CVD.[171-175]

Blood levels of fat-soluble vitamins A and E are usually normal or elevated, even without supplementation; therefore, supplementation is generally avoided.[176,177] Hypervitaminosis A can contribute to hypercalcemia in children with CKD and should be checked at least annually.[178] Although vitamin K is not cleared by the kidney or dialysis, deficiency is possible, especially for children with poor dietary intakes and those who receive frequent antibiotics. Vitamin K status plays an important role in bone health and is therefore of interest.

In the absence of a pediatric renal vitamin supplement in North America, a renal water-soluble vitamin preparation specifically formulated for adult patients undergoing dialysis is often used (see Chapter 17 for a comparison of renal multivitamin products). These preparations are designed to contain 100 mg or less of vitamin C to avoid complications of retention of oxalate, a vitamin C metabolite for which the kidney is the only route of excretion. Smaller doses (eg, ½ tablet) or less frequent dosing (eg, one tablet every 2 days) can be used for infants and young children. A crushed or dissolved tablet can be used for infants and children who have difficulty swallowing intact tablets or receive enteral feeding; alternatively, a liquid water-soluble vitamin product can be used, where available.

Children of all ages who receive an erythropoietin-stimulating agent to treat renal anemia usually require large amounts of supplemental iron. Iron supplements are prescribed based on the levels of serum ferritin and transferrin saturation and may be provided orally or intravenously.[179]

Dialysis

Children on dialysis have additional risk of vitamin and mineral deficiencies associated with increased losses during dialysis treatment. Three small studies of children on PD have demonstrated intakes of most vitamins below the recommended amounts for healthy children.[180-182] For this reason, a water-soluble vitamin supplement is suggested for children on dialysis. Children who eat a healthy amount and a variety of food, or who receive the majority of their nutrition from complete enteral feedings, particularly adult renal products, may meet 100% of the DRI and may not require supplementation.[11] Excess magnesium levels have been reported in children, especially in those receiving supplemental feedings.[80]

Transplant

Multivitamin supplementation is generally not necessary after a successful kidney transplant because dietary mineral and electrolyte restrictions are removed or liberalized and appetite significantly improves. However, if the transplanted kidney function declines, CKD nutrient recommendations may need to be resumed. Hypomagnesemia occurs early in patients treated with calcineurin inhibitors (ie, tacrolimus).[96] The amount of dietary magnesium needed to correct hypomagnesemia is rarely achievable, and supplements are usually required in the initial posttransplant period but are rarely needed in the long term.[183] Hypophosphatemia

is also often seen in the initial posttransplant period due to persistent elevated levels of parathyroid hormone (PTH) and fibroblastic growth factor 23. A healthy, high-phosphorus diet and potentially phosphorus supplementation, may be needed.[184] 25-hydroxyvitamin D levels should be monitored and maintained as well.

PHOSPHORUS, CALCIUM, AND VITAMIN D

In children, chronic kidney disease–mineral and bone disorder (CKD–MBD) is associated with poor growth, tissue calcification, bone deformities, fracture risk, and chronic pain.[185] Managing CKD–MBD is especially important for children with immature skeletal and cardiovascular systems in development.[186] The goal of nutrition therapy is to achieve normal levels of serum calcium, phosphorus (see Table 13.9); 25-hydroxyvitamin D; and 1,25-dihydroxyvitamin D.[186-188] Hypocalcemia, hyperphosphatemia, and hyperparathyroidism result from low activity of renal 1-α-hydroxylase and cause high-turnover bone disease. Overtreatment can result in hypercalcemia, hypophosphatemia, hypoparathyroidism, and adynamic bone disease. Both hypercalcemia and hyperphosphatemia have been shown to contribute to soft-tissue and cardiovascular calcifications, as well as CVD. Therefore, the management of calcium, phosphorus, and vitamin D requires careful monitoring and adjustment of therapies to keep serum levels within the desired ranges.[135,186-188]

TABLE 13.9 | Normal Ranges for Blood Levels of Ionized and Total Calcium and Phosphorus

Age	Ionized calcium (mmol/L)[a]	Total calcium (mg/dL)[a]	Phosphorus (mg/dL)[b]
0-5 mo	1.22-1.40	8.7-11.3	5.2-8.4
6-12 mo	1.20-1.40	8.7-11.0	5.0-7.8
1-5 y	1.22-1.32	9.4-10.8	4.5-6.5
6-12 y	1.15-1.32	9.4-10.3	3.6-5.8
13-20 y	1.12-1.30	8.8-10.2	2.3-4.5

[a] To convert ionized and total calcium: mg/dL × 0.25 = mmol/L
[b] To convert phosphorus: mg/dL × 0.323 = mmol/L
Reproduced with permission from National Kidney Foundation. KDOQI Clinical Practice Guidelines for nutrition in children with CKD: 2008 update. Am J Kidney Dis. 2009;53(suppl 2):S67.[11]

Hyperphosphatemia is associated with renal osteo-dystrophy in children with CKD, as well as with CVD in adults with CKD. In children with CKD stage 5, evidence of an association between hyperphosphatemia and vascular damage has been observed.[189,190] Even before serum phosphorus levels become elevated, typically in CKD stage 3, dietary phosphorus restriction can aid in the management of hyperparathyroidism. For this reason, it is suggested that when serum PTH is elevated, dietary phosphorus intake should be limited to equal to or less than 100% of the DRI for age (Table 13.10) when phosphorus levels are normal, and equal to or less than 80% of the DRI once phosphorus levels become elevated.[11] That said, it should be noted that the updated guidelines recommend treatment of overt hyperphosphatemia, aiming for normal serum phosphorus ranges, but not necessarily maintaining them.[191]

TABLE 13.10 | Suggested Maximal Oral and Enteral Phosphorus Intake, mg/d

| Age | Phosphorus DRI, mg/d | Maximal oral and enteral phosphorus intake, mg/d | |
		If PTH is high and phosphorus is normal[a]	If both PTH and phosphorus are high[b]
0-6 mo	100	≤100	≤80
7-12 mo	275	≤275	≤220
1-3 y	460	≤460	≤370
4-8 y	500	≤500	≤400
9-18 y	1,250	≤1,250	≤1,000

DRI = Dietary Reference Intake | PTH = parathyroid hormone.
[a] ≤100% of the DRI.
[b] ≤80% of the DRI.
Reproduced with permission from National Kidney Foundation. KDOQI Clinical Practice Guidelines for nutrition in children with CKD: 2008 update. *Am J Kidney Dis.* 2009;53(suppl 2):S1-S124.[11]

It bears repeating that normal phosphorus ranges are higher for infants and young children, reflecting the need for bone mineralization (see Table 13.9). Non–breastfed infants who are hyperphosphatemic (>7.8 mg/dL for infants over 6 months) may require a low-phosphorus formula (Similac PM 60/40; Good Start) (see Table 13.5), which may be continued after 1 year of age to delay introducing phosphorus-rich

cow's milk. Milk and milk products are usually limited to one serving per day, in combination with avoidance of other high-phosphorus foods. Plant-based, nondairy milks, creamers, cheeses, and frozen desserts, if low in phosphorus and without phosphorus additives, can be used in place of dairy products.

Protein and phosphorus are often found in the same foods, so the goal should be to ensure an adequate protein intake while minimizing phosphorus intake. Dietary recommendations should be individualized to the patient, but, in general, foods highest in bioavailable phosphorus should be avoided. Previously, it was recommended to identify foods with low phosphorus to protein content; favorable foods were identified as those with an upper limit of 12 mg phosphorus per gram of protein. However, further studies on this topic have revealed that intestinal absorption of phosphorus is lower for foods of plant origin and higher for meat, fish, poultry, and dairy products. Furthermore, meats are commonly "enhanced" with phosphorus additives, increasing their total bioavailable phosphorus content.[192]

Phosphate additives are nearly 100% bioavailable, and, therefore, foods with phosphate-containing preservatives should be avoided.[193] Labels rarely state phosphorus content, and the increasing use of phosphate food additives in processed and fast foods—especially meats, cheeses, dressings, beverages, and bakery products—makes dietary control of phosphorus in children particularly challenging.[193,194] In fact, phosphate additives can double dietary phosphorus intake, especially in individuals who rely on processed foods.[195] Even modest dietary education in avoiding phosphorus-containing food additives has been shown to decrease phosphorus levels.[196,197]

Dietary education should include limiting foods high in bioavailable phosphorus (ie, hard cheeses, yolks, and tree nuts), cooking methods to reduce phosphorus content (ie, boiling foods and discarding water), and identifying sources of hidden phosphate additives in packaged, commercial, and fast foods or beverages (ie, phosphate-containing beverages and dark sodas, processed meats, and commercial cheeses). Phosphate additives should be avoided, whenever possible, as they significantly increase phosphorus burden while adding little in terms of nutrition.[193]

Dietary phosphorus restriction alone is often insufficient to maintain normophosphatemia. Intestinal phosphorus absorption can be minimized with calcium or non-calcium-based phosphate binders given with meals, snacks, or enteral feedings. Phosphate binder dosages should be matched to the phosphorus content of each feeding and should be taken with the breast milk/formula, meal, or snack to maximize binding. Children and caregivers can be taught to adjust the timing of binders to coincide with feedings containing the most phosphorus.

Calcium-based phosphate binders are recommended as the first-line treatment for pediatric patients given their high calcium requirements.[135] The aim is to provide sufficient calcium intake, while avoiding excess. While inadequate calcium interferes with healthy skeletal mineralization, excessive intake, whether through diet, binders, or dialysate, is associated with severe soft-tissue and vascular calcification.[11] This is regardless of overt risk indicators such as hypercalcemia.[191]

Total calcium intake from diet and phosphate binders should be between one to two times the DRI for age (see Table 13.11).[11] Calcium acetate and calcium carbonate are the front-line phosphate binders used in pediatrics. Calcium acetate binds phosphorus more efficaciously and causes fewer hypercalcemic episodes than calcium carbonate at a similar dose.[198,199] Calcium acetate is suggested for children prone to calcium overload, and calcium carbonate is suggested for children with inadequate intake.[11] Calcium citrate is not recommended due to its propensity to increase aluminum absorption from the gut.[200]

If calcium intake exceeds twice the DRI for age or persistent hypercalcemia is noted, a nonabsorbable, calcium- and metal-free phosphate binder, sevelamer, has been safely and effectively used to reduce serum phosphorus and calcium levels.[201,202] Sevelamer can also be used to pretreat formula to lower its phosphorus content; however, this should be done cautiously as it may adversely affect the nutrient profile. Moreover, it is critical to note that combined simultaneous treatment of

TABLE 13.11 | Suggested Maximal Calcium Intake From Oral, Enteral, and Phosphate Binder Intake for Children With Chronic Kidney Disease Stages 2 Through 5 and 5D

Age	DRI, mg/d	Maximal intake[a] (mg/d)
0-6 mo	210	≤420
7-12 mo	270	≤540
1-3 y	500	≤1,000
4-8 y	1,000	≤1,600
9-18 y	1,300	≤2,500

DRI = Dietary Reference Intake
[b] ≤200% of the DR), to a maximum of 2,500 mg (tolerable upper intake level [UL] for healthy children aged 9 through 18 years)
Adapted with permission from National Kidney Foundation. KDOQI Clinical Practice Guidelines for nutrition in children with CKD: 2008 update. *Am J Kidney Dis.* 2009;53(suppl 2):S1-S124.[11]

formula with sevelamer and sodium polystyrene sulfonate (SPS) suspension may reduce the potassium binder's efficacy and is not recommended.[203-205] Lanthanum carbonate, also a calcium-free phosphate binder, has been used in adults to lower phosphorus levels; however, little is known about the long-term effects of lanthanum accumulation in the liver, kidney, and bone; therefore, it is not recommended for routine use in children.[11,206]

Finally, phosphorus supplementation for hypophosphatemia is generally reserved for a serum phosphorus below 2.0 mg/dL.[206]

Because calcium and phosphorus commonly occur together in foods, the calcium content of the diet may be lower than the recommended DRI.[167] Calcium intake may be supplemented with foods that are naturally rich in calcium or foods that are fortified with calcium, but many of these foods will also be high in phosphorus and, therefore, would be unsuitable in the child with hyperphosphatemia. Calcium-containing medications, including calcium-containing phosphate binders, may be prescribed between meals to maximize calcium absorption. Iron supplements should not be taken at the same time as calcium-containing products because they compete with calcium for absorption and limit the binding of phosphorus. Native vitamin D supplementation (ergocalciferol, D2 or cholecalciferol, D3) may be used to augment 1,25-dihydroxyvitamin D (active vitamin D) synthesis and improve intestinal calcium absorption, especially in early CKD.[11]

TABLE 13.12 | Criteria for Vitamin D Status in Children With Chronic Kidney Disease and Recommended Doses for Supplementation

Serum 25-hydroxyvitamin D level (ng/mL)[a]	Definition of vitamin D status deficiency	Dosing of cholecalciferol (D3) or ergocalciferol (D2)[b]	Duration of supplementation, months
<5	Severe	8,000 IU/d orally/enterally (or 50,000 IU/wk) × 4 wks; then 4,000 IU/d (or 50,000 IU 2 times/month) × 2 months	3
5–15	Mild	4,000 IU/d orally/enterally (or 50,000 IU every other week) × 12 weeks	3
16–30	Insufficiency	2,000 IU/d orally/enterally (or 50,000 IU once ~monthly)	3

[a] To convert serum vitamin D: ng/mL × 2.496 = nmol/L.
[b] Smaller doses are probably sufficient for children aged less than 1 year. The tolerable upper intake level (UL) for vitamin D in healthy infants is 1,000 IU.
Adapted with permission from National Kidney Foundation. KDOQI Clinical Practice Guidelines for nutrition in children with CKD: 2008 update. *Am J Kidney Dis.* 2009;53(suppl 2):S1-S124.[11]

In addition to calcium homeostasis, dietary vitamin D sufficiency may be needed in the prevention of common infectious, endocrine, cardiovascular, and autoimmune diseases. Even in the setting of kidney insufficiency, vitamin D is converted to the active form 1,25-dihydroxyvitamin D in various tissues of the body for localized use. Vitamin D is routinely prescribed to children with CKD, but nevertheless, deficiency is ubiquitous.[207-208] Possible causes include low intakes of vitamin D-rich foods such as fortified milk, a sedentary lifestyle that limits outdoor activity and exposure to sunlight, reduced synthesis of vitamin D3 in the skin of patients with uremia, and urinary losses of 25-hydroxyvitamin D and vitamin D-binding protein in patients with proteinuria.[11]

Since nutritional vitamin D deficiency contributes to hyperparathyroidism, bone demineralization, hypocalcemia, and osteomalacia, close monitoring and supplementation are imperative. Supplementation with vitamin D as D3 or D2 is suggested for all children with CKD stages 2 through 5 and 5D. Table 13.12 describes dosing recommendations which vary by age and vitamin D status.[11,191] When serum 25-hydroxyvitamin D levels are replete, continued supplementation with the DRI is suggested to maintain homeostasis.[11]

Active forms of vitamin D (eg, alfacalcidol and calcitriol) or synthetic active vitamin D analogs (eg, doxercalciferol and paricalcitol) should not be used to treat nutritional 25-hydroxyvitamin D deficiency. Calcitriol and vitamin D analogs are utilized to maintain calcium homeostasis and treat or prevent CKD–MBD. They are initiated and adjusted based on serum PTH, calcium and phosphorus, and 1,25-dihydroxyvitamin D levels, according to recommended guidelines.[187,191]

The optimal level of PTH for children is unknown and somewhat controversial. While current recommendations encourage maintaining PTH levels within two to three times the upper limit of the normal range (see Table 13.13), elevated PTH levels are associated with reduced bone mineralization and increased vascular calcification.[11,187,188] Conversely, PTH levels below lower acceptable limits can contribute to adynamic bone disease.

Dialysis

All forms of conventional dialysis, with the exception of nocturnal HD, are poor in clearing phosphorus, so hyperphosphatemia continues to be treated with a low-phosphorus diet and phosphate binders taken with feedings, meals, and snacks.[209] The calcium content of

TABLE 13.13 | Suggested Target Ranges for Serum Parathyroid Hormone Levels According to Chronic Kidney Disease Stages

CKD stage	GFR, mL/min/1.73 m²	Target serum PTH, pg/mL
3	30-59	35-70
4	15-29	70-110
5, 5D	<15	200-300

GFR = glomerular filtration rate
Adapted with permission from National Kidney Foundation. KDOQI Clinical Practice Guidelines for nutrition in children with CKD: 2008 update. *Am J Kidney Dis.* 2009;53(suppl 2):S1-S124.[11]

both PD and HD solutions can be adjusted to aid in the management of calcium balance.

Calcitriol or treatment with vitamin D analogs is generally required to maintain calcium absorption and PTH levels appropriate for the CKD stage.[210] A calcimimetic (eg, cinacalcet) may also be used to effectively lower calcium and PTH via allosteric regulation of the calcium receptor. Conservative use of calcimimetics is recommended in children due to the limited studies regarding long-term effects on growth and development.[206,210,211] In summary, PTH-lowering therapies must be used judiciously in children and hypocalcemia should be avoided.[210]

More research is needed to determine pediatric-specific recommendations for the prevention and the treatment of CKD–MBD and secondary hyperparathyroidism.[211]

Transplant

Children remain predisposed to progressive bone disease and osteoporosis after transplantation.[187,212] This is because of preestablished CKD-associated mineral bone disease, residual hyperparathyroidism, and an increased risk of bone demineralization from corticosteroid and calcineurin inhibitor immunosuppressant therapy.[187]

Hypophosphatemia is common in the early transplantation period because of increased urinary phosphate loss and persistent hyperparathyroidism; its prevalence decreases after several months, but mild hypophosphatemia may persist indefinitely among more than 50% of adult recipients.[213] Liberal dietary intake of dairy and other high-phosphorus products is encouraged but is often insufficient to achieve normal serum phosphorus levels, and early supplementation may be needed.[187]

Calcium and vitamin D intakes equal to or greater than 100% of the DRI are suggested for children with CKD stages 1 through 5T.[11] Kidney Disease Improving Global Outcomes (KDIGO) Guidelines suggest treatment with higher doses of calcium, calcitriol, or vitamin D analogs, and bisphosphonates to improve bone mineral density in kidney transplant recipients; however, due to the lack of biopsy data and efficacy in children, there is insufficient evidence to justify such therapy.[214] The use of steroid-free protocols theoretically

reduces the risk of bone mineral loss. Because transplantation is a continuum of CKD, KDOQI Clinical Practice Guidelines also suggest that the total calcium intake from oral, enteral, and phosphate binder sources for all children with transplants be kept to equal to or less than 200% of the DRI to avoid future risk of vascular and nonvascular calcifications.[11] Vitamin D supplementation may be needed until levels of serum calcium, phosphorus, and PTH normalize. Because children with transplants are advised to avoid direct sun exposure and because immunosuppressive therapy is associated with a higher risk of skin carcinomas, they are at particular risk of hypovitaminosis D.[215] Early reports of high proportions of adult patients with transplant experiencing vitamin D insufficiency and deficiency many years after transplantation suggest that vitamin D supplementation may be required for a long-term period, especially for children with chronic allograft nephropathy.[216,217]

Children may also be susceptible to calcium deficiencies because of limited sun exposure and corticosteroid therapy, which reduces intestinal calcium absorption and increases calcium resorption. Children with CKD stages 3 through 5T with mineral bone disorders should be managed similarly to children without transplants with similar eGFRs.

SODIUM

Sodium is directly linked to fluid balance. The need for sodium restriction varies with the primary kidney disease, RKF, and mode of KRT. Infants and children with polyuria and salt-wasting syndromes, such as renal dysplasia, may need sodium and free water supplements to promote growth and avoid chronic sodium and intravascular depletion.[11,13] Sodium supplementation in the range of 4 to 7 mmol/kg daily may be medically appropriate. A high-sodium formula may be preferable to a standard infant formula in specific instances.[11] Homemade sodium supplements are not recommended due to the risk of error in preparation.[11,218]

Dietary sodium restriction is an important component of an overall strategy for volume and blood pressure control.[153,219,220] Sodium restriction should be considered for children who have HTN (systolic and diastolic blood pressure ≥95th percentile) or prehypertension (systolic and diastolic blood pressure ≥90th and <95th percentiles).[221] Serum sodium reflects water balance and not total body sodium; hence, it is not an indicator of the need to limit sodium intake. The recommended degree of restriction is approximately 1 to 2 mmol/kg/d, which is relatively consistent with age-appropriate DRI for healthy children (Table 13.14).[11]

Most daily sodium intake (75%) comes from salt added by manufacturers during processing; salt added while cooking or at the table provides only 5% to 10%, and sodium naturally occurring in foods accounts for the final 10%.[223] Salty snacks, processed luncheon meats and cheeses, packaged entrees, and foods from fast food restaurants are typically hardest for children to avoid. Medications (eg, SPS, sodium bicarbonate and citrate, and some antacids, laxatives, and nonsteroidal anti-inflammatory agents) add to sodium intake. Children and their caregivers should be taught to read ingredient lists and nutrient content charts on food labels to identify salty foods. Foods containing up to 140 mg sodium per serving are considered low in sodium.[11,224] Salt substitutes containing potassium in place of sodium should be avoided if the patient is at risk for hyperkalemia due to renal dysfunction or drug–nutrient interactions.

Dialysis

Infants on PD are prone to substantial sodium losses because their high ultrafiltration requirements per kilogram body weight result in significant removal of sodium chloride.[225] The sodium content of breast milk and commercial infant formulas is too low to compensate for these losses, so sodium supplements should be considered for all infants on PD and should be individualized based on clinical symptomology, including serum levels of sodium and chloride, and hypotension.[11] Normal serum sodium levels do not rule out sodium depletion.

Sodium and fluid restrictions are generally more liberal in patients on PD compared with those on HD because dialysis is performed daily. In addition, dialysate dextrose concentration can be increased to improve flu-

TABLE 13.14 | Dietary Reference Intake for Sodium and Potassium Adequacy in Healthy Children[222,a]

Age	Sodium (mg/d) AI	Sodium (mg/d) CDRR[b]	Potassium (mg/d) AI	Potassium (mg/d) UL[c]
0-6 mo	110	ND	400	ND
7-12 mo	370	ND	860	ND
1-3 y	800	1,200	2,000	ND
4-8 y	1,000	1,500	2,300	ND
9-13 y	1,200	1,800	2,500 (males) 2,300 (females)	ND
14-18 y	1,500	2,300	3,000 (males) 2,300 (females)	ND

AI = Adequate Intake | CDRR = Chronic Disease Risk Reduction Intake | ND = not determined | UL = Tolerable Upper Intake Level
[a] This table provides a summary of updated sodium and potassium Adequate Intake values for healthy infants and children established by the National Academics of Sciences, Engineering, and Medicine (NASEM) in 2019, which served as an update to the previous 2005 Dietary Reference Intake values.
[b] The sodium CDRR represents the lowest level of intake for which there was sufficient strength of evidence to characterize chronic disease risk reduction in healthy populations.
[c] The committee notes that although no specific UL value was established for dietary potassium, evidence does suggest that even in healthy individuals, without kidney disease or altered urine excretion, high-dose supplemental potassium can lead to adverse outcomes, including death.

id removal, when necessary; however, routine use of dialysate with high dextrose concentrations is discouraged to avoid exacerbation of hypertriglyceridemia, undesirable weight gain, and to protect the peritoneum from scarring that could lead to peritoneal membrane failure.

Transplant

HTN and the need for antihypertensive medications are common post transplant. The prevalence of HTN and antihypertensive medication use in children are highest initially (80%), gradually decrease to approximately 70% by 1 year post transplant and 60% by 5 years post transplant. Corticosteroids, FK 506, and tacrolimus enhance sodium retention and cause HTN.[96] Sodium restriction is prescribed for children with HTN and can be liberalized as HTN subsides with decreases in immunosuppressant doses. Nonpharmacological antihypertensive therapies include lifestyle changes, such as diet modifications and exercise for weight loss.

POTASSIUM

Serum potassium levels, both high and low, affect all muscle function and can produce cardiac arrhythmias. Elevated serum levels can lead to cardiac arrest. Normal kidney potassium excretion typically occurs until advanced CKD stages; however, acidosis, urinary obstruction, rhabdomyolysis, hemolysis, or medications (eg, potassium-sparing diuretics, angiotensin-converting enzyme [ACE] inhibitors, angiotensin receptor blockers, or β blockers) also increase the risk of hyperkalemia.

Potassium intake should be limited for all children with CKD who have or who are at risk of hyperkalemia. Pediatric limits for potassium restriction have not been studied, and recommendations to limit intake to 40 to 120 mg/kg/d (1–3 mmol/kg/d) for infants and young children, and 30 to 40 mg/kg/d (0.8–1 mmol/kg/d) for older children and adolescents have been based on extrapolation from adult guidelines.[11] A tolerable upper limit for potassium has not been established for healthy children of any age.[226] Breast milk (524 mg/L), along with Similac PM 60/40 (541 mg/L) and Renastart (160 mg/L) formulas have the lowest potassium content compared to standard infant cow's milk formulas (700 mg/L to 730 mg/L) (see Table 13.5).

As of January 2021, potassium will now be required on packaged food labels.[227] As a general rule of thumb, foods containing less than 100 mg potassium per serving are considered low in potassium, whereas foods containing 200 to 250 mg or more per serving are considered high in potassium.[11] High-potassium foods favored by children (eg, french fries, potato chips, chocolate, tomato soups and sauces, bananas, and orange juice) should generally be discouraged. If a child's potassium is well controlled, they may be permitted to try some of these foods on a limited basis to enhance flavor or boost energy intake. Avoiding potassium additives in packaged and processed foods should be reviewed.

The RDN can help the child and family select low-potassium, nutritious foods, particularly fruits and vegetables that are often avoided by patients on renal diets. Furthermore, high-potassium foods can be incorporated into a child's daily potassium allowance, provided other foods eaten that day are low in potassium. If hyperkalemia persists, potassium exchange resins may be necessary. Currently, SPS or Kayexalate, approved by the Food and Drug Administration (FDA) in 1958, is the most widely used potassium binder in the United States.[228] Two new potassium-binding agents have recently been approved for usage by the FDA: sodium zirconium cyclosilicate and patiromer; however, their safety and efficacy have not been established in pediatric patients.[229]

Gastrointestinal and biochemical adverse effects (anorexia, nausea, vomiting, constipation, sodium retention, hypokalemia, and hypocalcemia) and their related clinical manifestations may occur with potassium binder usage.[228,229] Potassium binders have also been used successfully to pretreat infant formulas, breast milk, enteral feedings, and drinks to lower their potassium content.[230-232]

When a dietary source of hyperkalemia cannot be identified, nondietary causes should also be investigated, including constipation; spurious values (eg, hemolyzed blood sample); metabolic acidosis; inadequate dialysis; medications such as potassium-sparing diuretics, tacrolimus, ACE inhibitors, angiotensin receptor blockers, β blockers; and tissue destruction due to infection, chemotherapy, surgery, or catabolism.[119,233] Salt substitutes using potassium to replace sodium should be avoided.[234] Serum bicarbonate levels should be monitored and corrected, as metabolic acidosis precipitates an extracellular shift of potassium, essentially leading to hyperkalemia.[11]

Dialysis

Because PD occurs daily and in most types continually, children on PD seldom need dietary potassium restriction once they reach target exchange volumes (ie, 0.6–0.8 L/m² body surface area in infants and toddlers; 1.0–1.2 L/m² body surface area in children aged 2 years and older). Likewise, children on frequent HD (more than five sessions per week) usually do not need to restrict dietary potassium after they reach this target number of treatment sessions. Occasionally, children on PD or frequent HD may require a high-potassium diet, potassium supplementation or potassium added to their dialysate to maintain normal serum levels. In contrast, most children on standard HD, in particular, those with oligoanuria (urine output <1.0 mL/kg/h in infants and <0.5 mL/kg/h in children) need to carefully follow a low-potassium diet.

Transplant

In transplant recipients, hyperkalemia may occur in the early posttransplant period from FK 506 or tacrolimus therapy, especially when FK 506 or tacrolimus blood levels are above the target range.[96] Other medications used in the course of transplant may also contribute to hyperkalemia. Dietary potassium restriction is initiated only as serum levels dictate.

FLUIDS

Similar to sodium, the fluid requirements of individual children vary with their primary kidney disease, RKF, and mode of KRT. Infants and children with polyuria require high fluid intakes to prevent chronic dehydration and poor growth. Infants and children with oliguria or anuria need a fluid restriction to prevent complications of fluid overload, including HTN.[11] The accepted formula for determining fluid requirements is as follows (Table 13.15 explains insensible fluid losses):

total daily fluid intake = insensible fluid losses + 24-hour urine output + replacement of other losses (eg, vomiting, diarrhea, drainage, ostomy output, dialysis ultrafiltration) + amount to be deficited

Approximately 80% of total water intake comes from beverages, and the remainder comes from food. Liquids and foods that are liquid at room temperature (eg, gelatin, ice, flavored ice pops, ice cream, yogurt, pudding, and gravy) are considered in the total fluid intake. Many fruits and vegetables, and some foods that absorb water during cooking (eg, rice, couscous, and other grains), have high water content that may add to a child's fluid intake. Finally, restricting fluid intake without restricting sodium intake may not be optimal, as excessive sodium intake will stimulate thirst and additional fluid ingestion.[235]

TABLE 13.15 | Estimated Insensible Fluid Losses

Age	Loss
Preterm infants	40 mL/kg/d
Neonates	20-30 mL/kg/d
Children and adolescents	20 mL/kg/d or 400 mL/m²

Adapted with permission from National Kidney Foundation. KDOQI Clinical Practice Guidelines for nutrition in children with CKD: 2008 update. *Am J Kidney Dis.* 2009;53:S1-S124.[11]

Dialysis

Nutrition should never be compromised by fluid restrictions. More frequent dialysis is warranted if more volume for oral or enteral feeds is needed to meet nutritional goals. Regarding HD, the goals for maximum interdialytic (fluid) weight gain are individualized based on the patient's body size and tolerance of fluid removal and, except for the smallest children, are typically equal to or less than 5% of dry (or euvolemic) weight. Adult-sized adolescents may be able to tolerate 2- to 3-kg weight gain, similar to adults. When malnutrition is a concern, adolescents should not be discouraged from using oral nutrition supplements in order to avoid extra HD sessions.

Transplant

High fluid intakes are encouraged post transplant to maintain good perfusion of the transplanted kidney, replace high urine output, and avoid FK 506 or tacrolimus toxicity that can occur if children become dehydrated. Children are given an individualized minimum daily total fluid intake based on urine output and clinical and laboratory signs of fluid balance. Unless undernutrition is a concern, the suggested beverages are water and low-sugar, low-calorie drinks to avoid undesirable weight gain, dental caries, and hyperglycemia.[11]

Summary

Nutrition management of infants and children with CKD is a challenging process that requires frequent alterations in the nutrition care plan in response to changes in the child's age and stage of development, as well as changes in medical status and therapy. Promoting the benefits of diet and fluid modification and providing practical information relevant to the individual child goes a long way toward a successful adaptation to these changes by the child and family and the optimization of the child's nutritional status, growth, development, and health.

References

1. *North American Pediatric Renal Trials and Collaborative Studies. North American Pediatric Renal Trials and Collaborative Studies (NAPRTCS) 2011 Annual Dialysis Report.* NAPRTCS; 2011. Accessed 27 July 2022. https://naprtcs.org/system/files/2011_Annual_Dialysis_Report.pdf

2. Harambat J, van Stralen KJ, Kim JJ, Tizard EJ. Epidemiology of chronic kidney disease in children. *Pediatr Nephrol.* 2012;27(3):363-373. doi:10.1007/s00467-011-1939-1

3. Massengill SF, Ferris M. Chronic kidney disease in children and adolescents. *Pediatr Rev.* 2014;35(1):16-29. doi:10.1542/pir.35-1-16

4. Furth SL, Hwang W, Yang C, Neu AM, Fivush BA, Powe NR. Growth failure, risk of hospitalization and death for children with end-stage renal disease. *Pediatr Nephrol.* 2002;17(6):450-455. doi:10.1007/s00467-002-0838-x

5. Wong CS, Gipson DS, Gillen DL, et al. Anthropometric measures and risk of death in children with end-stage renal disease. *Am J Kidney Dis.* 2000;36(4):811-819. doi:10.1053/ajkd.2000.17674

6. Rees L. Long-term outcome after renal transplantation in childhood. *Pediatr Nephrol.* 2009;24(3):475-484. doi:10.1007/s00467-007-0559-2

7. Morel P, Almond PS, Matas AJ, et al. Long-term quality of life after kidney transplantation in childhood. *Transplantation.* 1991;52(1):47-53. doi:10.1097/00007890-199107000-00010

8. Gerson AC, Wentz A, Abraham AG, et al. Health-related quality of life of children with mild to moderate chronic kidney disease. *Pediatrics.* 2010;125(2):e349-e357. doi:10.1542/peds.2009-0085

9. Parekh RS, Flynn JT, Smoyer WE, et al. Improved growth in young children with severe chronic renal insufficiency who use specified nutritional therapy. *J Am Soc Nephrol.* 2001;12(11):2418-2426.

10. Ledermann SE, Shaw V, Trompeter RS. Long-term enteral nutrition in infants and young children with chronic renal failure. *Pediatr Nephrol.* 1999;13(9):870-875. doi:10.1007/s004670050718

11. KDOQI Clinical Practice Guideline for Nutrition in Children with CKD: 2008 update. Executive summary. *Am J Kidney Dis.* 2009;53(3 suppl 2):S11-S104. doi:10.1053/j.ajkd.2008.11.017

12. Kerzner B. Clinical investigation of feeding difficulties in young children: a practical approach. *Clin Pediatr (Phila).* 2009;48(9):960-965. doi:10.1177/0009922809336074

13. Rodriguez-Soriano J, Arant BS, Brodehl J, Norman ME. Fluid and electrolyte imbalances in children with chronic renal failure. *Am J Kidney Dis.* 1986;7(4):268-274. doi:10.1016/s0272-6386(86)80067-1

14. Ruley EJ, Bock GH, Kerzner B, Abbott AW, Majd M, Chatoor I. Feeding disorders and gastroesophageal reflux in infants with chronic renal failure. *Pediatr Nephrol.* 1989;3(4):424-429. doi:10.1007/BF00850220

15. Daschner M, Tönshoff B, Blum WF, et al. Inappropriate elevation of serum leptin levels in children with chronic renal failure. European Study Group for Nutritional Treatment of Chronic Renal Failure in Childhood. *J Am Soc Nephrol.* 1998;9(6):1074-1079.

16. Ravelli AM. Gastrointestinal function in chronic renal failure. *Pediatr Nephrol.* 1995;9(6):756-762. doi:10.1007/BF00868736

17. Ravelli AM, Ledermann SE, Bisset WM, Trompeter RS, Barratt TM, Milla PJ. Foregut motor function in chronic renal failure. *Arch Dis Child.* 1992;67(11):1343-1347. doi:10.1136/adc.67.11.1343

18. Rosen R, Vandenplas Y, Singendonk M, et al. Pediatric gastroesophageal reflux clinical practice guidelines: joint recommendations of the North American Society for Pediatric Gastroenterology, Hepatology, and Nutrition and the European Society for Pediatric Gastroenterology, Hepatology, and Nutrition. *J Pediatr Gastroenterol Nutr.* 2018;66(3):516-554. doi:10.1097/MPG.0000000000001889

19. World Health Organization. WHO Child Growth Standards. World Health Organization website. 2006. Accessed September 19, 2020. www.who.int/childgrowth/standards/en

20. CDC Growth Charts: United States 2000. Centers for Disease Control and Prevention website. September 9, 2010. Accessed September 19, 2020. www.cdc.gov/growthcharts

21. Bouma S. Diagnosing pediatric malnutrition. *Nutr Clin Pract.* 2017;32(1):52-67. doi:10.1177/0884533616671861

22. US Department of Health and Human Services Maternal and Child Health Bureau. Using the CDC growth charts for children with special health care needs. Electronic training module. HRSA website. 2001. Accessed January 21, 2019. http://depts.washington.edu/growth/cshcn/text/page1a.htm

23. Abitbol CL, Warady BA, Massie MD, et al. Linear growth and anthropometric and nutritional measurements in children with mild to moderate renal insufficiency: a report of the growth failure in children with renal diseases study. *J Pediatr.* 1990;116(2):S46-S54. doi:10.1016/s0022-3476(05)82925-7

24. Arnold WC, Danford D, Holliday MA. Effects of caloric supplementation on growth in children with uremia. *Kidney Int.* 1983;24(2):205-209. doi:10.1038/ki.1983.145

25. Betts PR, Magrath G. Growth pattern and dietary intake of children with chronic renal insufficiency. *Br Med J.* 1974;2(5912):189-193. doi:10.1136/bmj.2.5912.189

26. Norman LJ, Coleman JE, Macdonald IA, Tomsett AM, Watson AR. Nutrition and growth in relation to severity of renal disease in children. *Pediatr Nephrol.* 2000;15(3-4):259-265. doi:10.1007/s004670000465

27. Rosenkranz J, Reichwald-Klugger E, Oh J, Turzer M, Mehls O, Schaefer F. Psychosocial rehabilitation and satisfaction with life in adults with childhood-onset of end-stage renal disease. *Pediatr Nephrol.* 2005;20(9):1288-1294. doi:10.1007/s00467-005-1952-3

28. Stabler B, Clopper RR, Siegel PT, Stoppani C, Compton PG, Underwood LE. Academic achievement and psychological adjustment in short children. The National Cooperative Growth Study. *J Devel Behav Pediatr.* 1994;15(1):1-6. doi:10.1097/00004703-199402000-00001

29. Furth SL, Stablein D, Fine RN, Powe NR, Fivush BA. Adverse clinical outcomes associated with short stature at dialysis initiation: a report of the North American Pediatric Renal Transplant Cooperative Study. *Pediatrics.* 2002;109(5):909-913. doi:10.1542/peds.109.5.909

30. Mahan JD, Warady BA. Assessment and treatment of short stature in pediatric patients with chronic kidney disease: a consensus statement. *Pediatr Nephrol.* 2006;21(7):917-930. doi:10.1007/s00467-006-0020-y

31. Drube J, Wan M, Bonthuis M, et al. Clinical practice recommendations for growth hormone treatment in children with chronic kidney disease. *Nat Revs Nephrol.* 2019;15(9):577-589. doi:10.1038/s41581-019-0161-4

32. World Health Organization. *Who Child Growth Standards: Growth Velocity Based On Weight, Length and Head Circumference: Methods and Development.* World Health Organization; 2009.

33. Demir K, Ozen S, Konakci E, Aydin M, Darendeliler F. A comprehensive online calculator for pediatric endocrinologists: CEDD Cozum/TPEDS Metrics. *J Clin Res Pediatr Endocrinol.* 2017;9(2):182-184. doi:10.4274/jcrpe.4526

34. Mehta NM, Corkins MR, Lyman B, et al. Defining pediatric malnutrition: a paradigm shift toward etiology-related definitions. *JPEN J Parenter Enteral Nutr.* 2013;37(4):460-481. doi:10.1177/0148607113479972

35. Baumgartner RN, Roche AF, Himes JH. Incremental growth tables: supplementary to previously published charts. *Am J Clin Nutr.* 1986;43(5):711-722. doi:10.1093/ajcn/43.5.711

36. Fomon SJ, Haschke F, Ziegler EE, Nelson SE. Body composition of reference children from birth to age 10 years. *Am J Clin Nutr.* 1982;35(5 suppl):1169-1175. doi:10.1093/ajcn/35.5.1169

37. Defining Childhood Obesity. Centers for Disease Control and Prevention website. July 3, 2018. Accessed January 28, 2019. www.cdc.gov/obesity/childhood/defining.html

38. The Children's Hospital of Philadelphia. Welcome to pediatric *z*-score calculator. Children's Hospital of Philadelphia Research Institute website. January 2021. Accessed March 4, 2021. https://zscore.research.chop.edu

39. Abraham AG, Mak RH, Mitsnefes M et al. Protein energy wasting in children with chronic kidney disease. *Pediatr Nephrol.* 2014;29(7):1231-1238. doi:10.1007/s00467-014-2768-9

40. Becker PJ, Nieman Carney L, Corkins MR, et al. Consensus statement of the Academy of Nutrition and Dietetics/American Society for Parenteral and Enteral Nutrition: indicators recommended for the identification and documentation of pediatric malnutrition (undernutrition). *Nutr Clin Pract.* 2015;30(1):147-161. doi:10.1177/0884533614557642

41. Gao T, Leonard MB, Zemel B, Kalkwarf HJ, Foster BJ. Interpretation of body mass index in children with CKD. *Clin J Am Soc Nephrol.* 2012;7(4):558-564. doi:10.2215/CJN.09710911

42. On-site resources. PediTools website. Accessed December 3, 2018. www.peditools.org

43. Abdel-Rahman SM, Bi C, Thaete K. Construction of lambda, mu, sigma values for determining mid-upper arm circumference z scores in U.S. children aged 2 months through 18 years. *Nutr Clin Pract.* 2017;32(1):68-76. doi:10.1177/0884533616676597

44. Mwangome MK, Fegan G, Prentice AM, Berkley JA. Are diagnostic criteria for acute malnutrition affected by hydration status in hospitalized children? A repeated measures study. *Nutr J.* 2011;10(1):92. doi:10.1186/1475-2891-10-92

45. Hogan J, Schneider MF, Pai R, et al. Grip strength in children with chronic kidney disease. *Pediatr Nephrol.* 2020;35(5):891-899. doi:10.1007/s00467-019-04461-x

46. Larson-Nath C, Goday P. Malnutrition in children with chronic kidney disease. *Nutr Clin Pract.* 2019;34(3):349-358. doi:10.1002/ncp.10274

47. Foster BJ, Leonard MB. Measuring nutritional status in children with chronic kidney disease. *Am J Clin Nutr.* 2004;80(4):801-814. doi:10.1093/ajcn/80.4.801

48. Wong CS, Hingorani S, Gillen DL, et al. Hypoalbuminemia and risk of death in pediatric patients with end-stage renal disease. *Kidney Int.* 2002;61(2):630-637. doi:10.1046/j.1523-1755.2002.00169.x

49. Don BR, Kaysen G. Serum albumin: relationship to inflammation and nutrition. *Semin Dial.* 2004;17(6):432-437. doi:10.1111/j.0894-0959.2004.17603.x

50. Juarez-Congelosi M, Orellana P, Goldstein SL. Normalized protein catabolic rate versus serum albumin as a nutrition status marker in pediatric patients receiving hemodialysis. *J Ren Nutr.* 2007;17(4):269-274. doi:10.1053/j.jrn.2007.04.002

51. Silverstein DM, Sgambat K, Fragale M, Moylan K, McCarter RJ, Kher KK. Assessment of relationship between nutrition and growth in pediatric hemodialysis patients. *J Ren Nutr.* 2009;19(5):422-431. doi:10.1053/j.jrn.2009.01.024

52. Bickley, L. Patient assessment: comprehensive or focused. In: Firdaus U, ed. *Bates' Guide to Physical Examination and History Taking.* 11th ed. Lippencott Williams & Wilkins; 2013:3-5.

53. Green, CK. Nutrition-focused physical examination in pediatric patients. *Nutr Clin Pract.* 2015;30(2):203-209. doi:10.1177/0884533615572654

54. Secker DJ, Jeejeebhoy KN. How to perform subjective global nutritional assessment in children. *J Acad Nutr Diet.* 2012;112(3):424-431.e6. doi:10.1016/j.jada.2001.08.039

55. Goldberg LJ, Lenzy Y. Nutrition and hair. *Clin Dermatol.* 2010;28(4):412-419. doi:10.1016/j.clindermatol.2010.03.038

56. Radler DR, Lister T. Nutrient deficiencies associated with nutrition-focused physical findings of the oral cavity. *Nutr Clin Pract.* 2013;28(6):710-721. doi:10.1177/0884533613507284

57. Litchford MD. *Nutrition Focused Physical Assessment: Making Clinical Connections.* CASE Software & Books; 2012.

58. Academy of Nutrition and Dietetics. Nutrition Care Manual. Manual. October 2013. Accessed December 3, 2018. https://nutritioncaremanual.org/category.cfm?ncm_category_id=11

59. Mordoarski B, Wolff J. *Pediatric Nutrition Focused Physical Exam Pocket Guide.* Academy of Nutrition and Dietetics; 2015.

60. Carvalho-Salemi J, Salemi JL, Wong-Vega MR, et al. Malnutrition among hospitalized children in the United States: changing prevalence, clinical correlates, and practice patterns between 2002 and 2011. *J Acad Nutr Diet.* 2018;118(1):40-51.e7. doi:10.1016/j.jand.2017.02.015

61. Carrero JJ, Stenvinkel P, Cuppari L, et al. Etiology of the protein-energy wasting syndrome in chronic kidney disease: a consensus statement from the International Society of Renal Nutrition and Metabolism (ISRNM). *J Ren Nutr.* 2013;23(2):77-90. doi:10.1053/j.jrn.2013.01.001

62. Iorember FM. Malnutrition in chronic kidney disease. *Front Pediatr.* 2018;6:161. doi:10.3389/fped.2018.00161

63. Joint statement: Office of Inspector General Report on Hospital Inpatient Billing for Malnutrition. Association of Clinical Documentation Integrity Specialist website. August 25, 2020. Accessed February 20, 2021. https://acdis.org/resources/joint-statement-office-inspector-general-report-hospital-inpatient-billing-malnutrition

64. Evans DC, Corkins MR, Malone A, et al. The use of visceral proteins as nutrition markers: an ASPEN position paper. *Nutr Clin Pract.* 2021;36(1):22-28. doi:10.1002/ncp.10588

65. Marcason W. Should albumin and prealbumin be used as indicators for malnutrition? *J Acad Nutr Diet.* 2017;117(7):1144. doi:10.1016/j.jand.2017.04.018

66. *Texas Children's Hospital Pediatric Nutrition Reference Guide.* 12th ed. Texas Children's Hospital; 2019.

67. Phillips W, Becker PJ, Wong Vega M, et al. Comprehensive application of the Malnutrition Quality Improvement Initiative (MQII) toolkit to pediatric malnutrition care. *J Acad Nutr Diet.* 2021;121(6):1021-1034. doi:10.1016//j.jand.2020.08.091

68. Rodig NM, McDermott KC, Schneider MF, et al. Growth in children with chronic kidney disease: a report from the chronic kidney disease in children study. *Pediatr Nephrol.* 2014;29(10):1987-1995. doi:10.1007/s00467-014-2812-9

69. Rees L, Jones H. Nutritional management and growth in children with chronic kidney disease. *Pediatr Nephrol.* 2013;28(4):527-536. doi:10.1007/s00467-012-2258-x

70. Al-Uzri A, Matheson M, Gipson DS, et al. The impact of short stature on HRQoL in children with chronic kidney disease. *J Pediatr.* 2013;163(3):736-741. doi:10.1016/j.jpeds.2013.03.016

71. Vimalachandra D, Hodson EM, Willis NS, Craig JC, Cowell CT, Knight JF. Growth hormone for children with chronic kidney disease. In: *Cochrane Database of Systematic Reviews.* John Wiley & Sons, Ltd; 2006.

72. Haffner D, Schaefer F, Nissel R, Wühl E, Tönshoff B, Mehls O. Effect of growth hormone treatment on the adult height of children with chronic renal failure. *N Engl J Med.* 2000;343(13):923-930. doi:10.1056/NEJM200009283431304

73. Hokken-Koelega A, Mulder P, De Jong R, Lilien M, Donckerwolcke R, Groothof J. Long-term effects of growth hormone treatment on growth and puberty in patients with chronic renal insufficiency. *Pediatr Nephrol.* 2000;14(7):701-706. doi:10.1007/s004670000340

74. Nissel R, Lindberg A, Mehls O, Haffner D. Factors predicting the near-final height in growth hormone-treated children and adolescents with chronic kidney disease. *J Clin Endocrinol Metab.* 2008;93(4):1359-1365. doi:10.1210/jc.2007-2302

75. Fine RN, Stablein D, Cohen AH, Tejani A, Kohaut E. Recombinant human growth hormone post-renal transplantation in children: a randomized controlled study of the NAPRTCS. *Kidney Int.* 2002;62(2):688-696. doi:10.1046/j.1523-1755.2002.00489.x

76. Apostolou A, Karagiozoglou-Lampoudi T. Dietary adherence in children with chronic kidney disease: a review of the evidence. *J Ren Care.* 2014;40(2):125-130 doi:10.1111/jorc.12069

77. Davis MC, Tucker CM, Fennell RS. Family behavior, adaptation, and treatment adherence of pediatric nephrology patients. *Pediatr Neprhol.* 1996;10:160-166. doi:10.1007/BF00862061

78. Arts-Rodas D, Benoit D. Feeding problems in infancy and early childhood: identification and management. *Paediatr Child Health.* 1998;3(1):21-27. doi:10.1093/pch/3.1.21

79. Nguyen L, Levitt R, Mak RH. Practical nutrition management of children with chronic kidney disease. *Clinical Medicine Insights: Urology.* 2016;9:1-6. doi:10.4137/CMU.S13180

80. Nelms, CL. Optimizing enteral nutrition for growth in pediatric chronic kidney disease (CKD). *Front Pediatr.* 2018;6:214. doi:10.3389/fped.2018.00214

81. Sabath RJ. Exercise evaluation of children with end-stage renal disease. *Adv Ren Replace Ther.* 1999;6:189-194. doi:10.1016/s1073-4449(99)70051-8

82. Clark S, Denburg MR, Furth SL. Physical activity and screen time in adolescents in the chronic kidney disease in children (CKiD) cohort. *Pediatr Nephrol.* 2016;31(5):801-808. doi:10.1007/s00467-015-3287-z

83. Goldstein SL, Montgomery LR. A pilot study of twice-weekly exercise during hemodialysis in children. *Pediatr Nephrol.* 2009;24(4):833-839. doi:10.1007/s00467-008-1079-4

84. Chazot C, Kopple JD. Vitamin metabolism and requirements in renal disease and renal failure. In: Kopple J, Massry S, eds. *Nutritional Management of Renal Disease.* Lippincott Williams & Wilkins; 1997:415-477.

85. Mason NA, Boyd SM. Drug–nutrient interactions in renal failure. *J Ren Nutr.* 1995;5(4):214-222. doi:10.1016/1051-2276(95)90005-5

86. Becherucci F, Roperto RM, Materassi M, Romagnani P. Chronic kidney disease in children. *Clin Kidney J.* 2016;9(4):583-591. doi:10.1093/ckj/sfw047

87. Ellis, D. Pathophysiology, evaluation, and management of edema in childhood nephrotic syndrome. *Front Pediatr.* 2015;3:111. doi:10.3389/fped.2015.00111

88. Al-Bander H, Kaysen GA. Ineffectiveness of dietary protein augmentation in the management of nephrotic syndrome. *Pediatr Nephrol.* 1991;5(4):482-486. doi:10.1007/BF01453686

89. Chan JCM, Williams DM, Roth KS. Kidney failure in infants and children. *Pediatr Rev.* 2002;23(2):47-60. doi:10.1542/pir.23-2-47

90. South A, Fainman B, Sutherland SM, Wong CJ. Children tolerate intradialytic oral nutrition. *J Ren Care.* 2018;44(1):38-43. doi:10.1111/jorc.12226

91. Fischbach M, Terzic J, Menouer S, et al. Intensified and daily hemodialysis in children might improve statural growth. *Pediatr Nephrol.* 2006;21:1746-1752. doi:10.1007/s00467-006-0226-z

92. Geary DR, Piva E, Tyrrell J, et al. Home nocturnal hemodialysis in children. *J Pediatr.* 2005;147:383-387. doi:10.1016/j.jpeds.2005.04.034

93. Goldstein SL, Silverstein DM, Leung JC, et al. Frequent hemodialysis with NxStage™ system in pediatric patients receiving maintenance hemodialysis. *Pediatr Nephrol.* 2008;23:129-135. doi:10.1007/s00467-007-0649-1

94. Amaral, S, Sayed BA, Kutner N, Patzer RE. Preemptive kidney transplantation is associated with survival benefits among pediatric patients with end-stage renal disease. *Kidney Int.* 2016 Nov;90(5):1100-1108. doi:10.1016/j.kint.2016.07.028

95. Cashion AK, Hathaway DK, Stanfill A, et al. Pre-transplant predictors of one year weight gain after kidney transplantation. *Clin Transplant.* 2014 Nov;28(11):1271-1278. doi:10.1111/ctr.12456

96. McPartland KJ, Pomposelli JJ. Update on immunosuppressive drugs used in solid-organ transplantation and their nutrition implications. *Nutr Clin Pract.* 2007;22(5):467-473. doi:10.1177/0115426507022005467

97. Lau KK, Giglia L, Chan H, Chan AK. Management of children after renal transplantation: highlights for general pediatricians. *Transl Pediatr.* 2012;1(1):35-46. doi:10.3978/j.issn.2224-4336.2012.02.02

98. Qvist E, Marttinen E, Ronnholm K, et al. Growth after renal transplantation in infancy or early childhood. *Pediatr Nephrol.* 2002;17(6):438-443. doi:10.1007/s00467-002-0850-1

99. El Haggan W. Vendrely B, Chauveau P, et al. Early evaluation of nutritional status and body composition after kidney transplantation. *Am J Kid Dis.* 2002;40(3):629-637. doi:10.1053/ajkd.2002.34926

100. Franke D, Thomas L, Steffens R, et al. Patterns of growth after kidney transplantation among children with ESRD. *Clin J Am Soc Nephrol.* 2015;10(1):127-134. doi:10.2215/CJN.02180314

101. Li Y, Greenbaum LA, Warady BA, Furth SL, Ng DK. Short stature in advanced pediatric CKD is associated with faster time to reduced kidney function after transplant. *Pediatr Nephrol.* 2019;34(5):897-905. doi:10.1007/s00467-018-4165-2

102. de Aquino T, Avesani C, Brasileiro R, Carvalhaes J. Resting energy expenditure of children and adolescents undergoing hemodialysis. *J Ren Nutr.* 2008;18:312-319.

103. Shapiro A, Bandini L, Kurtin P. Estimating energy requirements for children with renal disease; a comparison of methods. *J Am Diet Assoc.* 1992;92:571-573.

104. Institute of Medicine. *Dietary Reference Intakes for Energy, Carbohydrates, Fiber, Fat, Protein, and Amino Acids (Macronutrients).* National Academies Press; 2002.

105. Shaw V, Polderman N, Renken-Terhaerdt J, et al. Energy and protein requirements for children with CKD stages 2–5 and on dialysis—clinical practice recommendations from the Pediatric Renal Nutrition Taskforce. *Pediatr Nephrol.* 2020;35(3):519-531. doi:10.1007/s00467-019-04426-0

106. Academy of Nutrition and Dietetics. Pediatric Nutrition Care Manual. Summary for pediatric weight management determination of total energy expenditure. Academy of Nutrition and Dietetics website. Accessed February 28, 2021. www.nutritioncaremanual.org

107. Spinozzi NS, Nelson PA. Nutrition support in the newborn intensive care unit. *J Ren Nutr.* 1996;6(4):188-197. doi:10.1016/S1051-2276(96)90065-5

108. Yiu VWY, Harmon WE, Spinozzi N, Jonas M, Kim MS. High-calorie nutrition for infants with chronic renal disease. *J Ren Nutr.* 1996;6(4):203-206. doi:10.1016/S1051-2276(96)90067-9

109. Fried MD, Khoshoo V, Secker DJ, Gilday DL, Ash JM, Pencharz PB. Decrease in gastric emptying time and episodes of regurgitation in children with spastic quadriplegia fed a whey-based formula. *J Pediatr.* 1992;120(4 Pt 1):569-572. doi:10.1016/s0022-3476(10)80003-4

110. Tolia V, Lin CH, Kuhns LR. Gastric emptying using three different formulas in infants with gastoesophageal reflux. *J Pediatr Gastroenterol Nutr.* 1992;15(3):297-301. doi:10.1097/00005176-199210000-00011

111. Woodley FW, Mousa H. Revisiting the effect of casein and whey on gastric emptying: do differences in protein source really matter? *J Neonatal-Perinatal Med.* 2008;1(2):111-117.

112. Bhatia J, Greer F, American Academy of Pediatrics Committee on Nutrition. Use of soy protein-based formulas in infant feeding. *Pediatrics.* 2008;121(5):1062-1068. doi:10.1542/peds.2008-0564

113. Rees L, Shaw V, Qizalbash L, et al. Delivery of a nutritional prescription by enteral tube feeding in children with chronic kidney disease stages 2–5 and on dialysis—clinical practice recommendations from the Pediatric Renal Nutrition Taskforce. *Pediatr Nephrol.* 2021;36(1):187-204. doi:10.1007/s00467-020-04623-2

114. Hobbs DJ, Gast TR, Ferguson KB, Bunchman T, Barletta GM. Nutritional management of hyperkalemic infants with chronic kidney disease using adult renal formulas. *J Ren Nutr.* 2010;20(2):121-126. doi:10.1053/j.jrn.2009.06.003

115. Rees L, Brandt ML. Tube feeding in children with chronic kidney disease: technical and practical issues. *Pediatr Nephrol.* 2010;25(4):699-704. doi:10.1007/s00467-009-1309-4

116. Kar JA, Gonzalez C, Ledermann SE, Shaw V, Rees L. Outcome and growth of infants with severe chronic renal failure. *Kidney Int.* 2000;57(4):1681-1687. doi:10.1046/j.1523-1755.2000.00013.x

117. Ramage IJ, Geary DF, Harvey E, Secker DJ, Balfe JA, Balfe JW. Efficacy of gastrostomy feeding in infants and older children receiving chronic peritoneal dialysis. *Perit Dial Int.* 1999;19(3):231-236.

118. Ramage IJ, Harvey E, Geary DF, Herbert D, Balfe JA, Balfe JW. Complications of gastrostomy feeding in children receiving peritoneal dialysis. *Pediatr Nephrol.* 1999;13(3):249-252. doi:10.1007/s004670050603

119. Dello Strologo L, Principato F, Sinibaldi D, et al. Feeding dysfunction in infants with severe chronic renal failure after long-term nasogastric tube feeding. *Pediatr Nephrol.* 1997;11(1):84-86. doi:10.1007/s004670050239

120. Tom A, McCauley L, Bell L, et al. Growth during maintenance hemodialysis: impact of enhanced nutrition and clearance. *J Pediatr.* 1999;134(4):464-471. doi:10.1016/s0022-3476(99)70205-2

121. Pugh P, Watson AR. Transition from gastrostomy to oral feeding following renal transplantation. *Adv Perit Dial.* 2006;22:153-157.

122. Warady BA, Kriley M, Belden B, Hellerstein S, Alan U. Nutritional and behavioral aspects of nasogastric feeding in infants receiving chronic peritoneal dialysis. *Adv Perit Dial.* 1990;6:265-268.

123. Mehrotra R, Nolph KD. Treatment of advanced renal failure; low-protein diets or timely initiation of dialysis? *Kidney Int.* 2000;58(4):1381-1388. doi:10.1046/j.1523-1755.2000.00300.x

124. Salusky IB, Fine RN, Nelson P, Blumenkrantz MJ, Kopple JD. Nutritional status of children undergoing continuous ambulatory peritoneal dialysis. *Am J Clin Nutr.* 1983;38(4):599-611. doi:10.1093/ajcn/38.4.599

125. de Boer AW, Schroder CH, van Vliet R, Willems JL, Monnens LA. Clinical experience with icodextrin in children: ultrafiltration profiles and metabolism. *Pediatr Nephrol.* 2000;15(1-2):21-24. doi:10.1007/s004670000406

126. Michallat AC, Dheu C, Loichot C, Danner S, Fishcbach M. Long daytime exchange in children on continuous cycling peritoneal dialysis: preservation of drained volume because of icodextrin use. *Adv Perit Dial.* 2005;21:195-199.

127. Juarez MD. Intradialytic parenteral nutrition in pediatrics. *Front Pediatr.* 2018;6:267. doi:10.3389/fped.2018.00267

128. Mitsnefes MM, Khoury P, McEnery PT. Body mass index and allograft function in pediatric renal transplantation. *Pediatr Nephrol.* 2002;17:535-539.

129. Meier-Kriesche HU, Arndorfer J, Kaplan B. The impact of body mass index on renal transplant outcomes: a significant independent risk factor for graft failure and patient death. *Transplant.* 2002;73(1):70-74. doi:10.1097/00007890-200201150-00013

130. Hanevold CD, Ho PL, Talley L, Mitsnefes MM. Obesity and renal transplant outcome: a report of the North American pediatric renal transplant cooperative study. *Pediatrics.* 2005;115(2):352-356. doi:10.1542/peds.2004-0289

131. Al-Uzri A, Stablein DM, Choh RA. Posttransplant diabetes mellitus in pediatric renal transplant recipients: a report of the North American pediatric renal transplant cooperative study (NAPRTCS). *Transplant.* 2001;72(6):1020-1024. doi:10.1097/00007890-200109270-00007

132. Foreman JW, Abitbol CL, Trachtman H, et al. Nutritional intake in children with renal insufficiency: a report of the growth failure in children with renal disease study. *J Am Coll Nutr.* 1996;15(6):579-585. doi:10.1080/07315724.1996.10718633

133. Ratsch IM, Catassi C, Verrina E, et al. Energy and nutrient intake of patients with mild-to- moderate chronic renal failure compared with healthy children: an Italian multicentre study. *Eur J Pediatr.* 1992;151(9):701-705. doi:10.1007/BF01957578

134. Wingen AM, Fabian-Bach C, Schaefer F, Mehls O. European Study Group for Nutritional Treatment of Chronic Renal Failure in Childhood. Randomised multicentre study of a low-protein diet on the progression of chronic renal failure in children. European Study Group for Nutritional Treatment of Chronic Renal Failure in Childhood. *Lancet.* 1997;349(9059):1117-1123. doi:10.1016/s0140-6736(96)09260-4

135. McAlister L, Pugh P, Greenbaum L, et al. The dietary management of calcium and phosphate in children with CKD stages 2–5 and on dialysis—clinical practice recommendation from the Pediatric Renal Nutrition Taskforce. *Pediatr Nephrol.* 2019;35(3):501-518. doi:10.1007/s00467-019-04370-z

136. Pagenkemper J. Planning a vegetarian renal diet. *J Ren Nutr.* 1995;5(4):234-238. doi:10.1016/1051 -2276(95)90009-8

137. Quan A, Baum M. Protein losses in children on continuous cycler peritoneal dialysis. *Pediatr Nephrol.* 1996;10:728-731. doi:10.1007 /s004670050200

138. Canepa A, Verrina E, Perfumo F, et al. Value of intraperitoneal amino acids in children treated with chronic peritoneal dialysis. *Perit Dial Int.* 1999;19(suppl 2):S435-S440.

139. Tjiong HL, Rietveld T, Wattimena JL, et al. Peritoneal dialysis with solutions containing amino acids plus glucose promotes protein synthesis during oral feeding. *Clin J Am Soc Nephrol.* 2007;2(1):74-80. doi:10.2215/CJN.01370406

140. Canepa A, Carrea A, Menoni S, et al. Acute effects of simultaneous intraperitoneal infusion of glucose and amino acids. *Kidney Int.* 2001;59(5):1967-1973. doi:10.1046/j.1523-1755.2001.0590051967.x

141. Tjiong HL, van den Berg JW, Wattimena JL, et al. Dialysate as food: combined amino acid and glucose dialysate improves protein anabolism in renal failure patients on automated peritoneal dialysis. *J Am Soc Nephrol.* 2005;16(5):1486-1493. doi:10.1681/ASN.2004050402

142. Edefonti A, Picca M, Damiana G, et al. Models to assess nitrogen losses in pediatric patients on chronic peritoneal dialysis. *Pediatr Nephrol.* 2000;15:25-30.

143. Mendley SR, Majkowski NL. Urea and nitrogen excretion in pediatric peritoneal dialysis patients. *Kidney Int.* 2000;58(6):2564-2570. doi:10.1046/j .1523-1755.2000.00442.x

144. Goldstein S. Hemodialysis in the pediatric patient: state of the art. *Adv Ren Replace Ther.* 2001;8(3):173-179. doi:10.1053/jarr.2001.26347

145. Asfaw M, Mingle J, Hendricks J, et al. Nutrition management after pediatric solid organ transplantation. *Nutr Clin Pract.* 2014;29(2):192-200. doi:10.1177/0884533614521242

146. Saland J, Ginsberg H. Lipoprotein metabolism in chronic renal insufficiency. *Pediatr Nephrol.* 2007;22:1095-1112.

147. Saland J, Ginsberg H, Fisher EA. Dyslipidemia in pediatric renal disease: epidemiology, pathophysiology, and management. *Curr Opin Pediatr.* 2002;14(2):197-204. doi:10.1097 /00008480-200204000-00009

148. National Kidney Foundations. KDOQI Clinical Practice Guidelines for chronic kidney disease: evaluation, classification, and stratification. *Am J Kidney Dis.* 2002;39(2 suppl 1):S1-S266.

149. Sland J, Pierce CB, Mitsnefes MM, et al. Dyslipidemia in children with chronic kidney disease. *Kidney Int.* 2010;78(11):1154-1163. doi:10.1038/ki.2010.311

150. Baek HS, Kim SH, Kang HG, et al. Dyslipidemia in pediatric CKD patients: results from KNOW-PedCKD (KoreaN cohort study for Outcomes in patients With Pediatric CKD). *Pediatr Nephrol.* 2020;35(8):1455-1461. doi:10.1007/s00467-020-04545-z

151. Thabet MA, Salcedo JR, Chan JC. Hyperlipidemia in childhood nephrotic syndrome. *Pediatr Nephrol.* 1993;7(5):559-566. doi:10.1007/BF00852550

152. Kavey RW, Allada V, Daniels RS, et al. Cardiovascular risk reduction in high-risk pediatric patients: a scientific statement from the American Heart Association Expert Panel on population and prevention science; the Councils on Cardiovascular Disease in the young, epidemiology and prevention, nutrition, physical activity and metabolism, high blood pressure research, cardiovascular nursing, and the kidney in heart disease; and the Interdisciplinary Working Group on Quality of Care and Outcomes Research: endorsed by the American Academy of Pediatrics. *Circulation.* 2006;114(24):2710-2738. doi:10.1161/CIRCULATIONAHA.106.179568

153. National Kidney Foundation. KDOQI Clinical Practice Guidelines for cardiovascular disease in dialysis patients. *Am J Kidney Dis.* 2005;45(4 suppl 3):S1-S154.

154. Foster BJ, McCauley L, Mak RH. Nutrition in infants and very young children with chronic kidney disease. *Pediatr Nephrol.* 2012;27:1427-1439. doi:10.1007/s00467-011-1983-x

155. Kari J, Shaw V, Vallance DT, Rees L. Effect of enteral feeding on lipid subfractions in children with chronic renal failure. *Pediatr Nephrol.* 1998;12(5):401-404. doi:10.1007/s004670050474

156. Gidding SS, Dennison BA, Birch LL, et al. Dietary recommendations for children and adolescents: a guide for practitioners: consensus statement from the American Heart Association. *Circulation.* 2005;112(13):2061-2075. doi:10.1161 /CIRCULATIONAHA.105.169251

157. Wanner C, Tonelli M; Kidney Disease: Improving Global Outcomes Lipid Guideline Development Work Group Members. KDIGO Clinical Practice Guideline for Lipid Management in CKD: summary of recommendation statements and clinical approach to the patient. *Kidney Int.* 2014;85(6):1303-1309. doi:10.1038/ki.2014.31

158. Chiu H, Wu P, Huang J, et al. There is a U shaped association between non high density lipoprotein cholesterol with overall and cardiovascular mortality in chronic kidney disease stage 3–5. *Sci Rep.* 2020;10(1):12749.doi:10.1038/s41598-020-69794-2

159. Sarnak MJ, Bloom R, Muntner P, et al. KDOQI US commentary on the 2013 KDIGO Clinical Practice Guideline for Lipid Management in CKD. *Am J Kidney Dis.* 2015;65(3):354-366. doi:10.1053/j .ajkd.2014.10.005

160. Anderson JLC, Bakker SJL, Tietge UJF. Triglyceride/HDL cholesterol ratio and premature all-cause mortality in renal transplant recipients. *Nephrol Dial Transplant.* 2021;36(5):936-938. doi:10.1093/ndt/gfaa321

161. Ateya AM, Sabri NA, Hakim IE, Shaheen SM. Effect of omega-3 fatty acids on serum lipid profile and oxidative stress in pediatric patients on regular hemodialysis: a randomized placebo-controlled study. *J Ren Nutr.* 2017;27(3):169-174. doi:10.1053 /j.jrn.2016.11.005

162. Omar ZA, Montser BA, Farhat MAR. Effect of high-dose omega-3 on lipid profile and inflammatory markers in chronic hemodialysis children. *Saudi J Kidney Dis Transpl.* 2019;30(3):634-639. doi:10 .4103/1319-2442.261337

163. Flanagan JL, Simmons PA, Vehige J, et al. Role of carnitine in disease. *Nutr Metab (Lond).* 2010;7:30. doi:10.1186/1743-7075-7-30

164. Verrina E, Caruso U, Calevo M, et al. Effect of carnitine supplementation on lipid profile and anemia in children on chronic dialysis. *Pediatr Nephrol.* 2007;22(5):727-733. doi:10.1007/s00467 -006-0408-8

165. Belay B, Esteban-Cruciani N, Walsh CA, et al. The use of levo-carnitine in children with renal disease: a review and a call for future studies. *Pediatr Nephrol.* 2006;21(3):308-317. doi:10.1007/s00467 -005-2085-4

166. Thorsteinsdottir H, Christensen JJ, Holven KB, et al. Cardiovascular risk factors are inversely associated with omega-3 polyunsaturated fatty acid plasma levels in pediatric kidney transplant recipients. *J Ren Nutr.* 2021;31(3):278-285. doi:10.1053/j.jrn .2020.06.002

167. Institute of Medicine. *Dietary Reference Intakes for Calcium, Phosphorus, Magnesium, Vitamin D, and Fluoride.* National Academies Press; 1997.

168. Institute of Medicine. *Dietary Reference Intakes for Thiamin, Riboflavin, Niacin, Vitamin B-6, Folate, Vitamins B-12, Pantothenic Acid, Biotin, and Choline.* National Academies Press; 1998.

169. Institute of Medicine. *Dietary Reference Intakes for Vitamin C, Vitamin E, Selenium, and Carotenoids.* National Academies Press; 2000.

170. Institute of Medicine. *Dietary Reference Intakes for Vitamin A, Vitamin K, Arsenic, Boron, Chromium, Copper, Iodine, Iron, Manganese, Molybdenum, Nickel, Silicon, Vanadium, and Zinc.* National Academies Press; 2002.

171. Feinstein S, Sela B, Drukker A, et al. Hyperhomocysteinemia in children on renal placement therapy. *Pediatr Nephrol.* 2002;17(7):515-519. doi:10.1007/s00467-002-0901-7

172. Kang H, Lee B, Hah H, et al. Reduction of plasma homocysteine by folic acid in children with chronic renal failure. *Pediatr Nephrol.* 2002;17:511-514.

173. Schroder CH, de Boer AW, Giesen AM, Monnens LA, Blom H. Treatment of hyperhomocysteinemia in children on dialysis by folic acid. *Pediatr Nephrol.* 1999:13:583-585. doi:10.1007/s004670050748

174. Jamison R, Hartigan P, Kaufman J, et al. Effect of homocysteine lowering on mortality and vascular disease in advanced chronic kidney disease and end-stage renal disease: a randomized controlled trial. *JAMA.* 2007;298(10):1163-1170. doi:10.1001 /jama.298.10.1163

175. Sunder-Plassmann G, Winkelmayer W, Fodinger M. Approaching the end of the homocysteine hype? *Am J Kidney Dis.* 2008;51:549-553. doi:10.1053/j .ajkd.2008.01.007

176. Farrington K, Miller P, Varghese Z, Baillod R, Moorhead J. Vitamin A toxicity and hypercalcaemia in chronic renal failure. *BMJ.* 1981;282:1999-2002. doi:10.1136/bmj.282.6281.1999

177. Norman L, Coleman JE, Watson AR, Waddell LJ, Evans J. Nutritional supplements and elevated serum vitamin A levels in children on chronic dialysis. *J Hum Nutr Diet.* 2003;9(4):257-262. doi:10 .1046/j.1365-277X.1996.00464.x

178. Manickavasagar B, McArdle AJ, Yadav P, et al. Hypervitaminosis A is prevalent in children with CKD and contributes to hypercalcemia. *Pediatr Nephrol.* 2015;30(2):317-325. doi:10.1007/s00467 -014-2916-2

179. National Kidney Foundation. KDOQI Clinical Practice Guidelines and clinical practice recommendations for anemia in chronic kidney disease. *Am J Kidney Dis.* 2006;47(5 suppl 3):S1-S145. doi:10.1053/j.ajkd .2006.03.010

180. Coleman JE, Watson AR. Vitamin, mineral and trace element supplementation of children on chronic peritoneal dialysis. *J Hum Nutr Diet.* 1991;4:13-17. doi:10.1111/j.1365-277X.1991.tb00071.x

181. Kriley M, Warady BA. Vitamin status of pediatric patients receiving long-term peritoneal dialysis. *Am J Clin Nutr.*1991;53:1476-1479. doi:10.1093/ajcn/53.6.1476

182. Warady BA, Kriley M, Alon U, Hellerstein S. Vitamin status of infants receive long-term peritoneal dialysis. *Pediatr Nephrol.* 1994;8(3):354-356. doi:10.1007/BF00866365

183. Ramos EL, Barri YM, Kubilis P, et al. Hypomagnesemia in renal transplant patients: improvement over time and association with hypertension and cyclosporine levels. *Clin Transplant.* 1995;9(3 Pt 1):185-189.

184. Haffner D, Leifheit-Nestler M. CKD-MBD post kidney transplantation. *Pediatric Nephrol.* 2021;36(1):41-50. doi:10.1007/s00467-019-04421-5

185. Hahn D, Hodson EM, Craig JC. Interventions for metabolic bone disease in children with chronic kidney disease. *Cochrane Database Syst Rev.* 2015(11):CD008327. doi:10.1002/14651858.CD008327.pub2

186. Wesseling-Perry K, Bakkaloglu S, Salusky IB. Chronic kidney disease mineral and bone disorder in children. *Pediatr Nephrol.* 2007;23(2):195-207.

187. National Kidney Foundation. K/DOQI clinical practice guidelines for bone metabolism and disease in chronic kidney disease. *Am J Kidney Dis.* 2003;42(4 suppl 3):S1-S201.

188. Klaus G, Watson A, Edefonti A, et al. Prevention and treatment of renal osteodystrophy in children on chronic renal failure: European guidelines. *Pediatr Nephrol.* 2006;21(2):151-159. doi:10.1007/s00467-005-2082-7

189. Oh J, Wunsch R, Turzer M, et al. Advanced coronary and carotid arteriopathy in young adults with childhood-onset chronic renal failure. *Circulation.* 2002;106(1):100-105. doi:10.1161/01.cir.0000020222.63035.c0

190. Shroff RC, Donald AE, Hiorns MP, et al. Mineral metabolism and vascular damage in children on dialysis. *J Am Soc Nephrol.* 2007;18(11):2996-3003. doi:10.1081/ASN.2006121397

191. Ketteler M, Block GA, Evenepoel P, et al. Executive summary of the 2017 KDIGO Chronic Kidney Disease–Mineral and Bone Disorder (CKD–MBD) Guideline Update: what's changed and why it matters. *Kidney Int.* 2017;92(1):26-36. doi:10.1016/j.kint.2017.04.006

192. Kalantar-Zadeh K, Gutekunst L, Mehrotra R, et al. Understanding sources of dietary phosphorus in the treatment of patients with chronic kidney disease. *Clin J Am Soc Nephrol.* 2010;5(3):519-530. doi:10.2215/CJN.06080809

193. D'Alessandro C, Piccoli GB, Cupisti A. The "phosphorus pyramid": a visual tool for dietary phosphate management in dialysis and CKD patients. *BMC Nephrol.* 2015;16:9. doi:10.1186/1471-2369-16-9

194. Uribarri J, Calvo MS. Hidden sources of phosphorus in the typical American diet: does it matter in nephrology? *Semin Dial.* 2003;16(3):186-188. doi:10.1046/j.1525-139x.2003.16037.x

195. Moon WH, Malzer JL, Clark HE. Phosphorus balances of adults consuming several food combinations. *J Am Diet Assoc.* 1974;64(4):386-390.

196. Uribarri J. Phosphorus additives in food and their effect in dialysis patients. *Clin J Am Soc Nephrol.* 2009;4(8):1290-1292. doi:10.2215/CJN.03950609

197. Sullivan C, Sayre SS, Leon JB, et al. Effect of food additives on hyperphosphatemia among patients with end-stage renal disease: a randomized controlled trial. *JAMA.* 2009;301(6):629-635. doi:10.1001/jama.2009.96

198. Sheikh MS, Maguire JA, Emmett M, et al. Reduction of dietary phosphorus absorption by phosphorus binders. A theoretical, in vitro, and in vivo study. *J Clin Invest.* 1989;83(1):66-73. doi:10.1172/JCI113886

199. Ring T, Nielsen C, Andersen SP, Bchrens JK, Sodemann B, Kornerup HJ. Calcium acetate versus calcium carbonate as phosphorus binders in patients on chronic haemodialysis: a controlled study. *Nephrol Dial Transplant.* 1993;8(4):341-346. doi:10.1093/oxfordjournals.ndt.a092467

200. Coburn JW, Mischel MG, Goodman WG, Salusky IB. Calcium citrate markedly enhances aluminum absorption from aluminum hydroxide. *Am J Kid Dis.* 1991;17(6):708-711. doi:10.1016/S0272-6386(12)80356-8

201. Pieper A-K, Haffner D, Hoppe B, et al. A randomized crossover trial comparing sevelamer with calcium acetate in children with CKD. *Am J Kid Dis.* 2006;47(4):625-635. doi:10.1053/j.ajkd.2005.12.039

202. Salusky IB, Goodman WG, Sahney S, et al. Sevelamer controls parathyroid hormone-induced bone disease as efficiently as calcium carbonate without increasing serum calcium levels during therapy with active vitamin D sterols. *J Am Soc Nephrol.* 2005;16(8):2501-2508. doi:10.1681/ASN.2004100885

203. Ferrara E, Lemire J, Reznik VM, Grimm PC. Dietary phosphorus reduction by pretreatment of human breast milk with sevelamer. *Pediatr Nephrol.* 2004;19(7):775-779. doi:10.1007/s00467-004-1448-6

204. Raaijmakers R, Willems HL, Houkes L, van den Heuvel LP, Schroder C, Monnens L. Pre-treatment of different dairy products with sevelamer: effective phosphorus reduction but also a rise in pH. *Pediatr Nephrol*. 2008;23(29):1604.

205. Taylor JM, Oladitan L, Carlson S, Hamilton-Reeves JM. Renal formulas pretreated with medications alters the nutrient profile. *Pediatr Nephrol*. 2015;30(10):1815-1823. doi:10.1007/s00467-015-3115-5

206. Hanudel MR, Salusky IB. Treatment of pediatric chronic kidney disease-mineral and bone disorder. *Curr Osteoporos Rep*. 2017;15(3):198-206. doi:10.1007/s11914-017-0365-0

207. Ali FN, Arguelles LM, Langman CB, Price HE. Vitamin D deficiency in children with chronic kidney disease: uncovering an epidemic. *Pediatrics*. 2009;123(3):791-796. doi:10.1542/peds.2008-0634

208. Shroff R, Wan M, Nagler EV, et al. Clinical practice recommendations for treatment with active vitamin D analogues in children with chronic kidney disease stages 2–5 and on dialysis. *Nephrol Dial Transplant*. 2017;32(7):1114-1127. doi:10.1093/ndt/gfx080

209. King RS, Glickman JD. Electrolyte management in frequent home hemodialysis. *Semin Dial*. 2010;23(6):571-574. doi:10.1111/j.1525-139X.2010.00792.x

210. Wesseling-Perry K, Salusky IB. Phosphate binders, vitamin D and calcimimetics in the management of chronic kidney disease–mineral bone disorders (CKD–MBD) in children. *Pediatr Nephrol*. 2013;28:617-625.

211. Kidney Disease: Improving Global Outcomes CKD–MBD Update Work Group. KDIGO 2017 clinical practice guideline update for the diagnosis, evaluation, prevention, and treatment of chronic kidney disease–mineral and bone disorder (CKD–MBD). *Kidney Int Suppl (2011)*. 2017;7(1):1-59. doi:10.1016/j.kisu.2017.04.001

212. Chan JC. Post-transplant metabolic bone complications and optimization of treatment. *Pediatr Transplant*. 2007;11(4):349-353. doi:10.1111/j.1399-3046.2007.00709.x

213. Levi M. Post-transplant hypophosphatemia. *Kid Int*. 2001;59(6):2377-2387.

214. Kidney Disease: Improving Global Outcomes Transplant Work Group. KDIGO clinical practice guideline for the care of kidney transplant recipients. *Am J Transplant*. 2009;9(suppl 3):S1-S155. doi:10.1111/j.1600-6143.2009.02834.x

215. Euvrard S, Kanitakis J, Claudy A. Skin cancers after organ transplantation. *N Engl J Med*. 2003;348(17):1681-1691. doi:10.1056/NEJMra022137

216. Ewers B, Gasbjerg A, Moelgaard C, Frederiksen AM, Marckmann P. Vitamin D status in kidney transplant patients: need for intensified routine supplementation. *Am J Clin Nutr*. 2008;87(2):431-437. doi:10.1093/ajcn/87.2.431

217. Stavroulopoulos A, Cassidy MJD, Porter CJ, Hosking DJ, Roe SD. Vitamin D status in renal transplant recipients. *Am J Transplant*. 2007;7(11):2546-2552. doi:10.111/j.1600-6143.2007.01978.x

218. Parekh R, Smoyer WE, Milne JL, et al. Letter from the authors of "Improved growth in young children with severe chronic renal insufficiency who use specified nutritional therapy." *JASN*. 2002;13(5):1421-1422.

219. Kidney Disease Outcomes Quality Initiative. K/DOQI clinical practice guidelines on hypertension and antihypertensive agents in chronic kidney disease. *Am J Kidney Dis*. 2004;43(5 suppl 1):S1-S290.

220. Hemodialysis Adequacy 2006 Work Group. Clinical practice guidelines for hemodialysis adequacy, update 2006. *Am J Kidney Dis*. 2006;48(suppl 1):S2-S90. doi:10.1053/j.ajkd.2006.03.051

221. National High Blood Pressure Education Program Working Group. The fourth report on the diagnosis, evaluation, and treatment of high blood pressure in children and adolescents. *Pediatrics*. 2004;114(2 suppl 4th Report):555-576.

222. National Academies of Sciences, Engineering, and Medicine; Health and Medicine Division. *Dietary Reference Intakes for Sodium and Potassium*. National Academies Press; 2019.

223. Mattes RD, Donnelly D. Relative contributions of dietary sodium sources. *J Am Coll Nutr*. 1991;10(4):383-393. doi:10.1080/07315724.1991.10718167

224. Klemm S. The basics of the nutrition facts label. Accessed February 11, 2019. eatRIGHT website. www.eatright.org/food/nutrition/nutrition-facts-and-food-labels/the-basics-of-the-nutrition-facts-label

225. Paulson WD, Bock GH, Nelson AP, Moxey-Mims MM, Crim LM. Hyponatremia in the very young chronic peritoneal dialysis patient. *Am J Kidney Dis*. 1989;14(3):196-199. doi:10.1016/s0272-6386(89)80070-8

226. Institute of Medicine. *Dietary Reference Intakes for Water, Potassium, Sodium, Chloride, and Sulfate*. National Academies Press; 2004.

227. Changes to the Nutrition Facts label. US Food and Drug Administration website. Accessed February 24, 2019. www.fda.gov/Food/GuidanceRegulation /GuidanceDocumentsRegulatoryInformation /LabelingNutrition/ucm385663.htm

228. Chaitman M, Dixit D, Bridgeman MB. Potassium-binding agents for the clinical management of hyperkalemia. P T. 2016;41(1):43-50.

229. US Food and Drug Administration. Accessed September 13, 2020. https://search.usa.gov /search?utf8=%%E2%9C%93&&affiliate==fda

230. Thompson K, Flynn J, Okamura D, Zhou L. Pretreatment of formula or expressed breast milk with sodium polystyrene sulfonate (Kayexalate(®)) as a treatment for hyperkalemia in infants with acute or chronic renal insufficiency. J Ren Nutr. 2013;23(5):333-339. doi:10.1053/j.jrn.2013.02.011

231. Rivard AL, Raup SM, Beilman GJ. Sodium polystyrene sulfonate used to reduce the potassium content of a high-protein enteral formula: a quantitative analysis. JPEN J Parenter Enteral Nutr. 2004;28(2):76-78. doi:10.1177/014860710402800276

232. Cameron JCF, Kennedy D, Feber J, et al. Pretreatment of infant formula with sodium polystyrene sulfonate. Pediatr Drugs. 2013;15(1):43-48. doi:10.1007/s40272-012-0003-3

233. Beto J, Bansal VK. Hyperkalemia: evaluating dietary and nondietary etiology. J Ren Nutr. 1992;2(1):28-29. doi:10.1016/S1051-2276(12)80166-X

234. Doorenbos CJ, Vermeij CG. Danger of salt substitutes that contain potassium in patients with renal failure. BMJ. 2003;326(7379):35-36. doi:10 .1136/bmj.326.7379.35

235. Tomson CRV. Advising dialysis patients to restrict fluid intake without restricting sodium intake is not based on evidence and is a waste of time. Nephrol Dial Transplant. 2001;16(8):1538-1542. doi:10.1093 /ndt/16.8.1538

CHAPTER 14

Nutrition Management of Kidney Stones

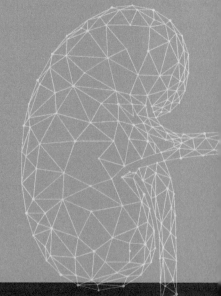

Haewook Han, PhD, RD, LDN, FNKF, Walter P. Mutter, MD, and Samer Nasser, MD, FASN

Introduction/Epidemiology

Nephrolithiasis or kidney stone disease is caused by the precipitation of stone-forming (lithogenic) substances in the urine. Kidney stones are common among adults and associated with significant morbidity and cost.[1,2] Unfortunately, the prevalence of nephrolithiasis is on the rise. The prevalence of kidney stones in the 2007 to 2010 National Health and Nutrition Examination Survey (NHANES) was 8.8% among all adults compared to 5.2% in 1994.[3,4] Kidney stones are more common in men than women with a lifetime risk of 12% and 6%, respectively.[5]

Both genetic and environmental risk factors likely contribute to stone risk. Some genetic risk factors are well defined and monogenetic (cystinuria, primary hyperoxaluria) while others, such as idiopathic hypercalcuria (IH), likely involve a complex interplay of genetic and environmental factors.[6] Epidemiologic studies show increased risk of nephrolithiasis among individuals with metabolic syndrome (MS), especially obesity.[7-9] Some experts have hypothesized that the increased incidence of nephrolithiasis may be related to the obesity epidemic in the United States. Living in warmer climates may also increase the risk. The prevalence of stone disease is as high as 50% in the southeastern compared to the northwestern United States. This may be due to increased fluid loss and decreased urine volume related to a higher mean annual temperature in the southern states, thus creating the "Stone Belt."[9,10]

Eighty percent of stones contain calcium, primarily calcium oxalate (CaOx) and less frequently calcium phosphate (CaP).[11] Among younger adults, CaP stones are more prevalent in female than male stone formers.[12] Uric acid stones account for 10% of stones and are more prevalent in individuals older than 50 years of age. The remaining 10% of stones are composed of a variety of substances including struvite, often associated with infection, and cysteine due to a genetic defect preventing reabsorption of cystine in the kidney.[13] Although each stone type has unique pathophysiologic features, stone formation usually requires concentration of its components at insoluble levels, also known as the urine supersaturation (SS) of the various components.

This chapter will discuss evaluation of patients with kidney stones, assessment of risk factors, and dietary and medical interventions for different types of stones.

Pathophysiology

Kidney stones develop when urine becomes supersaturated with insoluble compounds, such as CaOx, CaP, and uric acid. SS may result from decreased urine volume, overexcretion of these substances, or under excretion of inhibitors of stone formation, such as citrate. Low urine volume is considered the most easily modifiable risk factor for nephrolithiasis.[14] Over excretion can happen in genetic diseases (eg, cystinuria and primary hyperoxaluria [PH]) or in some disease states (eg, inflammatory bowel disease [IBD]), which results in secondary hyperoxaluria.[2,15] Hypocitraturia is found in 20% to 60% of stone formers and may be seen in patients with renal tubular acidosis (RTA) and those who consume high-protein diets.[16-18]

CRYSTALLIZATION

Nucleation is the first step of stone formation, and growth of crystals requires the presence of crystal-forming substances at concentrations above their solubility, termed SS.[19,20] The saturation status depends on the combined excretion of water and lithogenic material, which determines the concentration of the stone solutes. For uric acid and CaP stones, urine pH is also a factor. Normal urine pH is about 6. Uric acid is less soluble and more likely to precipitate in a lower or more acidic pH (<6) while CaP stones are formed in alkaline pH with pH greater than 6.2. SS for calcium and urate salts is determined by using urinary pH and 24-hour urine measured concentrations of calcium, oxalate, phosphate, and uric acid, as well as other urine substances that impact solubility.[21]

CRYSTALLIZATION INHIBITORS

Citrate, pyrophosphate, osteopontin, uromodulin, and glycosaminoglycan are known substances that inhibit nucleation, aggregation, and growth of calcium in vitro.[22,23] Citrate is the only inhibitor of clinical significance as it can be measured in the urine and prescribed as therapy. Citrate forms a complex with calcium, which lowers CaOx stone formation and also decreases non–calcium stone formation (especially uric acid) by increasing urine alkalization.[24]

Symptoms and Diagnosis

SYMPTOMS

Patients with kidney stones are often asymptomatic, and the stones are sometimes discovered incidentally on imaging done for other purposes. Patients who de-

velop renal colic are usually experiencing stone passage from the renal parenchyma into the ureter. The most common symptoms include ipsilateral flank pain, hematuria, nausea, vomiting, or urinary tract infection (UTI).[25] When pain becomes severe, patients can visit the emergency room for treatment that includes intravenous fluid and pain management with medication. If the stone does not pass spontaneously with medical management, urologic intervention is required.

DIAGNOSIS

Imaging

Computed tomography (CT), ultrasound, and plain film are the most commonly used imaging techniques to identify location, size, and type of stones. CT is generally considered the most sensitive but is associated with radiation exposure.[26] Magnetic resonance imaging does not involve radiation and is more sensitive than ultrasound or x-ray but less sensitive than CT.[26,27]

Ultimately, the decision should be guided by the patient's age, weight, medical history, pregnancy status, acuity of presentation, kidney function, and findings on physical exam. Ultrasound is a low-risk and low-cost modality that may be useful for following stones over time.[28]

24-Hour Urine Collection and Interpretation

Urine Collection A 24-hour urine collection is done to evaluate stone formation risk factors and help formulate medical and nutritional management for prevention. The collection will measure urine volume and pH as well as the concentration and SS of lithogenic substances, typically calcium, oxalate, sodium, citrate, and uric acid and the concentration of other nutrients that reflect dietary intake. Specific testing can be done if other stone types, such as cysteine, are suspected. A 24-hour urine collection should be obtained with stable kidney function and when the patient is feeling well with normal food and fluid intake.

The number of 24-hour urine collections performed during the initial evaluation is a matter of debate. For many years, the standard has been two 24-hour collections to ensure consistency between the collections, with a third collection performed if the results of the first two are markedly different. However, there is some thought that a well-collected first sample with patients on their standard diet can suffice.[29] Given the noted intrapatient variability in urine composition, missing a clinically significant metabolic abnormality may outweigh the inconvenience of multiple urine collections and two collections for the initial evaluation is ideal.[30] For follow-up of diet and medical therapy, one 24-hour urine collection suffices.

Adequacy of collection A 24-hour urine creatinine can be checked to verify adequacy of the sample. Men excrete 20 to 25 mg/kg/d and women excrete 15 to 20 mg/kg/d.[31] Values that are out of range should be interpreted carefully in a clinical setting. While low values indicate under collection, low 24-hour creatinine can point out decreased excretion as in acute kidney injury (AKI) or malnourishment due to low muscle mass. On the other end of the spectrum, a high level may indicate an over-collection or high muscle mass.

Interpretation of collection The 24-hour urine collection should at least include urine volume, calcium, phosphorus, oxalate, citrate, pH, sodium, and uric acid. These solutes provide an estimate of SS and risk of stone formation. It is important to note that measured substances may be present in "normal" quantities as determined by the laboratory, but those amounts may not be optimum for stone prevention in an individual patient.[17] Values can be trended with follow-up collections to determine the success of therapy. The 24-hour urine collection should be completed 6 weeks to 8 weeks after any urological procedure to minimize the effect of infection, blood, or AKI that may be present. Infections, for example, may change the pH and citrate levels. It is also very important for patients to continue with their usual diet and perform their regular activities during the collection period.

A 24-hour urine collection may also measure substances related to dietary risk factors, which include sodium, potassium, magnesium, sulfate, ammonia, and urea nitrogen. Sulfates come, for the most part, from animal protein (the acid ash diet) and may help determine protein intake. Urea nitrogen may also be used to estimate protein catabolic rate (PCR), which in the outpatient setting is usually indicative of dietary protein intake. Urinary sodium reflects dietary sodium intake in a steady state and is important because it alters calcium, potassium, and magnesium excretion.

The 24-hour urine collection is a starting point to evaluate dietary nutrient and fluid intake in an effort to provide guidance for management. For example, normal urinary calcium levels are less than 250 mg/d for men and less than 200 mg/d for women. High urinary calcium, hypercalciuria, can be caused by medical conditions such as IH, primary hyperparathyroidism, sarcoidosis, or a diet high in sodium or protein. Low urinary calcium, hypocalciuria, may be caused by malabsorption or underlying bone disease. Also, patients on thiazide diuretics may have low urinary calcium because they can increase reabsorption of calcium in the kidney. A high urinary oxalate may be due to a high oxalate diet, increased endogenous production, high vitamin C consumption, or IBD.[32] Acceptable urinary citrate excretion is greater than 450 mg/d for men and greater than 550 mg/d for women. A high consumption of animal protein or RTA can increase acid production and may lower urinary pH with citrate levels.[32]

For example, a 24-hour urine collection reporting 1,000 ml (1L) volume (goal >2.5 L), calcium greater than 250 mg (normal <200 mg/d for women and <250 mg/d for men), oxalate 60 mg (normal 20–40 mg/d), sodium 200 mEq (goal <150 mEq/d), citrate 45 mg (normal >550 mg/d for women and >450 mg/d for men), pH 5.2, and PCR 2 g/kg (normal 0.8–1.4 g/kg) would be consistent with a patient who has low fluid intake and low urinary citrate who consumes a high-protein, high-sodium diet with an increased risk of CaOx or uric acid stone formation.

Box 14.1 on page 292 provides a summary of the normal values of the 24-hour urine collection, with interpretation and causes of abnormal values.[32]

BOX 14.1 | Summary of the Normal Values for the 24-Hour Urine Collection, Interpretation, and Causes of Abnormal Values

URINE VOLUME (24-HOUR)

Reason for order	Assessment of daily urine flow
Normal value	>2,500 mL/d
Causes of abnormal values	↓ with low fluid intake

CREATININE (CR/KG)

Reason for order	Assessment of sample adequacy
Normal value	20 to 25 mg/kg/d for males
	15 to 20 mg/kg/d for females
Causes of abnormal values	↑ with more than 24-hour collection
	↓ with under collection

CALCIUM

Reason for order	Assessment of calcium stone risk
Normal value	<250 mg/d for males
	<200 mg/d for females
Causes of abnormal values	↑ idiopathic hypercalciuria, high-sodium diet (high urine sodium), high-protein diet, primary hyperparathyroidism
	↓ with bone disease

PHOSPHORUS

Reason for order	Assessment of primary hyperparathyroidism, malnutrition, or malabsorption
Normal value	0.6 to 1.2 g/d
Causes of abnormal values	↓ with bowel disease, malnutrition
	↑ with large amounts of dietary intake

pH

Reason for order	Assessment of risk for certain stones
Normal value	5.8 to 6.2
Causes of abnormal values	↓ Renal tubular acidosis (RTA,) urea splitting infection, acidosis, high animal-protein intake (high purine content), <5.5 increases uric acid stone risk
	↑ >6.5 increases calcium phosphate risk, vegetarian diet, and high citrus consumption

OXALATE

Reason for order	Assessment of calcium oxalate stone risk
Normal value	20 to 40 mg/d
Causes of abnormal values	↑ with high-oxalate diet, high vitamin C consumption; if >80 suspect intestinal (inflammatory bowel disease), malabsorptive states, or oxalosis

CITRATE

Reason for order	Assessment of calcium oxalate or uric acid stone risk
Normal value	>450 mg/d for males
	>550 mg/d for females
Causes of abnormal values	↓ RTA, hypokalemia, high animal protein diet, acidosis, diarrhea

URIC ACID

Reason for order	Assessment of uric acid stone risk
Normal value	<0.8 g/d for males
	<0.75 g/d for females
Causes of abnormal values	↑ with high nondairy animal protein diet (high purine), alcoholic beverages, overproduction, diabetes, and use of sodium-glucose cotransporter-2 inhibitors

MAGNESIUM

Reason for order	Magnesium binds oxalate
	Assessment of calcium stone risk
Normal value	30 to 120 mg/d
Causes of abnormal values	↓ with some laxatives, malnutrition, malabsorption, increase risk for calcium stones as more oxalate is available

SODIUM

Reason for order	Assessment of sodium intake
Normal value	50 to 150 mEq/d (1,150–3,450 mg/d)
Causes of abnormal values	↑ with high-sodium diet
	↓ with bowel disease

Continued on next page

Continued from previous page

POTASSIUM

Reason for order	Assess risk of hypocitraturia and follow medication compliance, if started on diuretics
Normal value	20 to 100 mEq/d
Causes of abnormal values	<20 with bowel disease, diuretics, laxatives

UREA NITROGEN

Reason for order	Assessment of total protein metabolism
Normal value	6 to 14 g/kg/d
Causes of abnormal values	↑ with high-protein diet

SULFATE

Reason for order	Assessment of protein intake, especially animal protein
Normal value	20 to 80 mEq/d
Causes of abnormal values	↑ with high-protein diet, especially animal protein

AMMONIUM

Reason for order	Assessment of infection and medical condition
Normal value	15 to 60 mmol/d
Causes of abnormal values	↑ pH >7: urea splitting bacterial infection ↓ pH <5.5: chronic kidney disease, uric acid stones, gout

PROTEIN CATABOLIC RATE (PCR)

Reason for order	Assessment of total protein intake to evaluate adequate amount
Normal value	0.8 to 1.4 g/kg/d
Causes of abnormal values	↑ with high-protein diet

SUPERSATURATION

Reason for order	Determines the risk of crystal formation in the urine
Normal value	Reference values vary with different labs—supersaturation of calcium oxalate, supersaturation of calcium phosphate, supersaturation of uric acid
Causes of abnormal values	↑ of each supersaturation: increase calcium oxalate, calcium phosphate, and uric acid stone risks

Adapted with permission from Asplin JR. Hyperoxaluric calcium nephrolithiasis. *Endocrinol Metab Clin North Am.* 2002;31(4):927.[32]

Risk Factors

GENETIC

Various inherited diseases can cause kidney stones. Many of these genetic diseases have several clinical findings, one of which is kidney stones. Examples of these diseases include distal RTA, variants of Bartter syndrome, familial hypomagnesemia with hypercalciuria and nephrocalcinosis, Dent disease, hypophosphatemic rickets with hypercalciuria, autosomal dominant hyperparathyroidism, and Lowe syndrome.[33] IH, PH, and cystinuria are examples of genetic diseases that mainly present with stone burden.

IH is the most common abnormality found in about 50% of calcium stone formers.[34] The genetics of this disorder are complex and not fully defined, but approximately 50% of patients have a family history of kidney stones.[6,34] IH involves abnormal calcium handling by the gut, kidney, and bone. Patients with IH often have elevated 1,25-dihydroxyvitamin D levels and increased intestinal absorption of calcium. The kidneys exhibit a decreased ability to reabsorb filtered calcium and, in turn, the urinary calcium is increased.[35]

PH is a genetic defect that leads to overproduction of oxalate in the liver. Hyperoxaluria increases urinary SS of CaOx and promotes calcium stone formation. Kidney stones are often present in multiples and may lead to obstruction. Due to the stone burden, patients may progress to end-stage kidney disease (ESKD).[36] Kidney failure is multifactorial and may be related to complications from tubular obstruction, but there may be direct renal toxicity. Oxalate is secreted and filtered into the proximal renal tubules and poses the threat of cortical crystal formation with cell loss and acute and chronic kidney failure.[37]

Cystinuria is a disease that usually presents early in life characterized by defects in cystine transporters, causing decreased reabsorption and increased urinary cystine. If untreated, cystinuria can lead to possible ESKD.[38]

ENVIRONMENTAL

Climate and geography are independent risk factors for kidney stone formation. Kidney stones appear to be more prevalent in warmer climates.[4,9,39] According to the Second Cancer Prevention Survey (CPS II), the highest prevalence of kidney stones in the United States is in six southeastern states: Tennessee, Alabama, Mississippi, Georgia, North Carolina, and South Carolina, which is known as the "Kidney Stone Belt." Inadequate fluid intake combined with increased sweating lead to decreased urinary volume and may be the driver of stone development.[40,41]

DIETARY FACTORS

Multiple dietary factors are believed to play a role in stone formation, including intake of calcium, sodium, oxalate, protein (especially animal protein), low dietary fiber, fructose, vitamin C, and amount of fluids. A variety of other nutrients may predispose to nephrolithiasis via a variety of mechanisms.

Fluid Intake

Increased fluid intake leads to higher urine volume and decreased urinary SS of any lithogenic substance and is particularly useful if the stone type is unknown. Fluid intake is probably the most important and easily modifiable risk factor among stone formers.[42-44]

Studies have found that increased consumption of any type of beverage, despite common previous perceptions that some beverages (eg, tea, coffee, beer, wine, soda, and orange juice) were associated with stone formation because of their contents, are associated with lower risk of nephrolithiasis.[43,45] However, orange juice and sweetened soda are not recommended due to sugar/fructose content, which can lead to increased excretion of CaOx and uric acid.[46] While caffeine has been shown to increase urinary calcium, a more recent study concluded that there is actually a decreased risk of kidney stone formation with coffee and tea consumption.[47] The mechanisms for the protective properties are probably from unmeasured components, such as phytochemicals in the coffee.[46]

Calcium

Misconceptions about the relationship between high calcium intake and increased risk of stone formation were debunked by multiple prospective studies. In a large cohort of male health care professionals, higher dietary calcium lowered the risk of nephrolithiasis after controlling for other risk factors.[48] Other studies confirmed the same findings in women.[44,49,50] In another randomized controlled trial, a normal calcium diet compared to a low-calcium diet in patients with IH and CaOx stones was associated with a 50% reduction in recurrent stones. Experts hypothesized that a low-calcium diet was associated with increased oxalate absorption and urinary excretion.[51] While higher dietary calcium intake (800–1,200 mg/d) has been associated with decreased stone formation, calcium supplements may increase the risk of stone formation, especially if taken without meals.[48,49,52] Thus far, there is consensus that a low-calcium diet promotes stone formation, but there is no agreement on the recommendation for a high calcium intake to reduce the risk of nephrolithiasis.

Oxalate

It is hard to assess the risk that dietary oxalate poses on CaOx stone formation because the urine oxalate levels are not always proportional to the amount of dietary oxalate.[53] Bioavailability of oxalate varies between different foods. While some foods are high in oxalate content, that does not necessarily mean that the oxalate is readily absorbable in the gastrointestinal (GI) tract. Moreover, oxalate absorption is increased in some patients with certain GI conditions such as IBD (especially Crohn's disease) and after gastric bypass surgery.[54,55] A low-oxalate diet is often recommended for stone formers, but reliable information on the oxalate content of foods is still lacking.[56-58] Furthermore, high-oxalate foods often overlap with heart-healthy foods, and clinical judgment is required when balancing risk and benefits of oxalate restriction.

Sodium

Hypercalciuria is common in IH and is especially sensitive to dietary sodium intake.[57,58] Multiple observational and experimental studies have demonstrated that calcium excretion increases more steeply in IH than in normal subjects for a given increase in sodium excretion.[59] Dietary sodium restriction decreases urinary calcium and decreases urinary citrate, lowering CaOx stone formation.[52] Encouraging lower sodium diets is an important strategy to prevent calcium stones, particularly in patients with IH.

Protein

High animal-protein intake increases calcium and uric acid excretion and decreases urinary citrate.[60] This, however, did not translate clinically into higher risk of stone formation, except in one prospective study on men with lower body mass index (BMI).[50] Protein restriction reduces hypercalciuria via multiple mechanisms, for the most part, through a decreased acid load, resulting in decreased bone resorption and urinary calcium excretion.[61] Urinary citrate also increases, which then increases urine pH. Therefore, protein restriction, especially animal protein (high in purine), may be of benefit for uric acid stone formers and CaOx stones.[52,60]

Potassium

High-potassium diets decrease calcium excretion and increase urinary citrate.[62] Studies have shown that dietary potassium supplementation decreases kidney stone risk in men and older women.[44,48,49]

Magnesium

Magnesium may decrease kidney stone risk by reducing oxalate absorption through complexing with oxalate in the GI tract. In urine, magnesium may also bind oxalate in a soluble form, acting as an inhibitor.[63,64] The effect of magnesium in studies on risk reduction has not been well established because of confounding factors, such as thiazide diuretics and citrate supplements.[5] Prospective studies on various nutrients have shown that magnesium may reduce risk in men but not in women.[44,49,50]

Phytate

Phytate in plants may also have an important role in stone prevention. Phytates are salts of inositol hexakiphosphate and are the main storage form of phosphate in plant tissues. They are abundant in cold cereal, dark bread, and beans. Urinary phytate levels were significantly lower in calcium stone formers compared with healthy controls, but the levels may be normalized with phytate supplementation.[65] Analysis of the Second Nurses' Health Study (NHS II) revealed that women with phytate intake had a 36% lower risk of stone formation.[44] The exact mechanism of phytate effect on stone reduction is not completely understood. Phytate may indirectly decrease urinary calcium excretion by forming insoluble complexes with calcium in the GI tract and preventing absorption.[44] This implies increased oxalate absorption from the GI tract, which makes the mechanism by inhibition of CaOx crystal formation in the urine more plausible.[66]

Vitamin and Herbal Supplements

Some vitamins may play a role in decreasing or increasing the risk of kidney stones. They are abundant in many over-the-counter supplements at several times the daily requirements and are easily overconsumed.

Vitamin C is one of the most widely used over-the-counter supplements or added vitamin to beverages. One of its metabolites is oxalate. A study showed that a twice daily regimen of 1,000 mg vitamin C supplement may increase urinary oxalate excretion by 20% in normal subjects and 33% in prior CaOx stone formers, independent of a pH change.[67] Observational studies show that supplemental and dietary vitamin C intake increase CaOx stone risk among men, but not women, probably due to gender difference of vitamin C metabolism.[50,68]

Vitamin D is a globally used vitamin in supplements and food. It has been implicated with increased risk of kidney stones because it increases calcium and phosphorus absorption. However, a small study of vitamin D repletion in healthy women did not increase urine calcium excretion.[69] A more recent study showed that stone formers with high serum 25-hydroxyvitamin D levels who took vitamin D supplements alone or with calcium may have an increase in urinary calcium excretion.[70] Therefore, vitamin D supplementation among stone formers should be individualized, and ensuring bone health may take priority over kidney stone prevention.

On the preventive end of the vitamin spectrum, experts have hypothesized that vitamin B6 decreases risk because it is a known cofactor in oxalate metabolism and may lower urinary oxalate excretion.[17] Observational data has shown that higher intake of vitamin B6 via supplements may reduce the risk of stone formation in women only, but the larger cohort (NHS I, NHS II, and Health Professional Follow-up Study [HPFS]) showed that vitamin B6 is not associated with decreased kidney stone incidence.[71-73]

Alternative therapies and supplements including herbs have been used for millenniums. According to Beto,[74] "These herbal formulas have multiple spectrums of intended action including analgesic, anti-inflammatory, antimicrobial, antispasmodic, anticalcifying, diuretic, or litholytic." "A comprehensive literature review of herbal use in the management of kidney stones found very few published studies of rigor and quality in humans."[74-77] There is concern among experts with respect to lack of regulation on the content of herbal supplements as well as the potential for impurities that may contribute to stone formation. Therefore, herbal supplements for stone prevention should be used very carefully.[78-80]

Box 14.2 summarizes the genetic, environmental, and dietary risk factors of kidney stones.

Medical Conditions

OBESITY, DIABETES MELLITUS, AND THE METABOLIC SYNDROME

Multiple studies have shown increased risk of stone formation in patients with obesity, diabetes mellitus (DM), and metabolic syndrome (MS). A large cross-sectional analysis of three cohorts with more than 200,000 participants (NHS I and II and the HPFS) revealed a relative risk of prevalent kidney stone formation ranging from 1.31 in men to 1.60 in younger women with DM

BOX 14.2 | Risk Factors for Kidney Stones

GENETIC AND OTHER DISEASE-RELATED

Genetic	Idiopathic hypercalciuria
	Hyperoxalosis
	Cystinuria
	Dent disease
Kidney disease-related	Medullary sponge kidney
	Polycystic kidney disease (10% develop stones)
	Horseshoe kidney
	Metabolic causes: hypercalcemia, hyperparathyroidism, diabetes mellitus, and obesity
Systemic disease	Gastrointestinal, inflammatory bowel diseases (oxalate and uric acid stones)
Primary hyperparathyroidism	Calcium phosphate stones
Renal tubular acidosis (RTA)	Hypercalcemic states, calcium phosphate stones
	Sjögren syndrome
Sarcoid	Hypercalciuria, calcium oxalate stones

ENVIRONMENTAL AND DIET-RELATED

Climate	Heat
	Water loss, sweating
Dietary	High sodium
	Oxalate
	Protein (mostly nondairy animal)
	Acid/alkaline-ash diet
	Fluid
	Potassium and citrate
	Vitamins (C, D)
	Calcium supplement
	Low-calcium diet
	High-protein weight loss diet

Adapted with permission from Han H, Seifte J. Nephrolithiasis. In: Byham-Gray L, Burrowes JD, Chertow GM, eds. *Nutrition in Kidney Disease*. 2nd ed. Humana Press; 2014:355-373.[81]

compared to controls. The relative risk of incident DM in subjects with a prior history of nephrolithiasis was also higher among the entire study population.[7]

Patients with DM and obesity tend to form uric acid stones in particular, possibly because insulin resistance in these patients leads to impaired ammonium excretion, which then causes a lower pH favoring uric acid stone formation.[82,83] Among uric acid stone formers, nearly 30% of those with DM reported stone formation compared to only 6.2% to 13% of those without DM with a greater difference detected in the female cohort.[82-85]

HYPERTENSION

The prevalence of nephrolithiasis is higher in hypertensive vs normotensive subjects.[41] A large prospective cohort revealed 79.5% reported that nephrolithiasis had occurred either prior to or concomitant with the diagnosis of hypertension (HTN), which suggests that the occurrence of nephrolithiasis might increase the risk of future HTN.[86] Patients with HTN are at risk of calcium and uric acid stones. HTN may be associated with impaired calcium homeostasis, as hypercalciuria is a common finding in essential HTN.[87-90] The evaluation of 24-hour urine collections among the three large cohorts also showed an independent association of HTN and hypocitraturia.[91] Hypertensive patients may be at risk for uric acid nephrolithiasis because childhood serum uric acid elevations have been associated with both childhood and adult HTN.[92]

ATHEROSCLEROSIS/CARDIOVASCULAR DISEASE

The association between cardiovascular disease (CVD) and nephrolithiasis was first reported in the early 1970s. An observational study out of Norway in 1973 noted an increased risk of myocardial infarction (MI) in patients with a history of kidney stones who were admitted to the hospital between 1892 and 1932.[93]

More recently, in a longitudinal study with a 20-year follow-up, a significant association was found between kidney stones and subclinical carotid atherosclerosis.[94] A population-based observational study of more than 5,000 White and Black participants ranging in age between 18 years and 30 years used ultrasound to determine carotid thickness and stenosis. This test showed an association between increased carotid thickness, particularly in the internal carotid artery, and symptomatic kidney stone formation. A case-control study of CaOx stone formers and normal controls reported that significantly more stone formers had a history of coronary artery disease vs controls.[95] Further data from the Rochester Epidemiology Project revealed a 31% increased risk of MI in stone formers, after adjustment for chronic kidney disease (CKD) and other comorbidities associated with MI.[96] A recent meta-analysis showed an increased risk of coronary heart disease (CHD) in patients with a history of kidney stones with a relative risk ratio (RR) of 1.23 (95% confidence interval [CI], 1.08–1.41), but this risk association was limited to women (RR, 1.43; 95% CI, 1.12–1.82). The authors also noted conflicting data with several studies showing no increased risk of CHD and other studies showing a more pronounced risk for women than men.[97]

CHRONIC KIDNEY DISEASE

Studies have shown an association between the development of CKD and nephrolithiasis. In case-control studies, kidney stone formation was found to be an independent risk factor for CKD and ESKD, after adjusting for the most common etiologies, including DM, HTN, and CVD.[98,99] In the NHANES III cohort, subjects with higher BMI (≥27) who formed stones were more likely to have lower glomerular filtration rate (GFR) than subjects with lower BMI. Furthermore, the investigators calculated that the probability of a GFR in the CKD stage 3 range (30–59 mL/min/1.73 m^2) in an overweight stone former was almost twice that of a similarly overweight non–stone former (RR, 1.87).[100] Despite these data, kidney stones are not a major cause of CKD unless obstruction remains untreated or the patient has a genetic abnormality like PH or cystinuria.

GASTROINTESTINAL DISEASE/ GASTRIC BYPASS SURGERY

Gastrointestinal Disease

GI diseases can cause increased GI losses through diarrhea and decreased intake, depending on the disease.[101] This leads to decreased urinary volume and concentrated urine, which increases the risk for kidney stone formation. Increased fluid intake is the hallmark of recommendations for reducing the recurrence of kidney stones and may be more important for those with GI disease or GI loss of fluids.[15,102,103]

GI disorders may also be associated with high urinary oxalate. Urinary oxalate comes from either an endogenous source as in PH or an exogenous source as in secondary hyperoxaluria. PH is a genetic disorder that is characterized by a hepatic enzyme deficiency leading to increased endogenous oxalate formation. Secondary hyperoxaluria, also known as enteric hyperoxaluria, is caused by increased oxalate absorption, which may be due to high dietary oxalate, fat malabsorption, alterations in the gut microbiome, or genetic variations in oxalate transporters in the gut.[101]

Absorption of oxalate from the gut is partially dependent on transporters; however, the exact mechanisms are unknown. The stomach is a site of oxalate uptake via transcellular transport. Increased oxalate absorption is observed when transit time through the stomach is slow. Under normal conditions, calcium binds to dietary oxalate in the distal intestine, forming a complex that is expelled in the stool. Other dietary factors (magnesium, fatty acids, and bile salts) may also affect the absorption of oxalates. CaOx stone formers seem to have a greater transient increase in the absorption of oxalate compared to normal individuals after an oxalate rich meal.[103] In fat malabsorption syndromes, increased oxalate is absorbed when calcium binds to malabsorbed fats rather than oxalate, increasing the amount of unbound oxalate. Inflammation increases the permeability of the intestinal mucosa, causing excess free oxalate absorption.[104] Research suggests that restriction of oxalates in the diet may also reduce the presence of *Oxalobacter formigenes* when it is deprived of its food source.[105] The loss of *O formigenes* colonization is associated with an increased risk of kidney stone formation.

Gastric Bypass Surgery

Malabsorption of fat as well as macronutrients, essential vitamins, and minerals may occur with substantial weight loss.[106] An increased incidence of kidney stones related to bariatric surgery has been observed similar to the risk of GI diseases.[107] Fat malabsorption, which may accompany some forms of bariatric surgery, decreases calcium and leaves less to bind to oxalate. A low-fat diet has been shown to lower urinary oxalate levels.[108] Vitamin deficiencies due to malabsorption include pyridoxine (vitamin B6, a cofactor in liver metabolism of glyoxalate), which could also lead to increased urinary levels of oxalate. Specific alterations in the microbiome after bariatric surgery are not well characterized; however, a decrease in oxalate-degrading bacteria in patients after gastric bypass was observed.[109]

Stone Type and Treatment

SURGICAL MANAGEMENT

Most urinary stones will spontaneously pass; however, between 10% to 20% of stone events will necessitate surgical intervention.[110,111] For struvite and staghorn stones, which are large and often associated with UTI, the primary treatment is surgical.

The most common reasons for stone surgery include intractable pain, kidney failure, infection associated with a kidney or ureteral stone, failure of a ureteral stone to pass, or management of a large kidney stone. There are a variety of techniques to surgically manage stones, including extracorporeal shock wave lithotripsy, ureteroscopy, and percutaneous nephrolithotomy.[112] In unusual situations, open surgical approaches are needed.[110,111,113]

MEDICAL AND DIET MANAGEMENT PER STONE TYPE

Patients are often referred to the nephrology and nutrition departments after they present with a symptomatic kidney stone or undergo a stone removal procedure. The indications for referral for medical stone prevention have been debated, but recurrent and multiple stones are common reasons. The primary purpose of medical and diet intervention is to prevent stone recurrence. All stone formers should be evaluated for medical conditions that might predispose to stones. A 24-hour urine collection is key to assess stone-forming risk factors and help guide nutritional risk factors. The American Urology Association (AUA) guidelines provide a useful reference for the standard treatment and prevention of kidney stones.[112]

GENERAL NUTRITION ASSESSMENT

Input from the registered dietitian nutritionist (RDN) is very important as changes in diet play a key role in stone prevention. The RDN should assess nutritional risk factors via diet intake assessment and provide medical nutrition therapy based on identified risks. Specifically, the RDN should evaluate for nutrient intake of dietary risk factors of stone formation and inhibition. Fluid intake is particularly important to quantify.

There are several methods for diet assessment: 24-hour recall, food record, and food frequency questionnaire. The RDN can instruct patients to keep food records including intake of foods, beverages, and dietary supplements (vitamin/mineral and other over-the-counter supplements) with portion size. The most appropriate diet assessment for kidney stones is the food record before and in conjunction with a 24-hour urine collection. The RDN should recommend that patients record 1 to 2 days prior to and during the urine collection periods to obtain an accurate analysis. Based on food intake and 24-hour urine assessment, the RDN provides nutritional advice that can be monitored and modified as needed based on future urine assessments. It is also helpful to question intake of high-oxalate foods that are typically only seasonally available (eg, rhubarb, beets, or spinach) and advise against excessive intake of these foods when they are in season.

CALCIUM STONES

Calcium stones are the most common type of stones, and patients can present to the RDN after incidental discovery or a symptomatic event. A study by Strohmaier[114] estimated that 10% of patients with calcium-type stones will have recurrence of symptomatic stones more than three times throughout their lives, with brushite stones being the most common. The majority of calcium stones are CaOx stones.

Calcium Oxalate Stones

Medical management Hypercalciuria is associated with the formation of calcium stones. However, low calcium intake was associated with increased formation of CaOx stones.[51] Restricting dietary calcium increases the availability of free oxalate to be absorbed from the GI tract. Additional calcium supplementation beyond adequate daily intake is associated with stone formation, and its usage in a stone former should be reviewed. Importantly, calcium intake needs to be considered in the context of the patient's bone health, which may take clinical priority. Dietary sodium restriction is important as it is associated with a reduction in urine calcium excretion, especially in IH.[115] All patients with calcium stones should follow a low-sodium diet. If a low-sodium diet does not improve urinary calcium excretion, medical management should be considered using thiazide diuretics. Thiazide diuretics can decrease calcium excretion but at the risk of hypercalcemia, hyperglycemia, hypokalemia, and low blood pressure, especially in patients who do not have HTN.[116]

Frequently, CaOx stone formers have low urine citrate with low urine pH. Potassium citrate is prescribed to increase citrate that competes with oxalate and forms a soluble compound with calcium. A common side effect with potassium citrate is upper GI disturbance.[117] Patients sometimes also complain about pill size. Sodium bicarbonate supplementation may increase urinary citrate levels and reduce CaOx SS but is not as effective as potassium citrate.[118] It also provides unwanted sodium. Studies using commercial fruit juices (such as orange, cranberry, and apple) have shown a significant increase in urinary citrate level.[119] However, patients with MS should pay attention to their intake of these juices due to their sugar content and possible high calorie contribution.

Prebiotic and probiotic supplementation is increasingly being recognized as a potential treatment option in obesity, DM, and IBD.[120-122] Probiotics have anti-inflammatory effects that may help lower intestinal permeability for excess oxalate absorption among patients with IBD, obesity, and gastric bypass surgery. However, there is not enough evidence to support use of probiotics for stone prevention.

As oxalate plays an important role in the formation of kidney stones, increased oxalate breakdown in the gut by certain bacteria may reduce oxalate gut absorption and subsequently reduce oxalate excretion in the kidney.[123] Another possible mechanism is that the gut microbiome may also play a role in influencing the net alkali absorption and may increase citrate concentration in the urine. These mechanisms may eventually reduce the rate of stone formation.[124] *O formigenes* uses oxalate as an energy source in the GI tract and lowers oxalate absorption. A study out of Boston, MA, observed a 70% reduction in recurrent stone formation in those colonized with *O formigenes*.[125] An initial small study in patients with PH suggested that *O formigenes* therapy reduced urinary oxalate significantly.[126] However, a subsequent 24-week randomized, placebo-controlled trial with PH did not show a difference in urinary oxalate excretion.[127] Therefore, clinical use of *O formigenes* for stone prevention is not clear at this time.

Nutritional Management

- ***Fluid*** The amount of fluid intake determines the urine volume, which in turn affects the concentration of stone-forming components in the urine. The AUA guidelines recommend enough fluid intake to produce 2.5 L urine daily with modifica-

tions based on the patient's clinical presentation.[112] The best way to consume a large quantity of fluid is to drink water after each void, but it can be individualized according to the patient's lifestyle. Coffee (both caffeinated and decaffeinated), tea, wine, and alcoholic beverages are associated with a lower risk of stones; however, sweetened beverages, grapefruit juice, and orange juice have positive association with stone risks, possibly because of their fructose content which has independently been associated with increased stone risk.[43,45,46,128,129] Although orange juice is high in citrate, it is not often recommended due to its high calorie content, and it is especially avoided in patients with DM. Most patients require 3 L or more of fluid intake per day to reach this urine volume goal, but this varies with patient-specific factors, including nonurine loss of fluids from sweating or GI loss.

- ***Calcium*** Assessment of calcium intake and excretion is important for treating CaOx and CaP stones. Low-calcium diets generally increase the risk of calcium stone formation possibly by lowering the availability of calcium to bind with dietary oxalate in the gut and subsequent excretion of CaOx in the stool. This may result in higher oxalate absorption and urinary excretion.[112] Sorensen and colleagues[130] showed a higher incidence of nephrolithiasis among individuals who consumed less than 800 mg calcium per day compared to consuming adequate dietary calcium, defined as 1,000 mg/d to 1,200 mg/d for most adults. Achieving the recommended intake of calcium with food alone may be difficult for some. Supplemental calcium is a reasonable intervention to address inadequate dietary intake; however, there is evidence that supplemental calcium may correlate with a higher risk of kidney stone formation in older women. In the Women's Health Initiative clinical trial, subjects who took supplements and exceeded the recommended upper limit of 1,200 mg daily for adults had a higher risk for kidney stones.[131,132] In addition to the dose of supplements, timing is an important consideration to prevent the formation of kidney stones. Experts recommend that adults not only take the supplements with meals in order to bind to the oxalate but also avoid exceeding the adequate range of approximately 1,000 to 1,200 mg total daily calcium intake from both diet and supplements. Assessing 24-hour urine collections for SS levels may help determine whether calcium supplements are beneficial or problematic for this patient group.[112]

- **Sodium** Calcium homeostasis is influenced substantially by dietary sodium. Increased urinary sodium causes hypercalciuria. Lower sodium paired with adequate calcium in the diet can reduce urinary calcium excretion in stone formers with hypercalciuria.[52] Based on the available evidence, the AUA recommends that dietary sodium should not exceed 100 mEq or 2,300 mg daily for most adult stone formers.[112] Nutrition strategies with reduction of dietary sodium are thus recommended for stone prevention. Dietary Approaches to Stop Hypertension (DASH), a heart-healthy diet, may be an appropriate strategy.[86] A DASH diet is low in sodium and nondairy animal protein, and higher in fruits, vegetables, nuts, legumes, whole grains, and dairy compared to a typical Western diet. Several observational studies have supported the DASH diet to reduce stone risks.[63,133]

- **Oxalate** Urinary oxalate may remain high, even with adding calcium to the diet. At that time, restricting oxalate in the diet may help further decrease urinary oxalate in patients with confirmed CaOx stones. Recently, the popularity of a gluten-free diet, even in those who do not have gluten enteropathy or irritable bowel syndrome, may introduce high oxalate-containing foods via substitutes for wheat/oat products (eg, nut bars, soy products, almond flour, and amaranth) which can greatly increase the oxalate consumption. Combination of adequate calcium consumption with small amounts of these high-oxalate foods can help lower oxalate absorption. The Harvard School of Public Health provides an extensive online oxalate database to help manage a lower-

oxalate diet.[112] Since dietary intake of oxalate is not the only factor influencing urinary oxalate, overly restrictive low-oxalate diets are not generally recommended as most high-oxalate foods provide other health benefits.[134,135] Table 14.1 shows examples of high-oxalate foods and content.

The reported values across oxalate references vary widely and may be confusing for both patients and providers when attempting a low-oxalate diet intervention. Multiple other conditions related to the plant's ripeness upon harvesting and soil characteristics may alter the oxalate content and make dietary advice challenging.[134,136] Thus, hyperoxaluria treatment is often focused on adequate calcium intake to decrease oxalate absorption, rather than decrease oxalate in the diet.[135,137] Adequate amount of calcium, lower nondairy animal protein and sodium, and high-

TABLE 14.1 | Oxalate Content of Commonly Known High-Oxalate Foods

Foods	Portion size	Oxalate content (mg)
Spinach (cooked)	½ cup	755
Spinach (raw)	1 cup	656
Rhubarb	½ cup	541
Almonds	1 ounce (22 nuts)	122
Miso soup	1 cup	111
Potato, baked with skin	1 medium	97
Bulgar, cooked	1 cup	86
Beets	½ cup	76
Navy beans	½ cup	76
Cocoa powder	4 teaspoon	67
Hot chocolate, homemade	1 cup	65
Okra	½ cup	57
Cashews	1 ounce (18 nuts)	49
Raspberries	1 cup	48
Dates	2 dates	48
Raisin Bran cereal	1 cup	46

Adapted with permission from Harvard T.H. Chan School of Public Health Nutrition Department. Available at https://regepi.bwh .harvard.edu/health/Oxalate/files

er amounts of fruits, vegetables, and plant-based proteins reduce the risk of CaOx stone formation and recurrence.[63] Although the DASH diet may be high in oxalate, it usually contains higher levels of fiber and phytate that help lower oxalate absorption in the GI tract. The vegetarian diet includes high oxalate content but a good calcium source (eg, almond milk or soy milk with calcium fortification) can have a similar effect on lowering oxalate absorption.

Patients with enteric hyperoxaluria (EH) absorb excessive amounts of oxalate. Predisposing conditions include gastric bypass surgery (eg, Roux-en-Y) and IBD where fat malabsorption is present, allowing calcium to bind to the malabsorbed fat rather than the oxalate.[101,138] Also, increased transit time in the bowel associated with these conditions does not allow for bacteria in the bowel to degrade oxalates. Since EH causes very high urinary oxalate excretion, a more restrictive oxalate diet may provide benefit. Higher calcium intake and lower fat intake may also help prevent increased oxalate absorption; calcium supplements provided with meals aid in promoting binding of free oxalate.

A variety of oral supplements may contribute to elevated urinary oxalate. Ascorbic acid from high-dose vitamin C supplements is metabolized to oxalate, and turmeric and cranberry supplements have been associated with higher oxalate levels in urine.[139-141] The AUA does not recommend vitamin C supplementation because of CaOx stone risk. Other supplements have been suggested as beneficial in reducing urinary oxalate in idiopathic CaOx stone formers. Probiotics, omega-3 fatty acids, vitamin B6, or pyridoxine have not been sufficiently studied at this point to justify recommendations by the AUA, but completing 24-hour urine studies before and after dietary interventions like these may provide guidance in specific situations.[112]

- ***Acid-Forming Foods and Protein*** Hypocitraturia, defined as urinary citrate less than 320 mg/d, is present in 20% to 60% of stone formers.[98] The average daily excretion of citrate is about 600 mg/d,

which is the minimal acceptable level for patients with kidney stones, according to the AUA guidelines.[112] Urinary citrate is an important inhibitor of calcium stone formation.[142] It is also used as a therapy to alkalinize the urine in patients with uric acid stones. A diet rich in foods with a high potential renal acid load (PRAL), including meat, eggs, and grain, can trigger acidosis as compared with fruits and vegetables, which have an alkali load.[143] Milk, yogurt, and dietary fat have a neutral PRAL.[144,145] The acidosis is buffered through the reabsorption of bicarbonate or citrate from the kidney, thus lowering the citrate in the urine. A study of 187 patients with calcium stones showed a negative correlation between PRAL and urinary citrate with no change in urinary calcium, oxalate, and urate.[145]

If a patient consumes high PRAL foods, which likely contribute to hypocitraturia, the patient may benefit from increasing fruits and vegetables and decreasing meats, fish, poultry, cheese, eggs, processed meats, and grains.

Animal protein sources appear to increase kidney stone risk (possibly because of the increased acid load) compared to plant-based proteins. The DASH diet is low in nondairy animal protein and higher in fruits, vegetables, nuts, legumes, whole grains, and dairy compared to a typical Western diet.[63]

A DASH diet plan provides about 4 oz to 6 oz animal protein per day, which is adequate for most people. The DASH diet has also shown potential benefit in reducing the risk of CKD, type 2 DM, CVD, and stroke.[133]

Increasing fruits and vegetables as a singular intervention may be adequate, but weight gain may ensue if other foods are not adjusted to balance calories.[146] Hypocitraturia may also be addressed with increased dietary citrate.[147]

Citrate from fruits and unsweetened juices may alleviate hypocitraturia similar to pharmacologic citrate.[128] The juice from two medium-sized fresh lemons consumed daily may provide a level of dietary citrate that is comparable to typical pharmacologic interventions at lower cost and without GI effects.[148]

Box 14.3 shows acid- and alkaline-ash foods.

Calcium Phosphate Stones

CaP stones comprise 20% of calcium stones. They occur when the SS of CaP is elevated. Alkaline pH (>6.2) and hypercalciuria increase the SS of CaP and enhance their formation. CaP stones are associated with certain diseases, such as primary hyperparathyroidism, sarcoidosis, and RTA. Treatment should focus on decreasing the SS of CaP by increasing fluid intake, decreasing urinary calcium, and treating the underlying cause. Although citrate is an inhibitor of stone formation, caution is advised when using citrate to treat hypocitraturia in patients with CaP stones, especially if the pH level is elevated. By further increasing the pH level, citrate may create an environment favorable for CaP crystal formation.[2,150] However, there are conflicting data emerging on this point as citrate has been shown to inhibit CaP stone formation in vitro. In vivo, it may depend if the citrate is given as potassium citrate, which provides an alkali load, and increases urinary citrate and pH (risking SS), or as citric acid which has a modest effect on urinary citrate but has less effect on raising urinary pH.[151]

Nutrition therapy may be the only needed intervention to prevent recurrence of calcium stones. However, medications (usually thiazide diuretics) are often required, especially for persistent hypercalciuria among patients with IH. Dietary management is usually the first intervention for stone management, and if that fails, pharmacological therapy is initiated to treat and prevent calcium stones.

URIC ACID STONES

The incidence of uric acid stones, which has increased in the United States in recent decades, represents approximately 10% of all stone disease. Elevation of uric acid in urine is associated with uncontrolled primary gout, obesity, DM, and MS. The population with these conditions also tends to have acidic urine with a pH less than

BOX 14.3 | Acid-Ash and Alkaline-Ash Foods

ACID-ASH FOODS

Meat	Meat, fish, fowl, shellfish, eggs
Dairy and other protein	All types of cheese
	Peanut butter
	Peanuts
Fat	Bacon, nuts (Brazil, filberts, walnuts)
Starch	All types, especially whole wheat
	Crackers, cereal, macaroni, spaghetti, noodles, rice
Vegetables	Corn, lentils
Fruits	Cranberries, plums, prunes
Desserts	Plain cakes, cookies

ALKALINE-ASH FOODS

Dairy	Milk and milk products
	Buttermilk
Fat	Nuts (almonds, chestnuts, coconuts)
Vegetables	All types, except corn and lentils
	Beets, beet greens, Swiss chard, dandelion greens, kale, mustard greens, spinach, turnip greens
Fruits	All types, except cranberries, plums, and prunes
Sweets	Molasses

Adapted with permission from Mahan LK, Escott-Stump S. *Krause's Food & Nutrition Therapy.* 12th ed. Saunders/Elsevier; 2008.[149]

6, which triggers uric acid stone formation.[152,153] Measurements of urinary calcium, uric acid, and postprandial urinary pH are used to assess uric acid stone disease.

Management strategies include increasing urinary volume, alkalinizing the urine, reducing uric acid excretion, or any of these combined. Uric acid stones tend to recur and may be multiple so that frequent monitoring is appropriate.

Medical Management

Urinary pH plays an important role in uric acid crystallization. Uric acid is soluble in alkaline pH greater than 6.5; therefore, keeping urinary pH greater than 6.5 is recommended to prevent uric acid stone formation.[154]

However, if urinary pH increases to 7.0 or more, there is a potential to promote CaP stone formation in predisposed patients.

Potassium citrate is the most commonly used drug for urinary alkalization for uric acid stone prevention. An average daily potassium citrate dose of 60 mEq divided three times daily usually showed an increase of urinary pH and citrate, and lowered recurrence of uric acid stones.[155] Treatment is sometimes limited by GI intolerance, pill burden, and cost. Another concern is hyperkalemia, particularly in patients with CKD and those taking renin angiotensin aldosterone system inhibitors, which increase serum potassium levels.[156] Dose adjustment of potassium citrate depends on the 24-hour urine test, urinary pH, and SS of uric acid. It is important to keep in mind that potassium citrate may predispose to CaP stone development.[2,150,157]

An alternative to potassium citrate is sodium citrate; however, the sodium load in this medicine can lead to increased calcium excretion and increased risk of calcium stone formation.[158] If uric acid stones are the result of diarrhea or other GI conditions resulting in volume depletion, sodium citrate may be preferable over potassium citrate for volume repletion and prevention.[159]

Sodium bicarbonate supplementation is another potential therapy for urinary alkalinization. However, high doses of sodium bicarbonate may cause elevation of urinary sodium, which can also elevate urinary calcium.[160]

Another therapeutic target is decreasing systemic uric acid production, which leads to hypouricosuria. Xanthine oxidase inhibitors, such as allopurinol, reduce xanthine and hypoxanthine conversion to uric acid. Usually used as gout prevention therapy, xanthine oxidase inhibitors lower serum uric acid production and eventually reduce uric acid excretion into the urine.[161] Interestingly, allopurinol has been shown to decrease the risk of calcium stones, serum uric acid, and urinary uric acid in a randomized controlled trial; however, the effect on preventing uric acid stone formation is less clear.[162,163] Allopurinol is generally used as a second-line treatment in individuals who continue to have uric acid stones, despite correction of urinary pH. Although extremely rare, allopurinol may cause severe allergic and life-threatening hypersensitivity reactions that should be highlighted to patients before starting this second-line therapy.[164,165]

Nutritional Management

The backbone of dietary intervention for uric acid stone prevention is urinary alkalization and weight loss. Low urinary pH is a very important risk factor for uric acid stones. Urinary uric acid is a product of exogenous and endogenous input with diet contributing about 30%, which comes, for the most part, from high purine animal sources in the typical Western diet.[166]

Healthy individuals consuming a typical Western diet produce about 300 to 400 mg/dL uric acid daily, and about two-thirds of the uric acid is excreted in the urine.[152,167] Nondairy animal protein, processed meat, and grains are high in purine, associated with PRAL, and become acid ash.[154,164,168] Therefore, moderate amounts of total protein, no more than 1.2 g/kg/d, is advised for uric acid stone formers.[168] Higher amounts of nondairy protein tend to result in acidic pH and increased uric acid excretion due to their high purine content.

Citrate prevents uric acid stones by increasing urinary pH and binding urinary calcium and, thus, reduces formation of calcium stones as well.

A vegetarian diet may be beneficial for preventing recurrence of uric acid nephrolithiasis because this type of diet is low in purine content and produces alkaline ash that increases urinary pH. It is also a good source of citrate. The DASH diet, which is abundant in citrate rich foods, can increase urinary citrate and, thus, generate an alkaline urine. In several studies, individuals who followed this diet had higher urinary citrate and pH levels.[63,153] However, the risk of kidney stones was not studied. The DASH diet may have additional benefits, as it is associated with weight loss and possible improvement in the MS, resulting in improved insulin sensitivity and higher urinary pH.

In terms of beverages with high citrate content, several studies have been performed to determine the effect of these beverages on urinary citrate. Kang et al[128] conducted a study to examine the effect of long-term use of lemonade compared with potassium citrate supplementation. The study showed that urinary pH was higher in the potassium citrate supplement group but that urinary citrate levels were within a good range in both groups (700 mg/d for lemonade, 800 mg/d for potassium citrate supplement group). The juices also provided a higher intake of fluids. One study compared the impact of 1 week of orange juice to lemonade consumption on kidney stone risk factors. Although orange juice showed a higher increase in urinary pH compared with lemonade, the caloric content in orange juice was of concern; therefore, it is not a recommended treatment for stone formers with DM.[169] We can conclude from these studies that citrate-containing beverages increase urinary citrate and pH; nonetheless, none of these studies had the end point of preventing uric acid stones.

Beer has high purine content, and it causes elevation of blood uric acid level.[170,171] Although alcohol was considered a risk factor for gout, no studies showed a positive association between alcohol consumption and nephrolithiasis.

Several studies examine the effects of different beverages on urinary uric acid. Choi and Curhan[172] monitored the effect of coffee, tea, and caffeine consumption on serum uric acid level. The serum levels were lower, but the urinary uric acid level was not measured. The high concentration of polyphenol and chlorogenic acid, which has insulin-sensitizing effects, are believed to be responsible for lowering the serum uric acid levels.[173,174] Mineral water with high amounts of bicarbonate also elevated urinary pH and citrate and lowered SS of uric acid among patients who consumed highly carbonated mineral water.[153,175] Few energy drinks have been studied with regard to their citrate content, but their high caloric content from fructose may raise uric acid levels.[176] Dietary fructose consumption is considered an independent risk factor of uric acid stone formation. High concentrated fructose corn syrup is used as a preservative; fructose produces purine that is converted to uric acid. Elevated uric acid in the urine was associated with increased fructose consumption among patients with gout.[177]

CYSTINE STONES

Cystine stones form in the rare genetic disease called cystinuria, which is largely a pediatric disease. Patients usually present with their first kidney stone in their early teens, and 80% of symptomatic patients have their first renal colic by the end of the second decade.[178-180] Patients tend to have more bilateral and larger stones as compared with other stone formers. Cystine stones are formed because the amino acid cystine is excreted in high amounts in the urine through genetically defective tubular transport.[181]

Cystinuria is diagnosed by measuring urinary cystine levels and should be suspected in young patients with numerous and recurrent stones. Workup should always include a 24-hour urine collection; urinary pH and volume are important risk factors since they are the most modifiable. Cystine is much more soluble in alkaline urine. The higher the pH and the higher the urine volume, the lower the concentration and more soluble is the cysteine in the urine.[182,183]

Medical Management

If left untreated, cystinuria may lead to recurrent kidney stones requiring multiple urological procedures and may eventually lead to HTN and CKD.[38,182,184] Since cystine stones are insoluble in an acidic pH, potassium citrate is used to alkalinize the urine.[185] When or if increasing volumes and urinary alkalization fail, patients are prescribed cystine-binding thiol drugs, which improve the solubility of cysteine; studies have shown that they lead to decreased stone size and even dissolution.[186,187] The two available thiol-binding agents are D penicillamine and tiopronin. The problem with these agents is the side effect profile and their frequent daily dosing, which makes adherence cumbersome in children.

Nutritional Management

The goal of nutritional management in cystinuria is to reduce urinary cystine concentration by increasing urine volume and decreasing production of cystine. High fluid intake of at least 3 to 4 L a day is the most important treatment in bringing the cystine concentration to below 250 mg/L. In order to keep the concentration low over 24 hours, patients are advised to hydrate well before bedtime and even sometimes in the middle of the night.

A low animal protein diet may have preventive effects. First, it helps increase the urinary pH, which decreases the SS of cystine; a diet rich in fruits and vegetables is recommended, as well in increasing the urinary pH.[146] Second, a low-protein diet reduces ingestion of methionine, the precursor of cystine production.[188] However, children and adolescents require normal protein intake for their overall growth, and limiting animal protein may not be a practical approach.

A low-sodium diet can help reduce urinary cystine concentration by a mechanism that remains unknown. A reduction in sodium intake to 150 mmol or 3,450 mg per day was effective in dropping the cystine excretion to 650 mmol/d, which is enough to lower the cystine concentration to a soluble level.[189]

STRUVITE/STAGHORN CALCULI

Struvite stones contain the compound struvite, which is composed of magnesium ammonium phosphate, and are associated with genitourinary infection. Struvite stones often form staghorn calculi, which are large branching calculi that fill the urinary space. One study found an infectious etiology in 59% to 68% of patients with higher rates up to 74% in women with bilateral staghorn calculi.[190,191] The 2005 AUA guidelines state that most staghorn calculi are composed of struvite and/or calcium apatite.[192] Recent data, however, suggest that staghorn calculi are not necessarily related to infection and that they do not necessarily contain struvite. One study looked at the composition of staghorn calculi in 48 patients and found that most (56%) were metabolic with the following breakdown: 56% CaP, 21% uric acid, 14% CaOx, and 10% cysteine. The remaining 44% were struvite (or infection stones).[191]

Struvite stones are more common in females by a factor of about 2:1, presumably because of the increased risk of UTI. Additional risk factors include urinary tract obstruction, indwelling catheters, neurogenic bladder, and immobility.[193,194]

The standard treatment of struvite and staghorn calculi is surgical, but metabolic evaluation may be warranted in some patients as struvite stones, even if occurring with infection, and may be associated with metabolic abnormalities. The use of antibiotics and documented clearance of infection are also important for the prevention of struvite stones; however, specific guidelines about the choice and the duration of antibiotics are lacking.[194,195]

Nutritional Management

The role of metabolic manipulation for the management and the prevention of struvite kidney stones is unknown. No dietary modification has proven effective at preventing or treating struvite stones. A diet that lowers urinary pH could potentially decrease stone formation, but there is no data to support this approach.

Metabolic evaluation has typically not been performed, as earlier data suggested few metabolic abnormalities in pure struvite stone formers.[196] However, for selected patients and mixed stone formers, metabolic evaluation with urine and serum chemistries may be reasonable.

Table 14.2 summarizes current nutritional goals and Box 14.4 summarizes medical and nutritional management of different types of stones. Box 14.5 presents an example of patient education on general guidelines for stone prevention.

TABLE 14.2 | Nutrient Recommendation for Kidney Stones

Nutrients	Recommendation
Calcium	1,000-1,200 mg/d
Oxalate	40-50 mg/d
Sodium	<2,300 mg/d
Protein	0.8-1.4 g/kg/d
Fluid	>3 L/d to produce >2.5 L urine output
Vitamin D	Low dose if vitamin D insufficiency or deficiency (1,000 IU/d)
Vitamin C	Dietary Reference Intake (DRI)

Reproduced with permission from Pearle MS, Goldfarb DS, Assimos DG, et al. Medical management of kidney stones: AUA guideline. *J Urol.* 2014;192(2):316-324.[197]

BOX 14.4 | Summary of Nutritional and Medical Recommendation of Different Types of Stones

TYPE OF STONE	MEDICAL MANAGEMENT	NUTRITIONAL MANAGEMENT
Calcium oxalate	Treatment of hypercalciuria Low urinary pH: potassium citrate Prebiotics/probiotics (depending on the clinical practice)	Fluid: >3 L to produce urine output >2.5 L; all types except soda/sugar-containing fluid Calcium: Calcium-rich foods 1,000 to 1,200 mg; avoid low calcium intake or high calcium supplement Low sodium: 2,300 mg Oxalate: avoid very high-oxalate foods; consume with calcium-rich foods at the same time Moderate amount of nondairy animal protein (acid-forming foods)
Calcium–phosphorus	Monitor primary hyperparathyroidism and renal tubular acidosis	High fluid intake Individualize with urinary calcium and medical condition
Uric acid	Urine alkalization Potassium citrate Sodium citrate Sodium bicarbonate Xanthine oxidase inhibitor	Fluid >3 L to produce urine output >2.5 L; includes mineral water and citrate rich sources Moderate protein, especially nondairy animal protein, to lower potential renal acid load Dietary Approaches to Stop Hypertension (DASH) diet Cut down on high fructose consumption More vegetable/fruit consumption
Cystine	Urine alkalization (pH higher is better) High urine volume Cystine-binding thiol agents	Fluid >3 to 4 L Low-to-moderate animal protein, especially low methionine Low sodium: 2,300 mg DASH/high fruit and vegetable intake
Struvite	Use of antibiotic to avoid infection	Fluid >3 L to produce urine output >2.5 L Low sodium: 2,300 mg

BOX 14.5 | General Diet Guidelines of Kidney Stone Prevention

Drink plenty of fluid: at least 3 L/d or more.	Any type of fluids (eg, water, coffee, and lemonade) except grapefruit juice and soda, have shown a beneficial effect. Produce less concentrated urine with good volume (at least 2.5 L/d).
Avoid or limit foods with high oxalate.	Spinach, lots of berries, chocolate, wheat bran, nuts, beets, and rhubarb should be limited or eliminated from the diet, if possible.
Consume adequate amounts of dietary calcium.	Three servings of dairy (or calcium-rich foods) consumption per day will help lower the risk of calcium stones by lowering absorption of oxalate. Consume with meals: timing is very important.
Avoid extra calcium supplements.	Calcium supplements should be individualized by the physician.
Avoid a high-protein diet.	With high protein intake, the kidneys will excrete more calcium and, therefore, will form more stones in the kidneys. Cut down most nondairy animal protein to lower potential renal acid load.
Avoid a high-salt diet.	A high-sodium diet can increase calcium in the urine, thus increasing stone risk. Blood pressure control is also important for stone formation, and a high-salt diet can lead to high blood pressure.
Avoid high doses of vitamin C supplements.	Recommend intake: US Dietary Reference Intake. Excess amount (1,000 mg/d) may produce more oxalate in the body.

Adapted with permission from H. Han (author) for patient education at the Department of Nephrology at Harvard Vanguard Medical Associates (Atrius Health).

Summary

Kidney stone formation is related to various genetic, environmental, and dietary risk factors. Most patients will have a recurrence of stones after their first episode. The risks of kidney stones are multiple and vary by individual; however, 24-hour urine collections provide information on specific risk factors, which can be measured and modified in order to prevent recurrence. Dietary factors play a very important role in the formation of kidney stones, and dietary changes can reduce the risk of recurrence. An increase in fluid intake to produce more than 2.5 L urine per day is the most important factor in preventing the recurrence of stones. Other dietary modifications include moderate protein intake (especially nondairy animal protein), low oxalate, low sodium, and adequate dietary calcium intake. Medical interventions using thiazide, citrate, and other medications will help with the prevention of kidney stone formation. Both dietary and medical treatment should be based on multiple 24-hour urine tests.

References

1. Saigal CS, Joyce G, Timilsina AR, Urologic Diseases in America Project. Direct and indirect costs of nephrolithiasis in an employed population: opportunity for disease management? *Kidney Int.* 2005;68(4):1808-1814. doi:10.1111/j.1523-1755.2005.00599.x

2. Worcester EM, Coe FL. Nephrolithiasis. *Primary Care.* 2008;35(2):369-391, vii. doi:10.1016/j.pop.2008.01.005

3. Scales CD Jr., Smith AC, Hanley JM, Saigal CS, Urologic Diseases in America Project. Prevalence of kidney stones in the United States. *Eur Urol.* 2012;62(1):160-165. doi:10.1016/j.eururo.2012.03.052

4. Stamatelou KK, Francis ME, Jones CA, Nyberg LM, Curhan GC. Time trends in reported prevalence of kidney stones in the United States: 1976–1994. *Kidney Int.* 2003;63(5):1817-1823. doi:10.1046/j.1523-1755.2003.00917.x

5. Curhan GC. Epidemiology of stone disease. *Urol Clin North Am.* 2007;34(3):287-293. doi:10.1016/j.ucl.2007.04.003

6. Moe OW, Bonny O. Genetic hypercalciuria. *J Am Soc Nephrol.* 2005;16(3):729-745. doi:10.1681/ASN.2004100888

7. Taylor EN, Stampfer MJ, Curhan GC. Diabetes mellitus and the risk of nephrolithiasis. *Kidney Int.* 2005;68(3):1230-1235. doi:10.1111/j.1523-1755.2005.00516.x

8. Taylor EN, Stampfer MJ, Curhan GC. Obesity, weight gain, and the risk of kidney stones. *JAMA.* 2005;293(4):455-462. doi:10.1001/jama.293.4.455

9. Brikowski TH, Lotan Y, Pearle MS. Climate-related increase in the prevalence of urolithiasis in the United States. *Proc Natl Acad Sci U S A.* 2008;105(28):9841-9846. doi:10.1073/pnas.0709652105

10. Pearle MS, Calhoun EA, Curhan GC, Urologic Diseases of America Project. Urologic diseases in America project: urolithiasis. *J Urol.* 2005;173(3):848-857. doi:10.1097/01.ju.0000152082.14384.d7

11. Costa-Bauza A, Ramis M, Montesinos V, et al. Type of renal calculi: variation with age and sex. *World J Urol.* 2007;25(4):415-421. doi:10.1007/s00345-007-0177-4

12. Lieske JC, Rule AD, Krambeck AE, et al. Stone composition as a function of age and sex. *Clin J Am Soc Nephrol.* 2014;9(12):2141-2146. doi:10.2215/CJN.05660614

13. Daudon M, Frochot V, Bazin D, Jungers P. Drug-induced kidney stones and crystalline nephropathy: pathophysiology, prevention and treatment. *Drugs.* 2018;78(2):163-201.

14. Borghi L, Meschi T, Schianchi T, et al. Urine volume: stone risk factor and preventive measure. *Nephron.* 1999;81(suppl 1):31-37. doi:10.1159/000046296

15. Moe OW. Kidney stones: pathophysiology and medical management. *Lancet.* 2006;367(9507):333-344. doi:10.1016/S0140-6736(06)68071-9

16. Zuckerman JM, Assimos DG. Hypocitraturia: pathophysiology and medical management. *Rev Urol.* 2009;11(3):134-144.

17. Curhan GC, Taylor EN. 24-h uric acid excretion and the risk of kidney stones. *Kidney Int.* 2008;73(4):489-496. doi:10.1038/sj.ki.5002708

18. Nicar MJ, Skurla C, Sakhaee K, Pak CY. Low urinary citrate excretion in nephrolithiasis. *Urology.* 1983;21(1):8-14. doi:10.1016/0090-4295(83)90113-9

19. Qiu SR, Wierzbicki A, Orme CA, et al. Molecular modulation of calcium oxalate crystallization by osteopontin and citrate. *Proc Natl Acad Sci U S A.* 2004;101(7):1811-1815. doi:10.1073/pnas.0307900100

20. Qiu SR, Orme CA. Dynamics of biomineral formation at the near-molecular level. *Chem Rev.* 2008;108(11):4784-4822. doi:10.1021/cr800322u

21. Werness PG, Brown CM, Smith LH, Finlayson B. EQUIL2: a BASIC computer program for the calculation of urinary saturation. *J Urol.* 1985;134(6):1242-1244. doi:10.1016/s0022-5347(17)47703-2

22. Aggarwal KP, Narula S, Kakkar M, Tandon C. Nephrolithiasis: molecular mechanism of renal stone formation and the critical role played by modulators. *Biomed Res Int*. 2013;2013:292953. doi:10.1155/2013/292953

23. De Yoreo JJ, Qiu SR, Hoyer JR. Molecular modulation of calcium oxalate crystallization. *Am J Physiol Renal Physiol*. 2006;291(6):F1123-F1132. doi:10.1152/ajprenal.00136.2006

24. Rimer JD, An Z, Zhu Z, et al. Crystal growth inhibitors for the prevention of L-cystine kidney stones through molecular design. *Science*. 2010;330(6002):337-341. doi:10.1126/science.1191968

25. Ingimarsson JP, Krambeck AE, Pais VM Jr. Diagnosis and management of nephrolithiasis. *Surg Clin North Am*. 2016;96(3):517-532. doi:10.1016/j.suc.2016.02.008

26. Brisbane W, Bailey MR, Sorensen MD. An overview of kidney stone imaging techniques. *Nat Rev Urol*. 2016;13(11):654-662. doi:10.1038/nrurol.2016.154

27. Fulgham PF, Assimos DG, Pearle MS, Preminger GM. Clinical effectiveness protocols for imaging in the management of ureteral calculous disease: AUA technology assessment. *J Urol*. 2013;189(4):1203-1213. doi:10.1016/j.juro.2012.10.031

28. Tzou DT, Usawachintachit M, Taguchi K, Chi T. Ultrasound use in urinary stones: adapting old technology for a modern-day disease. *J Endourol*. 2017;31(S1):S89-S94. doi:10.1089/end.2016.0584

29. Castle SM, Cooperberg MR, Sadetsky N, Eisner BH, Stoller ML. Adequacy of a single 24-hour urine collection for metabolic evaluation of recurrent nephrolithiasis. *J Urol*. 2010;184(2):579-583. doi:10.1016/j.juro.2010.03.129

30. Alruwaily AF, Dauw CA, Bierlein MJ, et al. How much information is lost when you only collect one 24-hour urine sample during the initial metabolic evaluation? *J Urol*. 2016;196(4):1143-1148. doi:10.1016/j.juro.2016.04.074

31. Reilly RF, Perazella MA. *Nephrology in 30 days*. 2nd ed. McGraw-Hill; 2014.

32. Asplin JR. Hyperoxaluric calcium nephrolithiasis. *Endocrinol Metab Clin North Am*. 2002;31(4):927-949. doi:10.1016/s0889-8529(02)00030-0

33. Vezzoli G, Terranegra A, Arcidiacono T, Soldati L. Genetics and calcium nephrolithiasis. *Kidney Int*. 2011;80(6):587-593. doi:10.1038/ki.2010.430

34. Coe FL, Parks JH, Moore ES. Familial idiopathic hypercalciuria. *N Engl J Med*. 1979;300(7):337-340. doi:10.1056/NEJM197902153000703

35. Worcester EM, Gillen DL, Evan AP, et al. Evidence that postprandial reduction of renal calcium reabsorption mediates hypercalciuria of patients with calcium nephrolithiasis. *Am J Physiol Ren Physiol*. 2007;292(1):F66-F75. doi:10.1152/ajprenal.00115.2006

36. Cochat P, Rumsby G. Primary hyperoxaluria. *N Engl J Med*. 2013;369:649-658. doi:10.1056/NEJMra1301564

37. Worcester EM, Evan AP, Coe FL, et al. A test of the hypothesis that oxalate secretion produces proximal tubule crystallization in primary hyperoxaluria type I. *Am J Physiol Renal Physiol*. 2013;305(11):F1574-F1584. doi:10.1152/ajprenal.00382.2013

38. Worcester EM, Coe FL, Evan AP, Parks JH. Reduced renal function and benefits of treatment in cystinuria vs other forms of nephrolithiasis. *BJU Int*. 2006;97(6):1285-1290. doi:10.1111/j.1464-410X.2006.06169.x

39. Soucie JM, Thun MJ, Coates RJ, McClellan W, Austin H. Demographic and geographic variability of kidney stones in the United States. *Kidney Int*. 1994;46(3):893-899. doi:10.1038/ki.1994.347

40. Robertson WG, Peacock M, Heyburn PJ, Hanes FA. Epidemiological risk factors in calcium stone disease. *Scand J Urol Nephrol Suppl*. 1980;53:15-30.

41. Soucie JM, Coates RJ, McClellan W, Austin H, Thun M. Relation between geographic variability in kidney stones prevalence and risk factors for stones. *Am J Epidemiol*. 1996;143(5):487-495.

42. Borghi L, Meschi T, Amato F, Briganti A, Novarini A, Giannini A. Urinary volume, water and recurrences in idiopathic calcium nephrolithiasis: a 5-year randomized prospective study. *J Urol*. 1996;155(3):839-843.

43. Curhan GC, Willett WC, Speizer FE, Stampfer MJ. Beverage use and risk for kidney stones in women. *Ann Intern Med*. 1998;128(7):534-540. doi:10.7326/0003-4819-128-7-199804010-00003

44. Curhan GC, Willett WC, Knight EL, Stampfer MJ. Dietary factors and the risk of incident kidney stones in younger women: Nurses' Health Study II. *Arch Intern Med*. 2004;164(8):885-891. doi:10.1001/archinte.164.8.885

45. Curhan GC, Willett WC, Rimm EB, Spiegelman D, Stampfer MJ. Prospective study of beverage use and the risk of kidney stones. *Am J Epidemiol*. 1996;143(3):240-247. doi:10.1093/oxfordjournals.aje.a008734

46. Ferraro PM, Taylor EN, Gambaro G, Curhan GC. Soda and other beverages and the risk of kidney stones. *Clin J Am Soc Nephrol*. 2013;8(8):1389-1395. doi:10.2215/CJN.11661112

47. Ferraro PM, Taylor EN, Gambaro G, Curhan GC. Caffeine intake and the risk of kidney stones. *Am J Clin Nutr*. 2014;100(6):1596-1603. doi:10.3945/ajcn.114.089987

48. Curhan GC, Willett WC, Rimm EB, Stampfer MJ. A prospective study of dietary calcium and other nutrients and the risk of symptomatic kidney stones. *N Engl J Med*. 1993;328(12):833-838. doi:10.1056/NEJM199303253281203

49. Curhan GC, Willett WC, Speizer FE, Spiegelman D, Stampfer MJ. Comparison of dietary calcium with supplemental calcium and other nutrients as factors affecting the risk for kidney stones in women. *Ann Intern Med*. 1997;126(7):497-504. doi:10.7326/0003-4819-126-7-199704010-00001

50. Taylor EN, Stampfer MJ, Curhan GC. Dietary factors and the risk of incident kidney stones in men: new insights after 14 years of follow-up. *J Am Soc Nephrol*. 2004;15(12):3225-3232. doi:10.1097/01.ASN.0000146012.44570.20

51. Bataille P, Charransol G, Gregoire I, et al. Effect of calcium restriction on renal excretion of oxalate and the probability of stones in the various pathophysiological groups with calcium stones. *J Urol*. 1983;130(2):218-223. doi:10.1016/S0022-5347(17)51073-3

52. Borghi L, Schianchi T, Meschi T, et al. Comparison of two diets for the prevention of recurrent stones in idiopathic hypercalciuria. *N Engl J Med*. 2002;346(2):77-84. doi:10.1056/NEJMoa010369

53. Holmes RP, Assimos DG. The impact of dietary oxalate on kidney stone formation. *Urol Res*. 2004;32(5):311-316. doi:10.1007/s00240-004-0437-3

54. da Silva Gaspar SR, Mendonca T, Oliveira P, Oliveira T, Dias J, Lopes T. Urolithiasis and Crohn's disease. *Urol Ann*. 2016;8(3):297-304. doi:10.4103/0974-7796.184879

55. Bhatti UH, Duffy AJ, Roberts KE, Shariff AH. Nephrolithiasis after bariatric surgery: a review of pathophysiologic mechanisms and procedural risk. *Int J Surg*. 2016;36(Pt D):618-623. doi:10.1016/j.ijsu.2016.11.025

56. Siener R, Honow R, Voss S, Seidler A, Hesse A. Oxalate content of cereals and cereal products. *J Agric Food Chem*. 2006;54(8):3008-3011. doi:10.1021/jf052776v

57. Lemann J Jr, Piering WF, Lennon EJ. Possible role of carbohydrate-induced calciuria in calcium oxalate kidney-stone formation. *N Engl J Med*. 1969;280(5):232-237. doi:10.1056/NEJM196901302800502

58. Muldowney FP, Freaney R, Moloney MF. Importance of dietary sodium in the hypercalciuria syndrome. *Kidney Int*. 1982;22(3):292-296. doi:10.1038/ki.1982.168

59. Coe F, Worcester EM. Idiopathic hypercalciuria. In: Coe F, Worcester EM, Lingeman JE, Evan AP, eds. *Kidney Stones: Medical and Surgical Management*. 2nd ed. Jaypee Brother Medical Publishers; 2018:276-302.

60. Breslau NA, Brinkley L, Hill KD, Pak CY. Relationship of animal protein-rich diet to kidney stone formation and calcium metabolism. *J Clin Endocrinol Metab*. 1988;66(1):140-146. doi:10.1210/jcem-66-1-140

61. Giannini S, Nobile M, Sartori L, et al. Acute effects of moderate dietary protein restriction in patients with idiopathic hypercalciuria and calcium nephrolithiasis. *Am J Clin Nutr*. 1999;69(2):267-271. doi:10.1093/ajcn/69.2.267

62. Lemann J Jr, Pleuss JA, Gray RW, Hoffmann RG. Potassium administration reduces and potassium deprivation increases urinary calcium excretion in healthy adults [corrected]. *Kidney Int*. 1991;39(5):973-983. doi:10.1038/ki.1991.123

63. Taylor EN, Fung TT, Curhan GC. DASH-style diet associates with reduced risk for kidney stones. *J Am Soc Nephrol*. 2009;20(10):2253-2259. doi:10.1681/ASN.2009030276

64. Taylor EN, Stampfer MJ, Mount DB, Curhan GC. DASH-style diet and 24-hour urine composition. *Clin J Am Soc Nephrol*. 2010;5(12):2315-2322. doi:10.2215/CJN.04420510

65. Grases F, March JG, Prieto RM, et al. Urinary phytate in calcium oxalate stone formers and healthy people—dietary effects on phytate excretion. *Scand J Urol Nephrol*. 2000;34(3):162-164. doi:10.1080/003655900750016526

66. Grases F, Garcia-Gonzalez R, Torres JJ, Llobera A. Effects of phytic acid on renal stone formation in rats. *Scand J Urol Nephrol*. 1998;32(4):261-265. doi:10.1080/003655998750015412

67. Traxer O, Huet B, Poindexter J, Pak CYC, Pearle MS. Effect of ascorbic acid consumption on urinary stone risk factors. *J Urol*. 2003;170(2 Pt 1):397-401. doi:10.1097/01.ju.0000076001.21606.53

68. Ferraro PM, Curhan GC, Gambaro G, Taylor EN. Total, dietary, and supplemental vitamin C intake and risk of incident kidney stones. *Am J Kidney Dis*. 2016;67(3):400-407. doi:10.1053/j.ajkd.2015.09.005

69. Penniston KL, Nakada SY, Hansen KE. Vitamin D repletion does not alter urinary calcium excretion in postmenopausal women. *J Urol*. 2008;179(4S):504-505. doi:10.1016/S0022-5347(08)61487-1

70. Letavernier E, Daudon M. Vitamin D, hypercalciuria and kidney stones. *Nutrients*. 2018;10(3):366. doi:10.3390/nu10030366

71. Curhan GC, Willett WC, Rimm EB, Stampfer MJ. A prospective study of the intake of vitamins C and B6, and the risk of kidney stones in men. *J Urol*. 1996;155(6):1847-1851.

72. Curhan GC, Willett WC, Speizer FE, Stampfer MJ. Intake of vitamins B_6 and C and the risk of kidney stones in women. *J Am Soc Nephrol.* 1999;10(4):840-845.

73. Ferraro PM, Taylor EN, Gambaro G, Curhan GC. Vitamin B_6 intake and the risk of incident kidney stones. *Urolithiasis.* 2018;46(3):265-270.

74. Beto J. Herbal use in the nutrition management of kidney stones. In: Han H, Mutter WP, Nasser S, eds. *Nutritional and Medical Management of Kidney Stones.* Humana Press/Springer Nature; 2019:255-260.

75. Ahmed S, Hasan MM, Mahmood ZA. Review: antiurolithiatic plants: formulations used in different countries and cultures. *Pak J Pharm Sci.* 2016;29(6):2129-2139.

76. Bahmani M, Baharvand-Ahmadi B, Tajeddini P, Rafieian-Kopaei M, Naghdi N. Identification of medicinal plants for the treatment of kidney and urinary stones. *J Renal Inj Prev.* 2016;5(3):129-133. doi:10.1517/jrip.2016.27

77. Clement YN, Baksh-Comeau YS, Seaforth CE. An ethnobotanical survey of medicinal plants in Trinidad. *J Ethnobiol Ethnomed.* 2015;11:67.

78. Kasote DM, Jagtap SD, Thapa D, Khyade MS, Russell WR. Herbal remedies for urinary stones used in India and China: a review. *J Ethnopharmacol.* 2017;203:55-68. doi:10.1016/j.jep.2017.03.038

79. Kieley S, Dwivedi R, Monga M. Ayurvedic medicine and renal calculi. *J Endourol.* 2008;22(8):1613-1616. doi:10.1089/end.2008.0020

80. Miyaoka R, Monga M. Use of traditional Chinese medicine in the management of urinary stone disease. *Int Braz J Urol.* 2009;35(4):396-405. doi:10.1590/s1677-55382009000400002

81. Han H, Seifte J. Nephrolithiasis. In: Byham-Gray L, Burrowes JD, Chertow GM, eds. *Nutrition in Kidney Disease.* 2nd ed. Humana Press; 2014:355-373.

82. Sakhaee K. Nephrolithiasis as a systemic disorder. *Curr Opin Nephrol Hypertens.* 2008;17(3):304-309. doi:10.1097/MNH.0b013e3282f8b34d

83. Sakhaee K. Epidemiology and clinical pathophysiology of uric acid kidney stones. *J Nephrol.* 2014;27(3):241-245. doi:10.1007/s40620-013-0034-z

84. Daudon M, Lacour B, Jungers P. High prevalence of uric acid calculi in diabetic stone formers. *Nephrol Dial Transplant.* 2005;20(2):468-469. doi:10.1093/ndt/gfh594

85. Pak CYC, Sakhaee K, Moe O, et al. Biochemical profile of stone-forming patients with diabetes mellitus. *Urology.* 2003;61(3):523-527. doi:10.1016/s0090-4295(02)02421-4

86. Madore F, Stampfer MJ, Willett WC, Speizer FE, Curhan GC. Nephrolithiasis and risk of hypertension in women. *Am J Kid Dis.* 1998;32(5):802-807. doi:10.1016/s0272-6386(98)70136-2

87. Cutler JA, Brittain E. Calcium and blood pressure. An epidemiologic perspective. *Am J Hypertens.* 1990;3(8 Pt 2):S137-S146. doi:10.1093/ajh/3.8.137

88. McCarron DA, Morris CD, Henry HJ, Stanton JL. Blood pressure and nutrient intake in the United States. *Science.* 1984;224(4656):1392-1398. doi:10.1126/science.6729459

89. Strazzullo P, Mancini M. Hypertension, calcium metabolism, and nephrolithiasis. *Am J Med Sci.* 1994;307(suppl 1):S102-S106.

90. Eisner BH, Porten SP, Bechis SK, Stoller ML. Hypertension is associated with increased urinary calcium excretion in patients with nephrolithiasis. *J Urol.* 2010;183(2):576-579. doi:10.1016/j.juro.2009.10.011

91. Taylor EN, Mount DB, Forman JP, Curhan GC. Association of prevalent hypertension with 24-hour urinary excretion of calcium, citrate, and other factors. *Am J Kidney Dis.* 2006;47(5):780-789. doi:10.1053/j.ajkd.2006.01.024

92. Alper AB Jr, Chen W, Yau L, Srinivasan SR, Berenson GS, Hamm LL. Childhood uric acid predicts adult blood pressure: the Bogalusa heart study. *Hypertension.* 2005;45(1):34-38. doi:10.1161/01.HYP.0000150783.79172.bb

93. Westlund K. Urolithiasis and coronary heart disease: a note on association. *Am J Epidemiol.* 1973;97(3):167-172. doi:10.1093/oxfordjournals.aje.a121497

94. Reiner AP, Kahn A, Eisner BH, et al. Kidney stones and subclinical atherosclerosis in young adults: Coronary Artery Risk Development in Young Adults (CARDIA) study. *J Urol.* 2011;185(3):920-925. doi:10.1016/j.juro.2010.10.086

95. Hamano S, Nakatsu H, Suzuki N, Tomioka S, Tanaka M, Murakami S. Kidney stone disease and risk factors for coronary heart disease. *Int J Urol.* 2005;12(10):859-863. doi:10.1111/j.1442-2042.2005.01160.x

96. Rule AD, Roger VL, Melton LJ III, et al. Kidney stones associate with increased risk for myocardial infarction. *J Am Soc Nephrol.* 2010;21(10):1641-1644. doi:10.1681/ASN.2010030253

97. Cheungpasitporn W, Thongprayoon C, Mao MA, O'Corragain OA, Edmonds PJ, Erickson SB. The risk of coronary heart disease in patients with kidney stones: a systematic review and meta-analysis. *N Am J Med Sci.* 2014;6(11):580-585. doi:10.4103/1947-2714.145477

98. El-Zoghby ZM, Lieske JC, Foley RN, et al. Urolithiasis and the risk of ESRD. *Clin J Am Soc Nephrol.* 2012;7(9):1409-1415. doi:10.2215/CJN.03210312

99. Rule AD, Bergstralh EJ, Melton LJ III, Li X, Weaver AL, Lieske JC. Kidney stones and the risk for chronic kidney disease. *Clin J Am Soc Nephrol.* 2009;4(4):804-811. doi:10.2215/CJN.05811108

100. Gillen DL, Worcester EM, Coe FL. Decreased renal function among adults with a history of nephrolithiasis: a study of NHANES III. *Kidney Int.* 2005;67(2):685-690. doi:10.1111/j1523-1755.2005.67128.x

101. Worcester EM. Stones from bowel disease. *Endocrinol Metab Clin North Am.* 2002;31(4):979-999. doi:10.1016/s0889-8529(02)00035-x

102. Fink HA, Akornor JW, Garimella PS, et al. Diet, fluid, or supplements for secondary prevention of nephrolithiasis: a systematic review and meta-analysis of randomized trials. *Eur Urol.* 2009;56(1):72-80. doi:10.1016/j.eururo.2009.03.031

103. Robijn S, Hoppe B, Vervaet BA, D'Haese PC, Verhulst A. Hyperoxaluria: a gut-kidney axis? *Kidney Int.* 2011;80(11):1146-1158. doi:10.1038/ki.2011.287

104. Tappenden KA. Pathophysiology of short bowel syndrome: considerations of resected and residual anatomy. *JPEN J Parenter Enteral Nutr.* 2014;38(1 suppl):14S-22S. doi:10.1177/0148607113520005

105. Noori N, Honarkar E, Goldfarb DS, et al. Urinary lithogenic risk profile in recurrent stone formers with hyperoxaluria: a randomized controlled trial comparing DASH (Dietary Approaches to Stop Hypertension)-style and low-oxalate diets. *Am J Kidney Dis.* 2014;63(3):456-463. doi:10.1053/j.ajkd.2013.11.022

106. Wong YV, Cook P, Somani BK. The association of metabolic syndrome and urolithiasis. *Int J Endocrinol.* 2015;570674. doi:10.1155/2015/570674

107. Nasr SH, D'Agati VD, Said SM, et al. Oxalate nephropathy complicating Roux-en-Y gastric bypass: an underrecognized cause of irreversible renal failure. *Clin J Am Soc Nephrol.* 2008;3(6):1676-1683. doi:10.2215/CJN.02940608

108. Lieske JC, Kumar R, Collozo-Clovell ML. Nephrolithiasis after bariatric surgery for obesity. *Semin Nephrol.* 2008;28(2):163-173. doi:10.1016/j.semnephrol.2008.01.009

109. Canales BK, Gonzalez RD. Kidney stone risk following Roux-en-Y gastric bypass surgery. *Transl Androl Urol.* 2014;3(3):242-249. doi:10.3978/j.issn.2223-4683.2014.06.02

110. Assimos D, Krambeck A, Miller NL, et al. Surgical management of stones: American Urological Association/Endourological Society Guideline, PART I. *J Urol.* 2016;196(4):1153-1160. doi:10.1016/j.juro.2016.05.090

111. Smith-Bindman R, Aubin C, Bailitz J, et al. Ultrasonography versus computed tomography for suspected nephrolithiasis. *N Engl J Med.* 2014;371(12):1100-1110. doi:10.1056/NEJMoa1404446

112. Pearle MS, Goldfarb DS, Assimos DG, et al. Medical management of kidney stones: AUA guideline. *J Urol.* 2014;192(2):316-324. doi:10.1016/j.juro.2014.05.006

113. Alivizatos G, Skolarikos A. Is there still a role for open surgery in the management of renal stones? *Curr Opin Urol.* 2006;16(2):106-111. doi:10.1097/01.mou.0000193379.08857.e7

114. Strohmaier WL. Course of calcium stone disease without treatment. What can we expect? *Eur Urol.* 2000;37(3):339-344. doi:10.1159/000052367

115. Nouvenne A, Meschi T, Prati B, et al. Effects of a low-salt diet on idiopathic hypercalciuria in calcium-oxalate stone formers: a 3-mo randomized controlled trial. *Am J Clin Nutr.* 2010;91(3):565-570. doi:10.3945/ajcn.2009.28614

116. Bergsland KJ, Worcester EM, Coe FL. Role of proximal tubule in the hypocalciuric response to thiazide of patients with idiopathic hypercalciuria. *Am J Physiol Renal Physiol.* 2013;305(4):F592-F599. doi:10.1152/ajprenal.00116.2013

117. Phillips R, Hanchanale VS, Myatt A, Somani B, Nabi G, Biyani CS. Citrate salts for preventing and treating calcium containing kidney stones in adults. *Cochrane Database Syst Rev.* 2015(10):CD010057. doi:10.1002/14651858.CD010057.pub2

118. Pinheiro VB, Baxmann AC, Tiselius HG, Heilberg IP. The effect of sodium bicarbonate upon urinary citrate excretion in calcium stone formers. *Urology.* 2013;82(1):33-37. doi:10.1016/j.urology.2013.03.002

119. Pachaly MA, Baena CP, Buiar AC, de Fraga FS, Carvalho M. Effects of non-pharmacological interventions on urinary citrate levels: a systematic review and meta-analysis. *Nephrol Dial Transplant.* 2016;31(8):1203-1211. doi:10.1093/ndt/gfv303

120. Barrett HL, Nitert MD, Conwell LS, Callaway LK. Probiotics for preventing gestational diabetes. *Cochrane Database Syst Rev.* 2014(2):CD009951. doi:10.1002/14651858.CD009951.pub2

121. Rapozo DCM, Bernardazzi C, Pereira de Souza HS. Diet and microbiota in inflammatory bowel disease: the gut in disharmony. *World J Gastroenterol.* 2017;23(12):2124-2140. doi:10.3748/wjg.v23.i12.2124

122. Seganfredo FB, Blume CA, Moehlecke M, et al. Weight-loss interventions and gut microbiota changes in overweight and obese patients: a systematic review. *Obes Rev.* 2017;18(8):832-851. doi:10.1111/obr.12541

123. Abratt VR, Reid SJ. Oxalate degrading bacteria of the human gut as probiotics in the management of kidney stone disease. In: Laskin AI, Sariaslani S, Gadd GM, eds. *Advances in Applied Microbiology*. Vol 72. Elsevier; 2010:63-87.

124. Lieske JC. Probiotics for prevention of urinary stones. *Ann Transl Med*. 2017;5(2):29. doi:10.21037/atm.2016.11.86

125. Kaufman DW, Kelly JP, Curhan GC, et al. Oxalobacter formigenes may reduce the risk of calcium oxalate kidney stones. *J Am Soc Nephrol*. 2008;19(6):1197-1203. doi:10.1681/ASN.2007101058

126. Hoppe B, Beck B, Gatter N, et al. Oxalobacter formigenes: a potential tool for the treatment of primary hyperoxaluria type 1. *Kidney Int*. 2006;70(7):1305-1311. doi:10.1038/sj.ki.5001707

127. Milliner D, Hoppe B, Groothoff J. A randomised Phase II/III study to evaluate the efficacy and safety of orally administered *Oxalobacter formigenes* to treat primary hyperoxaluria. *Urolithiasis*. 2018;46(4):313-323. doi:10.1007/s00240-017-0998-6

128. Kang DE, Sur RL, Haleblian GE, Fitzsimons NJ, Borawski KM, Preminger GM. Long-term lemonade based dietary manipulation in patients with hypocitraturic nephrolithiasis. *J Urol*. 2007;177(4):1358-1362. doi:10.1016/j.juro.2006.11.058

129. Johnson RJ, Perez-Pozo SE, Lillo JL, et al. Fructose increases risk for kidney stones: potential role in metabolic syndrome and heat stress. *BMC Nephrol*. 2018;19(1):315. doi:10.1186/s12882-018-1105-0

130. Sorensen MD, Kahn AJ, Reiner AP, et al. Impact of nutritional factors on incident kidney stone formation: a report from the WHI OS. *J Urol*. 2012;187(5):1645-1649.doi:10.1016/j.juro.2011.12.077

131. Jackson RD, LaCroix AZ, Gass M, et al. Calcium plus vitamin D supplementation and the risk of fractures. *N Engl J Med*. 2006;354(7):669-683. doi:10.1056/NEJMoa055218

132. Wallace RB, Wactawski-Wende J, O'Sullivan MJ, et al. Urinary tract stone occurrence in the Women's Health Initiative (WHI) randomized clinical trial of calcium and vitamin D supplements. *Am J Clin Nutr*. 2011;94(1):270-277. doi:10.3945/ajcn.110.003350

133. Rebholz CM, Crews DC, Grams ME, et al. DASH (Dietary Approaches to Stop Hypertension) diet and risk of subsequent kidney disease. *Am J Kid Dis*. 2016;68(6):853-861. doi:10.1053/j.ajkd.2016.05.019

134. Massey LK. Food oxalate: factors affecting measurement, biological variation, and bioavailability. *J Am Diet Assoc*. 2007;107(7):1191-1194. doi:10.1016/j.jada.2007.04.007

135. Taylor EN, Curhan GC. Determinants of 24-hour urinary oxalate excretion. *Clin J Am Soc Nephrol*. 2008;3(5):1453-1460. doi:10.2215/CJN.01410308

136. Attalla K, De S, Monga M. Oxalate content of food: a tangled web. *Urology*. 2014;84(3):555-559. doi:10.1016/j.urology.2014.03.053

137. Taylor EN, Curhan GC. Oxalate intake and the risk for nephrolithiasis. *J Am Soc Nephrol*. 2007;18(7):2198-2204. doi:10.1681/ASN.2007020219

138. Hylander E, Jarnum S, Nielsen K. Calcium treatment of enteric hyperoxaluria after jejunoileal bypass for morbid obesity. *Scand J Gastroenterol*. 1980;15(3):349-352. doi:10.3109/00365528009181482

139. Baxmann AC, Mendonca CDOG, Heilberg IP. Effect of vitamin C supplements on urinary oxalate and pH in calcium stone-forming patients. *Kidney Int*. 2003;63(3):1066-1071. doi:10.1046/j.1523-1755.2003.00815.x

140. Tang M, Larson-Meyer DE, Liebman M. Effect of cinnamon and turmeric on urinary oxalate excretion, plasma lipids, and plasma glucose in healthy subjects. *Am J Clin Nutr*. 2008;87(5):1262-1267. doi:10.1093/ajcn/87.5.1262

141. Terris MK, Issa MM, Tacker JR. Dietary supplementation with cranberry concentrate tablets may increase the risk of nephrolithiasis. *Urology*. 2001;57(1):26-29. doi:10.1016/s0090-4295(00)00884-0

142. Ryall RL. Urinary inhibitors of calcium oxalate crystallization and their potential role in stone formation. *World J Urol*. 1997;15(3):155-164. doi:10.1007/BF02201852

143. Adeva MM, Souto G. Diet-induced metabolic acidosis. *Clin Nutr*. 2011;30(4):416-421. doi:10.1016/j.clnu.2011.03.008

144. Remer T, Manz F. Potential renal acid load of foods and its influence on urine pH. *J Am Diet Assoc*. 1995;95(7):791-797. doi:10.1016/S0002-8223(95)00219-7

145. Trinchieri A, Lizzano R, Marchesotti F, Zanetti G. Effect of potential renal acid load of foods on urinary citrate excretion in calcium renal stone formers. *Urol Res*. 2006;34(1):1-7.doi:10.1007/s00240-005-0001-9

146. Meschi T, Maggiore U, Fiaccadori E, et al. The effect of fruits and vegetables on urinary stone risk factors. *Kidney Int*. 2004;66(6):2402-2410. doi:10.1111/j.1523-1755.2004.66029.x

147. Sakhaee K, Alpern R, Poindexter J, Pak CY. Citrauric response to oral citric acid load. *J Urol*. 1992;147(4):975-976. doi:10.1016/s0022-5347(17)37437-2

148. Aras B, Kalfazade N, Tugcu V, et al. Can lemon juice be an alternative to potassium citrate in the treatment of urinary calcium stones in patients with hypocitraturia? A prospective randomized study. *Urol Res.* 2008;36(6):313-317. doi:10.1007/s00240-008-0152-6

149. Mahan LK, Escott-Stump S. *Krause's Food & Nutrition Therapy.* 12th ed. Saunders/Elsevier; 2008.

150. Krieger NS, Asplin JR, Frick KK, et al. Effect of potassium citrate on calcium phosphate stones in a model of hypercalciuria. *J Am Soc Nephrol.* 2015;26(12):3001-3008. doi:10.1681/ASN.2014121223

151. Rimer JD, Sakhaee K, Maalouf NM. Citrate therapy for calcium phosphate stones. *Curr Opin Nephrol Hypertens.* 2019;28(2):130-139. doi:10.1097/MNH.0000000000000474

152. Wiederkehr MR, Moe OW. Uric acid nephrolithiasis: a systemic metabolic disorder. *Clin Rev Bone Miner Metab.* 2011;9(3-4):207-217. doi:10.1007/s12018-011-9106-6

153. Heilberg IP. Treatment of patients with uric acid stones. *Urolithiasis.* 2016;44(1):57-63. doi:10.1007/s00240-015-0843-8

154. Coe FL. Uric acid and calcium oxalate nephrolithiasis. *Kidney Int.* 1983;24(3):392-403. doi:10.1038/ki.1983.172

155. Pak CY, Sakhaee K, Fuller C. Successful management of uric acid nephrolithiasis with potassium citrate. *Kidney Int.* 1986;30(3):422-428. doi:10/1038/ki.1986.201

156. Wang L, Cui Y, Zhang J, Zhang Q. Safety of potassium-bearing citrate in patients with renal transplantation: a case report. *Medicine.* 2017;96(42):e6933. doi:10.1097/MD.0000000000006933

157. Kim D, Rimer JD, Asplin JR. Hydroxycitrate: a potential new therapy for calcium urolithiasis. *Urolithiasis.* 2019;47(4):311-320. doi:10.1007/s00240-019-01125-1

158. Sakhaee K, Nicar M, Hill K, Pak CY. Contrasting effects of potassium citrate and sodium citrate therapies on urinary chemistries and crystallization of stone-forming salts. *Kidney Int.* 1983;24(3):348-352. doi:10.1038/ki.1983.165

159. Rodman JS. Intermittent versus continuous alkaline therapy for uric acid stones and ureteral stones of uncertain composition. *Urology.* 2002;60(3):378-382. doi:10.1016/s0090-4295(02)01752-9

160. McKenzie DC. Changes in urinary pH following bicarbonate loading. *Can J Sport Sci.* 1988;13(4):254-256.

161. Anderson EE, Rundles RW, Silberman HR, Metz EN. Allopurinol control of hyperuricosuria: a new concept in the prevention of uric acid stones. *J Urol.* 1967;97(2):344-347. doi:10.1016/s0022-5347(17)63042-8

162. Ettinger B, Tang A, Citron JT, Livermore B, Williams T. Randomized trial of allopurinol in the prevention of calcium oxalate calculi. *N Engl J Med.* 1986;315(22):1386-1389. doi:10.1056/NEJM198611273152204

163. Becker MA, Schumacher HR Jr, Wortmann RL, et al. Febuxostat compared with allopurinol in patients with hyperuricemia and gout. *N Engl J Med.* 2005;353(23):2450-2461. doi:10.1056/NEJMoa050373

164. Abou-Elela A. Epidemiology, pathophysiology, and management of uric acid urolithiasis: a narrative review. *J Adv Res.* 2017;8(5):513-527. doi:10.1016/j.jare.2017.04.005

165. Arellano F, Sacristan JA. Allopurinol hypersensitivity syndrome: a review. *Ann Pharmacother.* 1993;27(3):337-343. doi:10.1177/106002809302700317

166. Bobulescu A, Moe OW. Renal transport of uric acid: evolving concepts and uncertainties. *Adv Chronic Kidney Dis.* 2012;19(6):358-371. doi:10.1053/j.ackd.2012.07.009

167. Maiuolo J, Oppedisano F, Gratteri S, Muscoli C, Mollace V. Regulation of uric acid metabolism and excretion. *Int J Cardiol.* 2016;213:8-14. doi:10.1016/j.ijcard.2015.08.109

168. Han H, Segal AM, Seifter JL, Dwyer JT. Nutritional management of kidney stones (nephrolithiasis). *Clin Nutr Res.* 2015;4(3):137-152. doi:10.7762/cnr.2015.4.3.137

169. Odvina CV. Comparative value of orange juice versus lemonade in reducing stone-forming risk. *Clin J Am Soc Nephrol.* 2006;1(6):1269-1274. doi:10.2215/CJN.00800306

170. Choi HK, Liu SM, Curhan G. Intake of purine-rich foods, protein, and dairy products and relationship to serum levels of uric acid: the Third National Health and Nutrition Examination Survey. *Arthritis Rheum.* 2005;52(1):283-289. doi:10.1002/art.20761

171. Yu K-H, See L-C, Huang Y-C, Yang C-H, Sun J-H. Dietary factors associated with hyperuricemia in adults. *Sem Arthritis Rheum.* 2008;37(4):243-250. doi:10.1016/j.semarthrit.2007.04.007

172. Choi HK, Curhan G. Coffee, tea, and caffeine consumption and serum uric acid level: the third National Health and Nutrition Examination Survey. *Arthritis Rheum.* 2007;57(5):816-821. doi:10.1002/art.22762

173. Dragan S, Andrica F, Serban M-C, Timar R. Polyphenols-rich natural products for treatment of diabetes. *Curr Med Chem.* 2015;22(1):14-22. doi:10.2174/0929867321666140826115422

174. Ghadieh HE, Smiley ZN, Kopfman MW, Najjar MG, Hake MJ, Najjar SM. Chlorogenic acid/chromium supplement rescues diet-induced insulin resistance and obesity in mice. *Nutr Metab (Lond).* 2015;12:19. doi:10.1186/s12986-015-0014-5

175. Karaguelle O, Smorag U, Candir F, et al. Clinical study on the effect of mineral waters containing bicarbonate on the risk of urinary stone formation in patients with multiple episodes of CaOx-urolithiasis. *World J Urol.* 2007;25(3):315-323. doi:10.1007/s00345-007-0144-0

176. Taylor EN, Curhan GC. Fructose consumption and the risk of kidney stones. *Kidney Int.* 2008;73(2):207-212. doi:10.1038/sj.ki.5002588

177. Rho YH, Zhu Y, Choi HK. The epidemiology of uric acid and fructose. *Semin Nephrol.* 2011;31(5):410-419. doi:10.1016/j.semnephrol.2011.08.004

178. Dello Strologo L, Pras E, Pontesilli C, et al. Comparison between SLC3A1 and SLC7A9 cystinuria patients and carriers: a need for a new classification. *J Am Soc Nephrol.* 2002;13(10):2547-2553. doi:10.1097/01.asn.0000029586.17680.e5

179. Lambert EH, Asplin JR, Herrell SD, Miller NL. Analysis of 24-hour urine parameters as it relates to age of onset of cystine stone formation. *J Endourol.* 2010;24(7):1179-1182. doi:10.1089/end.2010.0133

180. Rhodes HL, Yarram-Smith L, Rice SJ, et al. Clinical and genetic analysis of patients with cystinuria in the United Kingdom. *Clin J Am Soc Nephrol.* 2015;10(7):1235-1245. doi:10.2215/CJN.10981114

181. Fattah H, Hambaroush Y, Goldfarb DS. Cystine nephrolithiasis. *Transl Androl Urol.* 2014;3(3):228-233. doi:10.3978/j.issn.2223-4683.2014.07.04

182. Barbey F, Joly D, Rieu P, Mejean A, Daudon M, Jungers P. Medical treatment of cystinuria: critical reappraisal of long-term results. *J Urol.* 2000;163(5):1419-1423. doi:10.1016/s0022-5347(05)67633-1

183. Mattoo A, Goldfarb DS. Cystinuria. *Semin Nephrol.* 2008;28(2):181-191. doi:10.1016/j.semnephrol.2008.01.011

184. Prot-Bertoye C, Lebbah S, Daudon M, et al. CKD and its risk factors among patients with cystinuria. *Clin J Am Soc Nephrol.* 2015;10(5):842-851. doi:10.2215/CJN.06680714

185. Torres VE, Chapman AB, Devuyst O, et al. Tolvaptan in patients with autosomal dominant polycystic kidney disease. *N Engl J Med.* 2012;367(25):2407-2418. doi:10.1056/NEJMoa1205511

186. Castro Pereira DJ, Schoolwerth AC, Pais VM. Cystinuria: current concepts and future directions. *Clin Nephrol.* 2015;83(3):138-146. doi:10.5414/cn108514

187. Andreassen KH, Pedersen KV, Osther SS, Jung HU, Lildal SK, Sloth Osther PJ. How should patients with cystine stone disease be evaluated and treated in the twenty-first century? *Urolithiasis.* 2016;44(1):65-76. doi:10.1007/s00240-015-0841-x

188. Rodman JS, Blackburn P, Williams JJ, Brown A, Pospischil MA, Peterson CM. The effect of dietary protein on cystine excretion in patients with cystinuria. *Clin Nephrol.* 1984;22(6):273-278.

189. Jaeger P, Portmann L, Saunders A, Rosenberg LE, Thier SO. Anticystinuric effects of glutamine and of dietary sodium restriction. *N Engl J Med.* 1986;315(18):1120-1123. doi:10.1056/NEJM198610303151803

190. Resnick MI, Boyce WH. Bilateral staghorn calculi—patient evaluation and management. *J Urol.* 1980;123(3):338-341. doi:10.1016/S0022-5347(17)55924-8

191. Viprakasit DP, Sawyer MD, Herrell SD, Miller NL. Changing composition of staghorn calculi. *J Urol.* 2011;186(6):2285-2290. doi:10.1016/j.juro.2011.07.089

192. Preminger GM, Assimos DG, Lingeman JE, et al. Chapter 1: AUA guideline on management of staghorn calculi: diagnosis and treatment recommendations. *J Urol.* 2005;173(6):1991-2000. doi:10.1097/01.ju.0000161171.67806.2a

193. Gnessin E, Mandeville JA, Handa SE, Lingeman JE. Changing composition of renal calculi in patients with musculoskeletal anomalies. *J Endourol.* 2011;25(9):1519-1523. doi:10.1089/end.2010.0698

194. Healy KA, Ogan K. Pathophysiology and management of infectious staghorn calculi. *Urol Clin North Am.* 2007;34(3):363-374. doi:10.1016/j.ucl.2007.05.006

195. Chamberlin JD, Clayman RV. Medical treatment of a staghorn calculus: the ultimate noninvasive therapy. *J Endourol Case Rep.* 2015;1(1):21-23. doi:10.1089/cren.2015.29003.jdc

196. Lingeman JE, Siegel YI, Steele B. Metabolic evaluation of infected renal lithiasis: clinical relevance. *J Endourol.* 1995;9(1):51-54. doi:10.1089/end.1995.9.51

197. Pearle MS, Goldfarb DS, Assimos DG, et al. Medical management of kidney stones: AUA guideline. *J Urol.* 2014;192(2):316-324.

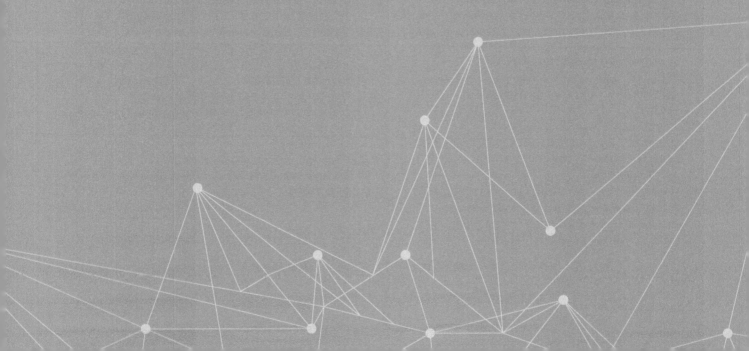

SECTION IV

Nutrition Support With Kidney Disease

CHAPTER 15

Enteral Nutrition and Kidney Disease

Mary Rath, MEd, RD, LD, CNSC, and Peggy Hipskind, MA, RD, LD

Introduction

When a patient can no longer meet their nutritional needs by mouth, an alternate means of nutrition support is warranted. Indications for enteral nutrition (EN) include, but are not limited to, patients who are expected to receive nothing by mouth (npo) for more than 5 to 7 days, critically ill patients, those with swallowing disorders, intestinal failure, severe malnutrition, and medical conditions that result in fatigue, nausea, and vomiting. Chronic kidney disease (CKD)-related malnutrition often results from insufficient calorie and protein intake due to anorexia and thereby leads to fat loss, muscle wasting, and/or weight loss. EN can be an effective intervention and should be considered with prolonged inadequate oral food and beverage intake to prevent catabolism.[1] In the hospital setting, the ideal time to implement EN can vary, depending on the degree of illness, nutrition status of the patient, as well as previously failed nutrition interventions such as oral supplement therapy or diet liberalization to stimulate increased oral intake. Presently, there is limited research on the timing of EN initiation for noncritically ill patients. However, the American Society of Parental and Enteral Nutrition (ASPEN) supports initiating early EN in a critically ill patient unable to maintain oral intake goals within 24 hours to 48 hours.[2] Nonetheless, when EN is used, feedings must be carefully monitored to prevent complications. Patient acceptance of EN support can be greatly influ-

enced by the knowledge and attitudes held by health care providers. The registered dietitian nutritionist (RDN) can help to facilitate implementation of EN not only through interactions with patients but also by providing education on the safety and the effectiveness of EN to other providers. This chapter will discuss feeding tube access, enteral formula selection, methods of delivery, and potential complications in order to provide optimum nutrition care to patients with CKD requiring nutrition support.

Tube Selection

The type of feeding tube and site of feeding are determined by the patient's clinical status. Key factors in determining the access device are duration of the enteral feeding (long-term vs short-term), gastrointestinal (GI) function, and underlying disease conditions affecting tube placement (see Table 15.1 on page 318).

NASOGASTRIC AND NASOENTERIC FEEDING TUBES

Nasogastric and nasoenteric (nasoduodenal and nasojejunal) feeding tubes are commonly used when less than 6 weeks of enteral feedings are anticipated.[3] Although not entirely risk free, large-bore nasogastric placement is preferred when the risk for aspiration is low as these tubes are quickly and easily inserted. Hospitalized critically ill patients are typically fed through

TABLE 15.1 | Enteral Feeding Tube Types[3]

Type	Duration	French (Fr) size[a]	Feeding pump	Contraindication in chronic kidney disease
Nasogastric Orogastric	<6 weeks	12-20	Not required	None
Nasoenteric	<6 weeks	8-14	Yes	None
Gastrostomy	>6 weeks	12-30 Percutaneous endoscopic gastrostomy (PEG) tube 12-30 Surgical gastrostomy 12-24 Low profile tubes	Not required	Peritoneal dialysis[b]
Jejunostomy	>6 weeks	8-14 Jejunostomy 8-10 Jejunal tube extension	Yes	Peritoneal dialysis[b]

[a] 1 French unit = 0.33 mm
[b] Except when PEG is preexisting

large-bore feeding tubes (nasogastric/orogastric). These tubes can be placed at the bedside without need for specialized training.[4,5] Small-bore nasoenteric feeding tubes are made of silicone or polyurethane. Trained practitioners can insert these tubes at the bedside using a blind technique, or (in some facilities) an assisted feeding tube insertion device is used for placement. Tube placement can also be accomplished fluoroscopically or via esophagogastroduodenoscopy when bedside placement is not feasible. Standard tube length is 110 cm, sufficient for placement into the stomach or small intestine. These small-bore tubes can accommodate standard or viscous fiber-containing formulas administered by pump, gravity drip, or syringe. As a general rule, when EN is expected to be long term, feeding via a gastrostomy or, in certain situations, enterostomy should be the preferred route.

GASTROSTOMY TUBES

Long-term feedings can be accomplished via either surgical or nonsurgical gastrostomy tube placement. Several different types of tubes are available, depending on the patient's needs and therapy chosen. Gastrostomy feedings are commonly used for long-term care for patients with adequate gastric emptying capacity and have the benefit of allowing for either continuous or bolus feeding. Nonsurgical long-term tube placement can be accomplished via a percutaneous endoscopic

gastrostomy (PEG). Feedings through a PEG are used less frequently in patients receiving peritoneal dialysis (PD) than in patients receiving hemodialysis (HD). Fein and colleagues[6] report that the initial placement of PEG tubes in patients on PD is associated with an increase in infectious complications, such as peritonitis. However, PEG tubes that were in place prior to the initiation of PD may be safe and can be used.[7] Maintaining patients on HD for at least 6 weeks and using antifungal prophylaxis appear to decrease the incidence of peritonitis but does not eliminate this risk.

JEJUNOSTOMY TUBES

Gastric feedings may be contraindicated in patients with some gastric disorders, such as gastroparesis, or those who may be at increased risk for aspiration as in patients who have had a stroke. In cases where patients with CKD may have one of these comorbid conditions, jejunostomy tube placement may be appropriate. Like gastrostomy tubes, jejunostomy tubes can be placed either surgically or endoscopically. Double-lumen tubes (eg, percutaneous gastrostomy with jejunal extension) are available and can be used to simultaneously decompress gastric contents and feed into the small intestine. These tubes are often placed in patients who have underlying GI disorders, such as severe gastroparesis. Jejunostomy tubes require pump assistance, which typically runs for 12 to 24 hours per day.

Enteral Formula Selection

Enteral formulas have been defined by the US Food and Drug Administration as[8]:

a food which is formulated to be consumed or administered enterally under the supervision of a physician and which is intended for the specific dietary management of a disease or condition for which distinctive nutrition requirements, based on recognized scientific principles are established by medical evaluation.

Formulas available on the market can differ in macronutrient and micronutrient composition, concentration, and fiber content, as well as addition of immune-modulating substances, such as arginine, glutamine, omega-3 fatty acids, and dietary nucleotides (see Box 15.1).[9] Retail cost of enteral formulas can vary, depending on formula type. Health care facilities often enter into buying contracts that can offer reduced prices for the cost of a more limited formulary. Cost containment is becoming an important component of health

BOX 15.1 | Categories, Nutrition Content, Indications, and Application of Enteral Products[10,11]

STANDARD, POLYMERIC	
Nutrition content	1 to 1.2 kcal/mL Moderate protein content (18% kcal)
Indication and contraindications	For most people requiring enteral feeding Monitor electrolytes and modify formula as needed
Stage of kidney disease/treatment modality considerations	Acute kidney injury (AKI) (not on dialysis) Peritoneal dialysis (PD)/Hemodialysis (HD) Kidney transplant (except in cases of delayed graft function and recurrence of chronic kidney disease [CKD])
FLUID-RESTRICTED FORMULAS	
Nutrition content	1.5 to 2 kcal/mL Moderate protein content (18% kcal)
Indication and contraindications	For patients with fluid restriction
Stage of kidney disease/treatment modality considerations	CKD or AKI with low urine output (electrolyte restriction not necessary)
FIBER-CONTAINING	
Nutrition content	1 to 1.5 kcal/mL Moderate protein content (18% kcal) Fiber content may vary by amount and type (soluble and insoluble)
Indication and contraindications	May help normalize bowel function in some patients; use with caution in critically ill patients on vasopressors due to concern for bowel ischemia Modify formula based on electrolytes
Stage of kidney disease/treatment modality considerations	AKI (not on dialysis) PD/HD CKD (not on dialysis) Kidney transplant
ELEMENTAL AND SEMIELEMENTAL	
Nutrition content	1.0 to 1.5 kcal/mL Moderate–high protein content (18%–25% kcal) Elemental contains amino acids Semielemental contains dipeptides and tripeptides

Continued on next page

Continued from previous page

Indication and contraindications	For patients with malabsorption and extreme gastrointestinal dysfunction
	Elemental formulas may be too hypertonic for use in jejunostomy tube
	More expensive
	Modify based on electrolytes
Stage of kidney disease/treatment modality considerations	PD/HD
	AKI/CKD on continuous renal replacement therapy (CRRT)
	Kidney transplant

GLUCOSE INTOLERANCE OR CARBOHYDRATE CONTROLLED, DIABETIC

Nutrition content	1.0 to 1.5 kcal/mL
	Moderate protein content (18% kcal)
	Lower carbohydrate content than standard formulas
Indication and contraindications	Consider a slow-release carbohydrate steady product when glucose levels are difficult to stabilize
	Modify based on electrolytes
Stage of kidney disease/treatment modality considerations	AKI
	CKD or AKI with low urine output
	PD/HD
	Kidney transplant

ELECTROLYTE RESTRICTED WITH LOW PROTEIN

Nutrition content	1.8 kcal/mL
	Low protein content (10% kcal)
	Electrolytes modified: sodium, potassium, phosphorus
	Modified complex carbohydrates
Indication and contraindications	For people prone to uremia
	For people with CKD who are not undergoing dialysis
Stage of kidney disease/treatment modality considerations	AKI (not on dialysis)
	CKD (not on dialysis)

ELECTROLYTE RESTRICTED WITH HIGH PROTEIN

Nutrition content	1.8 to 2.0 kcal/mL
	Moderate protein content (18% kcal)
	Electrolytes modified: sodium, potassium, phosphorus
Indication and contraindications	For people with increased needs on dialysis or CRRT
Stage of kidney disease/treatment modality considerations	AKI (CRRT or intermittent HD)
	PD/HD
	Kidney transplant (may be needed with acute/chronic rejection)

BLENDERIZED, WHOLE FOOD

Nutrition content	Nutrient content may vary (homemade vs commercial)
Indication and contraindications	Recommended that patients discuss with their primary care provider before transitioning/starting a blenderized tube feed regimen and work with a registered dietitian nutritionist to evaluate nutrition requirements and safety of delivery
	May not be appropriate for unstable patients or patients with high infection risk
Stage of kidney disease/treatment modality considerations	Product contents vary and need to be assessed for the patient's specific needs

care; therefore, it is important to choose the most cost-effective formula that will meet the patient's needs. Nutrition documentation is important for insurance coverage of enteral products and equipment. Insurance coverage varies widely, depending on whether the insurance is through a government program, such as Medicare and Medicaid, or from a private insurance agency. Each insurance agency has specific documentation requirements for reimbursement.

Cost containment in the delivery of EN products has health care facilities requiring practitioners to utilize formulary products while limiting specialized products. This may require practitioners to modify approaches using innovative measures to achieve optimal outcomes. Documentation of impaired nutrient utilization and altered GI function has become essential for securing the necessary products and equipment to deliver EN in special situations.

Several formulas have been developed specifically for use when patients have developed organ dysfunction (eg, liver disease or pulmonary failure), but there is no current evidence to support their usage. However, immune-enhancing formulas have been shown to be beneficial in critically ill surgical patients that require higher protein needs, such as patients on continuous renal replacement therapy (CRRT). In addition, for critically ill patients with acute kidney injury (AKI), experts recommend they be placed on a standard enteral formulation. If significant electrolyte abnormalities develop, a specialty formulation designed for kidney disease (with an appropriate electrolyte profile) may be considered.[2]

Due to modifications and revisions to product formulation, it is critical to stay abreast of the available research on kidney-specific enteral formulas and their indications for use by contacting respective manufacturers. For example, there are kidney-specific formulas that contain very low protein and electrolytes (sodium, phosphorus, and potassium) for people who have CKD but are not on dialysis. In addition, there are kidney-specific formulas that contain a higher amount of protein and lower electrolytes (sodium, potassium, and phosphorus) for those people that have CKD stage 5

and are on dialysis. Depending on the type of kidney disease, mode of kidney replacement therapy (KRT), and medical situation (outpatient, inpatient, or intensive care unit [ICU]), it is important to choose the most appropriate formula for that person.[9] Box 15.1 lists various categories of enteral formulas, including protein and electrolyte restricted formulas, for patients with CKD.

FLUID AND NUTRIENT CONSIDERATIONS OF ENTERAL FORMULAS

Fluid Concentration

Individuals with CKD or end-stage kidney disease (ESKD) on HD often must limit fluid intake. While most standard enteral formulas contain 1 kcal/mL and approximately 84% free water per liter of formula, calorie-dense renal-specific formulas are available that contain 1.8 to 2 kcal/mL, and thus less free water. Practitioners must consider that patients on EN are also typically prescribed a water flush for hydration, tube patency, and medication which should be included in the total fluid intake. Furthermore, some patients on EN may be allowed an oral diet as tolerated, such as clear liquids. Any additional fluid intake should be monitored to maintain daily goals for fluid restriction. It is important to follow interdialytic weight gains (IDWGs) to properly assess each patient's fluid needs. Not all patients on dialysis are anuric. Residual kidney function contributes to changes in electrolyte and fluid needs. Therefore, it is essential to monitor estimated dry weight and IDWG to assure euvolemia.

Protein Content

The current recommendations for protein intake for the patient with CKD depends on the stage of CKD and if KRT is necessary (refer to Chapters 3, 4, 5, 6, or 7). Protein content of the different categories of enteral formulas also vary, even the specific renal formulated products (see Box 15.1). Patients with CKD who are not receiving dialysis have lower protein requirements; therefore, they may require a lower protein, electrolyte-restricted formula. In contrast, other kidney-specific formulas may have higher protein content for those patients on dialysis who have increased protein needs. Protein modulars are also an option available for those patients requiring increased protein needs above the protein provision from the prescribed EN formula volume.

The sources of protein also differ within enteral formulas. Polymeric formulas contain proteins that are sodium and calcium caseinates. In contrast, semielemental formulas consist of enzymatically hydrolyzed whey protein, and elemental formulas contain free amino acids. Each formula has a unique patient application in clinical practice. With CKD, many of these formulas may not be appropriate. However, many of the semielemental formulas do have a higher protein content that may be beneficial to patients who require CRRT.

Electrolytes and Mineral Content

Other important considerations in choosing enteral formulas for patients with CKD include the electrolyte and mineral content. For those patients on EN following an oral diet, monitoring food and beverage selection is also encouraged to accurately evaluate serum electrolytes. Changes in the patient's condition, stage of CKD, and effectiveness of KRT may require adjusting electrolyte restrictions during illness. Electrolyte content of formulas varies widely. Most standard formulas are designed to provide adequate but not excessive amounts of potassium, sodium, and phosphorus. These formulas may be well tolerated by the patient with CKD who is stable and adequately dialyzed. Special kidney-specific formulas designed for patients with ESKD on dialysis that contain lower amounts of potassium and phosphorus are also available.

Administration of Enteral Feedings

The choice of feeding administration method will vary from patient to patient and may be guided by the patient's condition, need for time away from the feeding pump, type of feeding tube, and feeding tolerance. An RDN can work with the patient to help determine the best individualized plan.

DELIVERY SYSTEMS

The development of canned, sterile, nutritionally complete enteral formulas has allowed for standardized nutrient content as well as improved food safety. Bacterial contamination of feedings can be kept to a minimum when clinicians, patients, and caregivers use proper handling techniques, such as hand washing, cleaning the tops of cans before opening, using sterile equipment, including the use of disposable gloves during formula transfer to administration sets, and observing hang times.

Ready-to-use EN products come as either closed or open systems. Closed system feedings, in which formulas are purchased in ready-to-hang containers (1- to 1.5-L bottles), minimize contamination. Although closed systems offer the benefit of longer hang times (often up to 48 hours), there is potential for formula waste due to the manufacturer's recommendations for closed containers to be discarded after 24 hours.[12] The hang time of formula in an open system should be no longer than 4 hours for unsterilized formulas and 8 to 12 hours for sterilized formula (hospital = 8 hours; home = 12 hours).[13]

FEEDING SCHEDULES

Enteral feeding schedules should be individualized, especially after a patient is discharged from the hospital. If persons dependent on EN are discharged to a rehabilitation center, a long-term care facility, or a skilled nursing facility, they should have a feeding schedule that best fits their daily routine.

Cyclic feedings are often used during attempts to transition from an enteral to an oral diet. Feedings are typically administered nocturnally and are stopped 1 to 2 hours prior to the first meal of the day. This allows for a longer period free from feedings and may promote development of sensations of hunger and stimulation of increased voluntary oral intake.

Intermittent feedings are frequently seen in long-term care, rehabilitation centers, and home care settings with patients who have gastric feeding tubes. Intermittent or bolus feedings are not recommended with jejunostomy tubes (see Table 15.1). Intermittent feedings of EN provide time off from feedings for therapy, work, or other activities. This type of feeding schedule physiologically mimics regular mealtimes. The schedule can vary widely and can include from four to six or more feedings spaced throughout the day to meet nutritional requirements. Additionally, some medications (eg, phosphate binders) are more effective when administered with a feeding.

Diabetes is a common comorbidity with kidney disease. Diabetes may be better controlled with continuous EN, but some patients may have better insulin response with bolus feeds. The insulin regimen (rapid/intermediate/long-acting) must also be adjusted accordingly for the EN regimen.

Creative feeding schedules are often used for patients receiving HD. The total volume of formula required to meet the patient's needs and a feeding schedule that accommodates dialysis should be determined to ensure that the patient's nutritional goals are met. Typically, a patient on HD will not be allowed to eat or drink; therefore, EN should be held during this time.

Complications of Enteral Feeding

Clinicians must complete a comprehensive assessment of the patient before starting EN to identify and avoid potential problems. Educating the patient, family, or caregiver on the nutrition care plan can help to provide comfort and understanding when initiating and monitoring EN. Follow-up care is important in enterally fed patients to monitor for signs and symptoms of intolerance after the EN is initiated. The most common complications of enteral feeding can be classified as mechanical, GI, or metabolic (Box 15.2 on page 324).

MECHANICAL

Mechanical complications of EN include tube dislodgment and clogging. A dislodged tube may likely need replacement by the medical team. A clogged tube can be the result of administration of medications via the feeding tube; therefore, frequent and thorough flushing of tubes with warm water is the best method to ensure

tube patency. There is no evidence that the use of carbonated drinks, cranberry juice, or other liquids prevent tube clogging and can contribute to the clog. Whenever possible, replace crushed medications with a liquid equivalent to prevent tube occlusion. Acidic medication given through the tube should be diluted because the acidity of the medication may curdle the enteral formula and potentially lead to tube clogging.[14-16] Consult a pharmacist to assess the most appropriate dose, form, and route of delivery of medications for patients receiving enteral feedings. To treat a clogged feeding tube, enzymatic therapy can be considered. When a clogged tube fails to clear, the feeding tube should be replaced.

GASTROINTESTINAL

GI complications of EN include aspiration, constipation, diarrhea, nausea, and vomiting. Aspiration can be avoided using safe practices such as elevating the head of the bed greater than 30 degrees and using lower goal volume or postpyloric feeding tubes for high-risk patients, as medically appropriate.[17]

The cause of constipation or diarrhea involves a thorough assessment of medications, amount of fiber provided from the EN, or other underlying GI conditions. Additional free water may be warranted in patients who develop constipation (see Box 15.2).

Patients with underlying gastroparesis or pancreatitis may experience nausea and vomiting with initiation of EN. Adjusting the goal rate of the tube feeding and advancing the rate more slowly may help relieve nausea and vomiting. Gastric residual volume (GRV) has been used to assess EN tolerance; however, elevated GRVs do not necessarily correlate with intolerance. According to the ASPEN Critical Care guidelines, use of GRVs leads to increased changes of clogged feeding tubes and interruptions in EN infusion; requires additional nursing time; and, in turn, negatively affects outcomes through reduced volume of EN delivered.[2] Early identification of the GI concerns described may merit placement of a postpyloric feeding tube vs gastric feeding tube to optimize tolerance.

BOX 15.2 | Complications Associated With Enteral Nutrition

COMPLICATION	ETIOLOGY	TREATMENT
Mechanical		
Tube dislodgment	Patient dislodges	Replace tube
	Emesis	
Tube clog	Medications	Proper crushing of medications
	Lack of or insufficient free water flushes	Increase water flushes
		Consider enzymatic therapy and/or occlusion clearing system
Gastrointestinal		
Aspiration	Reflux and pulmonary aspiration as a result of reduced consciousness, dysphagia, disorders of the upper gastrointestinal tract	Elevate the head of the bed to >30 degrees
		Use low-volume EN
		Advance tube to postpyloric position
Constipation	Poor hydration	Adequate water flushes
	Lack of mobility	Increase mobility
	Lack of fiber	Fiber-containing formula or additive
	Pain medication	
Diarrhea	Hyperosmolar medications	Adjust medications (ie, avoid sugar alcohols) as able
	Not enough fiber	Fiber formula or fiber additive
	Too much fiber	Fiber free formula
	Malabsorption	Gastrointestinal workup
	Infectious diarrhea	Change to hypotonic enteral product
	Hypertonic enteral product	
Nausea/vomiting	Advancing EN too quickly	Slow EN to last tolerated rate and re-advance slowly
	Gastroparesis	Advance tip of tube into third or fourth duodenum portion
	Pancreatitis	Hold enteral feeding
	Ileus	
	Bowel obstruction	
	Malpositioned or dislodged tube	Confirm tip of tube location
Metabolic		
Refeeding syndrome	Rapid infusion rate	Identify at risk patients. Prevention is key. Recognize risk factors (malnutrition, prolonged nothing-by-mouth [npo] status, electrolyte disturbances)
		Advance EN rate slowly to goal over 2 to 4 days
		Monitor/replete electrolytes
		Assess thiamin/replete as warranted
Hyperglycemia	Medications (ie, corticosteroids, immunosuppressants)	Medically manage medications
		Adjust type/dose of insulin
	Critical illness	Reduce total calories from EN
	Diabetes mellitus type 1 or 2	
	Overfeeding	
Dehydration	Inadequate free water flush	Increase water flushes
	Low-volume EN formula	Change to a higher-volume formula, if medically appropriate

METABOLIC

Metabolic complications include hyperglycemia, hypoglycemia, refeeding syndrome, and dehydration. Hyperglycemia in enterally fed patients with CKD can be the result of underlying diabetes, metabolic stress, excessive carbohydrate intake, peripheral insulin resistance, and uptake of glucose from the dialysate solution. Hyperglycemia has been implicated in poor wound healing, as well as increased infectious complications after surgery, making it imperative that elevated blood glucose be identified and aggressively treated. Patients with kidney failure may have decreased insulin clearance, resulting in hypoglycemia. As CKD progresses, kidneys do not as effectively filter insulin out of the blood. This can lead to overdosing insulin (particularly intermediate and long-term insulin) and should be monitored.

RDNs should be aware of the signs of refeeding syndrome (RFS) in patients receiving EN. The reintroduction of nutrition to a starved or fasted individual results in a rapid increase in insulin, which stimulates the movement of extracellular potassium, phosphorus, and magnesium to the intracellular compartment.[18] Identifying high-risk patients prior to starting EN as well as knowing the symptoms are key to the prevention and treatment of RFS. Patients with CKD may have elevated potassium, magnesium, and phosphorus levels at the time of initiation of EN, which makes it difficult to assess if the patient is experiencing RFS. Following patients with CKD at high risk for RFS closely and advancing EN slowly to a goal rate over a 2- to 4-day period may be necessary.[19] Patients meeting the criteria for RFS, those with underlying malnutrition, and those with alcohol dependency will also benefit from thiamin supplementation before initiating EN. Thiamin is an essential coenzyme in carbohydrate metabolism. Deficiency in thiamin can lead to Korsakoff syndrome and Wernicke encephalopathy. The average dose for repletion is 100 mg thiamin daily for 5 to 7 days; however, in some cases, increased provision is needed.[2]

Patients with CKD may warrant a low-volume, electrolyte-restricted formula, which may result in dehydration because of inadequate free water. Dehydration can also result from acute illness with excessive GI fluid losses secondary to persistent vomiting and diarrhea. After discussion with the primary care team, make sure that the volume of the EN formula and free water flushes are adequate to meet the patient's needs. In addition, patients with kidney disease are often given diuretics, which may contribute to inadvertent over-diuresis, resulting in excessive loss of fluids and electrolytes.

Summary

EN is a safe and effective therapy for patients with CKD. The indications for EN in patients with CKD are no different from those in any other patient population; however, nutrient needs vary according to the stage of kidney disease, as well as the distinct metabolic implications and nutrient requirements of different KRT (see Chapters 3, 4, 5, 6, and 7). Standard enteral formulas may be appropriate for some patients with CKD, although special attention must be paid to the nutrient composition of feedings and individualized to the patient's nutritional goals.

References

1. Ikizler TA, Cano NJ, Franch H, Fouque D, Himmelfarb J, Kalantar-Zadeh K. Prevention and treatment of protein energy wasting in chronic kidney disease patients: a consensus statement by the International Society of Renal Nutrition and Metabolism. *Kidney Int.* 2013;84(6):1096-1107. doi:10.1038/ki.2013.147

2. McClave SA, Taylor BE, Martindale RG, et al; the Society of Critical Care Medicine and the American Society for Parenteral and Enteral Nutrition. Guidelines for the provision and assessment of nutrition support therapy in the adult critically ill patient: Society of Critical Care Medicine (SCCM) and American Society for Parenteral and Enteral Nutrition (A.S.P.E.N.). *JPEN J Parenter Enteral Nutr.* 2016;40(2):159-211. doi:10.1177/0148607115621863

3. Fang JC, Kinikini M. Enteral access devices. In: Mueller C, ed. *The A.S.P.E.N. Adult Nutrition Support Core Curriculum.* 3rd ed. American Society for Parenteral and Enteral Nutrition; 2017:251-264.

4. Miller K, McClave S, Kiraly L, Martindale R, Benns MV. Tutorial on enteral access in adult patients in the hospitalized setting. *JPEN J Parenter Enteral Nutr.* 2014;38(3):282-295. doi:10..1177/0148607114522487

5. Pash E. Enteral nutrition: options for short term access. *Nutr Clin Pract.* 2018;33(2):170-176. doi:10.1002/ncp.10007

6. Fein PA, Madane SJ, Jorden A, et al. Outcome of percutaneous endoscopic gastrostomy feeding in patients on peritoneal dialysis. *Adv Perit Dial.* 2001;17:148-152.

7. Lew SQ, Gruia A, Hakki F. Adult peritoneal dialysis patient with Tenckhoff and percutaneous endoscopic gastrostomy catheters. *Perit Dial Int.* 2011;31(3):360-361. doi:10.3747/pdi.2010.00249

8. Guidance for industry: frequently asked questions about medical foods. US Food and Drug Administration. May 2016. Accessed April 9, 2020. www.fda.gov/downloads/Food/GuidanceRegulation/GuidanceDocumentsRegulatoryInformation/UCM500094.pdf

9. Cano N, Fiaccadori E, Tesinsky P, et al. ESPEN guidelines on enteral nutrition: adult renal failure. *Clin Nutr.* 2006;25(2):295-310. doi:10.1016/j.clnu.2006.01.023

10. Epp L, Lammert L, Vallumsetla N, Hurt R, Mundi M. Use of blenderized tube feeding in adult and pediatric home enteral nutrition patients. *Nutr Clin Pract.* 2017;32(2):201-205. doi:10.1177//0884533616662992

11. Novak P, Wilson KE, Ausderau K, Cullinane D. The use of blenderized tube feedings. *ICAN: Infact, Child and Adolescent Nutrition*: 2009;1(1):21-23. doi:10.1177/1941406408329196

12. Phillips W, Roman B, Glassman K. Economic impact of switching from an open to a closed enteral nutrition feeding system in an acute care setting. *Nutr Clin Pract.* 2013;28(4):510-514. doi:10.1177/0884533613489712

13. Sewify K, Genena D. Open versus closed tube feeding in critically ill patients—which is the best? *J Nutr Food Sci.* 2017;7:621. doi:10.4172/2155-9600.1000621

14. Guenter P, Boullata J. Drug administration by enteral feeding tube. *Nursing.* 2013;43(12):26-33. doi:10.1097/01.NURSE.0000437469.13218.7b

15. Kurien M, Penny H, Sanders DS. Impact of direct drug delivery via gastric access devices. *Expert Opin Drug Deliv.* 2015;12(3):455-463. doi:10.1517/17425247.2015.966683

16. Boullata JI. Drug administration through an enteral feeding tube. *Am J Nurs.* 2009;109(10):34-43. doi:10.1097/01.NAJ.0000361488.45094.28

17. Boullata J, Carrera A, Harvey L, et al. ASPEN safe practices for enteral nutrition therapy. *JPEN J Parenter Enteral Nutr.* 2017;41(1):15-103. doi:10.1177/0148607116673053

18. Tresley J, Sheean P. Refeeding syndrome: recognition is the key to prevention and management. *J Am Diet Assoc.* 2008;108(12):2105-2108. doi:10.1016/j.jada.2008.09.015

19. Khan LUR, Ahmed J, Khan S, Macfie J. Refeeding syndrome: a literature review. *Gastroenterol Res Pract.* 2011;2011:410971. doi:10.1155/2011/410971

CHAPTER 16

Parenteral Nutrition and Kidney Disease

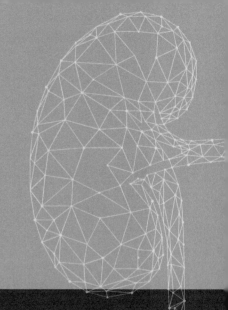

Marian Glick-Bauer, MS, RD, CDN, CSR, CNSC, and Eileen Moore, CNSC, RD, LD

Parenteral nutrition (PN) is an alternative feeding modality, delivered via a central vein or a peripheral vein with peripheral parenteral nutrition (PPN). When the gastrointestinal (GI) tract is nonfunctioning or when enteral nutrition (EN) is unable to provide adequate nutrition to meet the patient's nutrient requirements, PN or PPN can be used. PN may also be utilized as supplementary nutrition support for malnourished patients receiving kidney replacement therapy (KRT), either as intradialytic parenteral nutrition (IDPN) or intraperitoneal nutrition (IPN). This chapter includes discussion on the following four topics:

- PN in chronic kidney disease (CKD)
- PN in acute kidney injury (AKI)
- IDPN
- intraperitoneal amino acids (IPAA)/IPN

Parenteral Nutrition and Chronic Kidney Disease

Patients with CKD may require PN support if they are unable to tolerate adequate amounts of nutrients enterally. Depending on the patient's ability to transition to EN, the length of PN therapy may be short term (less than 3 months during recovery from injury) or long term (greater than 3 months or lifetime; Medicare criteria for "permanence" is 90 days). PN should be initiated after 7 days for well-nourished patients, within 3 to 5 days for those nutritionally at risk, and as soon as feasible for patients with moderate-to-severe malnutrition when these patients are unlikely to meet their needs via oral intake or EN.[1,2] The nutrient composition of the PN solution should be individualized based on the patient's requirements and tolerance. Nutritional requirements depend on clinical evidence of catabolic, proinflammatory, protein–energy wasting (PEW) markers, malnutrition–inflammation score (MIS), and subjective global assessment (SGA) score, comorbidities, activity/functional capacity or stress level, and stage of CKD.

Calculations for energy requirements should be based on the patient's edema-free, estimated dry, or target weight. If the patient is significantly underweight with body mass index (BMI) of less than 20, or if MIS/SGA scores show signs of catabolic muscle and fat wasting, additional energy can be provided to support gradual weight gain. Protein requirements are often based on the patient's ideal body weight (IBW) or standard body weight. Calorie requirements are met from amino acids, dextrose, and lipids, but contributions from intravenous (IV) medications, such as propofol, should be accounted for as well. In most cases, PN and PPN prescriptions include standard multivitamin and trace element preparations.[3] Box 16.1 on page 328 provides general guidelines for PN composition for patients with CKD.[4]

The nutrition assessment of patients who are candidates for PN should include determining indications

327

BOX 16.1 | Suggested Composition of Parenteral Nutrition Solution for Adults With Acute Kidney Injury or Chronic Kidney Disease[4-10]

COMPONENT	RECOMMENDATIONS
Macronutrients	
Energy	Chronic kidney disease (CKD) stages 1 through 5: 25 to 35 kcal/kg/d
	Acute kidney injury (AKI) stage 2: 25 to 35 kcal/kg/d
	AKI stage 3, stable/oral diet: 30 to 35 kcal/kg/d
	AKI stage 3, critically ill/ventilated: 20 to 30 kcal/kg/d
Amino acids[a]	CKD 3 through 5 not on hemodialysis (HD), without diabetes mellitus 0.55 to 0.6 g/kg/d; with diabetes mellitus 0.6 to 0.8 g/kg/d
	CKD on chronic dialysis or peritoneal dialysis (PD): 1.0 to 1.2 g/kg/d
	AKI: 0.8 to 1.0 g/kg/d, noncatabolic, without dialysis
	AKI: 1.0 to 1.5 g/kg/d, catabolic and intermittent HD
	AKI on continuous renal replacement therapy (CRRT): 1.7 to 2 g/kg/d to a maximum of 2.5 g/kg/d
Dextrose	Consider all sources of dextrose (intravenous fluids, dialytic therapy)
	AKI: less than 4 mg/kg/min
Lipids	Include propofol infusion (1.1 kcal/mL) in lipid sources
	Less than 1 g/kg/d, less than 0.11 g/kg/min, or 20% to 30% of total kcal
	Peripheral parenteral nutrition (PPN) lipid content should not exceed 60% total kcal
Fluid	Volume depends on patient tolerance/requirements, insensible losses, and urine output
Micronutrients	
Minerals	
May need to restrict for CKD not on HD or with intermittent HD; may need to restrict for AKI not on kidney replacement therapy (KRT); monitor serum levels and adjust accordingly	
Higher/lower needs may occur with CRRT; varies by dialysate mineral content	
Sodium	1 to 2 mEq/kg/d standard PPN
	May be removed from parenteral nutrition (PN) for CRRT
Potassium	1 to 2 mEq/kg/d standard PN
	May be removed from PN for CRRT
Phosphorus	20 to 40 mmol/d standard PN
	May need supplementation during CRRT
Calcium	10 to 15 mEq/d standard PN
	May need supplementation during CRRT
Magnesium	8 to 20 mEq/d standard PN
	May need supplementation during CRRT
Chloride and acetate	Proportions vary, depending on acid-base status and degree of kidney impairment

Continued on next page

Continued from previous page

COMPONENT	RECOMMENDATIONS
Vitamins	
May need to restrict for CKD not on HD or with intermittent HD; may need to restrict for AKI not on KRT; monitor serum levels and adjust accordingly	
A	990 mcg/d or 3,300 IU
D	5 mcg/d or 200 IU
E	10 mg/d or 10 IU
K	150 mcg/d
C	200 mg/d
Thiamin (B1)	6 mg/d
Riboflavin (B2)	3.6 mg/d
Niacin (B3)	40 mg/d
Pyridoxine (B6)	6 mg/d
Cyanocobalamin (B12)	5 mcg/d
Folate	600 mcg/d
Pantothenic acid	15 mg/d
Biotin	60 mcg/d
Trace elements	
Standard PN regimen typically contains multitrace element product	
Zinc	2.5 to 5 mg/d
Copper	0.3 to 0.5 mg/d
Chromium	10 to 15 mcg/d
Manganese	0.06 to 0.1 mg/d
Selenium	20 to 60 mcg/d

[a] Consider if patient is metabolically stable when determining protein needs.

Adapted with permission from Fuhrman MP. Parenteral nutrition in kidney disease. In: Byham-Gray L, Stover J, Wiesen K, eds. *A Clinical Guide to Nutrition Care in Kidney Disease.* 2nd ed. Academy of Nutrition and Dietetics; 2013:197-216.

and contraindications for PN, identifying line availability and the route of infusion (central or peripheral), calculating macronutrient and micronutrient requirements, identifying metabolic derangements, and setting nutritional goals and measurable desired outcomes. Indications for PN include a nonfunctioning or inaccessible GI tract. PN may also be indicated when a patient's total nutrient needs cannot be met with either

oral diet or tube feeding.[2,5] The 2020 Kidney Disease Outcomes Quality Initiative (KDOQI) Clinical Practice Guideline for Nutrition in CKD recommends a trial of PN for patients with CKD and PEW if nutritional requirements cannot be met with existing oral and energy intake. For patients with CKD on maintenance hemodialysis (HD), a combination of IDPN and oral intake is recommended.[5] Contraindications for PN include an inability to obtain IV access in addition to poor prognosis.[1,2]

COMPONENTS OF PARENTERAL NUTRITION

Macronutrient components of PN solutions are amino acids, dextrose, and lipids. The most concentrated form of each can be used in PN when the total volume must be minimized. The caloric contribution of each PN component is shown in Table 16.1.[11] The most concentrated source of PN calories is a 30% lipid solution providing 3 kcal/mL. However, this solution is not available in all facilities. A 20% lipid solution is more frequently used and provides 2 kcal/mL. Likewise, a 10% intravenous lipid emulsion (ILE) solution, including propofol, provides 1.1 kcal/mL. Of the dextrose and amino acid solutions, the most concentrated solutions are 70% dextrose, which provides 2.38 kcal/mL, and 20% amino acids, which provides 0.8 kcal/mL.

TABLE 16.1 | Calorie Contribution of Parenteral Nutrition Components[11]

Component	kcal/g	Concentration (%)	g/L	kcal/L	kcal/mL
Dextrose	3.4	50	500	1,700	1.7
		70	700	2380	2.38
Amino acids	4	10	100	400	0.4
		15	150	600	0.6
		20	200	800	0.8
Lipids	10	10	100	1,100[a]	1.1[a]
		20	200	2000	2
		30	300	3000	3

[a] Total calories in intravenous lipid emulsion are determined by the fat, phospholipid, and glycerin content.

Amino Acids

The amount of amino acids in PN is determined by the dialysis modality and the patient's comorbidities. KDOQI Guidelines recommend protein intake of 0.55 to 0.60 g/kg/d for metabolically stable adults with CKD stages 3 through 5 (without diabetes mellitus [DM]). Metabolically stable patients with CKD stage 5 on maintenance HD or peritoneal dialysis (PD) require 1.0 to 1.2 g/kg/d of protein, while higher protein levels may be appropriate for patients with DM or hyperglycemia.[5] The registered dietitian nutritionist (RDN) should use clinical judgment in determining the weight used (ideal, usual, current, or adjusted) and the need for increased calories and protein with critical illness, inflammation, hospitalization, infectious or consumptive diseases, or malnutrition. While high losses of peptides, amino acids, and protein have been reported during HD and PD, newer HD technology and the introduction of continuous ambulatory peritoneal dialysis (CAPD) may translate to lower losses. Recent studies have identified 12 g amino acid losses via the dialysate per HD session.[12] Another study found weekly protein losses of approximately 26 g for HD and 47 g for PD, but total nitrogen losses were similar for both HD and PD over the course of a week.[13] Amino acid losses from PD are estimated at approximately 8 g per day.[6] Experts do not recommend that patients on PD with PEW substitute conventional dextrose dialysate with IPN or IPAA unless nutritional needs cannot be met with existing oral and enteral intake.[5] In patients with DM receiving PD who have uncontrolled hyperglycemia, the substitution of IPAA for glucose in PD solutions may reduce the infused carbohydrate load and improve glycemic control.[5] Patients with CKD and protein loss in excess of 1.0 g/d due to proteinuria may need compensatory additional protein provision. The required compensatory protein intake can be calculated based on IBW as[14]:

$$\text{Required compensatory protein intake} = \text{kg} \times (0.6 \text{ to } 0.8) \times \text{proteinuria}$$

Dextrose

Dextrose monohydrate is the primary energy source in PN. Total glucose provision should not exceed 4 to 5 mg/kg/min in stable nonacute patients and should be less than 4 mg/kg/min in critically ill or trauma patients, those with sepsis, and those at risk for hyperglycemia to avoid exceeding the oxidative capacity of the liver to metabolize glucose.[7,15] Long-term patients on home PN often have compressed cycles less than 24 hours and may tolerate higher dextrose infusion rates, although it is recommended that carbohydrate content of the PN should not exceed 7 g/kg/d.[3] The delivery of adequate dextrose to meet energy requirements without precipitating or worsening hyperglycemia can be challenging, especially in patients with DM. Patients with CKD on CAPD may uptake 100 to 200 g/d of glucose from the peritoneal solution, further increasing the risk for hyperglycemia from excessive glucose provision.[14] Given both the serious risks from hypoglycemia (blood glucose [BG] <70 mg/dL), and the higher mortality rates among patients with a mean BG of 180 mg/dL or above, the recommended target BG for hospitalized patients on PN is 140 to 180 mg/dL.[6,16,17] Hyperglycemia is associated with poorer clinical outcomes as well as increased risk of infection and poor wound healing, while hypoglycemia may be life threatening.[18]

Insulin therapy for patients on PN with DM and without CKD is generally 0.1 unit regular insulin or more per gram dextrose in the PN solution. However, the presence of CKD reduces insulin clearance, which may decrease insulin requirements. Insulin can be provided as needed as an insulin drip, a subcutaneous injection, or an additive to PN. While the reported availability of insulin added to PN ranges from 44% to 95%, the steady availability of insulin within the PN may provide a smoother glycemic profile than IV or subcutaneous dosing. However, a stable BG and consistent PN prescription should be achieved prior to adding insulin to the PN, and BG must be monitored after an interruption in PN, as the lingering effects of insulin administration may result in dangerous hypoglycemia.[16,17]

Refeeding syndrome (RFS) is a concern when initiating PN, as the infusion of glucose can promote an intracellular shift of electrolytes in patients who have had an extended period of inadequate nutrition. During starvation, the body uses lipid as its primary source of fuel. When glucose is provided to a lipolytic metabolic system, it can result in RFS with hypokalemia, hypomagnesemia, hypophosphatemia, hyperglycemia, sodium and fluid retention, and thiamin deficiency.[6,19] If left untreated, RFS can result in cardiac failure and death. Serum levels of potassium, magnesium, and phosphorus should be monitored when initiating PN in patients at risk for RFS and repleted appropriately with consideration for kidney impairment.[20] Electrolytes should be monitored every 12 hours for the first 3 days in patients at high risk for RFS.[21] Other recommendations include thiamin supplementation, caloric restriction for the first 72 hours after initiation of nutrition support, and careful monitoring of fluid status.[6,19,21]

Lipids

Lipids are a source of energy and essential fatty acids. To prevent essential fatty acid deficiency (EFAD), 2% to 4% of total energy as lipid is sufficient.[3] More lipids can be added to offset the adverse effects of providing a high proportion of total energy as dextrose. Lipid infusion should not exceed 2.5 g/kg/d.[3,18] The American Society of Parenteral and Enteral Nutrition (ASPEN) guidelines recommend a lipid infusion rate of less than 1 g/kg/d soybean oil (SO)-based emulsion for critically ill/trauma/sepsis patients, and up to 1 g/kg/d for stable patients.[7] Dosing may vary for alternative ILEs; refer to the manufacturer's product literature. Lipids generally provide 20% to 30% of total calories.[3,4,22]

Conventional SO-based ILEs contain a high content of omega-6 long-chain polyunsaturated fatty acids (PUFA), which may be associated with adverse effects of immunosuppression, liver function impairment, and hyperlipidemia.[23] Alternative ILEs, which contain a higher proportion of omega-3 long-chain PUFAs and omega-9 monounsaturated fatty acids (MUFA), are now available in the United States. These include olive oil (OO)-based ILE, or a mixture containing SO, medium-chain triglycerides, OO, and fish oil (FO), referred to as SMOF ILE. OO- and SMOF-based ILE demonstrate nutritional benefits over traditional SO-based ILE, with test subjects demonstrating higher plasma concentrations of omega-9 oleic acid (ie, a MUFA), plasma α-tocopherol, eicosapentaenoic acid, and docosahexaenoic acid, when treated with these alternative ILEs.[24,25] Patients with CKD have unusually low levels of long-chain omega-3 PUFA and should benefit from alternative ILEs such as SMOF to address common conditions, such as dyslipidemia, HD access failure, and cardiac disease.[5] Numerous studies have supported the immunomodulatory and anti-inflammatory benefits of SMOF ILE, and treat SMOF lipid as the gold standard of PN, to improve both clinical outcomes and reduce treatment costs.[26] A 2020 international consensus statement on ILEs concluded that including omega-3 fatty acids as a component of PN offers benefits over the use of standard ILEs, including reductions in infection rates and length of hospital and ICU stay.[27] ILEs high in omega-3 fatty acids, such as SMOF lipid, may also be preferable for patients requiring long-term parenteral supplementation.[28] Research in this area remains ongoing.

Serum triglyceride levels should be monitored in patients receiving lipid-containing solutions to prevent severe disorders of fat metabolism and hyperlipidemia. Acute pancreatitis may result when triglyceride levels exceed 1,000 mg/dL.[29] Lipids in PN should be discontinued if serum triglycerides exceed 400 mg/dL, and ILE infusion rates should be limited to less than 0.11 g/kg/hour.[1] The lipid contribution from propofol may be a source of hypertriglyceridemia in vented patients, and total ILE provision should be adjusted accordingly if an alternative method of sedation is not feasible. If hypertriglyceridemia persists despite omission of lipids for more than 2 weeks and the patient is receiving no fat enterally, the patient should receive a minimum of 250 mL 20% lipids twice per week to prevent EFAD.[18]

Lipids should be evaluated for other possible contra-indications, including vitamin K1 content, phosphate content, and allergens. Refer to full prescribing information (available online) for ILEs. The vitamin K1 content of lipid emulsions varies from 20 mcg/L to greater than 360 mcg/L, depending on the oils used in the emulsion. The international normalized ratio (INR) should be monitored in patients on PN receiving lipids in conjunction with anticoagulation therapy.[3] Lipids also contain egg phospholipid, which contributes 15 mmol phosphate per liter. Recent research does not suggest holding lipids for refractory hyperphosphatemia, but clinical judgment should be used. Patients with an egg, soy, or peanut allergy should not receive lipids.[29] Similarly, SMOF- or OO-based ILE may be contraindicated for patients with a fish or OO allergy.

There is a risk of a patient experiencing an anaphylactic reaction to lipids. Lipid tolerance can be assessed by giving a test dose of 0.5 mL lipids per minute for 15 to 30 minutes and then increase to 1 mL/min with a maximum of 2.5 g lipid per kg.[30] An allergic reaction to lipids may include dyspnea, cyanosis, nausea, vomiting, headache, fever, flushing, sleepiness, or chest pain.[18,22]

Fluid, Electrolytes, and Minerals

The average adult with normal kidney function requires 30 to 40 mL/kg/d total fluid.[7,31] Although the volume of PN will be determined primarily by the patient's macronutrient requirements and the concentration of solutions available for compounding at the institution, other factors will play a role in the final volume determination. These factors include fluid allowance, output from urine, stool, gastric decompression, and fistula losses, and total fluid volume required for medication and electrolyte management. Medical conditions (eg, kidney failure, congestive heart failure, cirrhotic ascites, pulmonary disease, and syndrome of inappropriate antidiuretic hormone [SIADH]) may require fluid restrictions.[6]

The recommended average sodium provision in PN is 1 to 2 mEq/kg/d, provided as sodium chloride, sodium acetate, or sodium phosphate.[7] Making adjustments to the sodium in PN requires an understanding of the relationship between sodium and fluid balance.[31] Serum sodium does not reflect total body sodium, but rather is used to determine the intracellular fluid volume and the extracellular fluid volume (ECFV). If the ECFV volume contains excess sodium, fluid overload may result. Similarly, insufficient sodium in the ECFV results in fluid depletion.

Hypernatremia (serum sodium greater than 145 mEq/L) is a hypertonic state in which water moves from the intracellular fluid to the extracellular fluid, commonly due to excessive body fluid losses during critical illness. Hyponatremia (sodium less than 135 mEq/L) is a common electrolyte disorder, with many possible etiologies.[32,33] To assess the etiology of hyponatremia, the first step is to evaluate the serum osmolality. If the serum osmolality is normal (isotonic 280 to 295 mOsm/kg), the likely cause is hyperlipidemia or hyperproteinemia. If the serum osmolality is high (hypertonic greater than 295 mOsm/kg), the likely cause is hyperglycemia or mannitol. In these cases, better management of BG, lipids, and medications may help correct the apparent hyponatremia. Corrected sodium, in the setting of hyperglycemia, can be calculated as follows:

$$\text{Corrected sodium} = \text{Measured sodium} + 0.016 \times (\text{Serum glucose} - 100)$$

True (hypotonic) hyponatremia is identified by low serum osmolality (hypotonic less than 280 mOsm/kg) and may be classified as euvolemic, hypervolemic, or hypovolemic. To distinguish among these, it is necessary to obtain the urine osmolality and urine sodium. Urine osmolality can help distinguish between impaired water excretion (urine osmolality greater than 100 mOsm/kg), and hyponatremia with normal water excretion (urine osmolality less than 100 mOsm/kg). If urine osmolality is less than 100 mOsm/kg, the likely etiology is excessive fluid intake or low solute intake, and the diet, EN, or PN prescription may be modified accordingly. However, if the urine osmolality is greater than 100 mOsm/kg, the urine sodium must be measured to further identify the etiology. If the urine sodium is less than 30 mmol/L, this indicates low effective arterial blood volume, typically found in heart failure, liver cirrhosis, nephrotic syndrome, diarrhea/vomiting, or third spacing. If the urine sodium is greater than 30 mmol/L, etiologies may include diuretics, renal salt-wasting, cerebral salt-wasting, and SIADH, among other causes.[32,33]

Hypotonic hyponatremia (serum osmolality less than 280 mOsm/kg) can be further categorized by measuring urine sodium. Euvolemic hyponatremia is most commonly caused by SIADH and is, in part, identified by a urine sodium greater than 20 mEq/L. Treatment typically involves fluid restriction, diuretics, and medication. Acute cases may require 3% sodium chloride or salt tablets to raise serum sodium. A urine sodium less than 20 mEq/L may indicate excessive fluid intake (primary polydipsia), or other causes. Hypervolemic hyponatremia is seen in congestive heart failure, liver cirrhosis, and nephrotic syndrome (urine sodium less than 20 mEq/L), or in kidney failure (urine sodium greater than 20 mEq/L). Fluid restriction and loop diuretics are standard treatments for hypervolemic hyponatremia. Hypovolemic hyponatremia is associated with low plasma volume, may be acute or chronic, and may have kidney or nonkidney causes. A urine sodium greater than 20 mEq/L may be caused by diuretics, cerebral salt-wasting, or other causes. A urine sodium less than 20 mEq/L may be due to diarrhea and vomiting or third space losses. Treatment varies by etiology. A thorough review of sodium/fluid balance, the different etiologies of hyponatremia and hypernatremia, corresponding calculations and interventions, and decision trees for evaluating the etiology of hyponatremia can be found in other publications.[31-34]

Electrolyte and mineral metabolism are altered with CKD. Serum levels of phosphorus, potassium, and magnesium can increase as kidney function declines, particularly as CKD progresses to stages 3 through 5, and may need to be decreased in PN accordingly. KRT can effectively clear potassium and magnesium. Potassium content in the HD or continuous renal replacement therapy (CRRT) solution can be adjusted to

achieve a target serum level, so adjustments via the PN prescription may not be necessary.[35] Phosphorus is not well dialyzed—except with CRRT—and often requires restriction in the PN solution to control serum phosphorus levels. Abnormal potassium laboratory results may reflect an underlying cause, such as acid-base disorders, drug-induced hyperkalemia, or hyperkalemia in the setting of hyperglycemia. These conditions should be corrected and accounted for before adjusting potassium in PN.[5] Box 16.1 lists the amounts of electrolytes commonly added to PN for patients with CKD. The amount of each electrolyte added to PN should be individualized to meet the patient's needs and KRT modality.

Acid-Base Balance

Acid-base disturbances can be identified by evaluating bicarbonate (HCO_3^-), the primary buffer system in the ECFV (which is controlled by the kidneys) and the partial pressure of carbon dioxide (which is controlled by the lungs). Acidosis (pH <7.4) and alkalosis (pH >7.4) may be classified as respiratory or metabolic in nature.[31] Metabolic acidosis can be managed via PN by increasing acetate or decreasing chloride, while metabolic alkalosis can be managed by increasing chloride, potassium, magnesium, or total volume or by decreasing acetate. Respiratory acidosis can be addressed by avoiding overfeeding, while respiratory alkalosis cannot be resolved by adjusting the PN prescription.[34,36]

In adults with CKD, serum bicarbonate levels below 22 mmol/L are associated with worsening kidney function. Updated KDOQI guidelines recommend maintaining serum bicarbonate levels at 24 to 26 mmol/L.[5] Bicarbonate cannot be added to the PN because it forms insoluble calcium and magnesium salts within the solution.[3] Instead, acetate is added to PN solutions and is quickly metabolized to bicarbonate by the liver. The absolute amount of acetate and chloride that can be added to PN solutions depends on the amount of sodium and potassium added because chloride and acetate are given as sodium and potassium salts. Intrinsic amounts of chloride and acetate are also included in the amino acid solutions. Metabolic acidosis is associated with hyperkalemia, whereas metabolic alkalosis may be associated with hypokalemia. This relationship should be considered while correcting the patient's acidosis or alkalosis. For example, if the patient has a low serum potassium with metabolic acidosis, the patient may require additional potassium with correction of the acidosis.

Vitamins and Trace Elements

Micronutrient losses occur with acute and chronic dialysis. Patients with CKD should be assessed for deficiencies in thiamin, riboflavin, vitamin B6, vitamin C, vitamin K, and vitamin D.[5] In the patient receiving chronic dialysis, water-soluble vitamins lost during treatment can be replaced with an oral renal multivitamin. Vitamin C may be supplemented to meet the recommended intake of at least 90 mg/d for males and 75 mg/d for females.* Supplementation in excess of this recommendation may be contraindicated for oliguric patients with CKD, as vitamin C may be metabolized to oxalate crystals which precipitate in soft tissue.[37] Vitamin D may be prescribed in the form of cholecalciferol or ergocalciferol to correct 25-hydroxyvitamin D deficiency/insufficiency, which is prevalent in patients with CKD. Vitamins A and E should not be routinely supplemented due to the risk of toxicity.[5] Injectable multivitamins in PN contain vitamin A (retinol or palmitate) and vitamin E (DL-α-tocopheryl acetate). Patients receiving CKD on long-term PN should be monitored for potential vitamin A toxicity.[14,35] Folate, B12, or a B-vitamin complex may be prescribed for a deficiency based on clinical signs and symptoms. There is no evidence to support the benefit of routine selenium or zinc supplementation.[5]

Commercially available IV multivitamin products contain vitamins A, D, E, K, C, B1 (thiamin), B2 (riboflavin), B6 (pyridoxine), B12 (cyanocobalamin), niacinamide, dexpanthenol, biotin, and folic acid.[38] Patients receiving anticoagulation therapy should not receive vitamin K.[5] The current injectable adult multivitamin preparation is available with and without 150 mcg vi-

tamin K1. The combined vitamin K1 content of the injectable multivitamin and the lipid solution is within 2 to 4 mg vitamin K per week. Thus, it is important to monitor the INR level in patients on PN with CKD who are receiving anticoagulation therapy.[1,3]

Trace elements are protein bound, which reduces loss with dialytic therapy. Patients with CKD on PN should receive a standard daily trace element preparation, typically containing zinc, copper, chromium, manganese, and selenium, unless there is a risk of a deficiency or toxicity of a trace element.[3] Both copper and manganese require elimination via bile excretion and should, therefore, be decreased or omitted in the PN prescription for patients with significant hepatic dysfunction or cholestasis. A 2012 position paper recommended modifications to the standard multitrace elements for PN, including increasing selenium to 60 to 100 mcg/d, reducing manganese to 55 mcg/d, and decreasing copper to 0.3 to 0.5 mg/d. A chromium-free option was also recommended, due to significant parenteral contamination.[6]

Iron is not a component of standard trace element preparations. Iron dextran is the only iron supplement approved for addition to PN. Iron dextran should not be added to lipid-containing PN because it can destabilize the lipid emulsion. The addition of 25 to 50 mg iron dextran once monthly to lipid-free PN is estimated to meet the maintenance requirements for iron when there is no blood loss.[3] Patients should receive a test dose of iron dextran before it is added to PN. There is concern that iron supplementation could stimulate microorganism proliferation, especially in patients with infections.[39] Iron supplementation can be given outside of the PN infusion, to correct deficiency and support erythropoiesis in patients on HD.[37]

Levocarnitine

Levocarnitine (l-carnitine) is a compound involved in fatty acid metabolism, and is required to transport long-chain fatty acids into the mitochondria for oxidation. l-carnitine production is decreased in CKD, and lost

---

*Specific recommendations for transgender people were not provided.

during HD. While L-carnitine occurs naturally in the diet, deficiencies may occur in unsupplemented long-term patients on PN. Deficiency symptoms include hypertriglyceridemia, hyperglycemia, elevated liver function tests, and muscle weakness. The IV form of L-carnitine is used in patients on long-term PN and in patients with CKD requiring HD. L-carnitine dosing for patients receiving HD has been suggested at 15 mg/kg/d or 1 g/d, provided after dialysis treatments.[41] However, there is no strong evidence recommending routine L-carnitine supplementation in this population.[36]

ADMINISTRATION OF PARENTERAL NUTRITION

The ASPEN recommendations suggest appropriate PN dosing for adult patients at 20 to 30 kcal/kg/d total energy and 0.8 to 2.5 g/kg/d protein, as appropriate for the patient's weight, BMI, clinical status, and mode of KRT.[7] Limiting PN initially to 1,000 to 1,200 kcal and 100 to 150 g dextrose should be considered in patients at risk of RFS or hyperglycemia.[18] Any laboratory abnormalities should be corrected before increasing dosage toward the energy goal.

Patients with CKD who are hospitalized often receive short-term PN infused over 24 hours. However, patients in rehabilitation facilities, long-term care, or at home can have their PN cycled over a shorter period of time, such as 12 hours. This enables the patient to have "time off" the infusion for work, social activities, physical therapy, or medical appointments. The patient on chronic HD may prefer to cycle the PN at night or overlap the PN infusion time to coincide with the dialysis session, since the patient's mobility is already restricted for 3 to 4 hours on dialysis days. The cycle regimen will depend on the patient's tolerance to the total volume to be infused during the shortened time period.

PN can be tapered and then discontinued when the patient is able to meet more than 60% of estimated energy requirements from EN or an oral diet.[1] If PN requires abrupt discontinuation, reduce the PN infusion rate by half for 1 to 2 hours before stopping the

infusion. Tapering the PN infusion can be beneficial in preventing rebound hypoglycemia.[18] If PN infusion is inadvertently interrupted, BG levels should be monitored for 2 hours for potential rebound hypoglycemia, with appropriate treatment provided as needed with either oral glucose, or a 10% or 50% dextrose bolus for inpatient management, or oral glucose or intramuscular glucagon for outpatients.

MONITORING PATIENTS ON PARENTERAL NUTRITION

Table 16.2 on page 336 provides guidelines for monitoring patients while they receive PN therapy.[4] Parameters should be monitored more often in patients who are critically ill and more unstable. If possible, the monitoring of patients on long-term PN should coincide with the monthly assessment performed by the RDN in the dialysis unit.

Serum albumin has been used historically to monitor nutritional status. However, it is now known that serum albumin and other hepatic proteins respond more dramatically to acute and chronic inflammation than to nutrition.[41-43] Serum albumin, which has a long half-life of 20 days, will decrease in response to inflammatory cytokines, hepatic insufficiency, and kidney losses in the nephrotic syndrome.[44] Nutrition has been shown to change albumin by 0.1 to 0.3 g/dL, whereas inflammation can produce a precipitous drop.[45] Hypoalbuminemia is a prognostic indicator for increased morbidity and mortality.[42,43] Inflammation, the driving force for the declining albumin, contributes to malnutrition by decreasing appetite and increasing energy expenditure and catabolism. Serum prealbumin has a shorter half-life of 2 to 3 days, and may be a more useful indicator of changes in nutritional status. However, levels may be increased in the setting of kidney dysfunction or dehydration, and decreased during infection, hepatic insufficiency, and overhydration. Prealbumin should not be used as a nutrition prognostic indicator during an acute inflammatory state, when C-reactive protein levels exceed 15 mg/L.[44]

TABLE 16.2 | Guidelines for Monitoring Patients on Parenteral Nutrition

Parameter	Acute PN	Chronic PN	IDPN	IPAA/IPN
Weight	Daily	Daily	Every HD treatment	Daily
Intake and output	Daily	Daily	Daily	Daily
Appetite changes	Daily if consuming oral diet	Weekly if consuming oral diet	Weekly	Weekly
Diet records	N/A	Every 3-6 mo, if consuming oral diet	Every 3-6 mo	Every 3-6 mo
SGA	Daily	Every 6 mo	Every 6 mo	Every 6 mo
Anthropometrics	N/A	Monthly	Monthly	Monthly
BUN/electrolytes	Daily until stable, then 2-3 times/week	Monthly	Every dialysis treatment until stable, then monthly or as needed	Monthly
Calcium, phosphorus, magnesium	Daily until stable, then 2-3 times/week	Long-term: monthly	Every HD treatment until stable, weekly if low serum levels, then monthly	Monthly or at the discretion of the prescriber
Glucose	Initially 4-6 times/day, then as needed according to glycemic control	Weekly (more often with insulin therapy and hyperglycemia) Long-term: monthly	Prior to, during, and following the first 6 treatments; at the discretion of the prescriber for patient with DM	Daily for the first 6 treatments; at the discretion of the prescriber for patient with DM
Triglycerides	Initially, then weekly	Monthly	Before 1st and 2nd IDPN treatment with lipids, then quarterly, or at the discretion of the prescriber	Quarterly, or at the discretion of the prescriber
Liver enzymes and bilirubin	Initially, then weekly	Monthly	Monthly	Monthly
CBC[a]	Daily until stable, then 2-3 times/week	Monthly	Monthly	Monthly
Vitamin D, calcium, phosphorus, and PTH[b]	N/A	Monthly	Monthly	Monthly
Hepatic proteins	Weekly	Monthly	Monthly	Monthly

BUN = blood urea nitrogen | CBC = complete blood count | DM = diabetes | HD = hemodialysis | IDPN = intradialytic parenteral nutrition | IPAA = intraperitoneal amino acids | IPN = intraperitoneal parenteral nutrition | N/A = not applicable | PTH = parathyroid hormone | PN = parenteral nutrition | SGA = subjective global assessment

[a] Monitor for catheter-related infections and anemia.

[b] Monitor for metabolic bone disease.

Adapted with permission from Fuhrman MP. Parenteral nutrition in kidney disease. In: Byham-Gray L, Wiesen K, eds. *A Clinical Guide to Nutrition Care in Kidney Disease.* Academy of Nutrition and Dietetics; 2013:197-216.[4]

Long-term complications of PN include biliary and hepatic diseases, catheter-related infections, hyperoxaluria, intestinal hypoplasia, and metabolic bone disease. The patient should be monitored for the development of long-term PN complications. Meanwhile, every effort should be made to transition the patient to EN as soon as feasible. A more detailed discussion of long-term PN therapy complications can be found in other publications.[6,46]

Because aluminum is excreted by the kidneys, patients with CKD should be monitored for potential aluminum toxicity.[35] Sources of aluminum include medications such as antacids, phosphate binders, and sucralfate; intravenous fluids (IVF); and PN components.[3,47] Calcium and phosphate salts are major sources of aluminum in PN. The Food and Drug Administration labeling regulations for large-volume parenteral drug products mandate a statement that the product contains no more than 25 mcg/L aluminum.[3]

PERIPHERAL PARENTERAL NUTRITION

PPN is infused via a peripheral vein and is generally recommended for no longer than 14 days. Peripheral vein infusions are limited to 700 to 900 mOsm/L.[48] This limits the volume of hypertonic components (eg, dextrose and amino acids) that can be given peripherally. Lipids are fairly isotonic and have been used to provide a large proportion of total calories in PPN. The ASPEN guidelines recommend a lipid infusion rate less than 1 g/kg/d for critically ill/trauma/sepsis patients, and up to 1 g/kg/d for stable patients.[7] Lipids should be restricted to less than 30% of total energy in patients with an inflammatory process.[1] CKD and dialysis are associated with inflammatory processes and may indicate the need to reduce total fat provided in PN.[49] ILEs high in omega-3 fatty acids (eg, SMOF lipid) may be preferable for patients with inflammatory states, elevated liver function test results, and elevated triglyceride levels.[28] Sterile water is used as a component of PPN to dilute the osmolality of dextrose and amino acids. This can result in a final volume of 2 to 3 L/d. The large volume, high fat content, and inadequate energy and protein content limit the usefulness of PPN for patients with CKD.

Parenteral Nutrition and Acute Kidney Injury

Nutrition management of the patient with AKI focuses on the underlying disease or injury, with consideration given to the impact of the reduction or loss of kidney function, degree of existing malnutrition, and modality of KRT.[9,50-52] Patients who develop AKI may present with a multitude of comorbidities, such as trauma, sepsis, cardiovascular disease, liver disease, and multisystem organ failure. AKI is classified or staged according to abrupt changes in the serum creatinine level and urine output within a 48-hour period.[9,53] Hemodynamic instability, impaired GI motility, volume overload, and oliguria contribute to difficulties in providing consistent and adequate nutrition support in patients with AKI. A multinational cross-sectional study found that AKI occurred in more than half of ICU patients and was associated with increased mortality, even when controlling for the underlying disease and severity of illness.[54]

MALNUTRITION IN ACUTE KIDNEY INJURY

Gervasio and Cotton[50] reported that malnutrition negatively impacts kidney function and increases mortality, morbidity, and health care costs. Up to 42% of critically ill patients with AKI suffer from malnutrition.[55] The extent of preexisting malnutrition and the risk of iatrogenic malnutrition are dependent on the duration and the severity of the underlying disease and adequacy of nutrition. Factors that contribute to malnutrition with AKI include effects of inflammation on metabolic demand; metabolic alterations in amino acid, carbohydrate, and fat metabolism; and modality of KRT.[52] During severe metabolic stress, nutrient provision is often nil or sorely inadequate. Insufficient and inconsistent provision of nutrients contribute to poor wound healing, decreased immunocompetence, and catabolism of lean body mass. Hypercatabolism, demonstrated by negative nitrogen balance, is a predictor of higher mortality risk in patients with AKI.[56]

Identifying malnutrition in patients with AKI can be problematic using traditional nutritional parameters.[51] Weight is skewed by fluid shifts, complicating calculations for BMI and estimated energy and protein needs. As discussed earlier, hepatic protein levels reflect the inflammatory process and are neither reliable nor sensitive nutritional indicators.[50] However, PEW in chronic and acute kidney disease is often diagnosed by a combination of low serum biomarkers, including albumin, prealbumin, and cholesterol, along with low BMI, and reduced body mass and muscle mass. Together, these indices are used to predict 1-year mortality in patients with kidney failure.[44,56]

Insufficient nutrient intake may be the most accurate indicator that aggressive nutrition support is needed. Nutrition support can help sustain the patient during dialytic, medical, and surgical treatment to speed recovery. The route of nutrition support is selected based on the GI function of the patient. The indications for PN for patients with AKI are the same as for other critically ill patients.[1,2]

NUTRIENT REQUIREMENTS AND COMPONENTS OF PARENTERAL NUTRITION IN ACUTE KIDNEY INJURY

Energy and protein requirements in critically ill patients with AKI are estimated at 20 to 30 kcal/kg/d and 1.2 to 2 g/kg/d, respectively, with protein needs up to 2.5 g/kg/d for patients receiving frequent HD or CRRT.[1] Box 16.1 and Table 16.2 provide general guidelines for providing and monitoring PN in patients with AKI. The most concentrated sources of dextrose, amino acids, and lipids can be used to maximize calories in a limited total volume. Requirements should be estimated using edema-free weight.

Amino Acids

AKI and critical illness contribute to accelerated muscle catabolism and ineffective use of amino acids for protein synthesis, resulting in a negative nitrogen balance.[51] The insulin resistance and metabolic acidosis that accompany AKI contribute to protein breakdown and catabolism.[57] Protein recommendations for AKI range from 0.8 to 1.0 for noncatabolic patients without dialysis, to 1.0 to 1.5 g/kg/d for patients who are catabolic or require intermittent HD.[10] Hospitalized patients on CRRT may lose 10 to 15 g amino acids per day.[6] These patients may require 1.7 to 2.5 g/kg/d amino acids to compensate for losses.[10] Despite aggressive provision of nutrition support, negative nitrogen balance and protein catabolism often persist in patients with AKI. However, excessive protein provision in PN may increase catabolism of extra amino acids into urea and nitrogenous waste, resulting in worsening uremia, increasing dialysis requirements, and prolonging KRT duration.[58]

Carbohydrate

Hyperglycemia, a problem in critically ill patients, can be aggravated by concomitant AKI. Increased gluconeogenesis, insulin resistance, and glucose uptake from dialysate, along with decreased insulin clearance, decreased responsiveness to insulin, and decreased glycogen synthesis, impact glycemic control.[51] Patients on continuous venovenous hemofiltration (CVVH) may receive an additional 500 kcal per day from an acid citrate dextrose formula.[6] The amount of glucose transferred across the dialysis membrane in CRRT depends on the fluid glucose concentration, dialysis flow rate, and BG concentration. The dextrose content of replacement and dialysate solutions varies from 0 to 110 mg/dL, which could result in a net gain of energy or a net loss of glucose if a glucose-free fluid is used.[55] Energy obtained from CRRT can be calculated as follows[34]:

Energy obtained = Flow rate in L/h × 24 hours × Dextrose concentration in g/L × % uptake × 3.4 kcal/g

Where 3.4 kcal/g is the known energy from dextrose

Lipids

Lipid metabolism is adversely affected by critical illness and AKI.[59] AKI impairs lipolysis, with a resulting increase in serum triglycerides and a reduction in serum cholesterol, particularly high-density lipoprotein (HDL) cholesterol. Lipase enzyme activity is altered in AKI, and mobilization of fat from adipose tissue and clearance of triglycerides is impaired as well.[57] Lipid losses in CRRT are nonsignificant, so the lipid provision in PN should not need to be increased.[57,60] Lipid infusion in the critically ill patient with AKI should be 1 g/kg/d or less (every 500 mL of 20% lipid emulsion contains 100 g fat).[7,51]

Potential Nonparenteral Nutrition Sources of Energy

It is important to consider all potential sources of energy when determining the PN prescription. Carbohydrate sources of calories include IVF, medications, and KRT modalities, particularly hemodiafiltration and PD. Carbohydrate sources from CRRT fluids include citrate (3 kcal/g), glucose (3.4 kcal/g), and lactate (3.62 kcal/g). Both lactate and citrate may contribute significant calories, over 500 kcal/d.[55,57] Propofol, a sedative used in the ICU, is delivered in a 10% lipid solution that provides 1.1 kcal/mL. Blood products and albumin infusions are additional sources of nitrogen and protein. However, before adjusting the PN, consider that medications, IVF, and blood product infusions can be a temporary source of nutrients and may not have a significant impact on overall delivery of nutrition.

Fluid

Fluid management often becomes the focus of patient management in AKI. PPN, with its higher fluid and lipid content, is rarely used in oliguric or anuric patients. AKI with oliguria (urine output less than 500 mL/d) can result in the need to restrict PN solutions to 1,000 to 1,200 mL/d, in order to reflect the usual daily insensible water losses.[35,60] Fluids are not restricted in patients with nonoliguric AKI, except to address volume overload or hyponatremia.[35] The need for a severe volume restriction is often short term until AKI resolves or KRT is initiated. CRRT removes fluid and permits adequate provision of nutrients without fluid volume limitations. Urine output, as well as the patient's overall intake and output, should be closely monitored. Polyuria characterizes the recovery stage of AKI, with diuresis exceeding 150 to 200 mL/hour.[50]

Electrolytes and Minerals

Electrolyte and mineral requirements in AKI are affected by the underlying disease, urine output, type of KRT, and prescribed replacement fluid. Provision of potassium, magnesium, and phosphorus in PN is often limited with AKI. However, for patients requiring CRRT, the replacement fluid may play a greater role in electrolyte management than the PN. The appropriate dialysate is selected based on serum laboratory results and desired clearance of potassium and other electrolytes.[50,60] Sodium and potassium may need to be eliminated from the PN, as they are provided by the CRRT replacement fluid.[6] CRRT continuously clears phosphate from the blood, however, and close monitoring is required to avoid hypophosphatemia.[6,55,60] This is of particular importance if a phosphate-free dialysate is prescribed. Patients with AKI who are receiving PN and CRRT may also lose significant amounts of calcium and magnesium in the dialysate effluent.[6] Calcium levels should be maintained via the CRRT circuit and cannot be fully managed by adjustments to the PN. Clinicians should familiarize themselves with the dialysate fluids used at their institutions before making adjustments to the PN order. Table 16.3 on page 340 details ranges of electrolytes and other components in dialysate and replacement fluids.[55]

Hypocalcemia with decreased serum ionized calcium occurs with elevated calcitonin levels during AKI and sepsis. Provision of supplemental calcium in a patient with hyperphosphatemia increases the risk of precipitation of calcium phosphate in the blood, with subsequent deposition of calcium phosphate crystals in soft tissue. Patients with AKI on CRRT may require supplementation of magnesium and calcium beyond that which can be safely added to PN, due to the risk of calcium–phosphate precipitation.[61] In this case, supplemental electrolytes and minerals should be provided orally or intravenously as needed.

TABLE 16.3 | Components in Dialysate and Continuous Renal Replacement Therapy Replacement Fluids[54]

Component	Concentration
Sodium	136-140 mmol/L
Potassium	0-4 mmol/L
Calcium	0-3.5 mEq/L
Magnesium	0.5-1.5 mEq/L
Phosphate	0-1.25 mmol/L
Chloride	107.5-120.5 mmol/L
Bicarbonate	25-35 mmol/L
Lactate	0-38 mmol/L
Dextrose	0-110 mg/dL

Metabolic acidosis is a risk factor for the development of AKI, poor outcomes, and hospital mortality.[61] Patients often require a higher proportion of acetate salts compared to chloride salts in the PN. Treatment of metabolic acidosis may require the provision of sodium bicarbonate as a separate IV infusion. Hyperkalemia associated with metabolic acidosis will correct with treatment of acetate or bicarbonate.[6] If the patient is hypokalemic with metabolic acidosis, correction of acidosis should include potassium supplementation.

Vitamins and Trace Elements

Requirements for vitamins and trace elements in AKI are likely similar to that for HD. The standard PN preparations of multivitamins and trace elements are currently recommended for patients with AKI.[3,9] CRRT continuously clears small solutes, and this includes trace elements, vitamins, and other nutrients. Thiamin, pyridoxine, ascorbic acid, folic acid, zinc, and copper are readily dialyzed.[63,64] Patients may benefit from a renal multivitamin to correct deficiencies in water-soluble vitamins. Fat-soluble vitamins are not likely to demonstrate excess or deficiency, as AKI is typically a temporary disease state.[35]

Critically ill patients with AKI are at risk for hemosiderosis because of multiple blood product transfusions and decreased erythropoiesis.[39] Therefore, iron supplementation should be reserved for critically ill patients with a suspected or documented iron-deficiency anemia.

INFUSION AND MONITORING

Patients with AKI are often in the ICU and present as very complex patients. PN should be initiated at a low rate and advanced only when fluid, electrolyte, and glycemic controls are achieved at each increment of PN volume increase. Patients should be closely monitored for changes in clinical status, dialysis modality, and tolerance to PN.

Intradialytic Parenteral Nutrition

IDPN is a partial PN therapy meant to provide adjunctive nutrients and has been utilized for several decades. IDPN is administered via the venous chamber of the extracorporeal circuit during the patient's dialysis treatment. This therapy is indicated by failure to improve the nutritional status of a patient on HD via intensive counseling, liberalized diet, oral nutrition supplements (ONS), and enteral route of alimentation.[5] ONS can provide an additional 7 to 10 kcal/kg/d energy and 0.3 to 0.4 g/kg/d protein.[65] ONS has been demonstrated as effective in improving nutritional status, and, in two large recent studies, ONS has been beneficial in outcomes of survival and decreased hospitalization.[66-68] However, there remains a subset of patients for whom the oral or enteral route is not sufficiently effective to engender improvement of nutritional status. For those patients, IDPN is the consequent default interventional therapy.

EVOLUTION OF INTRADIALYTIC PARENTERAL NUTRITION FORMULATION COMPOSITION

The concepts behind traditional or historical formulation of IDPN are difficult to determine based on varied compositions utilized among studies, as shown in Table 16.4.[69-77] There were problems inherent to these traditional or historical formulations. The dextrose content could elevate BG levels and require the need for insulin provision.[78] Due to the inherent risk of rebound hypoglycemia, a snack was often provided prior

TABLE 16.4 | Intradialytic Parenteral Nutrition Studies Using Varying Compositions[69-77]

Study	Patient number	Protein (g)	Dextrose (g)	Lipid (g)
Korzets et al, 2008[69]	22	50-85	125-185	50-70
Cano et al, 2007[70]	98	Variable with formulations providing for oral intake deficit		
Cherry and Shalansky, 2002[71]	24	25-50	125	50
Blondin and Ryan, 1999[72]	45	63	91.5	18.4
Mortelmans et al, 1999[73]	16	35	125	50
Hiroshige et al, 1998[74]	10	14 EAA	100	40
Capelli et al, 1994[75]	81	50	50-125	20-50
Chertow et al, 1994[76]	1,679	1.2 g/kg	15 kcal/kg	
Goldstein and Strom, 1991[77]	Review	25-55	125-250	None (if intolerant) or 50

to treatment end.[77-79] Many patients on HD have the comorbidity of DM and/or insulin resistance, presenting challenges in glucose management.[49,77,78,80-83] The earlier formulations of IDPN also frequently contained IV lipid. Patients receiving dialysis are known to have lipid profile disorders and prevalence of elevated triglycerides. Studies have demonstrated that patients with CKD exhibit difficulty in clearing triglycerides from ILEs.[84-87] Nausea, vomiting, and diarrhea have been reported with lipid-containing IDPN.[76] Additional symptoms have also occurred with earlier IDPN formulations inclusive of muscle pain and muscle cramps, as well as nausea, vomiting, excess fluid gain, and hypotension.[70,71,73,84,88-91] Powers[91] noted patients experienced hypovolemia less frequently when using a 500-mL volume vs a 1,000-mL volume of IDPN. In 2008, weight-based formulations emerged designed in both consideration of these issues and earlier studies with IDPN that provided glucose and amino acids but lacked lipids. These studies demonstrated weight loss could be reversed and appetite improved (with consequent improved caloric intake) by correction of amino acid imbalances known to exist in patients on dialysis that could suppress appetite.[91-93] Thus, the protein component of the IDPN formulation was the critically important feature. In addition to lower dextrose content, recent formulations are weight based and utilize concentrated base components to minimize volume. Traditional moderate and higher dextrose formulations-containing lipid are still in use. Examples

of these formulations may be found in Table 16.5.[94] Generally, formulas containing lipid are reserved for patients who require additional calories.

APPROPRIATE USE AND INDICATIONS FOR INTRADIALYTIC PARENTERAL NUTRITION

The PEW syndrome, which is characterized by biochemical abnormalities, changes in nutrient intake, body weight, and muscle mass, is one of the strongest predictors of mortality in patients receiving dialysis and, therefore, interventions to prevent and treat PEW are

TABLE 16.5 | Recent Intradialytic Parenteral Nutrition Formulations[94]

Example: 60-kg patient requiring 3.5-hour hemodialysis				
Intradialytic parenteral nutrition formulation	70% dextrose (g)	20% amino acid (g)	20% lipid (g)	Total volume
Low dextrose No lipid	35	90	None	500 mL
Carbohydrate control (moderate dextrose) Lipid	74	96	38	776 mL
Standard (higher dextrose) Lipid	98	97	41	830 mL

Adapted with permission from Dukkipati R, Kalantar-Zadeh K, Kopple JD. Is there a role for intradialytic parenteral nutrition? A review of the evidence. *Am J Kidney Dis*. 2010;55(2):352-364. doi:10.1053/j.jrn.2012.08.013

imperative.[95-98] Kidney and nutrition support leaders, researchers, national associations, and consensus groups have provided support for IDPN. Through review of relevant literature, guidelines and recommendations for clinicians have been developed and published.[2,5,65,99] In the KDOQI Clinical Practice Guidelines for Nutrition in CKD: 2020 Update, Guideline 4 suggests a trial of IDPN in patients with CKD stage 5D on maintenance HD with PEW if nutritional requirements cannot be met with existing oral and enteral intake.[5] The following three criteria are provided: evidence of protein, energy, or protein–energy malnutrition and inadequate dietary protein and energy intake; inability to administer or tolerate adequate oral nutrition, including food supplements or enteral feeding; and finally, that protein and energy requirements can be met when IDPN is used in conjunction with oral intake or enteral feeding. Once patients are capable of ONS or enteral feeding upon observation of improvement in nutritional status (patient-specific criteria), IDPN should be discontinued. For those patients receiving IDPN in conjunction with oral intake where nutritional requirements cannot be achieved or for those patients with GI tract impairment, PN should be considered. Research experts in renal nutrition have developed an algorithm to guide clinician interventions. An adaption for patients undergoing dialysis can be found in Figure 16.1.[65] A similar algorithm was published in the 2013 Nutrition and Dialysis report that was developed and supported by the Chief Medical Officers of the 14 largest dialysis chains in the United States.[99] Recent consensus recommendations of ASPEN are based on the review of existing data and build on previous guidelines by providing support and indication for use of IDPN. Authors state that IDPN alone should not be used as the sole nutrition intervention for (adult or pediatric) patients with CKD who are malnourished but rather as a supplemental nutrition intervention in patients when oral intake and EN interventions have failed or are insufficient to reach nutritional goals.[2]

Clinical Criteria and Reimbursement Coverage of Intradialytic Parenteral Nutrition

The clinical criteria for IDPN for the patient on dialysis who has established malnutrition refractory to diet and oral supplementation and intolerance or refusal of enteral feeding are listed and reflect signs and symptoms of protein, energy, or protein–energy malnutrition. A study by Fuhrman[49] suggests that any combination of three or more of the following constitute protein, energy, or protein–energy malnutrition for consideration of IDPN:

- SGA "C" or "2"; serum albumin equal to or less than 3.4 g/dL (3-month rolling average)
- serum creatinine less than 8.0 mg/dL (3-month rolling average)
- weight less than 90% IBW
- weight loss: 10% IBW or 20% usual body weight over any period of time
- triceps skinfold values less than 6 mm (males) and less than 12 mm (females*)
- clinical examination consistent with moderate-to-severe malnutrition; protein catabolic rate less than 0.8 g/kg/d
- diet history of protein less than 0.8 g/kg and energy less than 25 kcal/kg

Reimbursement coverage criteria may vary by insurance provider. In the late 1990s, coverage under Medicare Part B required that a patient must have a severe and permanent pathology of the alimentary tract which did not allow absorption of sufficient nutrients to maintain weight and strength as the primary cause of malnutrition. In 2006, the Centers for Medicare & Medicaid Services recognized that certain types of PN (amino acids, dextrose, and lipid) that did not meet Medicare Part B would be covered drugs under Medicare Part D. In 2007, amino acid solutions were added to the Medicare Part D formulary.[100] Medicare Part D allows patients to be approved for therapy under a prior authorization

*Specific recommendations for transgender people were not provided.

FIGURE 16.1 | Nutritional care and intervention for the chronic kidney disease patient[1]

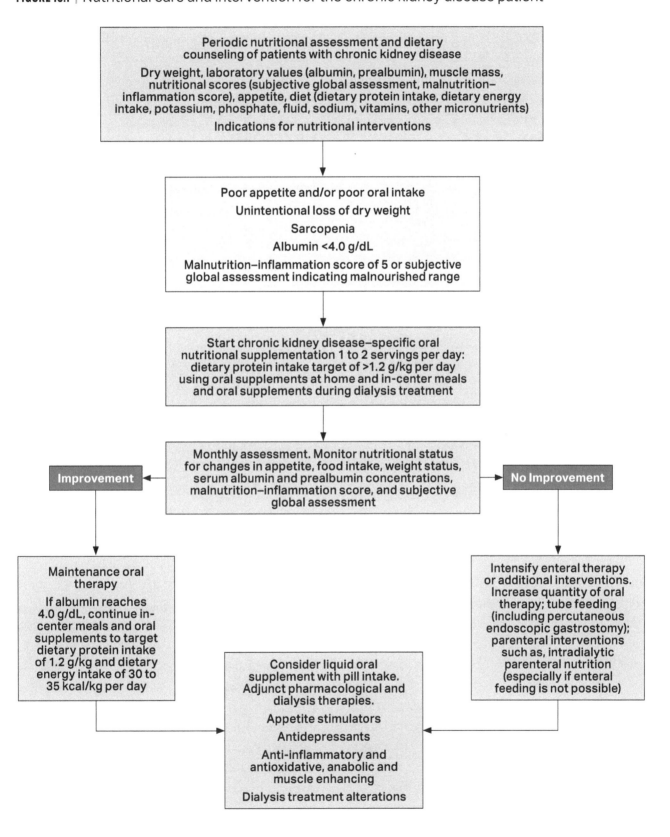

Periodic nutritional assessment and dietary counseling of patients with chronic kidney disease

Dry weight, laboratory values (albumin, prealbumin), muscle mass, nutritional scores (subjective global assessment, malnutrition–inflammation score), appetite, diet (dietary protein intake, dietary energy intake, potassium, phosphate, fluid, sodium, vitamins, other micronutrients)

Indications for nutritional interventions

Poor appetite and/or poor oral intake

Unintentional loss of dry weight

Sarcopenia

Albumin <4.0 g/dL

Malnutrition–inflammation score of 5 or subjective global assessment indicating malnourished range

Start chronic kidney disease–specific oral nutritional supplementation 1 to 2 servings per day: dietary protein intake target of >1.2 g/kg per day using oral supplements at home and in-center meals and oral supplements during dialysis treatment

Monthly assessment. Monitor nutritional status for changes in appetite, food intake, weight status, serum albumin and prealbumin concentrations, malnutrition–inflammation score, and subjective global assessment

Improvement

No Improvement

Maintenance oral therapy

If albumin reaches 4.0 g/dL, continue in-center meals and oral supplements to target dietary protein intake of 1.2 g/kg and dietary energy intake of 30 to 35 kcal/kg per day

Intensify enteral therapy or additional interventions. Increase quantity of oral therapy; tube feeding (including percutaneous endoscopic gastrostomy); parenteral interventions such as, intradialytic parenteral nutrition (especially if enteral feeding is not possible)

Consider liquid oral supplement with pill intake. Adjunct pharmacological and dialysis therapies.

Appetite stimulators

Antidepressants

Anti-inflammatory and antioxidative, anabolic and muscle enhancing

Dialysis treatment alterations

process. The criteria for coverage under Medicare Part D for protein malnutrition includes an average serum albumin level less than 3.5 g/dL over the last 3 months or reflection of inadequate protein intake, such as normalized protein catabolic rate (nPCR) or normalized protein nitrogen appearance (nPNA) less than 0.8 g/kg/d. The criteria for energy malnutrition under Medicare Part D are as follows: more than 5% weight loss over 3 months, more than 10% loss over 6 months, or more than 20% weight loss with no time frame and an IBW less than 90% or BMI under 18. Qualification also requires documentation that attempts have been made to increase energy and protein intake with intensive nutrition counseling and ONS for protein or calorie malnutrition.[83,100] Currently, reimbursement for IDPN is available from Medicare Part B or D, Fee for Service Medicaid (state dependent) and commercial health insurance plans. Depending on the plan, the deductibles, copays, medical policies, and coverage gaps will impact the coverage and benefit level of the therapy.

Administration and Management of Intradialytic Parenteral Nutrition

AMINO ACIDS

While a few small studies in the 1990s used essential amino acid formulations in IDPN, the predominant and currently utilized amino acid formulations are those consisting of essential and nonessential amino acids.[49,92,93,101] Amino acid solution concentrations of either 15% or 20% are utilized to minimize total volume of IDPN and generally provide 1.2 to 1.4 g/kg.[49,100,102] Higher amounts of protein can be provided and may be of benefit to an acutely ill patient undergoing dialysis. However, Kt/V (ie, dialysis clearance) may be impacted due to urea generation, which if persistent and significant may require either adjustments in dialysis treatment time or changes in formulation composition.[103-106] With administration of amino acid, serum bicarbonate

levels should be monitored and corrected to achieve the KDOQI recommended levels of 24 to 26 mmol/L. Sodium acetate can be added to the IDPN solution, if needed. Acidosis has been associated with oxidation of branched chain amino acids, increased protein degradation, and decreased albumin synthesis.[5]

DEXTROSE

Lower dextrose-containing IDPN solutions may be of benefit, particularly in patients with DM and insulin resistance. Whether using lower dextrose or traditional IDPN containing higher amounts of dextrose, temporary increases in glucose levels for some patients may be considered or may warrant the need for regular insulin. Based on a sliding scale, insulin is typically administered subcutaneously. It is important to consider a patient's current BG control regimen, which may impact glucose levels during IDPN infusion. The regimen may guide the use of regular insulin if hyperglycemia occurs during IDPN. Arterial or peripheral glucose levels should be checked prior to starting IDPN and 1 hour into the infusion. When required, 5 to 8 units of regular insulin per liter of IDPN has been suggested when serum glucose levels exceed 300 mg/dL.[49,83] Insulin can be increased incrementally by two units during subsequent dialysis treatments, if warranted, until desired glycemic control is achieved.[4] The potential for rebound hypoglycemia can be lowered by the provision of a snack 30 minutes before cessation of the IDPN infusion. The patient's peripheral BG level should be checked 1 hour after cessation of IDPN infusion. Tight glycemic control in IDPN has not been studied; however, CKD has been associated with reduced kidney gluconeogenesis and a prolonged half-life of commonly used diabetic medications predisposing the patient to hypoglycemia. In a large national cohort study of patients with CKD and with or without DM, it was determined that excessive mortality was associated with hypoglycemia, therefore identifying this complication as a significant threat to patient safety in those with CKD.[107] In consideration of these findings, it would appear that tight control of hyperglycemia may not be warranted.

LIPIDS

Lipids should not be given to patients with a known egg, soy, olive oil, fish, or peanut allergy, depending on the ILE used by the pharmacy. They should also be used with caution due to the potential for thrombocytopenia. Intolerance and clearance issues of ILE can be problematic with IDPN infusion. Dyslipidemia (elevated oxidized low-density lipoprotein and low/dysfunctional low HDL, and particularly elevated triglycerides) is present in patients on dialysis.[85] A reduced amount and partly inhibited function of lipase limits lipid breakdown, resulting in increased triglyceride concentration.[85,87] Serum triglycerides should be monitored prior to the first infusion and again before the second infusion of lipids to determine adequacy of lipid clearance. A serum triglyceride level of more than 400 mg/dL suggests poor lipid clearance.[49] Some OO-based ILEs contain vitamin K and have the potential of counteracting anticoagulant activity. ILE has been associated with the potential for thrombocytopenia, hepatic abnormalities, and free fatty acid toxicity in patients with low albumin levels.[49,101] Potential lipid intolerance symptoms include nausea, vomiting, headache, dizziness, fever, flushing, drowsiness, chest and back pain, eye pressure, and erythema at the infusion site. Some of these symptoms may be difficult to distinguish from the dialysis process or underlying disease.[48] Small studies of short duration have observed the use of alternative lipid emulsions (OO and FO); however, studies of longer duration are needed to determine the effects on nutritional status as well as plasma lipid, hematologic, oxidative, inflammatory, and immune parameters.[89,108,109] The optimal IDPN formulation is not known. Some patients may require and benefit from additional calories in the form of ILE; however, the use of lipid calories should be determined by assessment of total caloric intake of the individual patient and other factors that may be impeding response (eg, hospitalization and metabolic acidosis). No study has examined the need for lipid in IDPN.[110,111]

INFUSION AND MONITORING OF INTRADIALYTIC PARENTERAL NUTRITION

IDPN is ordered by a nephrology prescriber and managed/monitored by the unit clinical team. Dialysis chains may provide policy and protocols for IDPN administration and monitoring. Compounding pharmacies may provide manuals with suggested guidelines inclusive of administration and monitoring. In addition, providers offer internal assistance to unit clinicians on all aspects of the therapy from pharmacists and RDNs with IDPN expertise. IDPN is infused through the venous drip chamber of the extracorporeal circuit and, therefore, does not require additional IV access. IDPN is infused in typically less than a 1-L volume, which is calculated into the ultrafiltration rate for removal during the dialysis session in accordance with the clinical and physical assessment by the unit nurse. The initial rates of infusion and a regimen to reach goal rate are provided on the individual IDPN order form. In general, low volume of dextrose and amino acid is provided initially and is progressed with tolerance, as assessed by the clinical team.[94] At the discretion of the prescriber, predialysis serum levels of magnesium, potassium, and phosphorus may be monitored during initial IDPN and consequent sessions, where indicated. This is particularly important for those patients at risk of RFS.[49,102] Based on the laboratory data both during and consequent to the initial phase, adjustments can be made with oral medication, dialysate bath, or with the IDPN for low levels of magnesium, potassium, and phosphorus. The response to IDPN will guide monitoring frequency of laboratory parameters as influenced by metabolic condition(s) and comorbidities. Glycemic control is assessed and, where indicated, is treated and monitored per physician discretion and unit policy. If lipids are ordered, they are typically added after tolerance to amino acid and dextrose solution is observed.[94] Serum triglyceride levels should be monitored with adjustments or discontinuation, as indicated by serum levels. The addition of micronutrients is not standard practice; however, this can be added to IDPN by an individual determined need. Recommendations for the monitoring of nutrition support are presented in Box 16.2 on page 346.

BOX 16.2 | Nutrition Support Monitoring Guidelines in the Stable Dialysis Patient

MONITORING PARAMETER	INTRADIALYTIC PARENTERAL NUTRITION	INTRAPERITONEAL PARENTERAL NUTRITION
Transport proteins	Monthly	Monthly
Potassium/Phosphate/ Magnesium	Initially until stable per nephrology prescriber's discretion	Initially until stable per nephrology prescriber's discretion
	Monthly	Monthly
Fluids	Each treatment	Daily
Glucose	Initially: pre/mid/post (per nephrology prescriber's discretion)	Per nephrology prescriber's discretion
Lipids (triglycerides)	Initially: assess tolerance/clearance	Monthly
	Monthly	
Liver enzymes	Monthly	Monthly
Weight	Per treatment	Daily
Normalized protein nitrogen appearance /normalized protein catabolic rate	Monthly	Quarterly
Residual urine output	Quarterly	Quarterly
Subjective global assessment	Quarterly	Quarterly
Blood urea nitrogen/Kt/V	Monthly	Quarterly

Adapted with permission from McCann L, ed. *Pocket Guide to Nutrition Assessment of the Patient With Chronic Kidney Disease.* 6th ed. National Kidney Foundation; 2021.[10]

Intraperitoneal Amino Acids/ Intraperitoneal Nutrition

In PD, daily loss of protein is approximately 5 g (of which 4 g is albumin) and approximately 10 g per 24 hours for patients using automated PD and may be increased by dwell time and the number of nighttime exchanges. The losses are more frequent than HD losses, which are 1 g to 8 g or more per treatment.[112,113] The first demonstration that amino acids could be absorbed by the peritoneal cavity was in 1968.[114] The use of the peritoneal cavity providing glucose, amino acids, and lipids occurred in 1980 when substrates were administered intraperitoneally for 9 days (2,000 kcal/d), resulting in blood urea nitrogen (BUN) stabilization and reduced losses of 3 methyl histidine.[115] IPAA uses amino acids in place of some of the glucose (IPN) or all of the glucose (IPAA) as the osmotic gradient during PD, allowing both for the removal of toxins and as a means to replace and minimize loss of amino acids from the patient.[116] In the KDOQI 2020 update, Guideline 4 states that IPAA may cause mild acidosis in some patients. Although it

is readily treatable and in diabetic patients on PD with uncontrolled hyperglycemia, an immediate strategy for glycemic control could be the substitution of amino acid for glucose in PD solutions.[5] Amino acids provide approximately twice the osmotic load of glucose per gram. As with IDPN, IPN can provide significant amino acids to the patient on PD and can lead to normalization of serum amino acid abnormalities.[117-119] One of the primary concerns with PD solutions is the formation of glucose degradation products (GDPs) that result from heat sterilization and storage.[119] Long-term exposure to GDPs leads to increased vascularization of the peritoneal membrane, which increases surface area, and the absorption of low molecular weight solutes and loss of ultrafiltration.[120] GDPs induce formation of advanced glycation end products (AGEs), which bind to the peritoneal membrane and cause fibrosis and microvascular sclerosis. This can result in volume overload, poor solute clearance, rapid glucose absorption, and protein loss, which can have a significant impact on technique and patient survival.[120] Excess glucose absorption is thought to play an important role in dyslipidemia, hyperinsulinemia, insulin resistance oxidative stress, inflammation, and altered adipokine levels. Glucose-sparing strategies employed to reduce glucose load, thereby reducing the potential for metabolic and physical effects of standard PD solutions, include the use of icodextrin (a large glucose polymer) and amino acids.[121] Emerging biocompatible solutions are PD solutions stored within three chambered bags where the glucose component is kept separated from other electrolytes under acidic conditions. This minimizes the formation of GDPs during heat sterilization and storage.[122] Further research is needed to determine if these solutions exert effects on peritonitis, technique survival, and patient survival.

APPROPRIATE USE AND INDICATION FOR INTRAPERITONEAL AMINO ACIDS/ INTRAPERITONEAL NUTRITION: CONSENSUS STATEMENTS AND GUIDELINES

Guidance for IPAA/IPN is found in the nutritional supplementation section of the updated KDOQI guidelines.[5] It is suggested not to substitute conventional dextrose dialysate with amino acid dialysate as a general strategy to improve nutritional status in patients with PEW on PD. However, the guidelines do suggest that amino acid dialysate is a reasonable strategy to trial in attempts to improve nutritional status when nutritional requirements cannot be met with existing oral and enteral intake. In addition, as a strategy for PEW in patients undergoing PD, part of the rationale for amino acids described is that amino acids may reduce the infused carbohydrate load, lessening risk for hyperglycemia (immediate strategy for glycemic control in patients with diabetes and uncontrolled hyperglycemia on PD) and may reduce hypertriglyceridemia. Similar to IDPN, the guidelines suggest that IPAA should only be used if spontaneous protein and energy intakes, in conjunction with IPAA, are able to meet the required protein and energy targets. Otherwise, daily total or partial PN should be considered. In addition to the KDOQI recommendations, key nephrology nutrition

research leaders have also included IPN in their proposed algorithm (shown in Figure 16.1).[5,65]

CLINICAL CRITERIA AND REIMBURSEMENT COVERAGE OF INTRAPERITONEAL NUTRITION

Clinical criteria for IPN is similar to IDPN in that the patient on dialysis must have established malnutrition refractory to diet and oral supplementation and intolerance or refusal of enteral feeding. The criteria as listed for IDPN in the preceding section, which is reflective of protein, energy, or protein–energy malnutrition, may be used. Reimbursement for IPN differs from IDPN. PD dialysate and IPN are considered to be a supply relative to the dialysis facility, which falls into the prospective payment system and is therefore not separately billable.[100] They are considered a Medicare Part B compound not available under Medicare Part D. Reimbursement for IPN is available under commercial health insurance plans. Depending on the plan, the deductibles, copays, and medical policies will impact the coverage and benefit level of this therapy.

INTRAPERITONEAL AMINO ACIDS AND INTRAPERITONEAL NUTRITION FORMULATIONS: ADMINISTERING AND MONITORING

IPAA is also known as Nutrineal and is a commercial amino acid solution available outside the United States.[100] IPN is individually compounded in the United States by the removal of dextrose from a dialysate bag, which is then replaced with amino acids. It is utilized as a 1% to 2% weight/volume substitute for one 2-L exchange in CAPD providing 20 to 40 g amino acids. Selection of the IPN formulation is dependent on individual PD prescription and patient ultrafiltration needs or limitations. In CAPD, it is often used as the last dwell of the cycle and is left in the abdominal cavity for a 4- to 6-hour dwell. Approximately 80% to 90% of amino acids are absorbed within 6 hours.[123] IPN can also replace a cycler bag for patients on automated peritoneal dialysis (APD)/ continuous cycling peritoneal dialysis or can be used as a last fill option. As with CAPD, appropriate IPN formulation selection is dependent on individual PD prescription and ultrafiltration needs or limitations. Studies have demonstrated that approximately 50% of amino acids are absorbed in APD.[124] A prolonged dwell time increases the risk that some of the delivered amino acids will cross back into the peritoneal cavity and be lost when the waste-containing dialysate is removed. Absorption of amino acid is also dependent on transporter type and dialysis prescription. A comparison of CAPD vs APD IPN is presented in Table 16.6. It is important for the patient and caregiver to maintain aseptic technique when handling the amino acid solutions. Dialysis chains may provide policy and protocols for IPN administration and monitoring. Compounding pharmacies may provide manuals with suggested guidelines inclusive of administration and monitoring. Box 16.2 provides guidelines for monitoring patients while receiving IPN. A few studies in the 1990s noted issues with metabolic acidosis resulting in improved buffering of IPN solutions currently used.[117,118,125] Serum bicarbonate levels should be monitored and corrected per the nephrology prescriber and

may be added to the IPN. Acidosis has been associated with oxidation of branched chain amino acids, increased protein degradation, and decreased albumin synthesis.[5] Additional parameters may be monitored by the clinician as determined by individual patient comorbidity and metabolic conditions.

THERAPEUTIC EFFECTIVENESS OF INTRADIALYTIC PARENTERAL NUTRITION AND INTRAPERITONEAL NUTRITION

Monitoring the effectiveness of either IDPN or IPN therapy requires complete nutritional assessment, including laboratory parameters, appetite, total calorie and protein intake from all sources, and consideration of factors that influence inflammation and response such as hospitalization, infections, and comorbidities.[49,83] Published IDPN studies have demonstrated improvement in nutritional parameters, such as albumin, albumin and whole-body protein synthesis, nitrogen balance, prealbumin, amino acid profile, weight increase, and anthropometrics.[69-77,88-93,101,126-134] Studies related to IPAA and IPN show similar nutritional benefits as IDPN in demonstrating improved albumin levels, amino acid pattern/profile, anthropometrics, improved nitrogen balance, and protein synthesis.[114,116-118,124,125,135-144] Favorable lipid level improvements were also reported in several studies.[125,144]

TABLE 16.6 | Comparison of Intraperitoneal Nutrition in Continuous Ambulatory Peritoneal Dialysis vs Automated Peritoneal Dialysis

	Amino acids (g)	Amino acids absorbed (g)	Dextrose (g)
IPN CAPD option: 2-L bag compounded using 20% amino acid			
1% Amino acid	20	16-18	28.6
1.5% Amino acid	30	24-27	27.8
2% Amino acid	40	32-36	27
IPN APD option: 6-L bag compounded using 20% amino acid			
1% Amino acid	45	63	91.5
1.5% Amino acid	16	35	125
2% Amino acid	10	14 EAA	100

APD = automated peritoneal dialysis | CAPD = continuous ambulatory peritoneal dialysis | EAA = essential amino acid | IPN = intraperitoneal nutrition
Adapted with permission from Pentec Health Inc, Glen Mills, PA.

Protein–Energy Wasting and Outcomes: Role of Intradialytic Parenteral Nutrition/Intraperitoneal Nutrition

Large-scale randomized clinical trials of IDPN and IPN intervention on morbidity and mortality are lacking. Evidence-based reviews, systematic reviews, and general reviews on the subject of IDPN acknowledge numerous study flaws and limitations in experimental design, such as small numbers of patients, lack of adequate controls, uncontrolled or unmonitored oral intake, nonrandomized design, or short duration of study, and the inclusion of patients without PEW.[94,98,145] According to Cano and colleagues,[70] based on the results of the Finland Italy Netherlands Elderly (FINE) study, an adequately powered trial of IDPN would require 1,364 patients in two study groups to determine a difference in treatment. Such a large 2,700 patient study is unlikely to be planned in this area. Kovesdy[98] noted that the complex comorbidities of the patient with end-stage kidney disease would make it difficult to isolate the effects of a single intervention. Two randomized controlled trials, one retrospective intent-to-treat study, two nonrandomized retrospective studies, and one randomized prospective study have demonstrated improved survival with use of IDPN.[70,75,76,88,90,126] Three studies have demonstrated decreased hospitalization with use of IDPN.[70,72,88] Two long-term studies on IPN/IPAA have been published. One study demonstrated improved mortality and lower peritonitis rates in patients receiving IPAA vs glucose dialysate, and the other study demonstrated similar hospitalization and mortality between patients receiving IPAA or glucose dialysate. However, the IPAA group was better able to maintain albumin levels.[136,139] One retrospective analysis demonstrated improved mortality and hospitalization.[135] The proposed criteria for PEW include categories of low body weight, reduced body fat or weight loss, decreased muscle mass, low protein or energy intake, and biochemical indicators.[146] Studies have demonstrated an association between lower BMI with a higher mortality rate and higher muscle mass with lower mortality. The biochemical components of PEW, namely, low albumin, prealbumin, cholesterol and serum creatinine have demonstrated a strong association with high mortality, increased hospitalization rates, and poor quality of life.[98] Among these, albumin is the strongest predictor of mortality and poor outcomes when compared to any other risk factors.[97] Guideline 1 of the KDOQI update states that "serum albumin may

be used as a predictor of hospitalization and mortality, with lower levels associated with higher risk."[5] It is also stated that due to the influence by nonnutritional factors, serum albumin should not be used as a sole measure of nutritional status, but rather considered (among others) as a complementary tool.

Low albumin levels have been associated with increased mortality in very large studies on patients undergoing both HD and PD.[147-150] While interpretation of serum albumin as reflective of inflammation or a marker of nutrition has been debated, Kopple[151] notes "the negative correlation between serum albumin levels and serum markers of inflammation is not precise."

Three randomized controlled trials found that serum albumin is influenced by nutrition and that a correlation between albumin and markers of inflammation does not always show a relationship.[70,152,153] There are also observational studies elucidating that both inflammation and protein intake exert competing effects on serum albumin.[154,155] Regardless of the contributing factor(s) or cause(s) of low albumin levels in patients, in assessing and observing response to interventions for PEW, it should be kept in mind that an incremental increase or decrease in serum albumin concentration is associated with an increased or decreased survival rate in patients on HD and on PD, respectively.[147,149,150,156] In addition to inflammation, both serum albumin and body weight may be influenced by various factors, such as volume status, comorbid conditions, and metabolic derangements. Multiple parameters as well as nutritional intake should be used in both an individualized assessment of nutritional status of the patient on dialysis and in the assessment of response to therapies, such as IDPN or IPN.[5,36,83]

Summary

The use of PN should take into consideration disadvantages against the potential benefits. In patients with CKD and AKI, providing the adequate energy, protein, fluid, and electrolytes can be a challenge.

When PN provision is necessary, in a clinical setting or at home, these patients should be closely monitored to reduce the risk of PN infusion complications. Given the studies demonstrating the association of PEW with outcomes, the demonstrated improvements in nutritional markers with IDPN and IPN therapies have lent support and merit as potential interventions to help improve outcomes for patients on dialysis. It is important to consider patient outcomes and goals that support use of PN. PN should be used in the patient with CKD who is unable to receive adequate nutrition, either orally or enterally, to maintain weight and normal function.

References

1. McClave SA, Taylor BE, Martindale RG, et al. American Society for Parenteral and Enteral Nutrition. Guidelines for the provision and assessment of nutrition support therapy in the adult critically ill patient: Society of Critical Care Medicine (SCCM) and American Society for Parenteral and Enteral Nutrition (A.S.P.E.N.). *JPEN J Parenter Enteral Nutr*. 2016;40(2):159-211. doi:10.1177/0148607115621863

2. Worthington P, Balint J, Bechtold M, et al. When is parenteral nutrition appropriate? *JPEN J Parenter Enteral Nutr*. 2017;41(3):324-377. doi:10.1177/0148607117695251

3. Task Force for the Revision of Safe Practices for Parenteral Nutrition, Mirtallo J, Canada T, Johnson D, et al. Safe practices for parenteral nutrition. *JPEN J Parenter Enteral Nutr*. 2004;28(6):S39-S70. doi:10.1177/0148607104028006s39

4. Fuhrman MP. Parenteral nutrition in kidney disease. In: Byham-Gray L, Stover J, Wiesen K, eds. *A Clinical Guide to Nutrition Care in Kidney Disease*. 2nd ed. American Dietetic Association; 2013:197-216.

5. Ikizler TA, Burrowes JD, Byham-Gray LD, et al. KDOQI Clinical Practice Guideline for Nutrition in CKD: 2020 Update. *Am J Kidney Dis*. 2020;76(3 suppl 1):S1-S107. doi:10.1053/j.ajkd.2020.05.006

6. Mundi MS, Nystrom EM, Hurley DL, McMahon MM. Management of parenteral nutrition in hospitalized adult patients. *JPEN J Parenter Enteral Nutr*. 2016;41(4):535-549. doi:10.1177/0148607116667060

7. ASPEN. Appropriate Dosing for Parenteral Nutrition: ASPEN Recommendations. January 2019. Accessed April 20, 2020. www.nutritioncare.org/PNDosing

8. Vanek VW, Borum P, Buchman A, et al. A.S.P.E.N. position paper: recommendations for changes in commercially available parenteral multivitamin and multi-trace element products. *Nutr Clin Pract*. 2012;27(4):440-491. doi:10.1177/0884533612446706

9. Beemer Cotton A, Kalista-Richards M. Nutrition management in acute kidney disease. In: Byham-Gray L, Stover J, Wiesen K, eds. *A Clinical Guide to Nutrition Care in Kidney Disease*. 2nd ed. Academy of Nutrition and Dietetics; 2013:39-52.

10. McCann L, ed. *Pocket Guide to Nutrition Assessment of the Patient With Chronic Kidney Disease*. 6th ed. National Kidney Foundation; 2021.

11. Gasser E, Parekh N. Parenteral nutrition: macronutrient composition and requirements. *Support Line*. 2005;27(6):6-12.

12. Hendriks FK, Smeets JSJ, Broers NJH, et al. End-stage renal disease patients lose a substantial amount of amino acids during hemodialysis. *J Nutr*. 2020;150(5):1160-1166. doi:10.1093/jn/nxaa010

13. Salame C, Eaton S, Grimble G, Davenport A. Protein losses and urea nitrogen underestimate total nitrogen losses in peritoneal dialysis and hemodialysis patients. *J Ren Nutr*. 2018;28(5):317-323. doi:10.1053/j.jrn.2018.01.016

14. Cano NJM, Aparicio M, Brunori G, et al. ESPEN guidelines on parenteral nutrition: adult renal failure. *Clin Nutr*. 2009;28(4):401-414. doi:10.1016/j.clnu.2009.05.016

15. Malone AM. Parenteral nutrients and formulations. In: Charney P, Malone AM, eds. *ADA Pocket Guide to Parenteral Nutrition*. American Dietetic Association; 2007:52-75.

16. McCulloch A, Bansiya V, Woodward JM. Addition of insulin to parenteral nutrition for control of hyperglycemia. *JPEN J Parenter Enteral Nutr*. 2018;42(5):846-854. doi:10.1177/0148607117722750

17. Olveira G, Abuin J, Lopez R, et al. Regular insulin added to total parenteral nutrition vs subcutaneous glargine in non-critically ill diabetic inpatients, a multicenter randomized clinical trial: INSUPAR trial. *Clin Nutr*. 2020;39(2):388-394. doi:10.1016/j.clnu.2019.02.036

18. Kumpf VJ, Gervasio J. Complications of parenteral nutrition. In: Mueller CM, ed. *The A.S.P.E.N. Adult Nutrition Support Core Curriculum.* 3rd ed. American Society for Parenteral and Enteral Nutrition; 2017:346-360.

19. Friedli N, Stanga Z, Culkin A, et al. Management and prevention of refeeding syndrome in medical inpatients: an evidence-based and consensus-supported algorithm. *Nutrition.* 2018;47:13-20. doi:10.1016/j.nut.2017.09.007

20. Dotson B, Vulaj V. Electrolyte abnormalities in critically ill patients with end-stage renal disease receiving parenteral nutrition. *J Crit Care.* 2017;41:56-57. doi:10.1016/j.jcrc.2017.04.038

21. da Silva JSV, Seres DS, Sabino K, et al. ASPEN Consensus Recommendations for Refeeding Syndrome. *Nutr Clin Pract.* 2020;35(2):178-195. doi:10.1002/ncp.10474

22. Spray JW. Review of intravenous lipid emulsion therapy. *J Inf Nurs.* 2016;39(6):377-380. doi:10.1097/NAN.0000000000000194

23. Gottschlich MM. Selection of optimal lipid sources in enteral and parenteral nutrition. *Nutr Clin Pract.* 1992;7(4):152-165. doi:10.1177/0115426592007004152

24. Dai Y-J, Sun L-L, Li M-Y, et al. Comparison of formulas based on lipid emulsions of olive oil, soybean oil, or several oils for parenteral nutrition: a systematic review and meta-analysis. *Adv Nutr.* 2016;7(2):279-286. doi:10.3945/an.114.007427

25. Jones CJ, Calder PC. Influence of different intravenous lipid emulsions on fatty acid status and laboratory and clinical outcomes in adult patients receiving home parenteral nutrition: a systematic review. *Clin Nutr.* 2018;37(1):285-291. doi:10.1016/j.clnu.2016.12.026

26. Leguina-Ruzzi AA, Ortiz R. Current evidence for use of Smoflipid® emulsion in critical care patients for parenteral nutrition. *Crit Care Res Pract.* 2018:1-6. doi:10.1155/2018/6301293

27. Martindale RG, Berlana D, Boullata JI, et al. Summary of proceedings and expert consensus statements from the International Summit "Lipids in Parenteral Nutrition." *JPEN J Parenter Enteral Nutr.* 2020;44(suppl 1):S7-S20. doi:10.1002/jpen.1746

28. Mirtallo JM, Ayers P, Boullata J, et al. ASPEN lipid injectable emulsion safety recommendations, Part 1: Background and adult considerations. *Nutr Clin Pract.* 2020;35(5):769-782. doi:10.1002/ncp.10496

29. Ronchera-Oms, Peidro J. Stability of parenteral nutrition admixtures containing organic phosphates. *Clin Nutr.* 1995;14(6):373-380. doi:10.1016/S0261-5614(95)80055-7

30. Fresenius Kabi. SMOFLIPID (lipid injectable emulsion), for intravenous use. Food and Drug Administration website. May 2016. Accessed November 25, 2020. www.accessdata.fda.gov/drugsatfda_docs/label/2016/207648lbl.pdf

31. Kingsley J. Fluid and electrolyte management in parenteral nutrition. *Support Line.* 2005;27(6):13-22.

32. Sahay M, Sahay R. Hyponatremia: a practical approach. *Indian J Endocrinol Metab.* 2014;18(6):760-771. doi:10.4103/2230-8210.141320

33. Hoorn EJ, Zietse R. Diagnosis and treatment of hyponatremia: compilation of the guidelines. *J Am Soc Nephrol.* 2017;28(5):1340-1349. doi:10.1681/ASN.2016101139

34. Canada TW, Tajchman SK, Tucker AM, Ybarra JV. Chapter 4: Acid-Base Homeostasis and Disorders. In: *A.S.P.E.N. Fluids, Electrolytes, and Acid-Base Disorders Handbook.* American Society for Parenteral and Enteral Nutrition; 2015.

35. Sarav M, Csaba P. Renal disease. In: Mueller CM, ed. *The ASPEN Adult Nutrition Support Core Curriculum.* 3rd ed. American Society for Parenteral and Enteral Nutrition; 2017:565-586.

36. Ayers P, Dixon C, Mays A. Acid-base disorders: learning the basics. *Nutr Clin Pract.* 2015;30(1):14-20. doi:10.1177/0884533614562842

37. Hutson B, Stuart N. Nutrition management of the adult hemodialysis patient. In: Byham-Gray L, Stover J, Wiesen K, eds. *A Clinical Guide to Nutrition Care in Kidney Disease.* 2nd ed. Academy of Nutrition and Dietetics; 2013:53-68.

38. 2020 Parenteral Nutrition Multivitamin Product Shortage Considerations. American Society for Enteral and Parenteral Nutrition website. January 2020. Accessed November 17, 2020. www.nutritioncare.org/Guidelines_and_Clinical_Resources/Product_Shortages/2020_Parenteral_Nutrition_Multivitamin_Product_Shortage_Considerations

39. Burns DL, Mascioli EA, Bistrian BR. Parenteral iron dextran therapy: a review. *Nutrition.* 1995;11(2):163-168.

40. Mogensen K, Pfister D. Carnitine supplementation: an update. *Support Line.* 2013;35:3-9.

41. Friedman AN, Fadem SZ. Reassessment of albumin as a nutritional marker in kidney disease. *J Am Soc Nephrol.* 2010;21(2):223-230. doi:10.1681/ASN.2009020213

42. de Mutsert R, Grootendorst DC, Indemans F, et al. Association between serum albumin and mortality in dialysis patients is partly explained by inflammation, and not by nutrition. *J Ren Nutr.* 2009;19(2):127-135. doi:10.1053/j.jrn.2008.08.003

43. Fuhrman MP, Charney P, Mueller C. Hepatic proteins and nutrition assessment. *J Am Diet Assoc.* 2004;104(8):1258-1264. doi:10.1016/j.jada.2004.05.213

44. Keller U. Nutritional laboratory markers in malnutrition. *J Clin Med.* 2019;8(6):775. doi:10.3390/jcm8060775

45. Lacson E, Ikizler TA, Lazarus JM, Teng M, Hakim RM. Potential impact of nutritional intervention on end-stage renal disease hospitalization, death, and treatment costs. *J Ren Nutr.* 2007;17(6):363-371. doi:10.1053/j.jrn.2007.08.009

46. Davila J, Konrad D. Metabolic complications of home parenteral nutrition. *Nutr Clin Pract.* 2017;32(6):753-768. doi:10.1177/0884533617735089

47. Mulla H, Peek G, Upton D, Lin E, Loubani M. Plasma aluminum levels during sucralfate prophylaxis for stress ulceration in critically ill patients on continuous venovenous hemofiltration: a randomized, controlled trial. *Crit Care Med.* 2001;29(2):267-271. doi:10.1097/00003246-200102000-00008

48. Mirtallo JM. Overview of parenteral nutrition. In: Mueller CM, ed. *The ASPEN Adult Nutrition Support Core Curriculum.* 3rd ed. American Society for Parenteral and Enteral Nutrition; 2017:285-296.

49. Fuhrman MP. Intradialytic parenteral nutrition and intraperitoneal nutrition. *Nutr Clin Pract.* 2009;24(4):470-480. doi:10.1177/0884533609339072

50. Gervasio JM, Cotton AB. Nutrition support therapy in acute kidney injury: distinguishing dogma from good practice. *Curr Gastroenterol Rep.* 2009;11(4):325-331. doi:10.1007/s11894-009-0047-x

51. Druml W. Nutritional management of acute renal failure. *J Ren Nutr.* 2005;15(1):63-70. doi:10.1053/j.jrn.2004.09.012

52. Fiaccadori E, Parenti E, Maggiore U. Nutritional support in acute kidney injury. *J Nephrol.* 2008;21(5):645-656.

53. Mehta RL, Kellum JA, Shah SV, et al. Acute Kidney Injury Network: report of an initiative to improve outcomes in acute kidney injury. *Crit Care.* 2007;11(2):R31. doi:10.1186/cc5713

54. Hoste E, Bagshaw SM, Bellomo R, et al. Epidemiology of acute kidney injury in critically ill patients: the multinational AKI-EPI study. *Intensive Care Med.* 2015;41(8):1411-1423. doi:10.1007/s00134-015-3934-7

55. Nystrom EM, Nei AM. Metabolic support of the patient on continuous renal replacement therapy. *Nutr Clin Pract.* 2018;33(6):754-766. doi:10.1002/ncp.10208

56. Bufarah MNB, Costa NA, Losilla M, et al. Low caloric and protein intake is associated with mortality in patients with acute kidney injury. *Clin Nutr ESPEN.* 2018;24:66-70. doi:10.1016/j.clnesp.2018.01.012

57. Wiesen P, Overmeire LV, Delanaye P, Dubois B, Preiser J-C. Nutrition disorders during acute renal failure and renal replacement therapy. *JPEN J Parenter Enteral Nutr.* 2011;35(2):217-222. doi:10.1177/0148607110377205

58. Gunst J, Vanhorebeek I, Casaer MP, et al. Impact of early parenteral nutrition in metabolism and kidney injury. *J Am Soc Nephrol.* 2013;24(6):995-1005. doi:10.1681/ASN.2012070732

59. Druml W, Fischer M, Sertl S, Schneeweiss B, Lenz K, Widhalm K. Fat elimination in acute renal failure: long-chain vs medium-chain triglycerides. *Am J Clin Nutr.* 1992;55(2):468-472. doi:10.1093/ajcn/55.2.468

60. Wooley JA, Btaiche IF, Good KL. Metabolic and nutritional aspects of acute renal failure in critically ill patients requiring continuous renal replacement therapy. *Nutr Clin Pract.* 2005;20(2):176-191. doi:10.1177/0115426505020002176

61. Klein CJ, Moser-Veillon PB, Schweitzer A, et al. Magnesium, calcium, zinc, and nitrogen loss in trauma patients during continuous renal replacement therapy. *JPEN J Parenter Enteral Nutr.* 2002;26(2):77-93. doi:10.1177/0148607110202600277

62. Hu J, Wang Y, Geng X, et al. Metabolic acidosis as a risk factor for the development of acute kidney injury and hospital mortality. *Exp Ther Med.* 2017;13(5):2362-2374. doi:10.3892/etm.2017.4292

63. Brown RO, Compher C, A.S.P.E.N. Board of Directors. A.S.P.E.N. clinical guidelines: nutrition support in adult acute and chronic renal failure. *JPEN J Parenter Enteral Nutr.* 2010;34(4):366-377. doi:10.1177/0148607110374577

64. Kamel AY, Dave NJ, Zhao VM, Griffith DP, Connor MJ, Ziegler TR. Micronutrient alterations during continuous renal replacement therapy in critically ill adults: a retrospective study. *Nutr Clin Pract.* 2018;33(3):439-446. doi:10.1177/0884533617716618

65. Kalantar Zadeh K, Cano N, Budde K, et al. Diets and enteral supplements for improving outcomes in chronic kidney disease *Nat Rev Nephrol.* 2011;7(7):369-384. doi:10.1038/nrneph.2011.60

66. Lacson E Jr, Wang W, Zebrowski B, Wingard R, Hakim R. Outcomes associated with intradialytic oral nutritional supplements in patients undergoing maintenance hemodialysis: a quality improvement report. *Am J Kidney Dis*. 2012;60(4):591-600. doi:10.1053/j.ajkd.2012.04.019

67. Benner D, Brunelli S, Brosch B, Wheeler J, Nissenson A. Effects of oral nutritional supplements on mortality, missed dialysis treatments and nutritional markers in hemodialysis patients. *J Ren Nutr*. 2018;28(3):191-196. doi:10.1053/j.jrn.2017.10.002

68. Cheu C, Pearson J, Dahlerus C, et al. Association between oral nutritional supplementation and clinical outcomes among patients with ESRD. *Clin J Am Soc Nephrol*. 2013;8(1):100-107. doi:10.2215/CJN.13091211

69. Korzets A, Azoulay O, Ori Y, et al. The use of intradialytic parenteral nutrition in acutely ill haemodialysed patients. *J Ren Care*. 2008;34(1):14-18. doi:10.1111/j.1755-6686.2008.00005.x

70. Cano NJ, Fouque D, Roth H, et al. Intradialytic parenteral nutrition does not improve survival in malnourished hemodialysis patients: a 2-year multicenter, prospective, randomized study. *J Am Soc Nephrol*. 2007;18(9):2583-2591. doi:10.1681/ASN.2007020184

71. Cherry N, Shalansky K. Efficacy of intradialytic parenteral nutrition in malnourished hemodialysis patients. *Am J Health Syst Pharm*. 2002;59(18):1736-1741. doi:10.1093/ajhp/59.18.1736

72. Blondin J, Ryan C. Nutritional status: a continuous quality improvement approach. *Am J Kidney Dis*.1999;33(1):198-202. doi:10.1016/S0272-6386(99)70283-0

73. Mortelmans AK, Duym P, Vandenbroucke J, et al. Intradialytic parenteral nutrition in malnourished hemodialysis patients: a prospective long-term study. *JPEN J Parenter Enteral Nutr*. 1999;23(2):90-95. doi:10.1177/014860719902300290

74. Hiroshige K, Iwamoto K, Kabashima N, Mutoh Y, Yuu K, Ohtani A. Prolonged use of intradialysis parenteral nutrition in elderly malnourished chronic haemodialysis patients. *Nephrol Dial Transplant*. 1998;13(8):2081-2087. doi:10.1093/ndt/13.8.2081

75. Capelli JP, Kushner H, Camiscioli TC, Chen MS, Torres MA. Effect of intradialytic parenteral nutrition on mortality rates in end-stage renal disease care. *Am J Kidney Dis*. 1994;23(6):808-816. doi:10.1016/s0272-6386(12)80134-x

76. Chertow G, Ling J, Lew N, Lazarus JM, Lowrie EG. The association of intradialytic parenteral nutrition administration with survival in hemodialysis patients. *Am J Kid Dis*. 1994;24(6):912-920. doi:10.1016/S0272-6386(12)81060-2

77. Goldstein D, Strom J. Intradialytic parenteral nutrition: evolution and current concepts. *J Ren Nutr*. 1991;1(1):9-22. doi:10.1016/S1051-2276(12)80032-X

78. Chan A, Cochran C, Harbert G, Parker T, Foulks CJ, Lindley J. Use of intradialytic parenteral nutrition: an end-stage renal disease network perspective. *J Ren Nutr*.1994;4(1):11-14. doi:10.1016/S1051-2276(12)80126-9

79. Wolfson M, Jones MR, Kopple JD. Amino acid losses during hemodialysis with infusion of amino acids and glucose. *Kidney Int*. 1982;21(3):500-506. doi:10.1038/ki.1982.52

80. Pham H, Robinson-Cohen C, Biggs M, et al. Chronic kidney disease, insulin resistance, and incident diabetes in older adults. *Clin J Am Soc Nephrol*. 2012;7(4):588-594. doi:10.2215/CJN.11861111

81. Deger D, Sundell M, Siew E, et al. Insulin resistance and protein metabolism in chronic hemodialysis patients. *J Ren Nutr*. 2013; 23(3);59-66. doi:10.1053/j.jrn.2012.08.013

82. United States Renal Data System. 2018 USRDS Annual Data Report: Epidemiology of kidney disease in the United States. National Institutes of Health website. January 2020. Accessed November 26, 2020. www.usrds.org/annua l-data-report/previous-adrs

83. Moore E, Lindenfeld S. Intradialytic parenteral nutrition: a nutrition support intervention for high risk malnutrition in chronic kidney disease. *Support Line*. 2007;29:7-16.

84. Stegmayr B. Dialysis procedures alter metabolic conditions. *Nutrients*. 2017;9(6):548. doi:10.3390/nu9060548

85. Pandya V, Rao A, Chaudhary K, et al. Lipid abnormalities in kidney disease and management strategies. *World J Nephrol*. 2015;4(1):83-91. doi:10.5527/wjn.v4.i1.83

86. Russell G, Davies TG, Walls J. Evaluation of the intravenous fat tolerance test in chronic renal disease. *Clin Nephrol*. 1980;13(6):282-286.

87. Powers D. Considerations in the use of 3:1 intradialytic parenteral nutrition solutions containing long chain triglyceride. *Contemp Dial Nephrol*. 1990;29-34.

88. Foulks CJ. The effect of intradialytic parenteral nutrition on hospitalization rate and mortality in malnourished hemodialysis patients. *J Ren Nutr.*1994;4(1):5-10. doi:10.1016/S1051-2276(12)80125-7

89. Cano N, Saingra Y, Dupay AM, et al. Intradialytic parenteral nutrition: comparison of olive oil versus soybean oil-based lipid emulsions. *Br J Nutr.* 2006;95(1):152-159. doi:10.1079/bjn20051595

90. Marsen T, Beer J, Mann H, et al. Intradialytic parenteral nutrition in maintenance hemodialysis patients suffering from protein-energy wasting. Results of a multicenter, open, prospective, randomized trial. *Clin Nutr.* 2017;36(1):107-117. doi:10.1016/j.clnu.2015.11.016

91. Powers D. Prolonged experience with intradialytic hyperalimentation in marasmic chronic hemodialysis patients. *Contemp Dial Nephrol.* 1989;22-28.

92. Powers DV, Jackson A, Piraino AJ. Prolonged intradialysis hyperalimentation in chronic hemodialysis patients with an amino acid solution (RenAmin [amino acid] injection) formulated for renal failure. In: Kinney JM, Borum PR, eds. *Perspectives in Clinical Nutrition.* Urban & Schwarzenberg; 1989:191-205.

93. Piraino A, Firpo J, Powers D. Prolonged hyperalimentation in catabolic chronic dialysis therapy patients. *JPEN J Parenter Enteral Nutr.* 1981;5(6):463-477. doi:10.1177/0148607181005006463

94. Dukkipati R, Kalantar-Zadeh K, Kopple JD. Is there a role for intradialytic parenteral nutrition? A review of the evidence. *Am J Kidney Dis.* 2010;55(2):352-364. doi:10.1053/j.jrn.2012.08.013

95. Ikizler TA, Cano N, Franch H, et al. Prevention and treatment of protein energy wasting in chronic kidney disease patients: a consensus statement by the International Society of Renal Nutrition and Metabolism. *Kidney Int.* 2013;84(6):1096-1107. doi:10.1038/ki.2013.147

96. Obi Y, Qader H, Kovesdy CP, Kalantar-Zadeh K. Latest consensus and update on protein-energy wasting in chronic kidney disease. *Curr Opin Clin Nutr Metab Care.* 2015;18(3):254-262. doi:10.1097/MCO.0000000000000171

97. Mak R, Ikizler A, Kovesdy P, RaJ D, Stenvinkel P, Kalantar-Zadeh K. Wasting in chronic kidney disease. *J Cachexia Sarcopenia Muscle.* 2011;2(1):9-25. doi:10.1007/s13539-011-0019-5

98. Kovesdy CP. Malnutrition in dialysis patients—the need for intervention despite uncertain benefits. *Semin Dial.* 2016;29(1):28-34. doi:10.1111/sdi.12410

99. Parker T 3rd. Creating an open dialogue on improving dialysis care. *Nephrol News Issues.* 2013;27(10):14-16.

100. Medicare Prescription Drug Benefit Manual Chapter 6—Part D Drugs and Formulary Requirements. CMS website. January 2016. Accessed June 14, 2020. www.cms.gov/Medicare/Prescription-Drug-Coverage/PrescriptionDrugCovContra/Downloads/Part-D-Benefits-Manual-Chapter-6.pdf

101. Hiroshige K, Iwamoto K, Kabashima N, Mutoh Y, Yuu K, Ohtani A. Prolonged use of intradialysis parenteral nutrition in elderly malnourished chronic haemodialysis patients. *Nephrol Dial Transplant.* 1998;13(8):2081-2087. doi:10.1093/ndt/13.8.2081

102. Moore E, Celano J. Challenges of providing nutrition support in the outpatient dialysis setting. *Nutr Clin Pract.* 2005;20(2):202-212. doi:10.1177/0115426505020002202

103. Bergstrom J. Nutritional requirements of hemodialysis patients. In: *Nutrition in the Kidney.* Little Brown and Co; 1993.

104. Moore E, VanBolt G, Jaremowicz A. A superior proprietary IDPN formulation for malnourished patients with diabetes. *J Ren Nutr.* 2011;21(2):207. doi:10.1053/j.jrn.2011.01.004

105. McCann L, Feldman C, Hornberger J, et al. Effect of intradialytic parenteral nutrition on delivered Kt/V. *Am J Kidney Dis.* 1999;33(6):1131-1135. doi:10.1016/s0272-6386(99)70151-4

106. Dukkipati R, Moore E, VanBolt G, Kalantar-Zadeh K. Impact of IDPN on Kt/V. *Kidney Res Clin Pract.* 2012;31(2):A82. doi:10.1016/j.krcp.2012.04.583

107. Moen M, Zhan M, Hsu VD, et al. Frequency of hypoglycemia and its significance in chronic kidney disease. *Clin J Am Soc Nephrol.* 2009;4(6):1121-1127. doi:10.2215/CJN.00800209

108. Szklarek-Kubicka M, Fijalkowska-Morawska J, Zaremba-Drobnik D, Ucinski A, Czekalski S, Nowicki M. Effect of intradialytic intravenous administration of omega-3 fatty acids on nutritional status and inflammatory response in hemodialysis patients: a pilot study. *J Ren Nutr.* 2009;19(6):487-493. doi:10.1053/j.jrn.2009.05.007

109. Madsen T, Christensen JH, Toft E, Aardestrup I, Lundbye-Christensen S, Schmidt EB. Effect of intravenous omega-3 fatty acid infusion and hemodialysis on fatty acid composition of free fatty acids and phospholipids in patients with end stage renal disease. *JPEN J Parenter Enteral Nutr.* 2011;35(1):97-106. doi:10.1177/0148607110371807

110. Dong J, Ikizler TA. New insights into the role of anabolic interventions in dialysis patients with protein energy wasting. *Curr Opin Nephrol Hypertens.* 2009;18(6):469-475. doi:10.1097/MNH.0b013e328331489d

111. Sarav M, Friedman AN. Use of intradialytic parenteral nutrition in patients undergoing hemodialysis. *Nutr Clin Pract.* 2018;33(6):767-771. doi:10.1002/ncp.10190

112. Rippe B, Oberg CM. Albumin turnover in peritoneal dialysis and hemodialysis. *Semin Dial.* 2016;29(6):458-462. doi:10.1111/sdi.12534

113. Balafa O, Halbesma N, Struijk DG, Dekker F, Krediet R. Peritoneal albumin and protein losses do not predict outcome in peritoneal dialysis patients. *Clin J Am Soc Nephrol.* 2011;6(3):561-566. doi:10.2215/CJN.05540610

114. Gjessing J. Addition of amino acids to peritoneal-dialysis fluid. *Lancet.* 1968;292(7572):812. doi:10.1016/S0140-6736(68)92461-6

115. Giordano C, Capodicosa G, DeSanto NG. Artificial gut for total parenteral nutrition through the peritoneal cavity. *Int J Artif Organs.* 1980;3(6):326-330. doi:10.1177/039139888000300606

116. Wolk R. Intraperitoneal nutrition. *Hospital Nutrition.* 1992;27:893-905.

117. Arfeen S, Goodship T, Kirkwood A, Ward MK. The nutritional/metabolic and hormonal effects of 8 weeks continuous ambulatory peritoneal dialysis with 1% amino acid solution. *Clin Nephrol.* 1990;33(4):192-199.

118. Kopple JD, Bernard D, Messana J, et al. Treatment of malnourished CAPD patients with an amino acid based dialysate. *Kidney Int.* 1995;47(4):1148-1157. doi:10.1038/ki.1995.164

119. Chaudhary K, Khanna R. Biocompatible peritoneal dialysis solutions: do we have one? *Clin J Soc Nephrol.* 2010;5(4):723-732. doi:10.2215/CJN.05720809

120. Saxena R, West C. Peritoneal dialysis: a primary care perspective. *J Am Board Fam Med.* 2006;19(4):380-389. doi:10.3122/jabfm.19.4.380

121. Holmes C, Mujais S. Glucose sparing in peritoneal dialysis: implications and metrics. *Kidney Int Suppl.* 2006;103:S104-S109. doi:10.1038/sj.ki.5001924

122. Szeto CC, Johnson D. Low GDP solution and glucose-sparing strategies for peritoneal dialysis. *Semin Nephrol.* 2017;37(1):30-42. doi:10.1016/j.semnephrol.2016.10.005

123. Williams P, Marliss E, Anderson G, et al. Amino acid absorption following intraperitoneal administration in CAPD patients. *Perit Dial Int.* 1982;2:124-130. doi:10.1177/089686088100200309

124. Tjiong HL, Vanden Berg JW, Wattimena JL, et al. Dialysate as food: combined amino acid and glucose dialysate improves protein anabolism in renal failure patients on automated peritoneal dialysis. *J Am Soc Nephrol.* 2005;16(5):1486-1493. doi:10.1681/ASN.2004050402

125. Bruno M, Bagnis C, Marangella M, Rovera L, Cantaluppi A, Linari F. CAPD with an amino acid dialysis solution: a long-term, cross-over study. *Kidney Int.* 1989;35(5):1189-1194. doi:10.1038/ki.1989.109

126. Thabet AF, Moeen SM, Labiqe MO, Saleh MA. Could intradialytic nutrition improve refractory anaemia in patients undergoing haemodialysis? *J Ren Care.* 2017;43(3):183-191. doi:10.1111/jorc.12206

127. Cano N, Labastie-Coeyrehourq J, Lacombe P, et al. Perdialytic parenteral nutrition with lipids and amino acids in malnourished hemodialysis patients. *Am J Clin Nutr.* 1990;52(4):726-730. doi:10.1093/ajcn/52.4.726

128. Navarro JF, Mora C, Leon C, et al. Amino acid losses during hemodialysis with polyacrylonitrile membranes: effect of intradialytic amino acid supplementation on plasma amino acid concentrations and nutritional variables in nondiabetic patients. *Am J Clin Nutr* 2000;71(3):765-773. doi:10.1093/ajcn/71.3.765

129. Dezfuli A, Scholl D, Lindenfeld S, Kovesdy C, Kalantar-Zadeh K. Severity of hypoalbuminemia predicts response to intradialytic parenteral nutrition in hemodialysis patients. *J Ren Nutr.* 2009;19(4):291-297. doi:10.1053/j.jrn.2009.01.023

130. Bilbrey GL. IDPN is beneficial for selected dialysis patients. *Semin Dial.* 1993;6(3):168-170. doi:10.1111/j.1525-139X.1993.tb00288.x

131. Czekalski S, Hozejowski R, Malnutrition Working Group. Intradialytic amino acids supplementation in hemodialysis patients with malnutrition: results of a multicenter cohort study. *J Ren Nutr.* 2004;14(2):82-88. doi:10.1053/j.jrn.2004.01.007

132. Schulman G, Wingard R, Hutchinson R, Lawrence P, Hakim R. The effects of recombinant human growth hormone and intradialytic parenteral nutrition in malnourished hemodialysis patients. *Am J Kidney Dis.* 1993;21(5):527-534. doi:10.1016/s0272 -6386(12)80399-4

133. Pupim L, Flakoll P, Ikizler A. Nutritional supplementation acutely increases albumin fractional synthetic rate in chronic hemodialysis patients. *J Am Soc Nephrol.* 2004;15(7):1920-1926. doi:10.1097/01.ASN.0000128969.86268.c0

134. Pupim L, Flakoll P, Brouillette J, Levenhagen D, Hakim R, Ikizler TA. Intradialytic parenteral nutrition improves protein and energy homeostasis in chronic hemodialysis patients. *J Clin Invest.* 2002;110(4):483-492. doi:10.1172/JCI15449

135. Chertow G, Lazarus JM, Lyden ME, Caudry D, Nordberg P, Lowrie EG. Laboratory surrogates of nutritional status after administration of intraperitoneal AA based solutions in ambulatory peritoneal dialysis patients. *J Ren Nutr.* 1995;5(3):116-123. doi:10.1016/1051 -2276(95)90040-3

136. Taylor GS, Patel V, Spencer S, Fluck RJ, McIntyre CW. Long term use of 1.1% amino acid dialysis solution in hypoalbuminemic continuous ambulatory peritoneal dialysis patients. *Clin Nephrol.* 2002;58(6):445-450. doi:10.5414 /cnp58445

137. Faller B, Aparicio M, Faict D, et al. Clinical evaluation of an optimized 1.1% amino acid solution for peritoneal dialysis. *Nephrol Dial Transplant.* 1995;10(8):1432-1437.

138. Misra M, Ashworth J, Reaveley DA, Muller B, Brown EA. Nutritional effects of amino acid dialysate (Nutrineal) in CAPD patients. *Adv Perit Dial.* 1996;12:311-314.

139. Li FK, Yee Chan L, Yan Woo J, et al. A 3-year, prospective, randomized, controlled study on amino acid dialysate in patients on CAPD. *Am J Kidney Dis.* 2003;42(1):173-183. doi:10.1016/s0272 -6386(03)00421-9

140. Jones M, Hagen T, Boyle CA, et al. Treatment of malnutrition with 1.1% amino acid peritoneal dialysis solution: results of a multicenter outpatient study. *Am J Kidney Dis.* 1998;32(5):761-769. doi:10 .1016/s0272-6386(98)70131-3

141. Tjiong HL, Rietveld T, Wattimena JL, et al. Peritoneal dialysis with solutions containing amino acids plus glucose promotes protein synthesis during oral feeding. *Clin J Am Soc Nephrol.* 2007;2(1):74-80. doi:10.2215/CJN.01370406

142. Garibotto G, Sofia A, Canepa A, et al. Acute effects of peritoneal dialysis with dialysates containing dextrose or dextrose and amino acids on muscle protein turnover in patients with chronic renal failure. *J Am Soc Nephrol.* 2001;12(3):557-567.

143. Delarue J, Maingourd C, Objois M, et al. Effects of an amino acid dialysate on leucine metabolism in continuous ambulatory peritoneal dialysis patients. *Kidney Int.* 1999;56(5):1934-1943. doi:10.1046/j .1523-1755.1999.00723.x

144. Dibble J, Young G, Hobson S, Brownjohn AM. Amino-acid-based continuous ambulatory peritoneal dialysis (CAPD) fluid over twelve weeks: effects on carbohydrate and lipid metabolism. *Nephrol Dial Transplant.* 1990;10:71-77. doi:10.1177 /089686089001000119

145. Sigrist MK, Levin A, Tejani AM. Systematic review of evidence for the use of intradialytic parenteral nutrition in malnourished hemodialysis patients. *J Ren Nutr.* 2010;20(1):1-7. doi:10.1053/j.jrn.2009 .08.003

146. Fouque D, Kalantar-Zadeh K, Kopple J, et al. A proposed nomenclature and diagnostic criteria for protein-energy wasting in acute and chronic kidney disease. *Kidney Int.* 2008;73(4):391-398. doi:10 .1038/sj.ki.5002585

147. Kalantar-Zadeh K, Kilpatrick R, Kuwae N, et al. Revisiting mortality predictability of serum albumin in the dialysis population: time dependency, longitudinal changes and population-attributable fraction. *Nephrol Dial Transplant.* 2005;20(9):1880-1888. doi:10.1093/ndt/gfh941

148. Lacson E, Wang W, Hakim RM, Teng M, Lazarus M. Associates of mortality and hospitalization in hemodialysis: potentially actionable laboratory variables and vascular access. *Am J Kidney Dis.* 2009;53(1):79-90. doi:10.1053/j.ajkd.2008.07.031

149. Chiu PF, Tsai CD, Wu CL, et al. Trajectories of serum albumin predict survival of peritoneal dialysis patients: a 15-year follow-up study. *Medicine.* 2016;95(12):e3202. doi:10.1097/MD .0000000000003202

150. Mehrotra R, Duong U, Jiwakanon S, et al. Serum albumin as a predictor of mortality in peritoneal dialysis patients: comparisons with hemodialysis. *Am J Kidney Dis.* 2011;58(3):418-428. doi:10.1053/j .ajkd.2011.03.018

151. Kopple JD. Therapeutic approaches to malnutrition in chronic dialysis patients: the different modalities of nutritional support. *Am J Kidney Dis.* 1999;33(1):180-185. doi:10.1016/s0272 -6386(99)70280-5

CHAPTER 16 Parenteral Nutrition and Kidney Disease

152. Leon JB, Majerle A, Soinski J, Kushner I, Ohri-Vachaspati P, Sehgal A. Can a nutrition intervention improve albumin levels among hemodialysis patients? A pilot study. *J Ren Nutr*. 2001;11(1):9-15. doi:10.1016/s1051-2276(01)79890-1

153. Leon JB, Albert J, Gilchrist G, et al. Improving albumin levels among hemodialysis patients: a community-based randomized controlled trial. *Am J Kidney Dis*. 2006;48(1):28-36. doi:10.1053/j.ajkd.2006.03.046

154. Kaysen G, Chertow G, Adhikarla R, Young B, Ronco C, Levin N. Inflammation and dietary protein intake exert competing effects on serum albumin and creatinine in hemodialysis patients. *Kidney Int*. 2001;60(1):333-340. doi:10.1046/j.1523-1755.2001.00804.x

155. Kim Y, Molnar M, Rattanasompattikul M, et al. Relative contributions of inflammation and inadequate protein intake to hypoalbuminemia in patients on maintenance hemodialysis. *Int Urol Nephrol. 2013*;45(1):215-227. doi:10.1007/s11255-012-0170-8

156. Beddhu S, Kaysen GA, Yan G, et al. Association of serum albumin and atherosclerosis in chronic hemodialysis patients. *Am J Kidney Dis*. 2002;40(4):721-727. doi:10.1053/ajkd.2002.35679

Medication and Supplement Use in Kidney Disease

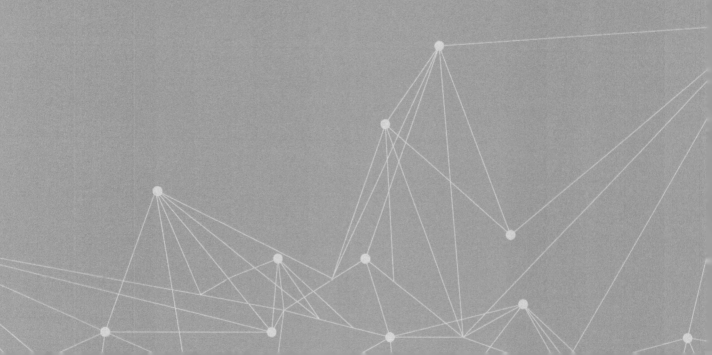

CHAPTER 17

Medications Commonly Prescribed in Kidney Disease

Desiree de Waal, MS, RD, CD, FAND

Introduction

The numerous medications needed to manage the complications of chronic kidney disease (CKD) and other comorbidities present a major challenge for the renal registered dietitian nutritionist and patients with all stages of CKD. The medication burden for those with CKD is significant. Some common side effects can interfere with dietary intake or nutrient adequacy. This chapter is not intended to present a comprehensive list of medications or their adverse effects but rather to serve as a reference for the more commonly prescribed medications for patients in all stages of CKD.

The medications in this chapter are categorized by common medical conditions. The adverse effects listed are limited, for the most part, to those that impact nutrition and gastrointestinal (GI) function. For a more complete review of medical adverse effects and mechanisms, consult other references, such as reliable internet resources and textbooks on medications and internal medicine. In this chapter, generic names of medications have been listed with one or two common brand names. Medication interactions were researched using their individual professional monographs and consumer information for each medication and medication

class. No attempt has been made to include alternative medications or their interactions in this chapter. Please see Chapter 19 for information on dietary supplements.

The following websites may be considered reliable resources on drug information:*

- Drugs.com (www.drugs.com)
- Medscape (www.medscape.com)
- Epocrates (www.epocrates.com)
- Physicians' Desk Reference (www.pdr.net)
- Up To Date (www.uptodate.com)

Anemia

One of the key functions of the kidney is the production of the hormone erythropoietin (EPO), which stimulates bone marrow to make red blood cells. In patients with CKD, EPO production is reduced, resulting in anemia. This is a common complication of CKD. Iron deficiency is also another major factor contributing to anemia in patients with CKD.[1,2] See Box 17.1 on page 360.

The signs and symptoms of anemia in patients with CKD may include the following[3]:

- weakness
- fatigue, or feeling tired
- headaches

* For general medication information, these websites were last accessed May 17, 2020.

- problems with concentration
- paleness
- dizziness
- difficulty breathing or shortness of breath
- chest pain

There are a number of nutrition-related factors that can cause hyporesponsiveness to anemia treatment, such as malnutrition, low blood iron/vitamin B12/folate levels, GI blood loss, and hyperparathyroidism. For more details, see Chapter 2 on anemia.

Cardiovascular Medications

Cardiovascular disease (CVD) is the leading cause of morbidity and mortality in patients with CKD. The prevalence of CVD has been reported to be tenfold higher in patients with CKD than in the general population. This CVD risk progressively increases as CKD progresses to end-stage kidney disease (ESKD). Ultimately, CVD accounts for about 50% of mortality in patients with ESKD.[5-9] See Box 17.2.

BOX 17.1 | Common Medications With Anemia and Chronic Kidney Disease

---

Erythropoietin-stimulating agents (ESAs)

ESAs promote red blood cell production and improve anemia associated with chronic kidney disease (CKD). Note: The use of ESAs can increase the risk for stroke, heart attack, heart failure, blood clots, and death. The manufacturer has revised the boxed Warnings and Precautions and Dosage and Administration sections of the labels for the ESAs to include this information.[4]

Darbepoetin alfa (Aranesp)	Nutrition implications	Dietary considerations
Epoetin alfa (Epogen, Procrit)	Potential gastrointestinal (GI) distress.	All hematologic parameters, as well as iron status, should be monitored regularly.
Methoxy polyethylene glycol-epoetin beta (Mircera)	Increased appetite. Increased blood pressure. Iron deficiency, low folate and vitamin B12 stores.	Iron supplementation is frequently required in conjunction with this therapy. Assess need for vitamins containing folate and vitamin B12.
Peginesatide (Omontys)		

Iron preparations

Iron preparations are used to treat iron-deficiency anemia caused by hemolysis, blood loss, lack of ESA production, and inadequate iron intake. Iron is necessary to support erythropoiesis. Iron available for erythropoiesis in patients with CKD is frequently decreased, compounded by a relative block in iron absorption from the intestines and reduced iron release from storage in macrophages and the liver.

ORAL

Ferrous fumarate (Nephro-Fer)	Nutrition implications	Dietary considerations
Ferrous sulfate (Feosol)	GI side effects include constipation, diarrhea, nausea, vomiting, altered taste, abdominal cramps, GI irritation, and dark stools.	To minimize the risk of various substances in foods binding to iron and preventing absorption, iron supplements should not be taken with meals.
Polysaccharide iron complex (Niferex, Nu-Iron)	With oral preparations, iron absorption is impaired if consumed at the same time as calcium, magnesium, fiber, phytates, tannins, certain sulfur-containing compounds, and cholesterol-lowering drugs.	If stomach upset occurs, iron may then be taken with some food. Oral iron supplements should be taken 1 hour apart from antacids and phosphate binders.
Heme iron polypeptide (Proferrin ES, Ferrimin)	Oral iron absorption may be enhanced by vitamin C, fructose, sorbitol, vitamin E, and certain organic acids, including succinic, lactic, pyruvic, and citric acids. Pica interferes with iron absorption.	Some iron supplements also contain vitamin C or B vitamin complex, which should be noted when considering vitamin recommendations for the CKD population. Slow-release iron preparations are not as well absorbed.

Continued on next page

Continued from previous page

INTRAVENOUS (IV)

Ferumoxytol (Ferraheme) **Sodium ferric gluconate (Ferrlecit)** **Iron sucrose (Venofer)**	**Nutrition implications** GI pain may be experienced, including nausea and cramps.	**Dietary considerations** No specific recommendations.

Iron-based phosphate binder

While reducing serum phosphorus levels, iron-based phosphate binders like ferric citrate increase serum iron levels.

Ferric citrate (Auryxia)	**Nutrition implications** GI side effects include diarrhea, constipation, nausea, vomiting, stomach pain, and darker bowel movements.	**Dietary considerations** Monitor blood levels of potassium, hemoglobin, transferrin saturation, and ferritin.

Hypoxia-inducible factor (HIF) prolyl hydroxylase inhibitor

HIFs are a new class of agents under development for the management of anemia in patients with CKD. HIFs act by stabilizing hypoxia-inducible factor through inhibition of the prolyl hydroxylase family of enzymes. New information has elucidated the critical role that stimulated endogenous response of the hypoxia-sensing system in mediating EPO synthesis and release.

Roxadustat **Vadadustat** **Daprodustat**	**Nutrition implications** HIF is approved in other countries but awaiting US Food and Drug Administration review at the time of this publication.	**Dietary considerations** Monitor potassium levels. Additional clinical side effects are pending trials.

BOX 17.2 | Common Medications With Cardiovascular Disease and Chronic Kidney Disease

Antithrombotic agents

Antithrombotic agents are used to treat and prevent blood clots that may occur in blood vessels. Examples of diseases and conditions that require anticoagulant treatment to reduce the risk of blood clots include heart attack, stroke, deep venous thrombosis, pulmonary embolism, and atrial fibrillation. Thrombolytic agents can be used to treat central venous catheter occlusions.

ANTICOAGULANTS

Factor Xa Inhibitors • **Edoxaban (Lixiana)** • **Apixaban (Eliquis)** **Heparin and derivatives (Lovenox)** **Dabigatran (Pradaxa)** **Fondaparinux (Arixtra)** **Rivaroxaban (Xarelto)**	**Nutrition implications** Gastrointestinal (GI) side effects may include abdominal pain, nausea, flatulence, and diarrhea. Other side effects include lethargy, dizziness, fever, anemia, bruises, bleeding, and headache.	**Dietary considerations** Monitor for GI side effects and help patient manage symptoms.

VITAMIN K ANTAGONISTS

Warfarin (Coumadin)	**Nutrition implications** Blocking vitamin K prevents easily forming blood clots by increasing the time it takes to make fibrin.	**Dietary considerations** Educate patient on diet consistent in food sources of vitamin K. Discourage vitamin K supplements.

ANTIPLATELET DRUGS

Clopidogrel (Plavix) **Aspirin** **Glycoprotein IIb/IIIa Inhibitors (tirofiban, eptifibatide, abciximab)**	**Nutrition implications** Chronic kidney disease (CKD) may increase antiplatelet drug effects. GI bleed is a common side effect.	**Dietary considerations** Some foods and supplements may increase effect (eg, garlic).

Continued on next page

Continued from previous page

THROMBOLYTIC DRUGS/FIBRINOLYTICS

| R-tPA (alteplase, tenecteplase) (TPA, Cathflo Activase) | **Nutrition implications**
GI bleed is a risk. | **Dietary considerations**
No specific recommendations. |

Antiarrhythmics

Antiarrhythmics are used to treat abnormal heart rhythms resulting from irregular electrical activity of the heart.

Amiodarone (Nexterone)	**Nutrition implications** Can include anorexia, abnormal taste and smell, salivation, nausea, vomiting, abdominal pain.	**Dietary considerations** Monitor for GI side effects and help patient manage symptoms. Since side effects increased with hypokalemia, manage potassium levels.
Digoxin (Digox)	Toxicity may occur in patients with low potassium and magnesium levels.	Maintain normal serum levels of potassium and magnesium.
Disopyramide phosphate (Norpace)	Hypotension is a common side effect.	Grapefruit juice may increase blood level of medication.
Flecainide acetate (Tambocor)	Can cause new or worsened supraventricular or ventricular arrhythmias.	No specific recommendations.

Diuretics

Diuretics are commonly prescribed in patients with CKD for volume management, hypertension, electrolyte management, and nephrolithiasis.

THIAZIDE OR "THIAZIDE-LIKE" DIURETICS

Thiazide-like diuretics reduce the reabsorption of sodium and chloride in the first half of the distal convoluted tubule of the nephron. Water follows the unabsorbed sodium.

| Bendroflumethiazide (Aldactide, Naturetin)
Chlorothiazide (Diuril)
Chlorthalidone (Thalitone)
Hydrochlorothiazide (HCTZ) (Microzide)
Hydroflumethiazide (Diucardin, Saluron)
Indapamide (Lozol)
Methyclothiazide (Enduron, Aquatensen)
Metolazone (Zaroxolyn)
Polythiazide (Renese) | **Nutrition implications**
Adverse effects include hyponatremia and hypokalemia.
There is a possibility of developing metabolic alkalosis, hyperglycemia, dry mouth, nausea, and vomiting. | **Dietary considerations**
Monitor serum sodium, potassium, magnesium, calcium, and uric acid levels.
Monitor glucose levels in patients with diabetes mellitus. |

LOOP DIURETICS

Loop diuretics inhibit the sodium, potassium, chloride (Na-K-2Cl) cotransporter on the luminal side of the thick ascending Loop of Henle, and salt and water excretion.

| Bumetanide (Bumex)
Ethacrynic acid (Edecrin)
Furosemide (Lasix)
Torsemide (Demadex) | **Nutrition implications**
Adverse effects may include hypokalemia, dry mouth, and hyperglycemia.
GI symptoms include anorexia, diarrhea, GI bleed, nausea, and vomiting. | **Dietary considerations**
Monitor blood potassium and glucose levels.
Monitor and address any GI symptoms. |

ALDOSTERONE ANTAGONISTS

Aldosterone antagonists (potassium-sparing agents) block the exchange of sodium with potassium and hydrogen ions in the distal half of the convoluted tubule. They are often used in combination with thiazide diuretics to reduce the risk of potassium retention.

| Amiloride hydrochloride (Midamor)
Spironolactone (Aldactone)
Triamterene (Dyrenium) | **Nutrition implications**
Adverse effects include hyperkalemia.
GI symptoms may include dry mouth, nausea, vomiting, diarrhea, constipation, abdominal cramps, dyspepsia, and gastritis. | **Dietary considerations**
Monitor potassium levels. Excessive potassium intake should be avoided.
Monitor and address any GI symptoms.
Encourage a diet adequate in folic acid. |

Continued on next page

Continued from previous page

Antiadrenergics

Antiadrenergics inhibit the function of adrenergic receptors. Adrenergic antagonists reverse the natural cardiovascular effect, based on the type of adrenoreceptor being blocked, and act as an antihypertensive medication.

CENTRAL α-AGONISTS

Central α-agonists function by blocking signals from the brain to the nervous system that speeds up the heart and narrows the veins and arteries.

Clonidine hydrochloride (Catapres) Guanabenz acetate (Wytensin) Guanfacine hydrochloride (Tenex) Methyldopa (Aldomet)	**Nutrition implications** May cause edema, constipation, diarrhea, dry mouth, loss of appetite, nausea, vomiting, flatulence, weight gain, and anemia.	**Dietary considerations** Monitor and address any GI side effects.

α-BLOCKERS

α-Blockers function by binding an α-blocker to α-receptors in the arteries and smooth muscle. Ultimately, depending on the type of α-receptor, this relaxes the smooth muscle or blood vessels, which increases fluid flow in these entities.

Doxazosin mesylate (Cardura) Prazosin hydrochloride (Minipres) Terazosin hydrochloride (Hytrin)	**Nutrition implications** Have a modest effect on reducing total cholesterol and low-density lipoprotein (LDL). May cause, nausea, vomiting, dry mouth, dizziness, fatigue, and headache.	**Dietary considerations** Monitor weight and appetite. Monitor and address any GI symptoms.

β-BLOCKERS

β-Blockers block sympathetic effects on the heart, resulting in reduced arterial pressure and cardiac output. Decrease release of renin hormone.

Acebutolol (Sectral) Atenolol (Tenormin) Betaxolol (Kerlone) Bisoprolol fumerate (Zebeta) Carteolol hydrochloride (Cartrol) Carvedilol (Coreg) Labetalol (Trandate) Metoprolol tartrate (Lopressor) Metoprolol succinate (Toprol XL) Nebivolol (Bystolic) Nadolol (Corgard) Penbutolol sulfate (Levatol) Sotalol (Betapace) Pindolol (Visken) Propranolol hydrochloride (Inderal; Inderal LA) Timolol maleate (Biocarden)	**Nutrition implications** May mask the early warning signs of hypoglycemia. Other adverse effects may include hyperkalemia. GI effects may include nausea, vomiting, constipation, diarrhea, and abdominal discomfort. Blood lipid changes: depressed high-density lipoprotein (HDL), increased total cholesterol, and increased triglycerides.	**Dietary considerations** Monitor blood sugars in people with diabetes mellitus. Monitor potassium levels. Excessive potassium intake should be avoided. Monitor and address any GI symptoms. Monitor blood lipid levels.

Vasodilators

Vasodilators dilate blood vessels. They cause the direct relaxation of vascular smooth muscle preventing the muscles from tightening and the walls from narrowing. As a result, blood flows more easily through the blood vessels and the heart does not need to pump as hard, reducing blood pressure (BP).

Hydralazine (Apresoline) Minoxidil (Lonite) Nitroprusside (Nitropress)	**Nutrition implications** Adverse effects may include nausea, vomiting, anorexia, diarrhea, edema, and weakness.	**Dietary considerations** Monitor and address any GI symptoms.

Continued on next page

Continued from previous page

Calcium channel blockers (Ca antagonists)

Ca antagonists lower BP by preventing calcium from entering the cells of the heart and arteries. Calcium causes the heart and arteries to contract more strongly. Ca antagonists allow blood vessels to relax and open. Some Ca antagonists have the added benefit of slowing one's heart rate, which can further lower BP, relieve chest pain, and control an irregular heartbeat.

Benzothiazepine derivatives: diltiazem (Cardizem SR or LA; Dilacor)	Nutrition implications	Dietary considerations
Diphenylalkylamine derivatives: verapamil (Calan; Isotin; Covera)	Possible side effects include dizziness, weakness, nausea, constipation, and diarrhea.	Monitor and address GI symptoms. In patients with diabetes, monitor blood glucose and help manage symptoms of gastroparesis.
Dihydropyridines: amlodipine, felodipine, isradipine, nicardipine, nifedipine, nisoldipine (Norvasc; Cardene; Procardia)	In patients with diabetes mellitus, Ca antagonists may cause an increase in serum glucose levels and also gastroparesis. Does not affect serum calcium concentrations.	

Angiotensin-converting enzyme (ACE) inhibitors

ACE inhibitors help relax veins and arteries to lower BP. ACE inhibitors prevent an enzyme from producing angiotensin II, a substance that narrows blood vessels. This narrowing can cause high BP and force the heart to work harder.

Benazepril hydrochloride (Lotensin)	Nutrition implications	Dietary considerations
Captopril (Capoten)	Renoprotective effect is prescribed for proteinuria.	Monitor potassium levels. Excessive potassium intake should be avoided.
Enalapril maleate (Vasotec)	Increase in serum potassium is possible.	Monitor magnesium levels.
Fosinopril sodium (Monopril)	Side effects may include dry, irritating cough, stomach pain, nausea, vomiting, diarrhea, and loss of taste.	Monitor and address any GI symptoms.
Lisinopril (Prinivil; Zestril)		
Moexipril (Univasc)		
Perindopril (Aceon)	May cause increased blood urea nitrogen and creatinine.	
Quinapril hydrochloride (Accupril)		
Ramipril (Altace)		
Trandolapril (Mavik)		

Angiotensin II receptor blockers (ARBs)

ARBs help relax veins and arteries to lower BP. ARBs block the action of angiotensin II, allowing the veins and arteries to dilate.

Candesartan (Atacand)	Nutrition implications	Dietary considerations
Eprosartan (Teveten)	Increase in serum potassium is possible.	Monitor potassium levels. Excessive potassium intake should be avoided.
Isbesartan (Avapro)	Side effects may include stomach pain, nausea, vomiting, and diarrhea.	Monitor and address any GI symptoms.
Losartan (Cozaar)		
Telmisartan (Micardis)		
Valsartan (Diovan)		

Cardiac glycosides (inotropic agents)

Inotropic agents primary action is the increase of intracellular (myocardial) sodium, which, in turn, increases cellular calcium intake and muscle contraction.

Digoxin (Lanoxin)	Nutrition implications	Dietary considerations
	Toxicity may occur in hypokalemia, hypercalcemia, and hypomagnesemia.	Monitor potassium, calcium, and magnesium levels.
	Adverse effects may include diarrhea, loss of appetite, lower abdominal pain, nausea, and vomiting.	Discourage herbs with digitalis effects (foxglove, dogbane, lily of the valley, and oleander).
	Rate of absorption, not amount of drug, is affected by concurrent food intake.	

Continued on next page

364

Continued from previous page

α-Adrenergic agonists

α-Adrenergic agonists cause blood vessels to tighten, which increases BP. It is used to treat orthostatic hypotension and are often used in patients with intradialytic hypotension to help with more effective volume removal during hemodialysis.

Midodrine (ProAmatine)	Nutrition implications	Dietary considerations
	GI side effects include stomach pain, dry mouth, nausea, and flatulence.	Monitor and address any GI symptoms.
	Other side effects include supine hypertension, itchiness, numbness, tingling, dizziness, rash, urination issues, slow heartbeat, fainting, headache, and blurry vision.	Monitor BP. Monitor kidney function laboratory results in patients with CKD. Monitor liver function laboratory results.
	Midodrine is removed by dialysis.	

Combination medications used in heart failure

Combination medications are used instead of an ACE inhibitor or an ARB in people with heart failure (HF) and a reduced left ventricular ejection fraction, alongside other standard therapies (eg, β blockers) for HF.

Sacubitril/valsartan (Entresto)	Nutrition implications	Dietary considerations
	Patients may experience hyperkalemia, angioedema, hypotension, or reduced kidney function.	Monitor potassium levels. Monitor kidney function.

Vasopressin V2-receptor antagonists

Vasopressin V2-receptor antagonist is used to treat hyponatremia in individuals with HF, and certain hormonal imbalances. Improves urine flow without causing the body to lose too much sodium. It is used to slow kidney function decline in adults who are at risk for rapidly progressing autosomal dominant polycystic kidney disease.

Tolvaptan (Jynarque)	Nutrition implications	Dietary considerations
	GI side effects include thirst, dry mouth, loss of appetite, abdominal pain, constipation, nausea, vomiting, or diarrhea.	Monitor liver function laboratory results (baseline transaminases and bilirubin, at 2 weeks and 4 weeks after initiation, then continuing monthly for the first 18 months and every 3 months thereafter).
	Other side effects include weakness, fatigue, dehydration, itchiness, jaundice, and dark urine.	Monitor sodium levels and kidney function laboratory results. Do not take with grapefruit.

Dyslipidemia

Dyslipidemia is one of the major risk factors of CVD and common in CKD. Dyslipidemia is an abnormal level of cholesterol and other lipids in the blood. High levels can increase your risk of having a heart attack or developing heart disease.[10]

ANTILIPIDS

Antilipids are used in pharmacologic treatment of dyslipidemias, in patients with/without diabetes and have been well proven to prolong patient survival and reduce the incidence of CVD events, including myocardial infarction and cardiovascular deaths.

HMG-CoA REDUCTASE INHIBITORS (STATINS)

Statins work by inhibiting a key step in hepatic cholesterol synthesis, leading to decreased levels of total cholesterol. Decreased total cholesterol may lead to an increased number of LDL receptors, increasing catabolism of LDL and clearing of LDL from blood circulation. In patients on dialysis, statins have little or no effect on CVD outcomes, despite LDL-lowering effect.[10]

Simvastatin (Zocor) Lovastatin (Mevacor) Fluvastatin (Livalo) Atorvastatin (Lipitor) Pravastatin (Pravachol)	Nutrition implications	Dietary considerations
	GI side effects include nausea, vomiting, constipation, and diarrhea.	Should not be taken with grapefruit juice.
	Other side effects include headache, rash, muscle pain, and rhabdomyolysis.	Monitor for elevation of liver · enzymes (alanine transaminase [ALT] and aspartate aminotransferase [AST]).
	Most serious (rare) side effect is liver failure.	

Continued on next page

Continued from previous page

FIBRIC ACID DERIVATIVES (FIBRATES)

Fibrates are a class of medications that lower blood triglyceride levels. Fibrates lower blood triglyceride levels by reducing the liver's production of very low-density lipoprotein (VLDL) (the triglyceride-carrying particle that circulates in the blood) and speeding up the removal of triglycerides from the blood.

Gemfibrozil (Lopid) **Clofibrate (Atromid-S)** **Fenofibrate (Antara, TriCor)**	**Nutrition implications** GI symptoms include nausea, stomach upset, and diarrhea. May irritate (inflame) the liver. May reduce potassium and blood sugar levels. May cause gallstones when used long term.	**Dietary considerations** Monitor and address GI symptoms. Monitor potassium levels. Monitor blood sugar in patients using oral antidiabetic agents.

CHOLESTEROL-LOWERING MEDICATIONS (NONSTATIN)

Nonstatins act on the brush border of the intestine by preventing the absorption of cholesterol in the intestine.

Ezetimibe (Zetia)	**Nutrition implications** GI side effects include diarrhea, loss of appetite, upset stomach, and fatty stools.	**Dietary considerations** Encourage lifestyle changes (eg, diet, weight loss, exercise).

ADENOSINE TRIPHOSPHATE-CITRATE LYASE (ACL) INHIBITOR

ACL inhibitors lower LDL cholesterol by inhibition of cholesterol synthesis in the liver.

Bempedoic acid (Nexletol) **Bempedoic acid and ezetimibe (Nexlizet)**	**Nutrition implications** GI symptoms include abdominal pain, nausea, constipation, and diarrhea. May increase blood uric acid levels and blood liver levels. Potential cholelithiasis, cholecystitis.	**Dietary considerations** Monitor uric acid levels. Monitor liver function tests.

ANTIHYPERLIPIDEMIC; OMEGA-3 FATTY ACID (EICOSAPENTAENOIC ACID [EPA])

EPA appears to reduce production of triglycerides in the liver and enhance the clearance of triglycerides from circulating VLDL.

Icosapent ethyl (Vascepa) **Omega-3 acid ethyl esters (Lovaza)**	**Nutrition implications** GI side effects include indigestion, altered taste, burping, constipation, throat pain, and dental pain. Other side effects include muscle joint pain; swelling of hands, legs, and feet; gout; atrial fibrillation; and increase in bleeding if on blood thinners. EPAs are not recommended for patients with fish or shellfish allergies.	**Dietary considerations** Monitor liver enzymes.

BILE ACID SEQUESTRANTS

Bile acid sequestrants bind with cholesterol-containing bile acids in the intestines and are eliminated in the stool.

Cholestyramine (Questran, Prevalite) **Colestipol (Colestid)** **Colesevelam (Welchol)**	**Nutrition implications** May prevent absorption of fat-soluble vitamins. Calcium absorption is decreased. GI side effects include constipation, heartburn, indigestion, nausea, vomiting, and stomach pain. May increase ALT, AST, alkaline phosphatase, phosphorus, and triglycerides. Reduced potassium levels.	**Dietary considerations** Consider monitoring for fat-soluble vitamin deficiencies. Supplemental vitamin K in patients with bleeding tendencies. Encourage adequate calcium intake. Monitor ALT, AST, alkaline phosphatase, phosphorus, and potassium laboratory values.

Continued on next page

Continued from previous page

NIACIN

Niacin (also known as nicotinic acid or vitamin B3 but does not include niacinamide form of this vitamin) is a vitamin that lowers total cholesterol and triglycerides at high doses and can also produce an increase in HDL.

Nicotinic acid (Niaspan)	Nutrition implications	Dietary considerations
	May raise glucose and uric acid levels.	Monitor blood glucose levels in patients with diabetes mellitus.
	May activate peptic ulcer or cause flushing.	Monitor uric acid levels.
	Can exacerbate hypotension.	Monitor liver function laboratory values.

Diabetes

Diabetes mellitus (type 1 and type 2) is one of the leading causes of CKD. A reduction in kidney function affects the clearance of several medications used to treat diabetes and can result in drug accumulation, which can lead to potential side effects and, in particular, a risk of hypoglycemia. High blood glucose levels may cause heart and blood vessel disease, stroke, kidney failure, and blindness.[11,12] See Box 17.3.

BOX 17.3 | Common Medications With Diabetes and Chronic Kidney Disease

Sulfonylureas

Sulfonylureas stimulate β cell production of insulin in type 2 diabetes mellitus. Onset of action is within 1.5 hours. This medication class is cleared in the urine. In patients with chronic kidney disease (CKD), there is a risk that this drug may build up in the body, which can cause lower blood sugar levels.

Chlorpropamide (Diabinese) Glimepiride (Amaryl) Glipizide (Glucotrol) Glyburide (Glynase, Micronase)	Nutrition implications	Dietary considerations
	May cause hypoglycemia.	Monitor blood sugars.
	Metabolized in the liver.	Monitor liver function tests.
	Dose adjustments needed in patients with CKD and is not recommended with glomerular filtration rate (GFR) <50 mL/min and in patients on dialysis.	Encourage positive lifestyle modifications, including diet and exercise.

Meglitinides

Meglitinides stimulate β cells of the pancreas. These medications have a quick onset with short action time and should be taken at mealtimes. They are effective on postprandial blood glucose and for individuals who have irregular meal patterns.

Nateglinide (Starlix) Repaglinide (Prandin)	Nutrition implications	Dietary considerations
	Possible weight gain.	Take 15 minutes before meals.
	May need dose adjustment in patients with CKD.	Encourage positive lifestyle modifications, including diet and exercise.

Biguanides

Biguanides may decrease hepatic glucose production and provide some increased peripheral sensitivity. They do not cause hypoglycemia.

Metformin (Glucophage, Riomet)	Nutrition implications	Dietary considerations
	Adverse effects include bloating, diarrhea, and flatulence.	Monitor for lactic acidosis.
	May need dose adjustment in patients with CKD. Avoid with GFR <30 mL/min.	Encourage positive lifestyle modifications, including diet and exercise.

Continued on next page

Continued from previous page

Thiazolidinediones (TZDs)

TZDs increase insulin sensitivity and are active only in the presence of insulin. TZDs may worsen heart failure (HF) by increasing fluid retention and may increase the risk of bone fractures.

| Pioglitazone (Actos)
Rosiglitazone (Avandia) | **Nutrition implications**
May lead to possible weight gain.
May alter blood lipid levels.
No dose adjustments needed in patients with CKD. | **Dietary considerations**
Monitor for fluid retention.
Monitor blood lipids.
Encourage positive lifestyle modifications, including diet and exercise. |

α-Glucosidase inhibitors

α-Glucosidase inhibitors delay the digestion and absorption of carbohydrates in the gastrointestinal (GI) tract.

| Miglitol (Glyset)
Acarbose (Precose) | **Nutrition implications**
Delay absorption of commonly used foods to correct for blood glucose.
No studies were conducted in patients with creatinine more than 2 mg/dL or GFR <25 mL/min. | **Dietary considerations**
In the event of hypoglycemia, use glucose for treatment.
Encourage positive lifestyle modifications, including diet and exercise. |

Dipeptidyl peptidase (DPP)-4 inhibitors

DPP-4 inhibitors work by blocking the action of DPP-4, an enzyme which destroys the hormone incretin. Incretins help the body produce more insulin only when it is needed and they reduce the amount of glucose being produced by the liver when it is not needed.

| Sitagliptin (Januvia)
Saxagliptin (Onglyza)
Linagliptin (Tradjenta) | **Nutrition implications**
Potential gastrointestinal issues include nausea, diarrhea, and stomach pain.
Other potential symptoms include headache, runny nose, sore throat, and skin reactions.
May need dose adjustments for patients with CKD. | **Dietary considerations**
Monitor and manage GI symptoms.
Encourage positive lifestyle modifications, including diet and exercise. |

Sodium-glucose cotransporter (SGLT)-2 inhibitors

SGLT-2 inhibitors work by preventing the kidneys from reabsorbing glucose back into the blood. This allows the kidneys to facilitate its excretion in the urine. As glucose is excreted, plasma levels fall, leading to an improvement in all glycemic parameters.

| Canagliflozin (Invokana)
Dapaglifozin (Forxiga)
Empagliflozin (Jardiance)
Erugliflozin (Steglatro)

Note: Dapaglifozin is being studied for CKD after promising results in Phase 3 HF trials. SGLT2 class may become the new standard of care in diabetes. | **Nutrition implications**
Kidney failure is a risk; make dose adjustments in patients with CKD and avoid if GFR <30 mL/min.
Patient may show signs of hyperkalemia, hypotension, or ketoacidosis. Patient may also have increased cholesterol levels or have a urinary tract infection. Patient may also exhibit clinical signs of dehydration.
Hypoglycemia may occur when SGLT-2 inhibitors are combined with insulin or medications that increase insulin production. | **Dietary considerations**
Monitor potassium levels.
Monitor for signs of dehydration.
Encourage positive lifestyle modifications, including diet and exercise. |

Continued on next page

Continued from previous page

Glucagon-like peptide-1 receptor agonists
Also called incretin mimetics, glucagon-like peptide-1 receptor agonists are used to treat patients with type 2 diabetes mellitus. They work by copying (or mimicking) the functions of the natural incretin hormones in the body that help lower postmeal blood glucose levels. They stimulate the release of insulin by the pancreas after eating.

| Exenatide (Bydureon, Byetta)
Lixisenatide (Adlyxin)
Liraglutide (Victoza, Saxenda)
Dulaglutide (Trulicity)
Semaglutide (Ozempic, Rybelsus) | **Nutrition implications**
GI side effects include diarrhea, constipation, nausea, vomiting, indigestion, and loss of appetite.
Other side effects: headaches, dizziness, and increased sweating. | **Dietary considerations**
Encourage positive lifestyle modifications, including diet and exercise. |

Insulin
Insulin is a hormone usually made by the pancreas that allows the body to use glucose from carbohydrates in food. In diabetes, the body is unable to make or use insulin correctly; so manmade insulin helps control blood sugar.

RAPID-ACTING

| *Can be used in insulin pumps:*
Insulin lispro (Humalog)
Insulin glulisine (Apidra)
Insulin aspart (Novolog) | **Nutrition implications**
Begins working within 15 minutes, peaks in 1 to 2 hours; has duration of about 3 to 4 hours. | **Dietary considerations**
Encourage positive lifestyle modifications, including diet and exercise.
Patient must eat immediately after insulin injection.
Monitor blood sugars and signs of hypoglycemia. |

SHORT-ACTING

| *Not used in insulin pumps:*
Regular (Novolin R)
Insulin human (Humulin R)
Can be used in insulin pumps:
Velosulin | **Nutrition implications**
Begins to lower blood glucose levels within 30 minutes, maximum effect 2 to 5 hours (regular), 1 to 2 hours (human), and has a duration of 5 to 8 hours (regular), 2 to 3 hours (human). | **Dietary considerations**
Patient needs to eat 30 minutes after injection.
Monitor blood sugar levels and signs of hypoglycemia. |

INTERMEDIATE-ACTING

| NPH Insulin (Novolin N)
Human isophane insulin (Humulin N) | **Nutrition implications**
Begins working in about 1 to 2 hours, peaks in 4 to 12 hours, and has a duration of about 18 to 24 hours.
Used with rapid- or short-acting insulin. | **Dietary considerations**
Monitor blood sugar levels and signs of hypoglycemia. |

LONG-ACTING

| Insulin glargine (Toujeo)
Insulin detemir (Levemir)
Insulin degludec (Tresiba) | **Nutrition implications**
No peak, steady level.
Begins in 1 to 2 hours, continuous release is effective for 24 hours.
Insulin degludec begins in 30 to 90 minutes and is effective for 24 hours. | **Dietary considerations**
Monitor blood sugar levels and signs of hypoglycemia. |

INSULIN MIXTURES

| 70/30
50/50
75/25 | **Nutrition implications**
Useful for patients unable to mix doses themselves. Often used in type 2 diabetes mellitus.
Premixed insulin combines specific amounts of intermediate- and short-acting insulin in one bottle or insulin pen. The numbers following the brand name indicate the percentage of each type of insulin. | **Dietary considerations**
These products are generally taken two or three times a day before mealtime.
Monitor blood sugar levels and signs of hypoglycemia. |

Continued on next page

Continued from previous page

ULTRA-RAPID-ACTING MEALTIME
Must be used with long-acting insulin in type 1 diabetes mellitus.

Inhaled human insulin powder (Afrezza)	Nutrition implications	Dietary considerations
	Enters the bloodstream in less than 1 minute. The time to first measurable effect is ~12 minutes. Peak at 30 to 60 minutes. Clears out of bloodstream within 1.5 to 3 hours.	Inhale when food arrives.
		To avoid coughing, take a sip of water before inhaling and inhale slowly.
	May be option to correct nighttime highs with less fear of hypoglycemia due to the faster offset.	Educate on the ability to have a flexible meal schedule.
	Risk of low blood sugar level (hypoglycemia) late after meals is much lower.	Individuals on a low-carbohydrate diet or who use low insulin doses may have difficulty with inhaled insulin.
	Side effects include cough, sore throat, hypoglycemia, and hypokalemia.	Monitor blood sugar levels and signs of hypoglycemia.
	Use with caution with lung disease, kidney disease, HF and co-use of TZDs.	Monitor potassium levels. Monitor for signs of fluid retention.

Gastrointestinal-Related Medications

Patients with CKD frequently experience upper GI symptoms, including dysgeusia, anorexia, hiccups, stomatitis, nausea, vomiting, and gastroparesis. Constipation and diarrhea represent the main lower GI tract symptoms associated with CKD. See Box 17.4.

BOX 17.4 | Common Medications With Gastrointestinal Disease and Chronic Kidney Disease

Dopaminergic-blocking agent
Dopaminergic-blocking agents inhibits gastric smooth muscle relaxation, accelerates intestinal transit and gastric emptying, and relaxes the upper small intestine, decreasing reflux into the esophagus and improving acid clearance from the esophagus. They are primarily used for diabetic gastroparesis and esophageal reflux.

Metoclopramide (Reglan)	Nutrition implications	Dietary considerations
	Gastrointestinal (GI) side effects include nausea, vomiting, and diarrhea.	May alter insulin requirements. Monitor blood sugars in diabetes.
	Other side effects include confusion and uncontrolled muscle movements (eg, tardive dyskinesia after long-term use).	Monitor and manage GI symptoms.

Histamine H2-receptor antagonists
Histamine H2-receptor antagonists are indicated for the treatment of pathological gastric hypersecretion (eg, gastroesophageal reflux [GERD], Zollinger-Ellison syndrome). Use if lifestyle measures do not work.

Cimetidine (Tagamet) Famotidine (Pepcid) Nizatidine (Tazac, Axid) Ranitidine (Zantac)	Nutrition implications	Dietary considerations
	GI side effects may include nausea, vomiting, dry mouth, constipation, diarrhea, anorexia, abdominal pain, and flatulence.	Encourage lifestyle measures. Monitor and manage GI symptoms. Monitor for increased levels of calcium and magnesium.
	Other side effects include dizziness, headache, irregular heartbeat, and alopecia.	
	Famotidine contains calcium and magnesium.	
	Ranitidine has been linked to a carcinogen in generic products.	

Continued on next page

Continued from previous page

Proton-pump inhibitors (PPI)

PPIs are used for the prevention of acid-related conditions (eg, stomach ulcers, GERD, erosive esophagitis, Zollinger-Ellison syndrome). They are also used in combination with antibiotics for treating *Helicobacter pylori* infections. It has been noted that PPI use is associated with a higher risk of incident chronic kidney disease (CKD).[13] Long-term use of PPIs has been linked to an increased risk of heart attacks, especially if the patient is on a blood thinner.[14]

Dexlansoprazole (Kapidex) **Esomeprazole (Nexium)** **Lansoprazole (Prevacid)** **Omeprazole (Prilosec)** **Pantoprazole (Protonix)** **Rabeprozole (Aciphex)**	**Nutrition implications** GI side effects include, nausea, constipation, and diarrhea. There is reduced absorption of iron, magnesium, and vitamin B12. PPIs are metabolized by the liver. Adverse side effects include headaches.	**Dietary considerations** Encourage lifestyle measures. Monitor and manage GI symptoms. Monitor iron, magnesium, and vitamin B12 levels.

Anorexia/appetite stimulants

Appetite stimulants are indicated for the treatment of anorexia, cachexia, or unexplained weight loss. They are also indicated as antiemetics.

Megestrol acetate (Megace) Not recommended for use in adults >65 years of age due to limited weight effects and increased risk of thrombotic events and death.[15]	**Nutrition implications** Side effects include diarrhea, dyspepsia, nausea, vomiting, and hyperglycemia. Blood clots can occur in sedentary individuals.	**Dietary considerations** Monitor dialysis clearance, weight, fluid retention, and appetite.
Dronabinol (Marinol)	**Nutrition implications** GI-related side effects include abdominal pain and dry mouth. Non-GI side effects include dizziness, seizures, euphoria, paranoia, tachycardia, central nervous system (CNS) effects, hypotension, and sleep disturbances.	**Dietary considerations** Monitor dialysis clearance, weight, fluid retention, and appetite.
Mirtazapine (Remeron)	**Nutrition implications** This medication is an antidepressant with increased appetite and weight gain as side effects. Side effects include constipation, dry mouth, dizziness, and abnormal dreams.	**Dietary considerations** Monitor dialysis clearance, weight, fluid retention, and appetite.

Medications to treat constipation

Constipation is common in patients with CKD. Physicians use various tests and procedures to diagnose the cause of chronic constipation. Several types of laxatives exist with each working somewhat differently to promote bowel movement ease.

FIBER SUPPLEMENTS

Fiber supplements add bulk to stool. Stools with greater bulk are softer and easier to pass.

Psyllium (Metamucil Psyllium) **Calcium polycarbophil (Equalactin, Fiber Tabs)** **Methylcellulose (Citrucel)**	**Nutrition implications** Fiber supplements have some effect within 12 to 24 hours, but their full effect usually takes 2 to 3 days to develop. Side effects include choking or trouble swallowing, severe stomach pain, cramping, nausea or vomiting, bloating, flatulence, rectal bleeding, or itchy skin rash. Calcium polycarbophil may cause hypercalcemia. Not recommended for patients on a fluid restriction.	**Dietary considerations** Take with sufficient fluid (8 oz per dose). Avoid taking within 2 hours before or 2 hours after other medicines as it may cause difficulty absorbing other medicines. Stop if constipation lasts beyond 7 days. Monitor calcium levels (with calcium polycarbophil).

Continued on next page

Continued from previous page

STIMULANT LAXATIVES
Increase the contractions/movement of the intestines, helping the stool to pass.

Bisacodyl (Dulcolax) **Sennosides (Senokot, ExLax)**	**Nutrition implications**	**Dietary considerations**
	Stimulant laxatives usually work within 6 to 12 hours.	Educate patient on lifestyle changes that may prevent or relieve constipation, including exercising, drinking enough water, and eating a proper diet with fiber-rich foods, such as whole grains, and fresh fruits and vegetables.
	GI issues include abdominal cramping/pain, diarrhea, nausea, and vomiting.	
	Other issues include rectal burning, vertigo, dizziness, weakness, muscle cramps, irregular heartbeat, decreased urination, and mental/mood changes (eg, confusion).	Monitor electrolyte levels.
		Monitor and manage GI symptoms.
	Sennosides may cause urine to turn reddish-brown.	
	Long-term use may lead to electrolyte and fluid imbalance that can cause heart function disorders, muscle weakness, liver damage, and other harmful effects.	

OSMOTIC LAXATIVES
Help stool move through the colon by increasing secretion of fluid from the intestines and helping to stimulate bowel movements. Cause the cells that line the intestines to secrete chloride, sodium, and water to help soften stools.

Magnesium hydroxide (Milk of Magnesia) **Magnesium citrate** **Lactulose** **Polyethylene glycol (Miralax)** **Linaclotide (Linzess)** **Lubiprostone (Amitiza)**	**Nutrition implications**	**Dietary considerations**
	Osmotic laxatives can take 2 to 3 days to have any effect, so they are not suitable for the rapid relief of constipation.	Educate patient on lifestyle changes that may prevent or relieve constipation, including exercising, drinking enough water, and eating a proper diet with fiber-rich foods, such as whole grains and fresh fruits and vegetables.
	GI side effects include nausea, vomiting, bloating, cramping, flatulence, fecal incontinence, and diarrhea.	Monitor electrolytes.
		Monitor magnesium.
		Monitor and manage GI symptoms.
		If nausea occurs, take with food and water.

SEROTONIN 5-HYDROXYTRYPTAMINE 4 RECEPTORS
Help move stool through the colon.

Prucalopride (Prudac, Motegrity)	**Nutrition implications**	**Dietary considerations**
	GI side effects include nausea, vomiting, diarrhea, stomach pain, bloating, and flatulence.	Monitor and manage GI symptoms.
	Other side effects include headache, dizziness, fatigue, and unusual changes in mood.	
	Not recommended with bowel perforation, intestinal obstruction, or serious conditions of the intestinal wall such as Crohn's disease, ulcerative colitis.	

Continued on next page

Continued from previous page

PERIPHERALLY ACTING MU-OPIOID RECEPTOR ANTAGONISTS (PAMORA)

For opioid-induced constipation (OIC), PAMORAs reverse the effect of opioids on the intestine to keep the bowel moving. They antagonize the peripheral mu-opioid receptor in the GI tract to decrease constipation without reversing the systemic analgesic effects of opiates.

Naloxegol (Movantik) Methylnaltrexone (Relistor)	Nutrition implications	Dietary considerations
	Naloxegol has a low risk of opioid withdrawal. Monitor for withdrawal symptoms, such as hyperhidrosis, rhinorrhea, anxiety, and chills. Contraindicated in patients with mechanical GI bowel obstruction and in those who are at increased risk for recurrent obstruction. With kidney or hepatic impairment, the dose of oral or injectable methylnaltrexone should be adjusted.	It is unlikely that dietary and lifestyle changes alone will prevent or treat OIC. Naloxegol should be taken on an empty stomach. Laxatives should be discontinued prior to PAMORA initiation; if adequate relief of constipation does not occur within 3 days, then laxatives may be reintroduced. When opioid therapy is discontinued, the PAMORA should also be discontinued.

STOOL SOFTENERS

Moisten the stool by drawing water from the intestines making them easier to pass. They aid by softening stools for people who should avoid straining during bowel movements because of heart conditions, hemorrhoids, and other problems.

Docusate sodium and dioctyl sodium sulfosuccinate (Docusate) Docusate calcium (Colace, Correctol) Dioctyl calcium sulfosuccinate (Colace)	Nutrition implications	Dietary considerations
	GI issues include stomach pain, intestinal cramps, nausea, vomiting, and swallowing difficulty. Other issues include throat irritation (from oral liquid), rash, and hives.	Educate patient on lifestyle changes that may prevent or relieve constipation, including exercising, drinking enough water, and eating a proper diet with fiber-rich foods, such as fresh fruits and vegetables. Monitor and manage GI symptoms.

ENEMAS AND SUPPOSITORIES

Aid in moving stool out of the body by providing lubrication and stimulation.

Enemas with or without soapsuds	Nutrition implications	Dietary considerations
	Potential side effects include hyponatremia and dehydration. Should produce a bowel movement within 2 to 15 minutes. Phosphate enemas can cause hyperphosphatemia and are not recommended in patients with kidney disease.	Educate on lifestyle changes that may prevent or relieve constipation, including exercising, drinking enough water, and eating a proper diet with fiber-rich foods, such as whole grains and fresh fruits and vegetables. Monitor and manage GI symptoms.
Glycerin or bisacodyl suppositories	Nutrition implications	Dietary considerations
	May cause rectal irritation/burning, abdominal discomfort/cramps, small amounts of mucus, severe/persistent stomach/abdominal pain, bloody stools, rectal bleeding, persistent urge to have a bowel movement, and persistent diarrhea.	Educate on lifestyle changes that may prevent or relieve constipation, including exercising, drinking enough water, and eating a proper diet with fiber-rich foods, such as whole grains and fresh fruits and vegetables. Monitor and manage GI symptoms.

LUBRICANTS

Enable stool to move through your colon more easily.

Mineral oil-oral	Nutrition implications	Dietary considerations
	Should not be taken with dysphagia, during pregnancy, or by patients who are ill, debilitated, or bedridden. Should produce a bowel movement within 6 to 8 hours. Common side effects may include diarrhea, flatulence, or stomach cramps.	Educate patient on lifestyle changes that may prevent or relieve constipation, including exercising, drinking enough water, and eating a proper diet with fiber-rich foods, such as whole grains and fresh fruits and vegetables. Monitor and manage GI symptoms.

Continued on next page

Continued from previous page

Antidiarrheal medications

Used to slow down or stop loose stools (diarrhea). These will not treat the underlying cause (such as infection or inflammation) but may help with the discomfort that comes from having repeated watery bowel movements. These may be harmful in certain types of inflammatory bowel diseases. If diarrhea lasts more than a few days, the cause should be investigated.

Loperamide (Imodium)	**Nutrition implications**	**Dietary considerations**
Slows the movement of food through the intestines, which lets the body absorb more liquid.	GI side effects include dry mouth, vomiting, constipation, stomach pain, discomfort, or bloating. Other side effects include dizziness, drowsiness, and fatigue.	Educate on lifestyle changes that may prevent or relieve diarrhea. Monitor and manage GI symptoms. In patients on dialysis, assess for fluid status. Provide education on fluid goals.
Bismuth subsalicylate (Bismuth)	**Nutrition implications**	**Dietary considerations**
Balances fluid movement through the digestive tract.	GI issues include abdominal pain, nausea, vomiting, discolored or sticky stools, constipation, diarrhea, indigestion, flatulence, sores in stomach lining, loss of appetite, taste changes, mild diarrhea, mouth pain, and dysphagia. Other issues include tongue changes (swollen, black or "hairy"), anal discomfort, anxiety, confusion, dark urine, depression, dizziness, GI bleed, headache, insomnia, itching, lightheadedness, muscle spasm, pain, rapid heart rate, tinnitus, shortness of breath, weakness, and jaundice.	Educate on lifestyle changes that may prevent or relieve diarrhea. Monitor and manage GI symptoms. In patients on dialysis, assess for fluid status. Provide education on fluid goals.

Antigout Agents

CKD can lead to gout, but gout may also increase the risk of CKD. Since uric acid is filtered through the kidneys, the two diseases are related. Uric acid is a waste product that is naturally found in blood, but with CKD, the kidneys cannot effectively filter uric acid. Too much uric acid accumulation in the body may cause gout.[16] See Box 17.5.

BOX 17.5 | Common Medications With Gout and Chronic Kidney Disease

Colchicine (Colcrys) **Probenecid (Probalan)**	**Nutrition implications**	**Dietary considerations**
Decreases swelling and lessens the accumulation of uric acid crystals that cause pain in the affected joint(s).	Renal excretion, which requires caution and dose adjustment in patients with chronic kidney disease (CKD). Gastrointestinal (GI) side effects include diarrhea, nausea, vomiting, cramping, and abdominal pain. Other side effects include urination changes, muscle weakness, mood changes, convulsions, easy bruising, or bleeding.	Nutrition recommendations include a balanced diet (Mediterranean, Dietary Approaches to Stop Hypertension), healthy weight goals, and to limit foods with purines (such as organ meats), sugar-sweetened beverages, and alcohol. Monitor kidney function. Avoid grapefruit.
Allopurinol (Zyloprim)	**Nutrition implications**	**Dietary considerations**
Decreases blood and urine uric acid levels by blocking xanthine oxidase, an enzyme that helps make uric acid.	GI side effects include diarrhea and nausea. Other side effects include skin rash. It is metabolized in liver, so there is a risk of hepatotoxicity gout flare-up.	Nutrition recommendations as above. Monitor liver function test.

Hyperkalemia

Hyperkalemia is common in patients with CKD and can be life threatening. High potassium levels can cause serious heart problems and sudden death. There are often no warning signs, meaning a person can have high potassium levels without knowing it. If symptoms do occur, they are often nonspecific, such as heart palpitations, nausea, weakness, or paresthesia.[17] See Box 17.6.

BOX 17.6 | Common Medications to Treat Hyperkalemia With Chronic Kidney Disease

Potassium-removing agents
Act to remove excess potassium from the body.

Sodium polystyrene sulfonate (Kayexalate)	Nutrition implications	Dietary considerations
Removes potassium from the body by an exchange of sodium ions with potassium ions, primarily in the large intestine.	Possible gastrointestinal (GI) side effects include gastric irritation, anorexia, nausea, vomiting, and constipation. When mixed with sorbitol, diarrhea is a common adverse effect. May cause fluid retention and should be used with caution in individuals who have intolerance to changes in blood pressure. May lower calcium and magnesium.	Monitor and manage GI symptoms. Monitor serum potassium levels carefully. Monitor calcium and magnesium levels. Consider further sodium restriction.
Patiromer (Veltassa)	**Nutrition implications**	**Dietary considerations**
Removes potassium from the body by an exchange of calcium for potassium in the GI tract, thereby increasing fecal potassium.	GI side effects include constipation, diarrhea, nausea, abdominal discomfort, and flatulence. May cause hypomagnesemia.	Monitor serum potassium levels carefully. Monitor calcium and magnesium levels.
Sodium zirconium cyclosilicate (Lokelma)	**Nutrition implications**	**Dietary considerations**
Nonabsorbed zirconium cyclosilicate preferentially captures potassium in exchange for hydrogen and sodium. It increases fecal potassium excretion through binding of potassium in the lumen of the GI tract; binding of potassium reduces the free potassium concentration in the GI lumen, thereby lowering serum potassium level.	May cause mild-to-moderate edema. Avoid with severe constipation or bowel obstruction or impaction, including abnormal postoperative bowel motility disorders; may worsen GI conditions.	Monitor serum potassium levels carefully. Monitor for constipation. Monitor for signs of edema in patients prone to fluid overload.

Chronic Kidney Disease– Mineral and Bone Disorder

Chronic kidney disease–mineral and bone disorder (CKD–MBD) is a systemic disorder of mineral and bone metabolism due to CKD manifested by either one or a combination of the following: abnormalities of calcium (Ca), phosphorus (P), parathyroid hormone (PTH), or vitamin D metabolism, abnormalities in bone turnover, mineralization, volume, linear growth (pediatrics), or strength.[18,19] See Box 17.7 on page 376.

BOX 17.7 | Common Medications With Mineral and Bone Disorder in Chronic Kidney Disease

---

Phosphate binders

Reduce phosphorus levels by reducing absorption of phosphorus in the gut. The goal is to maintain phosphorus within the normal range. Binders should be taken with or immediately after meals.

Calcium-based binders (also calcium supplements)

Calcium combines with dietary phosphate, forming an insoluble complex that is eliminated in the feces, resulting in reduced serum phosphorus concentration. Contraindicated in hypercalcemia (calcium >10.5) and low parathyroid hormone (PTH) levels. Per chronic kidney disease (CKD) guidelines, limit the use of calcium-based binders due to risk of poor outcomes (mortality and nonfatal cardiovascular disease events).

Calcium carbonate (TUMS)	Nutrition implications	Dietary considerations
	Decreased absorption/therapeutic effects of certain medications (tetracyclines, verapamil, quinolones [oral], levothyroxine). Max dose is 6,750 to 7,500 mg in dyspepsia, no renal dosing recommendations.	Monitor calcium, phosphorus, and PTH levels. Separate calcium-based binders from certain medications: • Separate from tetracyclines by 2 to 4 hours. • Separate from quinolones (oral) by 2 hours. • Separate from levothyroxine by 4 hours.
Calcium acetate (PhosLo–capsule or Phoslyra–liquid)	Nutrition implications	Dietary considerations
	Imparts a vinegar-like taste if chewed. Maximum dose is 8 to 12 capsules or 40 to 60 mL.	Monitor calcium, phosphorus, and PTH levels Separate calcium-based binders from certain medications: • Separate from tetracyclines by 2 to 4 hours. • Separate from quinolones (oral) by 2 hours. • Separate from levothyroxine by 4 hours.
Calcium, magnesium blends (Rolaids)	Nutrition implications	Dietary considerations
	Contains magnesium hydroxide. May act as a mild laxative. Some contain aluminum so are not recommended.	Monitor magnesium levels. Ensure choice does not have aluminum as ingredient.

Non–calcium-based phosphate binders

Recommended based on the Kidney Disease Improving Global Outcomes (KDIGO) guidelines to reduce risk of hypercalcemia, arterial calcification, and low PTH levels. Bound phosphorus is excreted in feces.

SEVELAMER TYPE

Binds dietary phosphate in gut and inhibits absorption from gut.

Sevelamer carbonate (tablets or powder) (Renvela) Sevelamer hydrochloride (Renagel)	Nutrition implications	Dietary considerations
	Contraindicated in bowel obstruction, dysphagia, or severe gastrointestinal (GI) motility disorders. GI side effects include nausea, vomiting, stomach pain, loss of appetite, upset stomach, flatulence, bloating, diarrhea, and constipation. Other side effects include fatigue, itching, and joint pain. Tablets should not be broken or crushed.	Monitor calcium, phosphorus, and PTH levels. Some GI symptoms are often dose related, so titrating dosing slowly may help. Separate from these medications by 2 hours: Ciprofloxine, Levothyroxine, Mycophenolate. Patients on antiarrhythmic and antiseizure medications were excluded in studies. Maximum dose studied: 16 to 17 tablets per day (equivalence in powder).
Lanthanum carbonate (tablets or powder) (Fosrenol)	Nutrition implications	Dietary considerations
	Must be fully chewed. Contraindicated in bowel obstruction, ileus, and fecal impaction. Precautions should be taken in GI disorders. GI side effects include nausea, vomiting, diarrhea, and abdominal pain.	Monitor calcium, phosphorus, and PTH levels. Powder can be sprinkled on food but must be consumed immediately. Separate from these medications by 2 hours: Ciprofloxine, Levothyroxine, Mycophenolate. Maximum dose is 3,750 mg/d.

Continued on next page

Continued from previous page

Ferric citrate (Auryxia)	Nutrition implications	Dietary considerations
	GI side effects include diarrhea, nausea, vomiting, constipation, and darkening of stools.	Monitor iron, ferritin, and transferrin saturation levels.
	Can lead to elevation in iron stores and elevations in serum ferritin and transferrin saturation.	Monitor calcium, phosphorus, and PTH levels. Separate dosing from:
	Not studied in inflammatory bowel disease or active GI bleeds.	• Doxycycline by 1 hour • Levodopa by at least 2 hours • Levothyroxine by 4 hours Avoid with quinolone antibiotics and methyldopa. Maximum dose is 12 tablets per day.
Sucroferric oxyhydroxide (Velphoro) Binds phosphorus in the aqueous environment of the GI tract by ligand exchange between hydroxyl or water groups on sucroferric oxyhydroxide and the phosphorus from diet.	**Nutrition implications** Does not affect serum iron levels as much as ferric citrate, but iron studies should be monitored. GI side effects include diarrhea, darkening of stools, nausea, dysgeusia, and tooth discoloration. Not recommended with levothyroxine, patients with GI disorders, hemochromatosis, hepatic disease or peritonitis (in patients on peritoneal dialysis).	**Dietary considerations** Monitor iron, transferrin saturation, and hemoglobin levels. Monitor calcium, phosphorus, and PTH levels. Maximum dose is 6 tablets/d.
Magnesium carbonate (MagneBind)	**Nutrition implications** GI side effects include abdominal discomfort, nausea, diarrhea, constipation. Other symptoms may include muscle weakness, numbness, and tingling. Magnesium can be toxic at high levels; however, some is removed by dialysis.	**Dietary considerations** Monitor calcium, phosphorus, PTH and magnesium levels.
Aluminum hydroxide (Amphojel, AlternaGEL)	**Nutrition implications** Not recommended due to the risk of high aluminum levels.	**Dietary considerations** No considerations.

Sodium/hydrogen exchanger 3 (NHE3) inhibitor

NHE3 inhibitors are a new class targeted for treatment of hyperphosphatemia in patients requiring dialysis. It acts in the gut to inhibit sodium/hydrogen exchanger 3 (NHE3), resulting in a conformational change of the epithelial cell junctions and reducing permeability specific to phosphate. Results in decreased phosphate absorption. Also reduces absorption of sodium from small intestine and colon resulting in increased water secretion and transit time in the intestine. Used to treat irritable bowel syndrome-colon.

Tenapanor (Ibsrela)	Nutrition implications	Dietary considerations
At time of this publication the medication was under review with the Food and Drug Administration for treatment of hyperphosphatemia.	GI side effects include diarrhea, abdominal distension, flatulence, and dizziness. Other side effects include hyperkalemia and dehydration.	Monitor potassium and phosphorus. Monitor for GI symptoms. Monitor for signs of dehydration. Take immediately prior to first meal of the day and prior to last meal of the day.

Vitamin D preparations

Vitamin D is an important regulator of calcium and phosphorus homeostasis and also has numerous extraskeletal effects on the cardiovascular system, central nervous system, endocrine system, immune system, etc, as well as on cell differentiation and cell growth. In patients with CKD, the mineral metabolism is progressively altered. Decreasing 25-hydroxyvitamin D and rising PTH levels occur early in the course of CKD.

NUTRITIONAL VITAMIN D

Declines in vitamin D levels have been found to be prevalent in the population with CKD. Vitamin D deficiency is considered when total 25-hydroxyvitamin D levels are less than 20 ng/mL; vitamin D insufficiency is determined when levels are between 20 and 29 ng/mL.

Continued on next page

Continued from previous page

Cholecalciferol (Vitamin D3) Ergocalciferol (Vitamin D2)	Nutrition implications	Dietary considerations
	In the general population, there appears to be some advantage of vitamin D3 over vitamin D2.	Monitor vitamin D levels. Recommendations should be based on the recommendations for the general population. However, consider individual response to vitamin D supplementation, and adjust as indicated.

VITAMIN D ANALOGS

Also known as active form of vitamin D, they are used for the treatment of secondary hyperparathyroidism. Since active vitamin D can also increase the absorption of calcium and phosphorus in the gut, concurrent management of serum calcium and phosphorus levels is imperative.

Calcitriol (Calcijex, Rocaltrol) Doxercalciferol (Hectorol) Paricalcitol (Zemplar)	Nutrition implications	Dietary considerations
	GI side effects include nausea, vomiting, and constipation. Mineral oil and cholestyramine impair intestinal absorption of oral vitamin D analogs.	Not recommended to be used when phosphorus levels are greater than 5.5 and calcium levels are greater than 10.5.

Calcimimetic agents

These bind with calcium sensing receptors found on the parathyroid gland, making them more sensitive to serum calcium levels, thus reducing the release of PTH. Calcimimetic agents are used most often when calcium levels are persistently greater than 10.2, PTH levels are high, and phosphorus levels are elevated, rendering treatment with vitamin D analogs not possible.

Cinacalcet HCl (Sensipar) Etelcalcetide (Parsabiv)	Nutrition implications	Dietary considerations
	GI side effects include nausea, vomiting, diarrhea, and GI bleed (gastritis, esophagitis, ulcers). Hypocalemia may cause paresthesia, myalgia, muscle spasms or cramps, seizures, and facial twitching. Cinacalcet HCl and etelcalcetide should not be used concurrently. Cinacalcet HCl is not removed by dialysis.	Monitor calcium levels carefully. Treatment should be discontinued if serum calcium level is less than normal. Treatment initiation is contraindicated if serum calcium level is less than the lower limit of the normal range. Should be held when PTH is low (<150 pg/mL). Monitor for GI symptoms. GI side effects tend to be dose related and resolve within a few days of starting or increasing the dose of the drug.

Other osteoporosis medications

These medications are prescribed with severe osteoporosis to increase bone mass. They act by inhibiting osteoclast formation, function, and survival decreasing bone resorption and increasing bone mass and strength in both cortical and trabecular bone.

Denosumab (Prolia)	Nutrition implications	Dietary considerations
	Contraindicated with use of calcimimetic agents. Will reduce calcium levels.	Monitor calcium, phosphorus, and magnesium levels. Encourage adequate intake of calcium and vitamin D.

Niacinamide

This is also known as vitamin B3 but not nicotinic acid. Inhibits intestinal phosphate uptake in the brush border cells of the small intestine (demonstrated in rats). In addition, it may have a protective effect on pancreatic function that is associated with improved insulin secretion and consequently a shift of phosphate to the intracellular space. No indication of effect on cardiovascular markers.

Doses of 500 to 1,000 mg daily were studied.	Nutrition implications	Dietary considerations
	Metabolism occurs in liver. May reduce platelet levels. Contraindicated if prescribed cytoxan or chemotherapy. Contraindicated with thrombocytopenia. GI side effects include diarrhea and GI irritation.	Monitor platelet count and discontinue if platelets drop to 100,000/mm^3 or lower.

Other Medications With Nutritional Implications

BOX 17.8 | Common Steroids Used With Chronic Kidney Disease

Anabolic-androgenic steroids

Anabolic-androgenic steroids are used to promote lean body mass and weight gain, especially in AIDS wasting syndrome. The action of these medications is to reverse catabolic processes and negative nitrogen balance by promoting anabolism and stimulating appetite. Prior to the development of erythropoietin-stimulating agents, these medications were used to treat anemia.

Oxymetholone (Anadrol-50)	**Nutrition implications**	**Dietary considerations**
	Gastrointestinal (GI) side effects include increased appetite, nausea, vomiting, diarrhea, and mild-to-moderate liver damage.	Monitor liver function tests.
		Monitor weight (increased dry weight gain).
	May increase effects of anticoagulants by alteration of procoagulant factor synthesis (prothrombin time may increase).	Monitor creatinine, triglycerides, blood urea nitrogen, fluid retention, and electrolytes (sodium, potassium, calcium, and phosphorus).

Corticosteroids

These steroid hormones are anti-inflammatory (suppress inflammation and immunity) and assist in the breakdown of fats, carbohydrates, and proteins or act as mineralocorticoids (salt retaining) that regulate the balance of salt and water in the body. They are often used posttransplant and for patients with lupus erythematosus.

Betamethasone (Celestone Soluspan, Sernivo)	**Nutrition implications**	**Dietary considerations**
Prednisone (Rayos, Deltasone)	GI side effects include colitis, peptic ulcers, and microbe/fungal overgrowth of GI tract.	Monitor weight and edema.
Prednisolone (Omnipred)		May require increased intake of potassium, calcium, zinc, pyridoxine, folate, and vitamins A, C, and D.
Triamcinolone methylprednisolone (Kenalog)	Other side effects include hyperglycemia, weight gain, sodium retention, hypertension, anxiety, depression, steroid-induced osteoporosis, and muscle wasting.	Monitor serum changes of triglycerides and cholesterol.
Dexamethasone (Ozurdex)		
Fludrocortisone (Florinef)		
Hydrocortisone (Cortef)		

Medications for Specific Kidney Diseases and Conditions

New medications have great potential to treat kidney disease and side effects that may occur. Listed below are some that have been approved, are under US Food and Drug Administration review, or remain in developmental stages. See Box 17.9.

BOX 17.9 | Additional Medications to Consider With Chronic Kidney Disease

---

Inherited kidney diseases

AUTOSOMAL DOMINANT POLYCYSTIC KIDNEY DISEASE (ADPKD)

Most common inherited kidney cystic disease characterized by the development of kidney cysts and various extra kidney manifestations.

ALPORT SYNDROME

Inherited disease caused by mutation changes in the protein collagen, important to the normal structure and function of the kidneys, causing damage by attacking the glomeruli.

Continued on next page

Continued from previous page

Tolvaptan (Jynarque)

Vasopressin V2 receptor-specific antagonist used to slow kidney disease progression and kidney growth.

US Food and Drug Administration (FDA) approved for ADPKD.

Nutrition implications

Increased thirst sensation and may experience fluid input and output of 5 to 6 L/d.

Risk of volume depletion is high as a result of fluid loss.

Dietary considerations

Need to maintain good hydration.

Monitor hepatic enzymes.

Avoid excessive use of acetaminophen or excess alcohol consumption.

Bardoxolone

Activator of the transcription factor Nrf2 that induces molecular pathways that promote the resolution of inflammation by restoring mitochondrial function, reducing oxidative stress, and inhibiting pro-inflammatory signaling. Can result in improved estimated glomerular filtration rate with a mean decrease in blood urea nitrogen, uric acid, and phosphorus.

Under investigation for Alport syndrome and ADPKD.

Nutrition implications

Gastrointestinal (GI) side effects include nausea, decreased appetite, and weight loss.

Other side effects include muscle spasms and pain.

Dietary considerations

Monitor blood magnesium levels.

Monitor weight and signs of fluid overload.

Venglustat (Ibiglustat)

Inhibitor of glucosylceramide synthase

Lixivaptan

Vasopressin 2 receptor antagonist

Tesevatinib

M receptor tyrosine kinase inhibitor

Nutrition implications

Undergoing clinical trials.

Dietary considerations

Not available.

LUPUS NEPHRITIS

Belimumab (Benlysta)

A human monoclonal antibody that inhibits the soluble form of a B-cell survival factor known as B-lymphocyte stimulator.

Approved to treat both systemic lupus erythematosus and active lupus nephritis in adults.

Nutrition implications

GI side effects include nausea and diarrhea.

Potential side effects are urinary infections, skin sores, fever, stuffy or runny nose and sore throat, persistent cough, trouble sleeping, leg or arm pain, depression, headache, and low blood pressure.

Dietary considerations

Monitor urine output for frequency or burning.

Voclosporin (Lupkynis)

A calcineurin inhibitor, to be used in combination with background immunosuppressive therapy to treat adults with active lupus nephritis.

Nutrition implications

GI side effects include diarrhea, abdominal pain, dyspepsia, decreased appetite, and mouth ulcerations.

Other side effects include hypertension, headaches, hyperkalemia, and potential neurotoxicities.

Dietary considerations

Monitor potassium levels.

Monitor liver and kidney function.

Diabetic kidney disease

This is a common complication of type 1 and type 2 diabetes mellitus. Over time, poorly controlled diabetes can cause damage to blood vessel clusters in the kidneys that help filter waste from the blood.

Finerenone (Kerendia)

A nonsteroidal mineralocorticoid receptor antagonist. Blocks the overactivation of the mineralocorticoid receptor, which is thought to contribute to fibrosis and inflammation.

FDA approval obtained in July 2021.

Nutrition implications

Found to reduce albuminuria.

Increased risk of hyperkalemia, hypotension and hyponatremia.

Dietary considerations

Monitor serum potassium and sodium levels.

Consider use of potassium binders for consistent hyperkalemia.

Monitor liver enzymes.

Continued on next page

Continued from previous page

Metabolic acidosis

The causes of metabolic acidosis in chronic kidney disease include impaired ammonia excretion, decreased tubular reabsorption of bicarbonate and insufficient production of bicarbonate in relation to the amount of acids synthesized in the body and ingested with food.

Sodium bicarbonate	Nutrition implications	Dietary considerations
Acid neutralizer	GI side effects include flatulence and bloating. Other side effects include hypocalcemia, hypernatremia, metabolic alkalosis, and hypokalemia.	Monitor blood levels of potassium, calcium, sodium, and bicarbonate. Monitor for signs of fluid overload.
Viverimer	**Nutrition implications**	**Dietary considerations**
A nonabsorbed polymer that selectively binds and removes hydrochloric acid from the GI lumen through feces resulting in an increase in serum bicarbonate. Undergoing clinical trials.	GI side effects include diarrhea, flatulence, nausea, and constipation.	Monitor blood potassium and bicarbonate levels. Manage any GI side effects.

Pruritis

Chronic kidney disease-associated pruritus (CKD-aP), previously called uremic pruritus, is a distressing symptom experienced by patients with mainly advanced chronic kidney disease. CKD-aP is associated with poor quality of life, depression, anxiety, sleep disturbance, and increased mortality. Though often suggested, antihistamines are ineffective for CKD-aP.

Gabapentin (Gralise, Horizant)	Nutrition implications	Dietary considerations
Anticonvulsant that affects chemicals and nerves involved in seizures and neuropathic pain.	GI side effects include nausea, vomiting, heartburn, diarrhea, constipation, dry mouth, and increased appetite. Other side effects include somnolence, dizziness, loss of balance, tremulousness, and anxiety.	Monitor weight and fluid retention. Manage any GI side effects.
Pregabalin (Lyrica)	**Nutrition implications**	**Dietary considerations**
Anticonvulsant that affects chemicals in the brain that send pain signals across nervous system.	GI side effects include dry mouth, constipation, and increased appetite. Other side effects include somnolence, dizziness, loss of balance, tremulousness, and headache.	Monitor weight and fluid retention. Manage any GI side effects.
Nalfurafine	**Nutrition implications**	**Dietary considerations**
Kappa-opiod receptor agonist	GI side effects include constipation, diarrhea, nausea, and vomiting. Additional side effects include insomnia and somnolence.	Taken after dialysis.
Difelikefalin (moderate to severe CKD-aP)	**Nutrition implications**	**Dietary considerations**
A kappa-opioid receptor agonist that inhibits ion channels responsible for afferent peripheral nerve activity and also acts as an anti-inflammatory mediator with immune system cells. Under priority FDA review at the time of this publication.	Side effects: diarrhea, dizziness, vomiting, and nasopharyngitis.	Monitor blood potassium levels. Taken after dialysis.

Renal Vitamins

Micronutrients are essential for metabolic function and, hence, maintaining these micronutrients is important. Some evidence indicates that patients with CKD are likely to be deficient in certain micronutrients. Several common reasons for this include insufficient dietary intake, dialysis procedures that may contribute to micronutrient loss, improper absorption of nutrients, use of certain medications, and illness. There is a paucity of good-quality evidence on micronutrient supplementation in patients with CKD, with goals often aligning with the recommended daily allowances for the general population (see Table 17.1). There is some evidence that patients undergoing hemodialysis may be deficient in thiamin, riboflavin, vitamin B6, vitamin C, vitamin K, and vitamin D. This has not been explored in other stages of CKD or in patients on peritoneal dialysis.

The recent KDOQI Clinical Practice Guideline for Nutrition in CKD: 2020 Update recommends the following opinion statements[20]:

- It is reasonable to recommend multivitamin supplementation in patients with CKD with inadequate intake.
- It is reasonable to consider supplementation with multivitamins, including all the water-soluble vitamins and essential trace elements to prevent or treat micronutrient deficiencies in patients on dialysis who exhibit inadequate dietary intake.
- Folic acid and vitamin B12 supplementation should be prescribed for deficiency/insufficiency based on clinical signs and symptoms.
- Vitamin D supplementation is based on supplementation guidelines when 25-hydroxyvitamin D insufficiency/deficiency exists. It is also reasonable to consider supplementation in patients with nephrotic range proteinuria.

TABLE 17.1 | Adult Dietary Guidelines for Micronutrients[21]

Vitamin	Units	Recommended Daily Allowances/Dietary Reference Intakes/Adequate Intake[a]	Upper Tolerable Intake Levels[a]
Folic acid	mcg	400	1,000
Thiamin (B1)	mg	1.1-1.2	ND
Riboflavin (B2)	mg	1.1-1.3	ND
Niacin (B3)	mg	14-16	35
Pantothenic acid (B5)	mg	5	ND
Pyridoxine (B6)	mg	1.3-1.7	100
Cobalamin (B12)	mcg	2.4	ND
Biotin	mcg	30	ND
Vitamin C	mg	75-90	2,000
Vitamin D3	mcg	15-20	100
	IU	600-800	4,000
Vitamin E	mcg	15	1,000
	IU	22.4	670
Zinc	mg	8-11	40
Copper	mcg	900	10,000
Selenium	mcg	55	400
Vitamin A	mcg	700-900	3,000
Vitamin K	mcg	90-120	ND

ND = not determined

[a] Developed by the National Academies of Sciences, Engineering, and Medicine; includes female/male ranges

- Vitamin C supplementation in patients with CKD at risk for deficiency should be considered, and it is reasonable to meet the recommended intake of at least 90 mg/d for men and 75 mg/d for women. Individualized decision-making for vitamin C supplementation or discontinuation of supplementation is required.
- Due to the potential for toxicity in patients receiving dialysis, it is reasonable not to routinely supplement with vitamins A and E.
- In patients on anticoagulant medications known to inhibit vitamin K activity (eg, warfarin compounds), it is reasonable for patients not to receive vitamin K supplements.
- There is little evidence that routine supplementation of selenium and zinc improves nutritional inflammatory or micronutrient status, and thus supplementation is not recommended.

There are a number of prescription and over-the-counter renal multivitamins. It is important to know which renal multivitamin your patient is taking as part of your assessment.

Table 17.2 presents a chart of the ranges of various nutrients found in a number of renal multivitamins.

TABLE 17.2 | Summary of Potential Nutrients in a Renal Multivitamin/Multimineral Supplement

Vitamin	Units	Ranges of nutrients found in renal vitamins
Folic acid	mcg	800-1,000, some as high as 5,000
Thiamin (B1)	mg	1.5
Riboflavin (B2)	mg	1.5-1.7
Niacin (B3)	mg	20
Pantothenic acid (B5)	mg	10
Pyridoxine (B6)	mg	10-50
Cobalamin (B12)	mcg	6-2,000
Biotin	mcg	150-300
Vitamin C	mg	60-100
Vitamin D	mcg	0-50
	IU	0-2,000
Vitamin E	mcg	0-20
	IU	0-30
Zinc	mg	0-50
Copper	mg	0-1.5
Selenium	mg	0-70

References

1. Kidney Disease: Improving Global Outcomes (KDIGO) Anemia Work Group. KDIGO clinical practice guideline for anemia in chronic kidney disease. *Kidney Int Suppl*. 2012;2:279-335. doi:10.1038/kisup.2012.37

2. Kliger AS, Foley RN, Goldfarb DS, et al. KDOQI US Commentary on the 2012 KDIGO clinical practice guideline for anemia in CKD. *Am J Kidney Dis*. 2013;62(5):849-859. doi:10.1053/j.ajkd.2013.06.008

3. Anemia in Chronic Kidney Disease. National Institute of Health: National Institute of Diabetes and Digestive and Kidney Diseases website. July 2014. Accessed August 7, 2020. www.niddk.nih.gov/health-information/kidney-disease/anemia

4. FDA Drug Safety Communication: Modified dosing recommendations to improve the safe use of Erythropoiesis-Stimulating Agents (ESAs) in chronic kidney disease. US Food and Drug Administration website. August 2017. Accessed August 7, 2020. www.fda.gov/drugs/drug-safety-and-availability/fda-drug-safety-communication-modified-dosing-recommendations-improve-safe-use-erythropoiesis

5. Kidney Disease: Improving Global Outcomes (KDIGO) Lipid Work Group. KDIGO clinical practice guideline for lipid management in chronic kidney disease. *Kidney Int Suppl*. 2013;3:259-305. doi:10.1038/kisup.2013.27

6. Sarnak MJ, Bloom R, Muntner P, et al. KDOQI US Commentary on the 2013 KDIGO clinical practice guideline for lipid management in CKD. *Am J Kidney Dis*. 2015;65(3):354-366. doi:10.1053/j.ajkd.2014.10.005

7. Obialo CI, Ofili EO, Norris KC. Statins and cardiovascular disease outcomes in chronic kidney disease: reaffirmation vs. repudiation. *Int J Environ Res Public Health*. 2018;15(12):2733. doi:10.3390/ijerph15122733

8. Kidney Disease: Improving Global Outcomes (KDIGO) Blood Pressure Work Group. KDIGO clinical practice guideline for the management of blood pressure in chronic kidney disease. *Kidney Int Suppl*. 2012;2:337-414. doi:10.1038/kisup.2012.46

9. Taler SJ, Agarwal R, Bakris GL, et al. KDOQI US Commentary on the 2012 KDIGO clinical practice guideline for management of blood pressure in CKD. *Am J Kidney Dis*. 2013;62(2):201-213. doi:10.1053/j.ajkd.2013.03.018

10. Mikolasevic I, Žutelija M, Mavrinac V, Orlic L. Dyslipidemia in patients with chronic kidney disease: etiology and management. *Int J Nephrol Renovasc Dis*. 2017;10:35-45. doi:10.2147/IJNRD.S101808

11. National Kidney Foundation. KDOQI clinical practice guideline for diabetes and CKD: 2012 Update. *Am J Kidney Dis*. 2012;60(5):850-886. doi:10.1053/j.ajkd.2012.07.005

12. Ferris H, Goldman S. Medication management for the older adult with diabetes. *On the Cutting Edge*. 2019;40(2):9-13.

13. Lazarus B, Chen Y, Wilson FP, et al. Proton pump inhibitor use and the risk of chronic kidney disease. *JAMA Intern Med*. 2016;176(2):238-246. doi:10.1001/jamainternmed.2015.7193

14. Lazarus B, Grams ME. Proton pump inhibitors in kidney disease. *Clin J Am Soc Nephrol*. 2018;13(10):1458-1459. doi:10.2215/CJN.10110818

15. 2019 American Geriatrics Society Beers Criteria® Update Expert Panel. American Geriatrics Society 2019 Updated AGS Beers Criteria® for potentially inappropriate medication use in older adults. *J Am Geriatr Soc*. 2019;67(4):674-694. doi:10.1111/jgs.15767

16. Vargas-Santos AB, Neogi T. Management of gout and hyperuricemia in CKD. *Am J Kidney Dis*. 2017;70(3):422-439. doi:10.1053/j.ajkd.2017.01.055

17. Bianchi S, Aucella F, De Nicola L, Genovesi S, Paoletti E, Regolisti G. Management of hyperkalemia in patients with kidney disease: a position paper endorsed by the Italian Society of Nephrology. *J Nephrol*. 2019;32(4):499-516. doi:10.1007/s40620-019-00617-y

18. Kidney Disease: Improving Global Outcomes (KDIGO) CKD-MBD Update Work Group. KDIGO 2017 clinical practice guideline update for the diagnosis, evaluation, prevention, and treatment of Chronic Kidney Disease–Mineral and Bone Disorder (CKD–MBD). *Kidney Int Suppl*. 2017;7:1-59. doi:10.1016/j.kisu.2017.04

19. Isakova T, Nikolas TL, Denburg M, et al. KDOQI US Commentary on the 2017 KDIGO clinical practice guideline update for the diagnosis, evaluation, prevention, and treatment of Chronic Kidney Disease–Mineral and Bone Disorder (CKD–MBD). *Am J Kidney Dis*. 2017;70(6):737-751. doi:10.1053/j.ajkd.2017.07.019

20. Ikizler TA, Burrowes JD, Byham-Gray LD, et al. KDOQI clinical practice guideline for nutrition in CKD: 2020 Update. *Am J Kidney Dis*. 76(3):S1-S107. doi:10.1053/j.ajkd.2020.05.006

21. Dietary Reference Intakes (DRIs): Recommended Dietary Allowances and Adequate Intakes, Vitamins; Food and Nutrition Board, Institute of Medicine, National Academies. National Institute of Health website. August 2020. Accessed May 17, 2020. https://ods.od.nih.gov/Health_Information/Dietary_Reference_Intakes.aspx

CHAPTER 18

Oral Nutrition Supplements in Kidney Disease

Wai Yin Ho, MSEd, MS, RDN, LD

Oral Nutrition Supplements in Patients on Dialysis

The causes of protein–energy wasting (PEW) in chronic kidney disease are multifactorial.[1] Inadequate oral dietary intake is only part of this complex presentation. For patients on dialysis who are at risk of or with PEW and are unable to meet their nutritional needs through oral intake, the updated Kidney Disease Outcomes Quality Initiative (KDOQI) nutrition guidelines recommend adding a 3-month trial of oral nutrition supplements (ONS) if dietary counseling alone does not meet the patients' nutritional needs or improve their nutritional status.[2] The International Society of Renal Nutrition and Metabolism (ISRNM) also endorses providing nutrition support during dialysis, citing benefits such as reduced mortality, improved nutrition-related biochemical measurements (albumin and prealbumin), prevention of acute catabolism, increased total dietary intake, and reduction of inflammation.[3] In the same consensus report, the authors also recognize the potential adverse effects of intradialytic nutrition deterring practitioners from adopting this practice more widely. Negative factors include postprandial hypotension, reducing Kt/V and urea reduction ratio, gastrointestinal symptoms, aspiration, staff burden, and food safety concerns.[3] While these guidelines give practitioners general recommendations, a knowledge gap has been identified in terms of practical outcomes and product comparison regarding ONS pro-

grams. While there are no shortages of clinical studies investigating the effectiveness of ONS programs, the variations on supplement protocols (type, dosage, and frequency of the nutrition supplement), participants' level of adherence, and outcomes measurements make clinical comparison difficult. The clinical evidence on ONS can be roughly divided into two main types: patients consuming a daily ONS at home, and the more widely adopted and systematic ONS programs administered at dialysis centers. The purpose of this chapter is to summarize the in-center ONS outcomes studies as well as provide a description of the most commonly used ONS products.

In-Center Oral Nutrition Supplement Programs

PROGRAM DESCRIPTION

Most of the major dialysis providers offer in-center ONS programs, and some also include this option for patients on home dialysis. Different programs are similar in nature but vary in details such as initiation or discontinuation criteria or ONS product offerings. A welcoming trend is that serum albumin-based inclusion criteria has been liberalized, allowing more patients to qualify for these programs. Some providers even extend their ONS programs to all incident patients, regardless of their baseline nutritional status.[4]

Most of the supplements used are kidney specific, but there are also standard, non–kidney-specific products being utilized in the in-center ONS programs. A summary of the kidney-friendly nutrition supplements can be found in Table 18.1 on page 388.

OUTCOMES STUDIES

Since 2009, a few large dialysis providers have systematically implemented in-center ONS programs across the nation, despite the lack of reimbursement from the Centers for Medicare & Medicaid Services. Dialysis providers such as Fresenius Kidney Care (FKC), Dialysis Clinic, Inc (DCI), DaVita Kidney Care, and Satellite Healthcare have all conducted retrospective outcome studies to evaluate their program effectiveness (see Table 18.2 on page 390).[5-8] The Fresenius Medical Care Health Plan (FMCHP), a participant of the Medicare Advantage Plans disease management program, has also implemented an ONS program for its beneficiaries who are on dialysis and qualify for malnutrition, with program criteria and outcomes being published.[5]

Similar to earlier studies conducted in the area of renal nutrition, the primary outcome measures of previous ONS studies focused on mortality risk and/or a singular nutrition indicator, such as serum albumin. More recent ONS studies have expanded the outcome measures to include other clinical outcomes (eg, hospitalization rates), missed treatments, and nutritional indicators (eg, normalized protein catabolic rate and body weight) (see Table 18.2).

MORTALITY

FKC was one of the early adopters of in-center ONS programs and was the first major dialysis provider to publish their outcomes. The outcomes studies from FKC, DCI, and DaVita Kidney Care were quite promising, as all found that ONS administration was significantly related to mortality reduction within the evaluated cohorts.[6-8]

NUTRITIONAL OUTCOMES

Most of the older ONS studies selected the singular nutrition indicator of serum albumin as the primary outcome measure. Serum albumin, however, did not show a significant improvement in the mortality rate with regard to ONS outcomes. The FKC study originally measured serum albumin as one of the end outcomes but decided to remove this measure when a systematic drop in serum albumin level was observed during the follow-up period. This observation was caused by a change in the laboratory serum albumin assay being used. The DCI study showed a slight improvement in albumin in both the ONS and control groups, but the overall difference was insignificant.[6] Similarly, the FMCHP study showed improvement in albumin in the beginning (month 1), but the effect subsided as time passed until the difference of albumin between the groups was no longer significant by month 12.[5] The DaVita study showed that the serum albumin level was lower among ONS patients than matched controls at the completion of the study.[8]

OTHER CLINICAL OUTCOMES

Using FKC's cohort data, Leonberg-Yoo et al[9] recently published their findings of the FKC ONS program's outcomes in terms of a 30-day hospital readmission rate. The readmission rate of the ONS group (19%) was half that of the control group (38.7%). DaVita's ONS cohort had a 23% lower missed treatment rate and 8% lower hospitalization rate compared to the control group.[8] In a poster presentation, Pace et al[4] describe the outcomes of Satellite Healthcare's ONS program extension to all incident hemodialysis patients, which resulted in a 6% reduction in hospitalization rate after 1 year of observation. A summary of the in-center ONS program outcome studies can be found in Table 18.1.*

---

* Organization-specific protocols may have been changed since the publication of the studies.

Other Evidence on Oral Nutrition Supplement Programs

In addition to the outcomes studies of in-center ONS programs by major dialysis providers, there are other clinical trials examining ONS effect. The results of many of the randomized controlled trials (RCT) on ONS with kidney disease that have been published since 2000 are summarized in Table 18.3 (see page 392). Most of the results show slight improvement in serum albumin, but the difference between the ONS and control groups was not significant statistically. The only RCT that shows significant improvement in serum albumin from the ONS is the Anti-Inflammatory and Anti-Oxidative Nutrition in Hypoalbuminemic Dialysis Patients (AIONID) study that provides Nepro in combination with an anti-inflammatory and antioxidant module (similar to the ingredients in Oxepa). In this study, the supplementation was provided to patients six times per week vs the three-times-a-week protocol in all of the in-center ONS programs.[10]

Outside of RCTs, there are smaller and nonrandomized studies examining the effects of ONS in patients on dialysis. These nonrandomized trials on ONS programs yield more favorable results on serum albumin levels.[11-19] However, they are usually smaller in scale and have a shorter intervention period. Moreover, there are wide variations in study design, nutrition supplement formula and protocol, subjects' inclusion and exclusion criteria, as well as patient compliance level. Therefore, it is difficult to have a fair comparison and draw a conclusion regarding the program effectiveness of ONS from these studies.

Implication on Practice

After review of the clinical evidence measuring the effectiveness of both in-center and daily ONS programs,

common clinical outcome indicators have primarily focused on measurements for serum albumin, hospitalization, and mortality. However, it is important to consider program effectiveness in other measures. For example, a comprehensive nutritional assessment can be represented quantitatively by using composite nutrition assessment scores such as the subjective global assessment (SGA) and malnutrition–inflammation score (MIS) recommended by the updated 2020 KDOQI Nutrition guidelines.[2] Other potential outcome measurements include a functional status evaluation, health-related quality of life measurements, self-reported appetite, overall well-being, and impact on dietary intake. A newer and ongoing clinical trial that examines the impact of ONS is called the Nutritional Outcomes From a Randomised Investigation of Intradialytic Oral Nutritional Supplements In Patients Receiving Haemodialysis (NOURISH) trial. This trial is designed to measure some of these aforementioned outcomes aside from the more traditional clinical and biometrical measurements.[20,21]

As the health care industry is more aware of the importance of patients' quality of life, so are researchers in focusing on and investigating studies with meaningful, patient-centered outcomes. Byham-Gray et al[22] recently updated the ISRNM 2008 PEW definition by incorporating patients' and clinicians' perspectives and affirming the importance of the proposed clinical outcomes. Besides survival, patients ranked avoiding hospitalization, increased activity (including traveling and volunteerism), and improving quality of life as their most important outcomes. Ideally, this new model will guide researchers to construct and conduct patient-centered outcomes research in the area of PEW and the effectiveness of nutrition interventions, such as ONS. This will, in turn, provide clinicians more meaningful and practical findings on nutrition-focused interventions.

TABLE 18.1 | Renal-Friendly Oral Nutrition Supplement Products

Name	Manufacturer	Type	Flavors available	Serving size
Nepro Carb Steady[23]	Abbott	Complete nutrition, liquid	Vanilla, mixed berry, butter pecan	8 fl oz (237 mL) can
Novasource Renal[24]	Nestlé	Complete nutrition, liquid	Vanilla	8 fl oz (237 mL) carton
Gelatein 20[25]	Medtrition	Protein, gelatin	Grape, fruit punch, lime, orange	4 fl oz (118 mL)
Liquacel	Global Health	Protein only liquid	Grape, lemonade, orange, peach mango, watermelon	1 fl oz (30 mL) 32-oz bottle, 64-oz bottle with pump or 1-oz packet
Prostat Renal[26]	Medical Nutrition USA	Protein only liquid	Citrus, grape, vanilla, cherry	1 fl oz (30 mL) or 32-oz bottle
Prosource[27]	Medtrition	Protein only liquid	Natural flavor	1 fl oz (30 mL) or 30-oz bottle
Proteinex Hydrolyzed Liquid Protein	Llorens	Protein only liquid	Unflavored	1 fl oz (30 mL)
Zone Bars	Zone Perfect	Protein bars	Multiple flavors, may include chocolate and nuts (consider allergies)	1 bar (50 g)
Procel Whey Protein[28]	Global Health	Protein powder	Unflavored (nutrition values based on unflavored, vanilla, chocolate)	5 g 10-oz can or single serving packet
ReGen BCAA	RSP Nutrition	Protein powder	Watermelon and fruit punch	8.8 g Comes in 264 g canister
Renal Support	Kate Farms, Inc.	Complete nutrition, liquid	Vanilla	8.45 oz (250 mL) carton

BCAA = branched chain amino acids | ND = no data

Total Kcal	Total protein (g) / Protein source	Fat (g) (total/saturated/ polyunsaturated/ monosaturated/ cholesterol) / Fat source	Carbohydrate (g) (total/fiber/sugar) / Main sugar source	Sodium (mg)	Potassium (mg)	Calcium (mg)	Phosphorus (mg)
425	19.1 / Milk protein isolate	22.7/2/4.1/16/6.5 / Safflower oil, canola oil	37.9/3/8.4 / Corn syrup solids, sugar	250	250	250	170
475	21.6 / Milk & soy proteins	23.8/ND / Canola oil	43.5/ND / Corn syrup, sugar	225	225	200	195
80-90	20 / Collagen hydrolyzate and whey protein isolate	0	2/1/0 / Sucralose	25-55	120-180	20-57	0-1
100	16 / Hydrolyzed collagen protein, L-arginine, whey protein isolate	0	9/0/0 / Glycerin	50	10	32	20
100	15 / Hydrolyzed collagen protein	0	10/ND / Glycerin	50	20	ND	50
100	15 / Collagen and whey protein isolate blend	0	16/0/8 / Maltodextrin, fructose	45	15	3	75
60	15 / Hydrolyzed collagen protein	0	0/0/0	5	8	ND	2
210	14 / Soy protein	7/4/ND/ND/<5 mg / Safflower oil	23/3/15 / Corn syrup, various ingredients such as chocolate, caramel, and marshmallow, depending on flavors	200	90	400	200
25	5 / Whey protein concentrate, soy lecithin	0.5/0/ND	0	12	35	80	ND
ND	6 g BCAA	ND	ND	47	105	ND	ND
450	20 / Pea protein	22/10/8/3.5 / Coconut oil, sunflower oil, flaxseed oil	43/4/12 / Brown rice syrup solids, agave	250	250	300	190

TABLE 18.2 | Oral Nutrition Supplements Program Outcomes Studies

Lead author	Year	N	Inclusion criteria	ONS type (provided 3 times per week)
Lacson[7] (Fresenius Kidney Care ONS program)	2012	AT:4,298 matched pairs ITT = 5,227 matched pairs	Albumin ≤3.5, stop when reach ≥4	4 products (Nepro, Prostat, Zone bar, Vital Protein bar): 14-20 g protein
Leonberg-Yoo[9] (data from Fresenius Kidney Care ONS program)	2019	Same cohort as above	Same as above	Same as above
Weiner[6] (evaluate Dialysis Clinic, Inc, ONS program)	2014	AT: 439 matched pairs ITT: 1,278 matched pairs	Albumin ≤3.5, stop when reach ≥4	Liquacel: 16 g protein Novasource Renal: 21.6 g protein
Kistler[3] (DaVita ONS program)	2017	3,374 matched pairs	Albumin ≤3.5	Liquacel: 16 g protein Novasource Renal: 21.6 g protein
Pace[4] (Satellite Healthcare)	2019	No details	New (first 90 days) patients in-center hemodialysis, regardless of nutritional status ONS provided for 30 days, follow existing ONS protocol afterward	Prostat 30 mL: 15 g protein
Cheu[5] (evaluate Fresenius Medical Care Health Plan disease management ONS program)	2013	470	Albumin <3.8; stop when 3 month avg albumin ≥3.8	Ensure Plus (13 g protein) Glucerna (14 g protein) 24 cans Ensure Plus or Glucerna per month. Patients were asked to consume 1 can/d.

AT = as treated | ITT = intention to treat | nPCR = normalized protein catabolic rate | ONS = oral nutrition supplements | OR = odds ratio

Outcomes	Serum albumin
Survival advantage of ONS group compared to control: +34% (AT); +9% (ITT analysis). Greatest effect of ONS on mortality observed in patients with lowest baseline albumin (albumin ≤3.2).	Did not use albumin as end outcome because change in laboratory assay skewed the results.
ONS treated group average 19% 30-day hospital readmission rate vs 38.7% in the control group. The individuals who did not receive ONS had more than double the odds of 30-day readmission (OR, 2.26) than those who received ONS. After adjusting for covariants and matching individuals' clinical and demographic backgrounds, the odds are still close to double (OR, 1.71).	
Mortality in the ONS group reduced by 25%-27% (ITT) and 26%-32% (AT) compared to the control group.	Both groups had small improvement in albumin (increased 0.015/mo [ONS] and increased 0.013/mo [control]) but no significant difference in change in albumin between groups in the AT model.
ONS group: 69% reduction in mortality, 33% fewer missed dialysis treatments. ONS group had lower albumin than control, but higher nPCR and postdialysis body weight.	Similar slightly upward trend in albumin in ONS and control groups. ONS group had lower starting albumin and remained lower than control group throughout the study (8 months).
89% of new patients qualified and received ONS. Hospitalization per patient year dropped from 1 per year for incident patients prior to this program to 0.94 per year 1 year after program implementation (6% reduction). Incident patients who did not receive ONS had 1.02 admissions per patient year.	Did not measure.
ONS group has significantly lower hospitalization (68.4%) than control group (88.7%). No significant reduction in mortality risk between the ONS and control group.	Albumin in ONS group was 0.058 higher than control group in month 1. This difference decreased by 0.001/mo to 0.052 at month 6. The difference between the groups is no longer significant by month 12.

TABLE 18.3 | Randomized Controlled Trial on Oral Nutrition Supplement Programs

Lead author	Year	Study design	N	Comparison	ONS type	ONS regimen
Cano[29]	2007	RCT 1 year	N = 186 ONS (93) ONS + IDPN (93)	ONS vs ONS + IDPN	ONS 500 kcal/25 g protein ONS – 5.9 kcal, 0.39 g protein/kg/d IDPN – 6.6 kcal, 0.26 g protein/kg/d	Every treatment 3×/wk × 1 year
Fouque[30]	2008	RCT 3 mo	N = 86	ONS vs standard care	Renilon (Netherlands) 500 kcal/18.75 g protein	125 mL 2×/d every day × 3 mo
Moretti[31]	2009	RCT 1 yr	N = 49	ONS vs control (crossover design)	Proteinex (15 g protein)	1 oz every treatment 3×/wk × 6 mo (HD) 1 oz given daily 7×/wk (PD)
Rattanasompattikul[10]	2013	RCT 4-mo intervention period + 1-month follow-up	N = 93	A: (n = 19) Nepro + AIAO + PTX B: (n = 22) Nepro + AIAO C: (n = 22) PTX D: (n = 21) placebo	Nepro (2 cans) + AIAO + PTX (38.2 g protein)	6 days/wk supplementation
Beddhu[32]	2015	Prospective 24-week longitudinal study	N = 50	Baseline vs intervention phase vs observation phase	45 g protein	45 g liquid protein every treatment × 24 wks
Tomayko[33]	2015	RCT (6-mo intervention)	N = 38	Whey vs soy protein nutrition supplement	Whey protein (27 g protein) and soy protein (27 g protein) vs placebo	1 drink pretreatment every treatment × 6 mo
Sahathevan[34]	2018	RCT 6-mo intervention	N = 126	Whey protein supplement + dietary counseling vs dietary counseling only	Whey protein powder (27.4 g protein)	2 packs of whey protein powder to be dissolved in water daily for 6 mo

AIAO = anti-inflammatory antioxidant | BMI = body mass index | CRP = C-reactive protein | HD = hemodialysis | IBW = ideal body weight | IDPN = intradialytic parenteral nutrition | IL-6 = interleukin-6 | MAMC = mid-arm muscle circumference | MIS = malnutrition–inflammation score | nPNA = normalized protein nitrogen appearance | ONS = oral nutrition supplement | PD = peritoneal dialysis | PNA = protein nitrogen appearance | PTX = pentoxifylline | QoL = quality of life | RCT = randomized control trial | SGA = subjective global assessment

Subjects qualifiers	Outcomes	Serum albumin
HD Any 2 of these: BMI <20 Weight decrease >10% in 6 mo Albumin <3.5 Prealbumin <30	No significant difference in mortality rate between groups. After 3 months, increases seen with BMI, albumin, and prealbumin in both groups. Increase in prealbumin of >30 within 3 mo predicts improved 2-year survival, hospital rate, and Karnofsky score.	Albumin levels increase from baseline of ~3.1 to ~3.3 in 3 mo in both groups; then the rate of increase slowed down and was maintained at around 3.38 at mo 12 in the ONS group but drops back down to 3.3 in the ONS + IDPN group.
HD Albumin <4 BMI <30 nPNA <1 exclude CRP >20	Significant increase in daily kcal/protein intake in the ONS group compared to the control group. Significant improvement in SGA and Qo in the ONS group compared to the control group. Serum phosphorus level was not affected by ONS consumption.	No difference between albumin and prealbumin between groups.
HD and PD Did not describe qualifications criteria	When ONS ended, weight decreased significantly for those with BMI <20. Hospital days decreased in both groups.	In the ONS group, albumin increased from 3.49 to 3.53. The control group had a significant decrease in albumin (from 3.35 to 3.29) after discontinuing ONS.
HD Albumin <4	All 3 intervention groups had an improvement in albumin, but only the ONS group without PTX was significant. No significant decline in inflammatory markers non-serum leptin.	Albumin increased by 0.21 (B), 0.18 (A), 0.14 (C), and 0.03 (D).
HD CRP >3 mg/L	PNA increased by 0.13 g/kg/d in intervention period compared with baseline. No clinically or statistically significant effects on MAMC, plasma albumin, BMI, physical or mental composite scores.	Baseline mean serum albumin = 3.8. No significant change after intervention period.
HD (no clinical or nutritional criteria)	IL-6 significantly decreased in both protein groups compared with control. Downward trend in CRP in both protein groups but insignificant difference. Gait speed and shuttle walk test performance significantly improved in both protein supplement groups. No change in body composition.	No significant change in albumin between protein supplement and control groups.
PD Dialysis vintage ≥6 mo Albumin <4, BMI of <24	Significantly higher proportion of patients achieved dietary protein intake goal of 1.2 g/kg IBW in the intervention group (59.5%) than in the control group (16.2%). Although statistically nonsignificant, the intervention group also had greater increase in postdialysis weight and MAMC. More patients in the intervention group (42.9%) improved their MIS score than the control group (29.7%). Insignificant between-group differences were observed in the following parameters: CRP, QoL, and handgrip strength.	Insignificant difference between groups.

References

1. Fouque D, Kalantar-Zadeh K, Kopple J, et al. A proposed nomenclature and diagnostic criteria for protein–energy wasting in acute and chronic kidney disease. *Kidney Int.* 2008;73(4):391-398. doi:10.1038/sj.ki.5002585

2. Ikizler T, Burrowes J, Byham-Gray L, et al. KDOQI Nutrition in CKD Guideline Work Group. KDOQI Clinical practice guideline for nutrition in chronic kidney disease: 2020 Update. *Am J Kidney Dis.* 2020;76(3 suppl 1):S1-S107. doi:10.1053/j.ajkd.2020.05.006

3. Kistler BM, Benner D, Burrowes JD, et al. Eating during hemodialysis treatment: a consensus statement from the International Society of Renal Nutrition and Metabolism. *J Ren Nutr.* 2018;28(1):4-12. doi:10.1053/j.jrn.2017.10.003

4. Pace R, Reiterman M, Sun S, Abra G, Schiller B. Impact of nutrition supplements on hospitalization rates in incident hemodialysis patients. *J Ren Nutr.* 2019;29(3):262. doi:10.1053/j.jrn.2019.03.070

5. Cheu C, Pearson J, Dahlerus C, et al. Association between oral nutritional supplementation and clinical outcomes among patients with ESRD. *Clin J Am Soc Nephrol.* 2013;8(1):100-107. doi:10.2215/CJN.13091211

6. Weiner DE, Tighiouart H, Ladik V, Meyer KB, Zager PG, Johnson DS. Oral intradialytic nutritional supplement use and mortality in hemodialysis patients. *Am J Kidney Dis.* 2014;63(2):276-285. doi:10.1053/j.ajkd.2013.08.007

7. Lacson E Jr, Wang W, Zebrowski B, Wingard R, Hakim RM. Outcomes associated with intradialytic oral nutritional supplements in patients undergoing maintenance hemodialysis: a quality improvement report. *Am J Kidney Dis.* 2012;60(4):591-600. doi:10.1053/j.ajkd.2012.04.019

8. Benner D, Brunelli SM, Brosch B, Wheeler J, Nissenson AR. Effects of oral nutritional supplements on mortality, missed dialysis treatments, and nutritional markers in hemodialysis patients. *J Ren Nutr.* 2018;28(3):191-196. doi:10.1053/j.jrn.2017.10.002

9. Leonberg-Yoo AK, Wang W, Weiner DE, Lacson E Jr. Oral nutritional supplements and 30-day readmission rate in hypoalbuminemic maintenance hemodialysis patients. *Hemodial Int.* 2019;23(1):93-100. doi:10.1111/hdi.12694

10. Rattanasompattikul M, Molnar MZ, Lee ML, et al. Anti-Inflammatory and Anti-Oxidative Nutrition in Hypoalbuminemic Dialysis Patients (AIONID) study: results of the pilot-feasibility, double-blind, randomized, placebo-controlled trial. *J Cachexia Sarcopenia Muscle.* 2013;4(4):247-257. doi:10.1007/s13539-013-0115-9

11. Kalantar-Zadeh K, Cano NJ, Budde K, et al. Diets and enteral supplements for improving outcomes in chronic kidney disease. *Nat Rev Nephrol.* 2011;7(7):369-384. doi:10.1038/nrneph.2011.60

12. Patel MG, Kitchen S, Miligan PJ. The effect of dietary supplements on the nPCR in stable hemodialysis patients. *J Ren Nutr.* 2000;10(2):69-75. doi:10.1016/s1051-2276(00)90002-5

13. Bronich L, Te T, Shetye K, Stewart T, Eustace JA. Successful treatment of hypoalbuminemic hemodialysis patients with a modified regimen of oral essential amino acids. *J Ren Nutr.* 2001;11(4):194-201. doi:10.1016/S1051-2276(01)70037-4

14. Caglar K, Fedje L, Dimmitt R, Hakim RM, Shyr Y, Ikizler TA. Therapeutic effects of oral nutritional supplementation during hemodialysis. *Kidney Int.* 2002;62(3):1054-1059. doi:10.1046/j.1523-1755.2002.00530.x

15. Hiroshige K, Sonta T, Suda T, Kanegae K, Ohtani A. Oral supplementation of branched-chain amino acid improves nutritional status in elderly patients on chronic haemodialysis. *Nephrol Dial Transplant.* 2001;16(9):1856-1862. doi:10.1093/ndt/16.9.1856

16. Holley JL, Kirk J. Enteral tube feeding in a cohort of chronic hemodialysis patients. *J Ren Nutr.* 2002;12(3):177-182. doi:10.1053/jren.2002.33514

17. Oguz Y, Bulucu F, Vural A. Oral and parenteral essential amino acid therapy in malnourished hemodialysis patients. *Nephron.* 2001;89(2):224-227. doi:10.1159/000046072

18. Poole R, Hamad A. Nutrition supplements in dialysis patients: use in peritoneal dialysis patients and diabetic patients. *Adv Perit Dial.* 2008;24:118-124.

19. Scott MK, Shah NA, Vilay AM, Thomas J 3rd, Kraus MA, Mueller BA. Effects of peridialytic oral supplements on nutritional status and quality of life in chronic hemodialysis patients. *J Ren Nutr.* 2009;19(2):145-152. doi:10.1053/j.jrn.2008.08.004

20. Jackson L, Cohen J, Sully B, Julious S. NOURISH, Nutritional OUtcomes from a Randomised Investigation of Intradialytic oral nutritional Supplements in patients receiving Haemodialysis: a pilot randomised controlled trial. *Pilot Feasibility Stud.* 2015;1:11. doi:10.1186/s40814-015-0007-1

21. Jackson L, Sully B, Cohen J, Julious S. Nutritional outcomes from a randomised investigation of intradialytic oral nutritional supplements in patients receiving haemodialysis, (NOURISH): a protocol for a pilot randomised controlled trial. *SpringerPlus*. 2013;2:515. doi:10.1186/2193-1801-2-515

22. Byham-Gray LD, Peters EN, Rothpletz-Puglia P. Patient-centered model for protein–energy wasting: stakeholder deliberative panels. *J Ren Nutr*. 2020;30(2):137-144. doi:10.1053/j.jrn.2019.06.001

23. Nepro® Carb Steady. Abbott website. January 2020. Accessed August 30, 2019. https://abbottnutrition.com/nepro-with-carbsteady

24. Novasource Renal. Nestlé Health Science Medical Hub website. January 2020. Accessed August 30, 2019. www.nestlehealthscience.us/brands/novasource/novasource-renal-hcp

25. Gelatein 20. Medtrition website. January 2021. Accessed February 27, 2021. https://medtrition.com/product/gelatein-20

26. Pro-Stat Sugar Free Liquid Protein. Vitality Medical website. January 2020. Accessed August 21, 2020. https://vitalitymedical.com/pro-stat-sugar-free-liquid-protein.html

27. Prosource Liquid Protein. Medtrition website. January 2021. Accessed February 27, 2021. https://medtrition.com/product/prosource-liquid-protein

28. ProCel Unflavored Whey Protein. Global Health Products, Inc website. January 2020. Accessed August 30, 2019. https://globalhp.com/shop/procel-whey-protein

29. Cano NJ, Fouque D, Roth H, et al. Intradialytic parenteral nutrition does not improve survival in malnourished hemodialysis patients: a 2-year multicenter, prospective, randomized study. *J Am Soc Nephrol*. 2007;18(9):2583-2591. doi:10.1681/ASN.2007020184

30. Fouque D, McKenzie J, de Mutsert R, et al. Use of a renal-specific oral supplement by haemodialysis patients with low protein intake does not increase the need for phosphate binders and may prevent a decline in nutritional status and quality of life. *Nephrol Dial Transplant*. 2008;23(9):2902-2910. doi:10.1093/ndt/gfn131

31. Moretti HD, Johnson AM, Keeling-Hathaway TJ. Effects of protein supplementation in chronic hemodialysis and peritoneal dialysis patients. *J Ren Nutr*. 2009;19(4):298-303. doi:10.1053/j.jrn.2009.01.029

32. Beddhu S, Filipowicz R, Chen X, et al. Supervised oral protein supplementation during dialysis in patients with elevated C-reactive protein levels: a two phase, longitudinal, single center, open labeled study. *BMC Nephrol*. 2015;16:87. doi:10.1186/s12882-015-0070-0

33. Tomayko EJ, Kistler BM, Fitschen PJ, Wilund KR. Intradialytic protein supplementation reduces inflammation and improves physical function in maintenance hemodialysis patients. *J Ren Nutr*. 2015;25(3):276-283. doi:10.1053/j.jrn.2014.10.005

34. Sahathevan S, Se CH, Ng S, et al. Clinical efficacy and feasibility of whey protein isolates supplementation in malnourished peritoneal dialysis patients: a multicenter, parallel, open-label randomized controlled trial. *Clin Nutr ESPEN*. 2018;25:68-77. doi:10.1016/j.clnesp.2018.04.002

CHAPTER 19

Commonly Used Dietary Supplements in Patients With Kidney Disease

Aida L. Moreno-Brown, MS, RD, LD

Introduction

A law passed by US Congress in 1994 called the Dietary Supplement Health and Education Act (DSHEA) provided our current definition of a dietary supplement.[1] According to DSHEA, a dietary supplement is a product that acts in the following manner:

- It is intended to supplement the diet.
- It contains one or more ingredients inclusive of vitamins, minerals, herbs or botanicals, amino acids, and certain other substances.
- It is taken by mouth in the form of a tablet, capsule, powder, gel cap, or liquid.
- It is labeled as a dietary supplement.

Herbal supplements are one type of dietary supplement. The term botanical is often used as another name for an herb. An herb is a plant or plant part (ie, leaves, flowers, seeds, or root) that is used for its flavor, scent, and therapeutic properties.

The use of complementary and alternative medicine (CAM) therapies is growing at a remarkable rate worldwide. Botanicals and dietary supplements are a subset of CAM therapies that have grown faster than any other CAM therapy in the United States. However, the prevalence of use among individuals with chronic kidney disease (CKD) is unknown and thought to be underreported to health care providers. In 2004, Burrowes and Van Houten[2] conducted a survey of renal registered dietitian nutritionists to better understand the prevalence of botanical and dietary supplement use among patients receiving dialysis in the United States. A list of 45 botanicals and dietary supplements was generated.[2] More recently, Nowack et al[3] conducted a survey regarding the use of dietary supplements among patients with CKD stage 5 and kidney transplant recipients in Germany. The results revealed a total of 41 different products that were being consumed by patients with CKD.[3] This chapter reviews 22 of the most commonly reported botanicals and dietary supplements used by patients with CKD based on these two studies. (Note: Hereafter, botanicals will be referred to as *dietary supplements*.)

There are numerous concerns regarding the use of dietary supplements in the population with CKD. Some concerns are due to direct toxicity to the kidney (those containing aristolochic acid being the most well known) and other concerns are due to an indirect effect in the population with CKD.[4-6] Dietary supplements contain many pharmacologically active compounds that may interact with medications or other dietary supplements commonly taken by individuals with CKD. The active and inactive ingredients in dietary supplements can build up to toxic levels because of reduced kidney function. The purity of dietary supplements is not guaranteed and, thus, products may contain contaminants harmful to patients with CKD (eg, aluminum, lead, and mercury).[7] Finally, various products may contain potassium and/or phosphorus in amounts sufficient to cause hyperkalemia and hyperphosphatemia.[4] Given these various concerns, in their 2012 guideline regarding the evaluation and management of patients with CKD, the Kidney Disease Improving Global Outcomes (KDIGO) work group recommends that these patients do not use herbal remedies.[8] To avoid potential harm from use of dietary supplements, kidney health care providers need to initiate discussions with their patients about the appropriate use of dietary supplements. It is important to establish a level of trust and rapport to place the patient at ease and promote open communication concerning dietary supplement use.

The content for each dietary supplement is organized as follows: background information; scientific evidence for use based on a grade of either A (strong) or B (good) (those indications graded C, D, or F are not included) (see Box 19.1); dosage; safety considerations; interactions with drugs and other dietary supplements; and implications for use in patients with CKD.

BOX 19.1 | Strong and Good Grade Defined[9]

Strong (A): Statistically significant evidence of benefit from more than two properly randomized controlled trials (RCTs), or evidence from one properly conducted RCT and one properly conducted meta-analysis, or evidence from multiple RCTs with a clear majority of the properly conducted trials showing statistically significant evidence of benefit and with supporting evidence in basic science, animal studies, or theory.

Good (B): Statistically significant evidence of benefit from one or two properly conducted RCTs, or evidence of benefit from at least one properly conducted meta-analysis, or evidence of benefit from more than one cohort/case control/non-RCT and with supporting evidence in basic science, animal studies, or theory. This grade applies to situations in which a well-designed RCT reports negative results but stands in contrast to the positive efficacy results of multiple other less well-designed trials or a well-designed meta-analysis while awaiting confirmatory evidence from an additional well-designed RCT.

Ascorbic Acid (Vitamin C)

BACKGROUND

Ascorbic acid (vitamin C) is a vitamin the body needs to form blood vessels, cartilage, muscle, and collagen in bones and plays an integral role in the body's healing process. As an antioxidant, vitamin C may help protect cells against the effects of free radicals. Vitamin C can also facilitate the body's ability to absorb and store iron.

Ascorbic acid is used to prevent or treat low levels of vitamin C in individuals who do not get enough of the vitamin from their diets. Most people who eat a varied diet do not need additional ascorbic acid. Low levels of vitamin C can result in a condition called scurvy.

SCIENTIFIC EVIDENCE

Evidence for vitamin C is good (B). Research on the use of vitamin C for specific conditions shows the following:

- A diet rich in fruits and vegetables may lower the risk of several types of cancer, such as breast, colon, and lung cancers. It is unclear, however, whether the protective effect of these foods is related solely to their vitamin C content as taking oral vitamin C supplements does not appear to offer the same benefit.

- Taking vitamin C supplements does not prevent the common cold. However, when those who regularly take vitamin C supplements get a cold, there is some evidence that the illness lasts fewer days and the symptoms are less severe. Taking a vitamin C supplement only after developing a cold offers no benefits.

- Taking vitamin C supplements in combination with other vitamins and minerals seems to prevent age-related macular degeneration (AMD) from progressing.[10]

DOSAGE

The recommended dietary allowance (RDA) of vitamin C for adult males is 90 mg/d and for adult females is 75 mg/d*.[11]

*Specific recommendations for transgender people were not provided.

SAFETY

Allergies

This product may contain inactive ingredients (such as peanut/soy) that can cause allergic reactions.

Adverse Effects and Warnings

When taken at appropriate doses, oral vitamin C supplements are generally considered safe for the general population. Individuals with CKD should only take the amount of supplemental vitamin C that is present in the typical renal multivitamin supplement.

Side effects tend to be dose related. Oral vitamin C supplements can cause nausea, vomiting, heartburn, esophagitis, intestinal obstruction, stomach cramps, fatigue, headache, sleepiness, diarrhea, skin flushing, and insomnia. Oral use of vitamin C can cause kidney stones in certain individuals. Long-term daily use of greater than 2,000 mg increases the risk of significant side effects.[10]

INTERACTIONS WITH DRUGS AND DIETARY SUPPLEMENTS

Possible interactions include the following:

- There might be increased absorption of aluminum from medications and dietary supplements containing aluminum.
- Vitamin C during chemotherapy might reduce the drug's effect.
- Vitamin C with oral contraceptives or hormone replacement therapy might increase estrogen levels.
- Use of vitamin C might reduce the effect of protease inhibitors.
- Vitamin C with niacin could reduce niacin's effect.
- High doses of vitamin C might reduce response to warfarin (Coumadin) and Jantoven.[10]

IMPLICATIONS FOR USE IN PATIENTS WITH CHRONIC KIDNEY DISEASE

Vitamin C is partially metabolized to oxalate, which can lead to secondary oxalosis in patients with CKD.

Oxalate can be deposited in many organs, including the kidneys, in tissues (eg, eye, skin, and cardiac muscle), and within joints. The dose of supplemental vitamin C at which this occurs is unknown; thus, patients with CKD are typically advised to not exceed the dose commonly found in renal multivitamins.[12]

Anemia is common in patients receiving dialysis. Administration of supplemental vitamin C (either intravenously or orally) can, in some cases, mitigate this concern, as vitamin C contributes to necessary iron delivery. The safety of this practice requires careful evaluation to determine which vitamin C dosage is effective while also avoiding complications of oxalosis.[13]

Aloe vera (Aloe barbadensis), Burn Plant, Lily of the Desert, Elephant's Gall

BACKGROUND

Aloe vera's use can be traced back 6,000 years to early Egypt. Known as the "plant of immortality," aloe was presented as a funeral gift to pharaohs. Aloe, a cactus-like plant, has been used to treat wounds, hair loss, and hemorrhoids and has also been used as a laxative. Two substances, gel and latex, are contained in the aloe plant. The gel is a clear, jelly-like substance found in the inner leaf, and the latex is a yellow-colored substance found just under the plant's skin. The clear gel and the yellow latex are used in health products. Aloe gel is primarily used topically as a remedy for skin conditions, such as burns, frostbite, psoriasis, and cold sores, but it may also be taken orally for conditions including osteoarthritis, bowel diseases, and fever. Aloe latex is taken orally, usually for constipation.

SCIENTIFIC EVIDENCE

Some scientific evidence exists for the topical use of aloe; however, there is not enough evidence regarding the efficacy for any of its other uses.[14]

DOSAGE

In research, oral doses of aloe gel at 15 mL/d have been prescribed for 42 days. Twice daily application is generally recommended for topical use.[15]

SAFETY

Allergies

Contact dermatitis is possible with topical use.

Adverse Effects and Warnings

Topical use of aloe gel is generally safe when used as directed. Oral consumption of aloe gel is considered "possibly safe" when used appropriately and for only short periods of time. Oral intake of aloe latex or the whole-leaf extract containing latex is "possibly unsafe" at any dose and deemed "likely unsafe" at high doses.[15] Aloe latex can cause stomach pain and cramps. High doses of aloe latex may cause diarrhea, kidney problems, hematuria, hypokalemia, muscle weakness, weight loss, and heart disturbances. Use of aloe latex of 1 g/d for several days can be fatal.[14]

INTERACTIONS WITH DRUGS AND DIETARY SUPPLEMENTS

Aloe should not be taken with digoxin (Lanoxin), and caution should be applied for use with medications for diabetes (DM), sevoflurane (Ultane), stimulant laxatives, warfarin (Coumadin), and diuretic drugs. When taken orally, preparations containing aloe latex act as a stimulant laxative that can decrease potassium levels. Low potassium levels can increase the risk of side effects from digoxin and result in hypokalemia when taken with diuretic drugs that also lower potassium levels. This stimulant laxative when taken with other stimulant laxatives can increase bowel transit time to the point that dehydration and low electrolytes are a concern. The resulting increase in bowel transit (eg, diarrhea) can increase the effects of warfarin and thus the risk of bleeding. Aloe might also decrease blood clotting which can be of concern during surgery when anesthetic medications such as sevoflurane are used, which also decrease

the clotting of blood (see Box 19.2 on page 402). Aloe can also lower blood glucose (BG) levels which can be problematic when taken with DM medications.[14]

IMPLICATIONS FOR USE IN PATIENTS WITH CHRONIC KIDNEY DISEASE

Oral intake of aloe products is contraindicated in patients with kidney concerns as it is associated with electrolyte imbalance and medication interactions.[16]

Biotin (Vitamin B7)

BACKGROUND

Biotin, also called vitamin B7 and formerly known as vitamin H or coenzyme R, is a water-soluble B vitamin. Biotin is involved in many metabolic processes related to the utilization of fats, carbohydrates, and amino acids. It can be found in eggs, milk, and bananas. Biotin is commonly used for hair loss, brittle nails, and nerve damage, as well as many other conditions.

Biotin deficiency can be caused by inadequate dietary intake or inheritance of an inborn genetic disorder that affects biotin metabolism. Deficiency can cause mild symptoms, such as hair thinning or a skin rash typically on the face. Neonatal screening for biotinidase deficiency began in the United States in 1984, with many other countries testing for this disorder at birth as well. Individuals born prior to 1984 are unlikely to have been screened, obscuring the true prevalence of the disorder.

SCIENTIFIC EVIDENCE

Taking biotin can help treat low blood levels. Low blood levels of biotin can cause thinning of the hair and rash around the eyes, nose, and mouth. Other deficiency symptoms might include depression, hallucinations, and tingling in the arms and legs. People who are pregnant, malnourished, have received long-term enteral feeding, have undergone rapid weight loss, or who have a specific inherited condition (eg, biotinidase deficiency) can have low biotin levels. Cigarette smoking can also cause low blood levels of biotin.

Biotin is often recommended as a dietary supplement for hair loss and brittle nails despite the fact that scientific data supporting these outcomes are weak.

There is an inherited disorder called biotin-thiamin-responsive basal ganglia disease that affects the brain and nervous system. Individuals with this condition experience episodes of altered mental status and muscle problems. According to early research, taking thiamin alone is more preventive than taking a combination of biotin and thiamin. However, when episodes of altered mental state and muscle problems occur, a combination of biotin and thiamin may shorten the length of the episode.[17]

For persons with DM, some early research shows that taking biotin along with chromium might lower blood glucose levels. Also, early research shows that taking biotin by mouth or as an injection might reduce leg nerve pain in individuals with DM.

People receiving dialysis have a tendency to develop muscle cramps. Early research shows that taking biotin by mouth might reduce muscle cramps in these individuals.

For individuals with multiple sclerosis, early research shows that taking high-dose biotin might improve vision and reduce partial paralysis.

More evidence, however, is needed to rate biotin for these uses.[18]

DOSAGE

Biotin does not have an RDA; however, the adequate intake (AI) for biotin is 30 mcg for adults and pregnant people, and 35 mcg for parents who breastfeed. Up to 10 mg daily has been used for persons with biotin deficiency.[18]

SAFETY

Allergies

An allergic reaction to biotin will often include nausea, a rash, or swelling of the throat and face. Commonly,

people who are allergic to vitamin B12 are allergic to biotin as well. Too much biotin might cause acne on the chin and jawline.[19]

Adverse Effects and Warnings

Biotin is likely safe for people when taken by mouth in appropriate doses or applied to skin as with cosmetic products containing 0.0001% to 0.6% biotin. Biotin is well tolerated when used at the recommended dosages.

Taking biotin supplements might interfere with the results of many different blood laboratory tests. Biotin can cause falsely high or falsely low test results, which might lead to a missed or incorrect diagnosis. Most multivitamins, including renal multivitamins, contain low doses of biotin which are not likely to interfere with blood tests.[18]

INTERACTIONS WITH DRUGS AND DIETARY SUPPLEMENTS

Biotin might increase how quickly the liver breaks down certain medications. Taking biotin along with some medications that are metabolized by the liver might decrease the effects of these medications. Examples of such medications include clozapine (Clozaril), cyclobenzaprine (Flexeril), fluvoxamine (Luvox), haloperidol (Haldol), imipramine (Tofranil), mexiletine (Mexitil), olanzapine (Zyprexa), pentazocine (Talwin), propranolol (Inderal), tacrine (Cognex), theophylline, zileuton (Zyflo), and zolmitriptan (Zomig).[18]

IMPLICATIONS FOR USE IN PATIENTS WITH CHRONIC KIDNEY DISEASE

Biotin can interfere with a number of test results, but of particular concern for the population with CKD is its potential effect on the results of parathyroid hormone and 25-hydroxyvitamin D (calcifediol) immunoassays as well as electrolyte assays.[20] When taken in high doses, patients should be advised to stop taking biotin a few days before their routine blood work is completed to avoid an erroneous laboratory value resulting from over-supplementation.

Black Cohosh (*Cimicifuga racemosa*), Baneberry, Black Snakeroot, Bug Root

BACKGROUND

Black cohosh, which is native to North America, is used as an alternative to prescription hormonal therapy to treat menopausal symptoms, such as hot flashes, night sweats, vaginal dryness, migraine headaches, sleep disturbances, perspiration, and mood disturbances. Black cohosh has also been used in people who experience menopausal symptoms and when estrogen replacement therapy is contraindicated. The exact mechanism of action and particular active components of this dietary supplement are not fully understood. However, several studies have reported improvements in menopausal symptoms for up to 6 months.[1,2,21]

SCIENTIFIC EVIDENCE

There are no indications for the use of black cohosh based on strong or good scientific evidence. A double-blind, placebo-controlled study funded by the National Center for Complementary and Alternative Medicine (NCCAM) found that black cohosh, whether used alone or in combination with other dietary supplements, failed to relieve hot flashes and night sweats in 351 perimenopausal and postmenopausal women*.[21]

DOSAGE

The black cohosh stems (fresh or dried) are commonly used to make strong teas (infusions) and are also available as capsules, tablets, or liquid extracts. There is no proven effective dose for black cohosh.

Studies on black cohosh for the management of menopausal symptoms have used 20 or 40 mg Remifemin tablets (ie, brand name for the standardized black cohosh root and rhizome extract supplement containing 1 or 2 mg 27-deoxyactein) twice daily or 40 drops of a liquid extract. Isopropanolic black cohosh has also been used at a dose of 40 mg/d for 12 weeks.[22]

SAFETY

Allergies

Black cohosh should be used with caution in people allergic to aspirin or other salicylates, as in nature black cohosh does contain small amounts of salicylic acid. It is not known how much, if any, salicylate acid is present in commercial products.[22]

Adverse Effects and Warnings

Black cohosh is generally well tolerated in recommended doses, but safety and efficacy beyond 6 months have not been proven. Frontal headaches, dizziness, perspiration, or visual disturbances can occur when taken in high doses. Other possible adverse effects that can occur while taking black cohosh include constipation, intestinal discomfort, loss of bone mass, irregular or slow heartbeat, low blood pressure (BP), muscle damage, nausea, and vomiting. Hepatitis and liver failure have been reported with the use of black cohosh-containing products. In fact, the US Pharmacopeia suggests that women should discontinue use of black cohosh and consult a health care provider if they have a liver disorder or develop symptoms of liver trouble while taking this dietary supplement. Black cohosh should also be used with caution in patients with a history of blood clots, seizure disorder, or high BP.[22]

INTERACTIONS WITH DRUGS AND DIETARY SUPPLEMENTS

Because of the potential estrogenic effects of black cohosh, caution is warranted in females and people taking estrogen or other dietary supplements which may have hormonal effects. Black cohosh may lower BP and should be used cautiously with other antihypertensive agents or similar dietary supplements. Other potential interactions include pain relievers, anesthetics, anti-inflammatory agents, cholesterol-lowering drugs, antiplatelet agents, and antiseizure medications. It may interfere with the absorption of medications and dietary supplements that have antidepressant, antihista-

Study participants were described as women. Gender was not further specified.

mine, or antioxidant effects. Interactions with St John's Wort (SJW) are also possible.[22]

IMPLICATIONS FOR USE IN PATIENTS WITH CHRONIC KIDNEY DISEASE

Studies regarding the use of black cohosh in patients with CKD are lacking; thus, its safety for use in the population with CKD is unknown. Because of its potential to interact with antihypertensive and antiplatelet medications, black cohosh use must be monitored closely in patients with CKD taking these medications.

Chamomile (*Matricaria recutita*)

BACKGROUND

Chamomile has been widely used medicinally for thousands of years to treat conditions, such as sleep disorders, anxiety, gastrointestinal (GI) disorders, and skin concerns. In the United States, it is most commonly found in herbal tea preparations.

SCIENTIFIC EVIDENCE

There are no indications for use based on strong or good scientific evidence.

DOSAGE

When consumed as a tea, 1 to 4 c/d (from tea bags) is a common dose. Capsule doses used in research studies range from 220 to 1,600 mg. No standard dose for chamomile has been established.[23]

SAFETY

Allergies

There are multiple reports of serious allergic reactions to chamomile, including anaphylaxis, throat swelling, and shortness of breath. People with allergies and sensitivities to other plants in the Asteraceae family (eg, chrysanthemums, ragweed, marigolds, or daisies) should avoid chamomile.[24]

Adverse Effects and Warnings

Chamomile may cause drowsiness or sedation; therefore, caution should be used when driving or operating heavy machinery. Based on case reports of chamomile use, this dietary supplement may increase the risk of bleeding because of its coumarin content.[23]

INTERACTIONS WITH DRUGS AND DIETARY SUPPLEMENTS

Chamomile may increase drowsiness caused by interactions with drugs such as benzodiazepines (eg, lorazepam and diazepam), narcotics, some antidepressants, and alcohol. Due to its coumarin content, chamomile may increase the risk of bleeding when used with medications or dietary supplements that increase this risk (see Box 19.2).[24] Chamomile may interfere with the way the body metabolizes certain medications through the cytochrome P450 (CYP450) enzyme system (eg, oral contraceptives, antiepileptics, anti-inflammatories, antidepressants, antivirals, anticoagulants, antirejection,

---

BOX 19.2 | Examples of Drugs and Dietary Supplements That May Increase the Risk of Bleeding

DRUGS

Aspirin

Anticoagulants (eg, warfarin and heparin)

Antiplatelets (eg, clopidogrel [Plavix])

Nonsteroidal anti-inflammatory drugs (NSAIDS) (eg, ibuprofen [Motrin, Advil] and naproxen [Naprosyn, Aleve])

DIETARY SUPPLEMENTS

Aloe

Chamomile

Fish oil

Flaxseed

Garlic

Ginkgo biloba

Ginseng

Glucosamine

Saw palmetto

Vitamin E

and benzodiazepines). As a result, serum or plasma levels of these medications may be unexpectedly high or low and may cause potentially serious outcomes. More research, however, is needed to determine the clinical relevance.[25] In experimental and laboratory research, constituents in chamomile may lower BG and BP (ie, flavonoid glucoside, chamaemeloside, and apigenin, respectively).[24] Therefore, caution should be taken with medications or dietary supplements that affect BG levels or BP. Chamomile may also interact with medications or dietary supplements that act as cardiac depressants, central nervous system depressants, calcium channel blockers, cardiac glycosides, and respiratory depressants. This dietary supplement may interact with antibiotics, antifungals, antihistamines, and diuretics, as well as medications used for treating elevated serum cholesterol, ulcers, diarrhea, or GI disorders. Chamomile may also have antiestrogenic effects and interact with dietary supplements like red clover or soy. No specific amount of chamomile is known which can cause these interactions, but caution is recommended.

IMPLICATIONS FOR USE IN PATIENTS WITH CHRONIC KIDNEY DISEASE

Studies regarding the use of chamomile in patients with CKD are lacking; thus, its use and safety are unknown. Because of the potential for increased bleeding, chamomile may be contraindicated in patients receiving maintenance hemodialysis (HD) and heparin during each dialysis treatment, as well as patients with CKD taking medications that increase the risk for bleeding.

Chamomile can interfere with the metabolism of antirejection medications taken by patients with kidney transplant.[26]

Cinnamon (*Cinnamomum verum*)

BACKGROUND

Cinnamon has been used as a spice for centuries and comes from the bark of the cinnamon tree. Cinnamon

and its constituents may have anti-inflammatory, antibacterial, antifungal, and antioxidant properties.[27] Cinnamon may also help lower BG levels in people with DM. A 2016 study of 25 individuals concluded that cinnamon may provide benefits for those with poorly controlled DM. Participants were given 1 g cinnamon for 12 weeks, which resulted in a 17% reduction in fasting BG levels.[28] Cinnamon is safe for most people with DM.

SCIENTIFIC EVIDENCE

There are no indications for cinnamon use as a sole treatment for any condition based on strong or good scientific evidence.

DOSAGE

There are no proven effective medicinal doses for cinnamon. Suggested dose is ½ to 1 teaspoon (2–4 g) of powder per day. Doses of above 6 g might be toxic.[27]

SAFETY

Allergies

Cinnamon should be avoided in people with a known allergy or hypersensitivity to cinnamon or its constituents.

Adverse Effects and Warnings

Cinnamon is likely safe when taken by mouth over a short-term period. Unfortunately, little is known about the long-term use of cinnamon.[1] Cinnamon bark may cause a decrease in platelet counts. Cinnamon may lower BG levels and, thus, should be used with caution in patients taking insulin or antidiabetic medications. Cinnamon may enhance the effects of antibiotics and antiarrhythmic drugs. People should also consider using a Ceylon cinnamon rather than Cassia cinnamon. Cassia cinnamon contains coumarin, which may be hepatotoxic, especially in high doses.

INTERACTIONS WITH DRUGS AND DIETARY SUPPLEMENTS

Cinnamon may interact with antibacterial, antidiabetic, anticoagulant, antifungal, antispasmodic, and antiviral medications and dietary supplements. Therefore, caution should be applied when these products are taken with cinnamon because of possible additive effects. Cinnamon may also interfere with the way the body processes certain medications and dietary supplements that are metabolized through the CYP450 system (eg, oral contraceptives, antiepileptics, anti-inflammatories, antidepressants, antivirals, anticoagulants, and benzodiazepines). As a result, the level of these substances in the blood may be altered.

IMPLICATIONS FOR USE IN PATIENTS WITH CHRONIC KIDNEY DISEASE

Cinnamon appears to be safe when used in the amounts typically added to foods. Short-term use of cinnamon supplements in small doses may be appropriate for patients with CKD, but further research is needed for verification.

Cobalamin (Vitamin B12)

BACKGROUND

Vitamin B12, also called cobalamin and one of eight B vitamins, is a water-soluble vitamin that plays an essential role in the metabolism of every cell in the human body. It is a cofactor in DNA synthesis and in both fatty acid and amino acid metabolism. It is also involved in red blood cell production and proper functioning of the nervous system.

Vitamin B12 consists of a class of chemically related compounds called vitamers. It also contains the biochemically rare element cobalt, hence, the name cobalamin.[29] Only certain bacteria produce vitamin B12.

There are no naturally occurring vegetable sources with significant amounts of this vitamin, so vegans and vegetarians should take a supplement and consume foods fortified with vitamin B12. Other than vegans or vegetarians, people in developed countries generally obtain enough vitamin B12 from the animal products they consume, which include meat, milk, eggs, and fish.[29]

Symptoms of low vitamin B12 levels can include fatigue, numbness or tingling in hands and feet, headaches, and moodiness.

SCIENTIFIC EVIDENCE

Older individuals are at risk of vitamin B12 deficiency because absorption depends on intrinsic factor and normal gut function, which is often impaired in this age group. Vitamin B12 deficiency in young adults, however, may be more prevalent than previously thought. The Framingham Offspring Study found that the percentage of participants in three age groups (26–49 years, 50–64 years, and 65 years and older) with deficient blood levels of vitamin B12 were similar. The study also showed that individuals who took a vitamin B12 supplement or consumed a fortified cereal more than four times per week were much less likely to be deficient.[30] By slowing down the release of acid into the stomach, proton pump inhibitors can interfere with vitamin B12 absorption. It is unclear to what degree this occurs, but it would be prudent to monitor the vitamin B12 status of individuals who take these medications long term.[29]

Insufficient intake of vitamin B12 may lead to increased homocysteine levels. Elevated homocysteine levels have been associated with arterial damage and thrombosis. Supplementation with B complex vitamins (eg, B6, B12, and folic acid) can reduce homocysteine levels. Studies, however, have been unable to prove a decrease in vascular events as a result of vitamin supplementation. These studies were small and of short duration; therefore, further research is warranted to determine whether vitamin supplementation can be beneficial in this regard.[31]

DOSAGE

Vitamin B12 supplements are available as either a single agent or as part of multivitamin tablets. This vitamin can also be given by intramuscular (IM) injection.

Recommended intake for vitamin B12 is as follows[32]:

- 0 to 6 months of age Adequate Intake (AI): 0.4 mcg/d
- 7 to 12 months of age AI: 0.5 mcg/d
- 1 to 3 years of age RDA: 0.9 mcg/d

- 4 to 8 years of age RDA: 1.2 mcg/d
- 9 to 13 years of age RDA: 1.8 mcg/d
- 14 years of age and over RDA* for:
  - males and females: 2.4 mcg/d
  - pregnant people: 2.6 mcg/d
  - lactating people: 2.8 mcg/d

The RDA is the recommended level of supplementation for patients with CKD and end-stage kidney disease (ESKD) receiving dialysis.[33]

When treating a patient with vitamin B12 deficiency, an individual's ability to absorb this vitamin must be evaluated because this will determine whether doses should be delivered orally or intravenously. Typically, vitamin B12 deficiency is treated via IM injection as this delivery method will bypass any potential absorption barriers.[29] Dosage is based on the specific medical condition being treated as well as the individual's response to treatment.

SAFETY

Allergies

A very serious allergic reaction to this supplement is rare.

Adverse Effects and Warnings

Side effects when taking vitamin B12 can include diarrhea, nausea, stomach upset, itching, rash, headache, dizziness, and weakness. When given IM, side effects around the injection site can include pain, redness, swelling, and irritation.

Symptoms of high vitamin B12 levels include restenosis (recurrence of narrowing of a blood vessel) after stent placement, high BP, acne, rash, itchy or burning skin, pink or red skin discoloration, facial flushing, and urine discoloration.

INTERACTIONS WITH DRUGS AND DIETARY SUPPLEMENTS

Certain medications, such as colchicine, metformin, extended-release potassium products, some antibiotics, antiseizure medications, and medications to treat heartburn, can decrease the absorption of vitamin B12.

IMPLICATIONS FOR USE IN PATIENTS WITH CHRONIC KIDNEY DISEASE

Patients receiving dialysis are at an increased risk of deficiency of water-soluble vitamins due to losses during dialysis and the potentially restrictive nature of the diet. The Kidney Disease Outcomes Quality Initiative (KDOQI) nutrition guidelines suggest that adults with CKD stages 1 through 5D be prescribed vitamin B12 to correct for deficiency or insufficiency based on clinical signs and symptoms.[34] Doses should be individualized based on clinical findings. Vitamin B12 content of the typical renal multivitamin is 6 mcg but can vary.[33] It is important to determine if oral supplementation is adequate because those without sufficient intrinsic factor may require IM administration to provide adequate dosing for repletion.

Patients with CKD and ESKD have higher homocysteine levels, as it is not metabolized well.[35] While supplementation with B vitamins inclusive of B12 can lower homocysteine in these patients, more studies are required to determine the absolute benefit of vitamin B12 supplementation and its impact on homocysteine levels.[36]

Coenzyme Q10

BACKGROUND

The human body produces coenzyme Q10 (CoQ10) which is necessary for the proper functioning of cells via synthesis of adenosine triphosphate (ATP). It is also a potent lipophilic antioxidant. CoQ10 levels decrease with age and can be low in patients with heart failure, DM, cancer, neurodegenerative diseases, fibromyalgia, mitochondrial diseases, muscular diseases, and those who take statin medications. Organ meats, fish, meat, nuts, and some oils are good sources of CoQ10.[37] The adult reference interval for plasma CoQ10 is approximately 0.5 mmol/L to 1.7 mmol/L. There is a strong correlation between plasma CoQ10 and lipid concentrations. Consequently, lipids should be considered when measuring plasma CoQ10 such that the ratio of CoQ10 to total or low-density lipoprotein (LDL) cholesterol is reported.[38]

*Specific recommendations for transgender people were not provided.

SCIENTIFIC EVIDENCE

CoQ10 deficiency Evidence for supplementation in COQ10 deficiency is strong (A). CoQ10 deficiency may occur in patients with reduced synthesis of CoQ10 resulting from nutrient deficiencies or statin use as well as increased utilization by the body due to chronic disease.[38] Depending on the cause of the deficiency, supplementation with CoQ10 or increased dietary intake of food sources that contain CoQ10 and the vitamins and minerals needed to produce CoQ10 (eg, riboflavin and niacinamide, just to name a few) may be required. CoQ10 is fat-soluble and should be taken with a meal containing fat for effective absorption.

Hypertension (HTN) Evidence for supplementation in HTN is strong (A). Research studies suggest that CoQ10 causes small decreases in systolic and perhaps diastolic BP. Low blood levels of CoQ10 have been found in people with HTN; however, it is unclear whether a CoQ10 deficiency is the cause of high BP and whether it affects antihypertensive medications or BP-lowering supplements.[39]

Congestive heart failure CoQ10 supplements, in addition to standard therapy, is associated with reduced symptom burden and adverse cardiovascular events.[37]

Migraines Clinical trials have shown that daily use can reduce the frequency, severity, and duration of headaches in migraine sufferers.[37]

DOSAGE

CoQ10 is typically sold in capsules or tablets in dosages of 100 or 200 mg per capsule or tablet. Although an ideal dose of CoQ10 has not been established, the typical daily dosage is 100 to 200 mg.[40]

SAFETY

Allergies

Allergic reactions to supplements containing CoQ10 may occur, such as itching or rash.

Adverse Effects and Warnings

There are few serious adverse effects of CoQ10. Possible reactions are usually mild and brief and include nausea, vomiting, loss of appetite, upper abdominal pain, and diarrhea. More rare adverse effects include dizziness, headache, irritability, fatigue, insomnia, and itching or skin rashes.[41]

INTERACTIONS WITH DRUGS AND DIETARY SUPPLEMENTS

CoQ10 may reduce the effectiveness of warfarin or other blood-thinning agents and may limit or prevent effective anticoagulation.[41] CoQ10 has been shown to lower fasting BG levels and should be used cautiously with DM or in those who experience hypoglycemia.[42] CoQ10 may lower BP and should be used with caution in individuals using antihypertensive medications.[37]

IMPLICATIONS FOR USE IN PATIENTS WITH CHRONIC KIDNEY DISEASE

Studies regarding the use of CoQ10 in patients with CKD are limited; thus, its use and safety are unknown. Because of its potential to interfere with anticoagulation, lower BP, and lower BG levels, use in patients with CKD who take these medications must be monitored closely.

Echinacea (*Echinacea angustifolia DC, Echinacea pallida, Echinacea purpurea*), Purple Coneflower

BACKGROUND

The echinacea plant is commonly referred to as the purple coneflower herb. It was originally used by Indigenous Americans to treat or prevent colds, flu, or other infections. The roots and above-ground parts of the plant may have immune-stimulating properties. Oral preparations are popular to prevent and treat upper respiratory infections. The most potent species for this indication is *Echinacea purpurea*. Sales of echinacea represent 34.9% of the global dietary supplement market.[43] The German Commission E discourages use of echinacea in patients with autoimmune disorders. This recommendation is based on theoretical considerations, not on human data.

SCIENTIFIC EVIDENCE

Evidence for prevention of upper respiratory tract infections with echinacea is good (B). Preliminary studies suggest that echinacea is not helpful for common cold prevention in adults.

Evidence for treatment of upper respiratory tract infections with echinacea is good (B). Multiple low-grade studies have suggested that taking echinacea by mouth when cold symptoms begin may reduce the length and the severity of symptoms. Goel et al[44] showed that standardized extracts of the herb lowered daily symptom scores of the common cold by 23.1% when compared with a placebo. However, Barrett et al[45] in a randomized, placebo-controlled trial did not find that reported symptom improvement was statistically significant. Another study by Yale and Liu[46] was also unable to replicate the findings of other studies touting the benefit of echinacea. It is important to note that there are different species of echinacea and different parts of the plant used in studies, which may, in part, explain conflicting findings in the literature.

DOSAGE

There is no proven effective dose for echinacea. It is available commercially as capsules, expressed juice, extract, tincture, and tea. A common dosing range in studies is 500 to 1,000 mg in capsule form taken by mouth, three times a day, for 5 to 7 days.[47] Long-term use of echinacea is not recommended.

SAFETY

Allergies

People with allergies to ragweed, chrysanthemums, marigolds, and daisies are theoretically more likely to have an allergic reaction to echinacea. People with asthma or other allergies can experience allergic reactions, such as itching, rash, wheezing, facial swelling, and anaphylaxis.

Adverse Effects and Warnings

Few adverse effects are reported when echinacea is used as recommended. Reported complaints include stomach discomfort, nausea, sore throat, rash, drowsiness, headache, dizziness, and muscle aches. Use of echinacea by people with conditions that affect the immune system (eg, HIV/AIDS, cancer, multiple sclerosis, tuberculosis, and rheumatologic diseases) are discouraged by some experts, although there is a lack of scientific evidence in this area. Long-term use of echinacea may cause leukopenia.[48]

INTERACTIONS WITH DRUGS AND DIETARY SUPPLEMENTS

Use of echinacea may lead to liver inflammation, although there is not sufficient laboratory or human studies to support this claim. Nevertheless, caution should be used when combining echinacea with other medications or dietary supplements that can harm the liver (eg, anabolic steroids, methotrexate, acetaminophen, antifungal medications, and kava). In addition, echinacea may affect the way certain medications or dietary supplements are metabolized by the liver. In theory, the ability of echinacea to stimulate the immune system may interfere with medications that suppress the immune system, such as cyclosporine and prednisone. Echinacea may also be used in combination products that are thought to stimulate the immune system. However, there is insufficient evidence that these products provide added benefits.

IMPLICATIONS FOR USE IN PATIENTS WITH CHRONIC KIDNEY DISEASE

Studies regarding the use of echinacea in patients with CKD are lacking; thus, its safety and use in this population is unknown. Echinacea can interfere with the metabolism of antirejection medications taken by patients with a kidney transplant.[26]

Fish Oil, Omega-3 Fatty Acids, and α-Linolenic Acid

BACKGROUND

Dietary sources of omega-3 fatty acids include fish oil and certain plant/nut oils. Fish oil is a rich source of omega-3 fatty acids, docosahexaenoic acid (DHA), and eicosapentaenoic acid (EPA), while some nuts (English walnuts) and vegetable oils (canola, soybean, flax seed/linseed, olive) contain α-linolenic acid (ALA), a precursor to EPA and DHA. EPA and DHA are precursors to eicosanoids, which have antiatherogenic and anti-inflammatory properties.[49] In 2004, the Food and Drug Administration (FDA) approved a limited health claim for labeling on omega-3 fatty acid supplements regarding coronary heart disease.[49] A 3- to 4-oz serving of fatty fish (eg, mackerel, salmon, herring, or anchovy) consumed twice a week provides approximately 3 g fish oil.

SCIENTIFIC EVIDENCE

Hypertension Evidence for using omega-3 for HTN is strong (A). Multiple trials report small reductions in BP (2–5 mm Hg) with intake of omega-3 fatty acids; the effects appear to be dose dependent. A high intake of omega-3 fatty acids a day may be necessary to obtain clinically relevant effects; however, at doses exceeding 3,000 mg/d, there is an increased risk of bleeding.[50]

Hypertriglyceridemia Evidence for using omega-3 for hypertriglyceridemia is strong (A). There is strong evidence that omega-3 fatty acids from fish or fish oil supplements significantly reduce serum triglyceride levels. A dose of 4 g daily of prescription omega-3 fatty acid medication has been shown to reduce serum triglyceride levels. Benefits appear to be dose dependent. Fish oil supplements also appear to cause minimal increases in high-density lipoprotein cholesterol levels; however, 5% to 10% increases in LDL cholesterol levels have been observed.[50]

Secondary cardiovascular disease (CVD) prevention Evidence for using omega-3 for prevention of CVD is strong (A). Several well-conducted, randomized controlled trials report that in people with a history of myocardial infarction, regular consumption of oily fish or fish oil or 2 g/d omega-3 fatty acid supplements reduce the risk of nonfatal heart attack, fatal heart attack, sudden death, and all-cause mortality. Most patients in these studies were also using conventional cardiac medications, suggesting that the benefits of fish oils may be additive. Furthermore, it is reported that 850 mg/d omega-3 fatty acids can reduce the risk of a heart attack.[50]

Primary CVD prevention Evidence for using omega-3 for primary CVD prevention is good (B). Several large studies report a significantly lower rate of death from heart disease in men and women who regularly eat fatty fish. The evidence suggests benefits of regular consumption of fish oil. Omega-3 fatty acid supplementation of 2 g/d may help to prevent the risk of primary CVD.[50]

Protection from cyclosporine toxicity in patients with organ transplant Evidence for using omega-3 for protection from cyclosporine toxicity is good (B). There are multiple studies of heart and kidney transplant recipients taking cyclosporine and fish oil supplements concurrently. The majority of trials report improvements in kidney function and fewer incidence of high BP compared with patients not taking fish oil. Adding 4 to 6 g/d omega-3 fatty acids from fish oil helped reduce high BP in patients with organ transplant.[50]

Rheumatoid arthritis Evidence for using omega-3 for rheumatoid arthritis is good (B). Multiple randomized, controlled trials report regular intake of fish oil supplements for up to 3 months improved morning stiffness and joint tenderness, but effects after 3 months have not been thoroughly studied. The recommended dose of omega-3 fatty acid for rheumatoid arthritis is 1 to 3 g/d.[50]

DOSAGE

There are currently no estimated average requirement recommendations for omega-3 fatty acid intake in the United States. Instead there are AI recommendations for ALA based on intake in healthy populations (ie, 1.6 g for adult males and 1.1 g for adult females*). ALA is the only omega-3 fatty acid that has an established AI as it is the only one that is essential.[49] The average American consumes about 1.6 g omega-3 fatty acids per day, of which about 1.4 g is from ALA and only 0.1 to 0.2 g is from EPA and DHA. The average individual consumes about ten times more omega-6 fatty acids than omega-3 fatty acids. These two fatty acids compete with each other for conversion to active metabolites in the body. Therefore, the benefits can be achieved either by decreasing intake of omega-6 fatty acids or by increasing intake of omega-3 fatty acids. The ALA form of omega-3 fatty acid is not created in human bodies. It needs to be acquired from diet or supplementation. ALA is good, but EPA is best for inflammation. DHA is good for brain and eye health. ALA can be converted to EPA and then to DHA, which occurs primarily in the liver, but the conversion rate is low, less than 15%.[49] For a healthy adult with no history of cardiac disease, the American Heart Association (AHA) recommends eating fatty fish at least twice a week. AHA also recommends consumption of plant-derived sources of ALA, such as tofu/soybeans, walnuts, flaxseed oil, and canola oil. Various health organizations offer recommendations for EPA and DHA intake for healthy individuals, but their opinions vary considerably. In general, a minimum of 250 to 500 mg of combined EPA and DHA per day is recommended.[51]

SAFETY

Allergies

People with allergy/hypersensitivity to fish should avoid fish oil or omega-3 fatty acid products derived from fish. People with allergy/hypersensitivity to nuts should avoid ALA or omega-3 fatty acid products derived from the types of nuts to which they react.

Adverse Effects and Warnings

Low intake (one 4-oz serving of fatty fish two times per week) of omega-3 fatty acids from fish is generally recognized as safe. However, caution is warranted in

people with DM because of potential increases in BG levels, those at risk of bleeding, or those with high levels of LDL cholesterol. Large intake of omega-3 fatty acid fish oil of 3,000 mg/d or more may increase the risk of hemorrhagic stroke. High doses have also been associated with nosebleeds and hematuria. Fish oils appear to decrease platelet aggregation, prolong bleeding time, and increase fibrinolysis. Potentially harmful contaminants, such as methyl mercury, accumulate in fish flesh more than fish oil. Fish oil supplements appear to contain almost no mercury. Certain species such as tilefish (Gulf of Mexico), swordfish, shark, king mackerel, and certain tunas contain the highest levels of mercury.[52] GI symptoms (eg, diarrhea, increased burping, acid reflux/heartburn/indigestion, abdominal bloating, and abdominal pain) are common with the use of fish oil supplements. These GI adverse effects can be minimized if fish oils are taken with meals and if doses are started low and increased gradually. Long-term use of fish oil may cause vitamin E deficiency; therefore, vitamin E is added to many commercial fish oil products. Regular use of vitamin E-enriched products may lead to elevated serum levels of vitamin E. Fish liver oil contains the fat-soluble vitamins A and D; thus, cod liver oil may increase the risk of vitamin A or D toxicity.

INTERACTIONS WITH DRUGS AND DIETARY SUPPLEMENTS

Omega-3 fatty acids may increase the risk of bleeding when taken with certain drugs and dietary supplements (see Box 19.2). They may lower BP and possibly add to the effects of other medications and dietary supplements taken to decrease BP. Fish oil supplements may lower BG levels; therefore, practitioners should use caution when suggesting fish oil use with other antidiabetic medications or dietary supplements. Omega-3 fatty acids may add to the triglyceride-lowering effects of agents, such as niacin/nicotinic acid, fibrates, and resins. However, it may work against the LDL-lowering properties of statins, barley, garlic, psyllium, or soy.[50]

---

*Specific recommendations for transgender people were not provided.

IMPLICATIONS FOR USE IN PATIENTS WITH CHRONIC KIDNEY DISEASE

When consumed in recommended amounts, the benefits of omega-3 fatty acids from dietary sources far outweigh the risks. Early studies show benefit for use of omega-3 fatty acids in treating patients with CKD-related pruritis. Until the most efficacious dose is determined, the AHA dose recommendation of 1 g EPA plus DHA per day is a safe place to start.[53] Use of omega-3 fatty acids significantly reduced the risk of ESKD and was also associated with a lower risk of proteinuria, perhaps because omega-3 fatty acids might be involved in BP control, as HTN is a strong risk factor for the progression of kidney disease.[54]

Current KDOQI nutrition guidelines do not recommend routine supplementation of omega-3 fatty acids to decrease the risk of cardiovascular events, mortality, and allograft rejection episodes or improve patency rates of arteriovenous (AV) grafts or AV fistulas. It, however, may be beneficial to prescribe this supplementation to improve the lipid profile for those with CKD stages 3 through 5 as well as those receiving HD or peritoneal dialysis. Recommended intake is approximately 2 g/d for the earlier stages of CKD and 1.3 to 4 g/d for those on dialysis.[34]

Use of omega-3 fatty acids significantly increases sirolimus exposure in patients with a kidney transplant on calcineurin inhibitor-free immunosuppression regimens, ultimately requiring a decrease in dose to maintain patients in trough concentration goal.[55]

Flaxseed and Flaxseed Oil (*Linum usitatissimum*)

BACKGROUND

Flaxseed has been cultivated for more than 5,000 years in Central Asia. It is now found throughout North America, Asia, and Europe. Omega-3 fatty acids (ie, ALA), lignans (phytoestrogens or plant estrogens), and fiber are compounds found in flaxseed.[56] Flaxseed is a rich source of heart healthy ALA and its lignin con-

tent may have anticancer benefits.[57] The oil derived from flaxseed is also a rich source of ALA but does not contain the fiber or lignin components of the seed. Although omega-3 fatty acids have been associated with improved cardiovascular outcomes, there is no substantial evidence from human trials to show that flaxseed products are effective for coronary artery disease or hyperlipidemia. Flaxseed oil may share the purported lipid-lowering properties of flaxseed, but not for the suggested laxative or anticancer abilities, as it does not contain fiber or lignan.

SCIENTIFIC EVIDENCE

There are no indications for use based on strong or good scientific evidence.

DOSAGE

Flaxseed is available in a whole, crushed, or powdered form (ie, meal or flour). Flaxseed oil is available as a liquid or in a capsule. Ground flaxseed and flaxseed oil are unstable at room temperature and must be refrigerated in airtight, opaque containers. Whole or ground flaxseed can be mixed with liquid or food and taken by mouth. As with other sources of fiber, flaxseed should be taken with plenty of water. A common dose is 1 tablespoon per day.[56] Up to 2 g flaxseed oil per day has been used for up to 6 months. Evidence is lacking for long-term use.[58]

SAFETY

Allergies

Severe allergic reactions are known for persons allergic to flaxseed or flaxseed derivatives.

Adverse Effects and Warnings

Flaxseed and flaxseed oil supplements in recommended doses appear to be well tolerated. Unripe flaxseed pods should not be eaten as they can be poisonous. Raw flaxseed or the flaxseed plant may increase blood levels of cyanide when taken in excess amounts. The laxative effects of flaxseed can cause diarrhea, increased number of bowel movements, and abdominal discomfort.

Individuals with diarrhea, irritable bowel syndrome, diverticulitis, or inflammatory bowel disease should avoid raw flaxseed. Large amounts of flaxseed (>250 mg/d) by mouth may cause the intestines to stop working. Other conditions where raw flaxseed should be avoided include narrowing of the esophagus or intestine, ileus, or bowel obstruction as well as those who are on fluid restrictions.

INTERACTIONS WITH DRUGS AND DIETARY SUPPLEMENTS

Consumption of raw flaxseed by mouth (not flaxseed oil) may reduce the absorption of other medications or dietary supplements. Therefore, these substances should be taken 1 hour before or 2 hours after raw flaxseed to prevent decreased absorption. Flaxseed may lower BP, decrease BG levels, increase the risk of bleeding (see Box 19.2), and decrease blood cholesterol levels. Therefore, medications and dietary supplements that have similar effects should be used with caution when taking flaxseed.[55] Laxatives, stool softeners, and other dietary supplements with laxative effects may enhance the effects of flaxseed. Since raw flaxseed (not flaxseed oil) is a rich source of lignans, it may possess estrogen-like properties and alter the effects of birth control pills or hormone replacement therapies. Flaxseed may also interact with muscle relaxants and drugs used for acid reflux or prostaglandins. Caution should be used when combining flaxseed with mood-altering dietary supplements, such as SJW, kava, or valerian.

IMPLICATIONS FOR USE IN PATIENTS WITH CHRONIC KIDNEY DISEASE

Given the need for adequate fluid intake when consuming flaxseed, its use may be contraindicated in patients with CKD stage 5 on dialysis requiring a fluid restriction. However, in patients with CKD who are not on a fluid restriction (eg, CKD stages 1 through 4), flaxseed may be appropriate in recommended amounts.

Because of the potential for increased bleeding, flaxseed and flaxseed oil may be contraindicated in patients on maintenance HD who receive heparin during each dialysis treatment as well as in patients with CKD taking medications that increase risk for bleeding.

Flaxseed contains phosphorus and is, thus, a potential contributor to hyperphosphatemia.[4]

Garlic (*Allium sativum*)

BACKGROUND

Garlic is one of the top-selling dietary supplements in the United States. For more than 5,000 years, garlic has been cultivated for medicinal and culinary purposes. Garlic is used to promote heart health and prevent cancer, as well as other diseases and infection. The cardioprotective benefits associated with garlic are generally attributed to the various sulfur compounds that can be isolated from the raw clove, such as alliin. There have been numerous controlled trials which have examined the effects of garlic on serum lipids, but the long-term effects on lipids and cardiovascular morbidity and mortality remain unknown. Some studies have shown that individuals who consume garlic routinely in their diet may be less likely to develop certain cancers, namely, stomach and colon cancers. Use as a dietary supplement has not proven to be effective in this regard. Enteric-coated preparations and raw garlic have not been well studied.

SCIENTIFIC EVIDENCE

Evidence of using garlic for hypercholesterolemia is good (B). Multiple human studies have reported small reductions in total serum cholesterol and LDL cholesterol during 4- to 12-week periods with consumption of garlic. It is unclear whether the benefits are sustained after this time period. A randomized clinical trial was conducted on the safety and effectiveness of fresh garlic, dried powdered garlic tablets, and aged garlic extract tablets for lowering serum cholesterol levels. The trial found no effect.[59]

DOSAGE

Use of 4 to 12.3 mg garlic oil daily by mouth has been reported. Other sources of garlic (eg, steam-distilled oils, oil from crushed garlic, and aged garlic in alcohol) may be less effective for some uses, particularly as a blood thinner. Noncoated, dehydrated garlic powder in doses of 600 to 900 mg/d, divided in three doses and standardized to 1.3% allicin content, has been used in human studies. The European Scientific Cooperative on Phytotherapy recommends 3 to 5 mg allicin per day, which is 1 clove or 0.5 to 1 g dried powder, to prevent atherosclerosis. The World Health Organization (WHO) recommends 2 to 5 g fresh garlic, 0.4 to 1.2 g dried garlic powder, 2 to 5 mg garlic oil, 300 to 1,000 mg garlic extract or any other form of garlic that is equivalent to 2 to 5 mg allicin daily.[60]

SAFETY

Allergies

People with a known allergy to garlic or other members of the Liliaceae family (eg, hyacinth, tulip, onion, leek, and chives) should avoid garlic. Allergic reactions have been reported to occur when garlic is taken by mouth, inhaled, or applied to the skin.

Adverse Effects and Warnings

For most individuals, garlic is likely safe in the amount typically consumed via food. Most commonly, the adverse effects of garlic are bad breath and body odor. Other reported adverse effects include dizziness, increased sweating, headache, itching, fever, chills, asthma flares, and a runny nose. A potentially serious adverse effect of garlic is bleeding, either after surgery or spontaneous bleeding (see Box 19.2). Garlic should be discontinued at least 7 days before surgical or dental procedures.[61] Several cases of bleeding have been reported, due either to the effects of garlic on blood platelets or to the increased breakdown of fibrin. Sev-

eral studies suggest that garlic does not alter the international normalized ratio (INR) values that are used to measure the effect of warfarin on blood thinning. Dehydrated garlic preparations or raw garlic taken by mouth may cause burning of the mouth, bad breath, abdominal pain or fullness, poor appetite, flatulence, belching, nausea, vomiting, irritation of the stomach lining, changes in the bacteria in the gut, heartburn, diarrhea, or constipation. Garlic should cautiously be used by people with stomach ulcers or who are prone to stomach irritation.[62]

INTERACTIONS WITH DRUGS AND DIETARY SUPPLEMENTS

Garlic may increase the risk of bleeding and lowering BP. Therefore, caution should be used when combining garlic with other medications and dietary supplements with similar effects. Garlic may alter levels of antiviral, anti-DM, and anticancer medications, or dietary supplements. It may also alter levels of certain medications and dietary supplements that are metabolized by the CYP450 enzyme system.

IMPLICATIONS FOR USE IN PATIENTS WITH CHRONIC KIDNEY DISEASE

Garlic may be safe in patients with CKD when used as recommended. However, because of its potential to increase bleeding and lower BP, use of garlic for long periods of time in the population with CKD, especially those who are on dialysis and receive heparin with each treatment, should be monitored closely by a physician.

Large doses (≥3.6 g/d) of garlic should be avoided in transplant recipients who are taking immunosuppressants due to its potential to interfere with the metabolism of these medications.[26]

Garlic also contains potassium and, thus, is a potential contributor to hyperkalemia.[4]

Ginkgo (*Ginkgo biloba*)

BACKGROUND

Ginkgo biloba has been used medicinally for thousands of years. It is one of the top-selling dietary supplements in the United States. The leaves of the ginkgo plant contain flavonoids, sesquiterpenes, and diterpenes (ginkgolides) that have been identified as possible active ingredients. Ginkgo is used effectively in the management of intermittent claudication, dementia secondary to Alzheimer disease, and multi-infarct and cerebral insufficiency. There is early promising evidence that may support the use of ginkgo for memory enhancement in healthy subjects, altitude sickness, symptoms of premenstrual syndrome, and reduction of chemotherapy-induced end-organ vascular damage.

SCIENTIFIC EVIDENCE

Claudication Evidence for using ginkgo for claudication is strong (A). Ginkgo causes a small improvement in claudication symptoms when taken by mouth. However, ginkgo may not be as beneficial for this condition as exercise therapy or prescription medications.

Dementia Evidence for using ginkgo for dementia is strong (A). Ginkgo may have benefits for people with early-stage Alzheimer disease and multi-infarct dementia, and it may be as beneficial as medication used to treat these disorders. However, the NCCAM funded a clinical trial known as the Ginkgo Evaluation of Memory Study and found that ginkgo was ineffective in lowering the overall incidence of dementia and Alzheimer disease in more than 3,000 elderly volunteers who were monitored for approximately 6 years.[63] In another randomized trial of 118 elderly subjects at high risk for cognitive decline, *Ginkgo biloba* extract did not appear to protect against a decline in memory function when taken for 42 months. However, in a secondary analysis where medication adherence was considered, there was a protective effect on the progression of the Clinical Dementia Rating scores from 0 to 0.5 as well as a smaller decline in memory scores.[64] Results from a larger prevention trial are needed to further clarify the effectiveness of ginkgo.

Cerebral insufficiency Evidence for using ginkgo for cerebral insufficiency is good (B). Many clinical trials have evaluated the effectiveness of ginkgo for the treatment of cerebral insufficiency, which is a syndrome that includes symptoms such as poor concentration, confusion, absent-mindedness, decreased physical performance, fatigue, headache, dizziness, depression, and anxiety. Cerebral insufficiency is thought to be caused by decreased blood flow to the brain due to clogged blood vessels. There are insufficient data findings indicating that ginkgo may or may not improve cerebral sufficiency.[65]

DOSAGE

Gingko is available as a capsule, tablet, extract, or tea. Studies have used 80 to 240 mg of a 50:1 standardized leaf extract taken daily by mouth in two to three divided doses (standardized to 24% to 25% ginkgo flavone glycosides and 6% terpine lactones). Dosing recommendations are dependent on the specific form used. It is advisable to start at a lower dose (no more than 120 mg/d) to avoid GI upset.[66]

SAFETY

Allergies

Allergy or hypersensitivity to Gingko may occur in sensitive individuals. A severe reaction, Stevens-Johnson syndrome, which includes skin blistering and sloughing, has been reported with the use of a combination product that contains ginkgo leaf extract, choline, vitamin B6, and vitamin B12.[67] There may be cross-sensitivity to ginkgo in people allergic to urushiol (eg, mango rind, sumac, poison ivy, poison oak, and cashews).

Adverse Effects and Warnings

Ginkgo leaf extract, which is used in most commercial products, appears to be well tolerated in most healthy adults at recommended doses for up to 6 months. Minor symptoms include headache, nausea, and intestinal complaints. Reports of bleeding ranging from a nosebleed to life-threatening bleeding have been associated with the use of ginkgo when taken by mouth. Ginkgo should be discontinued about 7 days prior to most surgical or dental procedures to avoid bleeding problems associated with any postsurgery/procedures. Eating ginkgo seeds is potentially toxic and should be avoided.[68]

INTERACTIONS WITH DRUGS AND DIETARY SUPPLEMENTS

Controlled trials of ginkgo report few adverse effects. It is suggested that use of ginkgo with medications and dietary supplements that cause bleeding may further increase the risk of bleeding (see Box 19.2). Ginkgo may also affect BG levels so caution is advised when using ginkgo with medications or dietary supplements that may lower BG levels. *Ginkgo biloba* leaf extract and nifedipine should not be ingested at the same time.[65] Ginkgo may alter drugs and dietary supplements that are metabolized through the CYP450 system.

IMPLICATIONS FOR USE IN PATIENTS WITH CHRONIC KIDNEY DISEASE

Studies regarding the use of ginkgo in patients with CKD are lacking; thus, its use and safety in this population are unknown.

Because of the potential for increased bleeding, large dosages of ginkgo for prolonged periods of time may be contraindicated in patients receiving maintenance HD who receive heparin during each dialysis treatment as well as patients with CKD taking medication that increases the risk for bleeding.

Ginseng, Korean Ginseng or Asian Ginseng (*Panax ginseng*), American Ginseng (*Panax quinquefolius*)

BACKGROUND

Ginseng is the collective term used to describe several species of plants belonging to the genus *Panax*. The roots of this slow-growing plant have been valued in Chinese medicine for more than 2,000 years. The two most commonly used species are Asian ginseng (*Panax ginseng*) and American ginseng (*Panax quinquefolius*). Asian ginseng is nearly extinct in its natural habitat, but it is still cultivated. American ginseng is both harvested from the wild and cultivated. *Panax ginseng* should not be confused with Siberian ginseng (*Eleutherococcus senticosus*), which does not contain ginsenosides—the active ingredients found in the *Panax* genus.

SCIENTIFIC EVIDENCE

Heart conditions Evidence is good (B) for use of ginseng for heart conditions. Some studies state that ginseng has antioxidant effects and can be of benefit to people with cardiovascular problems. Further studies state that ginseng can reduce oxidation of LDL cholesterol and brain tissue.

Type 2 diabetes mellitus/hyperglycemia/glucose intolerance Evidence for using ginseng for glucose intolerance and hyperglycemia in type 2 DM is good (B). Ginseng may lower BG levels in individuals with type 2 DM. Long-term effects are unclear, and the effective or safe dose is unknown. Persons diagnosed with DM should use more proven therapies, rather than ginseng. The effects of ginseng in persons with type 1 DM have not been adequately explored.

Immune system enhancement There is good (B) evidence that ginseng supports the immune system. Ginseng may boost the immune system. It can enhance the body's response to flu vaccines. It may also augment the effectiveness of antibiotics.[69]

DOSAGE

Ginseng is available in capsules, tablets, extracts, powders, and teas. Many different doses of ginseng have been traditionally used. However, after using ginseng continuously for 2 to 3 weeks, it is recommended that individuals refrain from using it for 1 to 2 weeks due to concerns about the development of adverse effects. Long-term dosing should not exceed 1 g dry root daily.

Capsules containing a standardized ginseng extract (4% ginsenosides), 100 to 200 mg, have been taken by mouth once or twice daily for up to 12 weeks. Dry ginseng root (0.5 to 2 g) taken by mouth in divided doses daily has also been used. A decoction of 1 to 2 g added to 150 mL water has been taken by mouth daily. A 1:1 (g/mL) liquid extract has been taken as 1 to 2 mL by mouth daily. A tincture of 5 to 10 mL (about 1–2 teaspoons) of a 1:5 (g/mL) ratio has been taken by mouth daily. *Panax ginseng* tea may be made by soaking about 3 g chopped fresh root or 1.5 g dried root powder in about 5 oz of boiling water for 5 to 15 minutes and then straining the tea. Some sources suggest consuming ginseng tea via this method three to four times per day for 3 to 4 weeks to achieve the reported effects.[69]

SAFETY

Allergies

Allergic reactions from ginseng may include severe rash, itching, or shortness of breath. Inhaling ginseng root dust has been associated with immediate- and late-onset asthma.[69]

Adverse Effects and Warnings

When used at recommended doses, *Panax ginseng* is likely safe when taken for a duration of less than 6 months.[70] There is limited evidence regarding adverse effects with long-term use, but those effects reported include skin rash, itching, diarrhea, sore throat, loss of appetite, excitability, anxiety, depression, or insomnia. It may increase or decrease BP. Seizures have been reported after high consumption of energy drinks containing caffeine, guarana, and dietary supplements, including ginseng. Ginseng should be avoided in patients with hormone-sensitive conditions, such as breast cancer and fibroids.[69]

INTERACTIONS WITH DRUGS AND DIETARY SUPPLEMENTS

American ginseng may reduce the anticoagulant effects of warfarin. It may also increase the risk of bleeding when taken with other medications or dietary supplements that increase the risk of bleeding (see Box 19.2). Ginseng may lower BG levels; thus, caution must be exercised when used with medications or dietary supplements that lower BG levels. Headache, tremors, mania, or insomnia may occur if ginseng is combined with antidepressant agents. Ginseng can also alter the effects of cardiac and BP medications. Theoretically, ginseng could interfere with medication and dietary supplement metabolism through the CYP450 enzyme pathway. Consequently, the levels of these substances may be increased in the blood and may cause increased effects or potentially serious adverse effects. Other substances in which ginseng may negatively interact with are sedative, cholesterol-lowering, anticancer, anti-inflammatory, antiviral, antipsychotic, steroid, erectile dysfunction, immunomodulator, and glucocorticoid medications and caffeine.[69]

IMPLICATIONS FOR USE IN PATIENTS WITH CHRONIC KIDNEY DISEASE

In patients receiving maintenance HD, ginseng may be contraindicated because of the increased risk of bleeding when taken with heparin as well as in patients with CKD taking medication that increases the risk for bleeding.

Asian ginseng can interfere with the metabolism of antirejection medications taken by patients with a kidney transplant.[26]

American ginseng contains potassium and phosphorus and, thus, is a potential contributor to hyperkalemia and hyperphosphatemia.[4]

Glucosamine and Chondroitin Sulfate

BACKGROUND

Glucosamine is an amino–polysaccharide (a combination of glutamine and glucose). It is a natural compound that is found in healthy cartilage. Chondroitin is currently manufactured either from natural sources (ie, shark/beef cartilage or bovine trachea) or by synthetic means. Glucosamine and chondroitin are usually taken in combination, although no information currently exists to suggest that when they are taken in combination, they are superior to either of the products consumed alone at the proper dosage. Glucosamine and chondroitin, taken alone or in combination, typically take 1 to 3 months to exert noticeable effects (eg, reduced pain and stiffness) in individuals with mild-to-moderate degrees of osteoarthritis.

SCIENTIFIC EVIDENCE

Knee osteoarthritis (mild-to-moderate) Evidence for using glucosamine for mild-to-moderate knee osteoarthritis is strong (A). There is good evidence to support the use of glucosamine sulfate in the treatment of mild-to-moderate knee osteoarthritis, but not severe osteoarthritis. A prospective, randomized clinical trial supported by the NCCAM and the National Institute of Arthritis and Musculoskeletal and Skin Diseases (Glucosamine/Chondroitin Arthritis Intervention Trial) found that glucosamine and chondroitin sulfate, alone and in combination, did not produce better results compared with the placebo group for treating cartilage loss in knee osteoarthritis.[71] Similar results were found by Clegg et al.[72] An analysis done by Reichenback et al in 2007 found that trial quality was low and that the symptomatic benefits of chondroitin are minimal or nonexistent.[73] Therefore, use of chondroitin should be discouraged.[73]

Osteoarthritis Evidence for using chondroitin with osteoarthritis is strong (A) and evidence for using glucosamine for osteoarthritis is good (B). Most studies have reported significant benefits in relief of symptoms, increased function, and reduced medication requirements when chondroitin is used for 6 to 24 months. The effects longer than 24 months are unclear. For glucosamine, the evidence supporting these benefits is not as convincing as it is for knee osteoarthritis.

Bladder control Evidence for use of chondroitin for bladder control is good (B). Studies have shown promise for using chondroitin for interstitial cystitis. This dietary supplement can also be used for overactive and unstable bladder.

DOSAGE

Glucosamine is available in tablets, capsules, or powders as glucosamine sulfate, glucosamine hydrochloride, or N-acetyl-D-glucosamine. In most studies, 500 mg glucosamine sulfate taken by mouth as tablets or capsules three times per day for 30 to 90 days was used. Once daily dosing of 1.5 g as tablets or capsules has also been used. Chondroitin sulfate is available in capsules in doses of 200 to 400 mg and taken by mouth two to three times per day or 800 to 1,200 mg once daily. It is unclear what dose of the combined glucosamine and chondroitin product is optimal or whether the combined product is as effective as or more effective than either agent alone.

SAFETY

Allergies

People with a shellfish allergy may have an allergic reaction to glucosamine and chondroitin products.

Adverse Effects and Warnings

Glucosamine sulfate is likely safe when taken as directed. Adverse effects may include heartburn, nausea, diarrhea, and constipation. Less commonly reported adverse effects include drowsiness, headache, and skin reactions. Early research suggested that glucosamine sulfate may increase both BG and BP. More recent research, however, shows that its use does not seem to affect either BG or BP.[74]

INTERACTIONS WITH DRUGS AND DIETARY SUPPLEMENTS

Glucosamine sulfate with or without chondroitin may increase the risk of bleeding when taken with warfarin (Coumadin) (see Box 19.2).[74]

IMPLICATIONS FOR USE IN PATIENTS WITH CHRONIC KIDNEY DISEASE

Glucosamine and chondroitin in combination appear to be safe in patients with CKD stages 1 and 2 when taken in recommended amounts for a specified period of time. Since glucosamine is removed by the body through the kidneys, people with CKD stages 3 through 5 should use this dietary supplement with caution. In patients on maintenance HD receiving heparin, glucosamine and chondroitin may be contraindicated because of the potential for increased risk of bleeding.

Green Tea (*Camellia sinensis*)

BACKGROUND

Green tea is the second most consumed beverage in the world; it is second only to water. Green, black, and oolong tea are all derived from the same plant (*Camellia sinensis*). The variety of tea reflects its growing region, form, and the way in which it is processed. The fresh leaves from the *C sinensis* plant are steamed and then dried to produce green tea. Green tea's potent antioxidant activity comes from polyphenols, also known as catechins. Tannins (large polyphenol molecules) form the bulk of the active compounds with catechins comprising approximately 90%. Green tea contains significant quantities of catechins, most notably epigallocatechin gallate (EGCG), epicatechin, and epicatechin gallate. EGCG is the most potent of the catechins, comprising 50% of the total quantity of catechins.[75] Catechins are antioxidants and, thus, fight cell damage.

SCIENTIFIC EVIDENCE

Green tea has been touted to improve cognitive performance, decrease cardiovascular risk factors, and lower cancer risk. There is evidence for increased mental alertness which would be expected, given its caffeine content. Study results for green tea and cancer have been inconsistent and, thus, the National Cancer Institute is not recommending it to reduce cancer risk. There have been some long-term studies investigating the benefit of green tea on cardiac disease. Limited evidence suggests that green tea may help with risk factors such as BP and cholesterol.[76]

DOSAGE

Green tea extract is available in capsules. In the capsule form, there is considerable variation in the amount of green tea extract; it may vary anywhere from 100 to 750 mg per capsule. Currently, there is no established recommended dose for green tea extract capsules. For the most part, studies have used green tea in a beverage form instead of capsules, by brewing 1 teaspoon tea leaves in 8 oz of water. One cup of tea contains approximately 50 mg caffeine and 80 to 100 mg polyphenols, depending on tea strength and cup size. Two to 5 cups per day is generally recommended.[47]

SAFETY

Allergies

People with known allergies/hypersensitivity to caffeine or tannins should avoid green tea.[76]

Adverse Effects and Warnings

Studies of the adverse effects relating to the consumption of green tea are limited. However, green tea has been found to be safe for most adults when used in the suggested amounts. Green tea and green tea extract contain caffeine, for which adverse reactions or effects have been reported (eg, insomnia, anxiety, irritability, diuresis, GI problems, and increased BP and heart rate). Caffeine toxicity is possible with high doses of green tea. Chronic use can result in tolerance and psychological dependence and may be habit-forming. Abrupt discontinuation may result in withdrawal symptoms, such as headache, irritation, and nervousness. Drinking tannin-containing beverages like tea may contribute to iron deficiency.[77]

INTERACTIONS WITH DRUGS AND DIETARY SUPPLEMENTS

Studies of the interactions of green tea with medications and dietary supplements are limited. However, green tea is a source of moderate amounts of caffeine, for which multiple interactions have been documented. Caffeine may potentiate the effects and adverse effects of other stimulants like nicotine, β-antagonists, or other methylxanthines. In contrast, caffeine can counteract lorazepam and diazepam due to their drowsiness and sluggish effects. Some medications, when taken with caffeine, may increase blood levels or the duration of the caffeine effect. These medications include birth control pills, hormone replacement therapy, ciprofloxin, cimetidine, and verapamil. Caffeine has also been shown to increase the headache-relieving effects of other pain relievers (eg, acetaminophen, aspirin, codeine, or ibuprofen). As a diuretic, caffeine increases urine and sodium losses through the kidney. Green tea, when consumed in large quantities, can reduce the blood-thinning effects of warfarin. Calcium, iron, and monoamine oxidase inhibitors (MAOIs) may also interact with green tea.[78]

IMPLICATIONS FOR USE IN PATIENTS WITH CHRONIC KIDNEY DISEASE

In general, brewed green tea appears to be safe for use by individuals with CKD when used at recommended amounts. Those who receive dialysis and must limit their fluid intake will need to limit their consumption of brewed green tea due to its fluid content.

For patients with CKD taking warfarin, green tea can be a significant source of vitamin K, thus decreasing its effectiveness.

Milk Thistle (*Silybum marianum*), Lady's Thistle

BACKGROUND

Milk thistle has been used medicinally for more than 2,000 years, most commonly for the treatment of liver cirrhosis, chronic hepatitis, and gallbladder disorders.[79] A flavonoid complex called silymarin can be extracted from the seeds (fruit) of the milk thistle plant. Silymarin is believed to be the biologically active component of the plant. The seeds are used to prepare capsules, extracts, and infusions.

SCIENTIFIC EVIDENCE

Preliminary research shows attenuation of proteinuria in patients with DM and overt nephropathy when silymarin was given in addition to renin-angiotensin system blockades. Although this was a randomized, double-blind, placebo-controlled trial, it was of short duration and the sample size was small; therefore, further trials of longer duration and increased sample size are required to determine efficacy and long-term safety.[80]

Chronic hepatitis Evidence for use of milk thistle for chronic hepatitis is good (B). Several studies of oral milk thistle taken for hepatitis caused by viruses or alcohol, report improvements in liver function tests (LFTs).

Liver cirrhosis Evidence for use of milk thistle for liver cirrhosis is good (B). Multiple studies suggest positive benefits with the use of oral milk thistle for cirrhosis. In experiments with up to 5 years of follow-up, milk thistle improved liver function and decreased the number of deaths that occurred in patients with cirrhosis.

DOSAGE

Milk thistle products are available as capsules, powders, and extracts. Silymarin (Legalon) in 230 to 600 mg/d divided into two to three doses has been studied. Silipide 160 to 480 mg/d in silybin equivalents has also been studied.

SAFETY

Allergies

People with allergies to plants in the Asteraceae family (eg, daisies, marigolds, ragweed, and chrysanthemums) or to any of the constituents in milk thistle may have allergic reactions to this dietary supplement. Anaphylactic shock from milk thistle tea or tablets has also been reported.

Adverse Effects and Warnings

Milk thistle appears to be well tolerated in recommended doses for up to 6 years. Some patients have experienced stomach upset, headache, and itching. Milk thistle may lower BG levels. Therefore, caution is advised in individuals with DM (on insulin or antidiabetics) or hypoglycemia.[81] Theoretically, because milk thistle plant extract may have estrogenic effects, females with hormone sensitive conditions (eg, fibroids or breast cancer) should avoid the above-ground parts of the milk thistle plant, but more research is needed.[82]

INTERACTIONS WITH DRUGS AND DIETARY SUPPLEMENTS

Experimental studies suggest that milk thistle may interfere with the way the body metabolizes drugs or dietary supplements through the CYP450 enzyme system. As a result, the levels of these substances may be increased in the blood and may cause increased adverse effects or reactions. Other medications and dietary supplements that milk thistle may interact with may be antidiabetics, hormonal, antiretroviral, or antioxidants.

IMPLICATIONS FOR USE IN PATIENTS WITH CHRONIC KIDNEY DISEASE

Studies regarding the use of milk thistle in patients with CKD are lacking; thus, its use and safety in patients with CKD are unknown.

Milk thistle contains phosphorus and, thus, is a potential contributor to hyperphosphatemia.[4]

Noni (*Morinda citrifolia*)

BACKGROUND

Noni is a traditional folk medicinal plant that has been used for more than 2,000 years. Few clinical trials have been conducted regarding its use. Based on scientific analysis and review of available information regarding claims of benefit, the European Commission Health and Consumer Protection Directorate-General Scientific Committee on Food provided no evidence for spe-

cial nutritional benefits of Tahitian noni juice.[83] While laboratory research has shown noni to have antioxidant, immune-stimulating, and tumor-fighting properties, it has not been well studied in people who have health conditions.

SCIENTIFIC EVIDENCE

There are no indications for use based on strong or good scientific evidence. When the content of noni products has been analyzed, wide variability of nutrient and phytochemical composition has been found. Given the lack of standardization of formulation, it is difficult to draw valid conclusions regarding the potential benefit of noni.[84] It should be noted that the FDA has issued many warnings to manufacturers of noni products about health claims made that are not supported by research.[85]

DOSAGE

Noni is commonly sold as a juice prepared from ripened Tahitian noni fruit. While dosing in research studies varies, a common dose ranges from 30 mL per day to 60 mL twice daily.[86] There is no proven safe or effective dose of noni for adults. Noni is likely safe when taken orally from preparations of fruits and leaves of the noni plant or when less than 10 g ripe noni fruit extract is taken daily for up to 28 days. Noni is possibly unsafe when more than 10 g ripe noni fruit extract is taken daily for more than 28 days.

SAFETY

Allergies

Avoid in individuals with a known allergy/hypersensitivity to noni or its constituents.

Adverse Effects and Warnings

Overall, noni has had few reported adverse effects. Noni juice may cause an increase in LFTs, possibly due to the anthraquinone content. The root of the noni plant as well as other parts such as the leaf and seed are known to contain liver-damaging anthraquinones. Recent research indicates that noni fruit puree made from ripe fruit where the seed and leaf materials are removed prior to processing contained no detectable amounts of anthraquinones.[86]

Potassium concentrations of the noni juice samples (56.3 mEq/L) were found to be similar to potassium levels in orange and tomato juice.[87] Therefore, patients with kidney disease and on a potassium-controlled diet should avoid noni products. Effects in individuals with normal kidney function are unknown.

Noni should be avoided in patients with GI disorders as it may decrease gastric transit time.

INTERACTIONS WITH DRUGS AND DIETARY SUPPLEMENTS

Since noni may decrease gastric transit time, individuals taking any medication or dietary supplement by mouth should consult with their pharmacists for any possible interactions. Given its high potassium content, noni juice should be very cautiously combined with medications such as angiotensin-converting enzyme inhibitors, angiotensin receptor blockers, or potassium-sparing diuretics that are known to increase serum potassium levels as this may result in hyperkalemia. Noni may also be hepatotoxic, and caution is advised when combining it with other potentially liver-damaging medications and dietary supplements. Interactions with warfarin could decrease its effectiveness and might possibly lead to a likelihood of blood clotting.[85]

IMPLICATIONS FOR USE IN PATIENTS WITH CHRONIC KIDNEY DISEASE

Use of noni is contraindicated in patients with CKD, particularly for those on a potassium-controlled diet due to its high potassium content, as well as potential interaction with medications commonly used in this patient population.[85]

Saw Palmetto (*Serenoa repens*)

BACKGROUND

Saw palmetto is native to the southern regions of North America. The berries of the plant were used in the early part of the 20th century to treat conditions such as cystitis and bronchitis. Today, saw palmetto is used primarily for urinary symptoms associated with benign prostatic hypertrophy (BPH). It is the most popular herbal treatment for this condition. Saw palmetto appears to possess 5-α-reductase inhibitory activity, thereby preventing the conversion of testosterone to dihydrotestosterone, a hormone implicated in prostate enlargement.

SCIENTIFIC EVIDENCE

Evidence for use of saw palmetto with enlarged prostate/BPH is strong (A). Early research showed that saw palmetto improved symptoms of BPH (eg, nighttime urination, urinary flow, and overall quality of life), although it may only have a minimal effect in reducing the size of the prostate. The effectiveness of saw palmetto may be similar to the medication finasteride (Proscar), but with the benefit of fewer adverse effects.[88] In 2006, however, the NCCAM and the National Institute of Diabetes and Digestive and Kidney Diseases cofunded a study that included 225 men with moderate-to-severe BPH and, after 1 year, found no improvement with 320 mg saw palmetto daily compared to the placebo group.[89] In 2012, a subsequent Cochrane review of 32 randomized controlled trials found that saw palmetto, even at two to three times the recommended dose, did not improve urinary flow in men with BPH.[90] More recent studies have found that saw palmetto when combined with selenium and lycopene was not inferior to tadalafil 5 mg with respect to improving the International Prostate Symptom Score and urinary flow rate in men with BPH.[91]

DOSAGE

Saw palmetto is available as an extract, capsule, tablet, tincture, or tea. The ripe fruit of the saw palmetto can be used in a variety of forms, including ground and as a dried fruit or a whole berry. For BPH, a dose of 320 mg/d in one or two divided doses (80% to 90% liposterolic content) has been used in numerous studies. Reports suggest that 160 mg once daily may be as effective as twice-daily dosages. When brewing tea using the saw palmetto berries, the active ingredient may not dissolve in water, making the tea less effective than other forms.

SAFETY

Allergies

Few allergic symptoms have been reported with saw palmetto.

Adverse Effects and Warnings

There are few severe effects with saw palmetto. The most common complaints involve the GI tract. Symptoms include upset stomach (this symptom can be reduced if taken with food), nausea, vomiting, bad breath, constipation, and diarrhea. Individuals with health concerns involving the stomach, liver, heart, or lungs should use saw palmetto with caution. Caution is also advised for individuals who require surgery or dental work, those with bleeding disorders, and those who take medications or supplements that affect bleeding as there may be an increased risk of bleeding when taking saw palmetto (see Box 19.2). Theoretically, saw palmetto may lower prostate-specific antigen (PSA). As a result, there may be a delay in diagnosis of prostate cancer or interference with PSA trends during treatment or ongoing monitoring in men with known prostate cancer.[92]

INTERACTIONS WITH DRUGS AND DIETARY SUPPLEMENTS

Do not take saw palmetto with medications and dietary supplements that affect the levels of androgens. Tannins in saw palmetto may inhibit iron absorption.[92]

IMPLICATIONS FOR USE IN PATIENTS WITH CHRONIC KIDNEY DISEASE

Studies regarding the use of saw palmetto in patients with CKD are lacking; thus, its use and safety in the population with CKD are unknown.

Because of the potential for increased bleeding, saw palmetto may be contraindicated in patients receiving maintenance HD who receive heparin during each treatment as well as patients with CKD taking medications that increase the risk for bleeding.

St John's Wort (*Hypericum perforatum*)

BACKGROUND

SJW is a yellow flowering plant that is plentiful in California and southern Oregon. Hypericin is the active ingredient found in SJW and its primary excretion is via the kidney.[93] Recently, the most common use of SJW is the treatment of mild-to-moderate depression. SJW appears to be helpful in approximately 50% to 60% of these types of patients, but similar to the treatment with prescription antidepressants, the full effect takes about 4 to 6 weeks to manifest. SJW should never be used for the treatment of severe depression (eg, feelings of suicide, extreme irritability, severe anxiety, or extreme fatigue). The mechanism by which SJW might improve depression is unknown. One thought is that it may increase serotonin levels similar to serotonin reuptake inhibitors. It may also inhibit reuptake of monoamines, dopamine noradrenaline, and neurotransmitters GABA and glutamate.

SCIENTIFIC EVIDENCE

Evidence for use of SJW for depressive disorder (mild-to-moderate) is strong (A). Short-term studies (1–3 months) suggest that SJW is more effective than a placebo. It is equally effective as tricyclic antidepressant medications in the short-term treatment of mild-to-moderate depression. A randomized controlled trial sponsored by the NCCAM showed that SJW was no more effective than the placebo in treating major depression of moderate severity.[94]

DOSAGE

SJW is available in various forms, including teas, powders, tablets, and capsules. It is also commonly added to products that contain valerian root, kava, or black cohosh. Clinical trials have used a range of doses, including 0.17 to 2.7 mg hypericin by mouth and 900 to 1,800 mg SJW extract daily by mouth.

SAFETY

Allergies

Infrequent allergic skin reactions are reported in human studies.

Adverse Effects and Warnings

SJW is generally well tolerated in recommended doses for up to 1 to 3 months. The most common adverse effects include GI upset, skin reactions, fatigue, restlessness or anxiety, sexual dysfunction, dizziness, headache, and dry mouth. Several recent studies suggest that adverse effects occur in 1% to 3% of patients taking SJW, and the number of adverse events may be similar to placebo results (and even less when compared with standard antidepressant drug therapy). It has been reported that SJW may cause psychiatric symptoms such as suicidal and homicidal thoughts. In some instances, SJW may be life threatening when interacting with other medications.[95]

INTERACTIONS WITH MEDICATIONS AND DIETARY SUPPLEMENTS

SJW interferes with the way the body metabolizes many medications and dietary supplements through the CYP450 enzyme system. As a result, the levels of these drugs and dietary supplements may be increased in the blood over a short-term period, causing potentiated effects or potentially serious reactions. The levels may also be decreased in the blood over a long-term pe-

riod, which can reduce the intended effects. The FDA suggests that patients with HIV/AIDS who are taking protease inhibitors or non-nucleoside reverse transcriptase inhibitors avoid taking SJW. Case reports exist of significant reductions in cyclosporine, tacrolimus, and mycophenolic acid drug levels, and possible organ rejections in individuals with transplants who are taking SJW. Reports also exist of altered menstrual flow, bleeding, and unwanted pregnancies in people taking birth control pills and SJW at the same time. SJW may interact with digoxin or digitoxin, resulting in a decrease in digoxin blood concentrations. Taking SJW with other antidepressants or dietary supplements with antidepressant activity may lead to increased adverse effects. In addition, using SJW with MAOIs may increase the risk of severely increased BP. SJW may lead to increased risk of sun sensitivity when taken with antibiotics, birth control pills, capsaicin, or other photosensitizing products. It may also interact with anesthetic medications, triptan-type headache medications, and certain chemotherapy agents. In higher doses, SJW has been shown to decrease blood concentrations of omeprazole, tolbutamide, caffeine, dextromethorphan, fexofenadine, carbamazepine, and cimetidine, among other medications. No relevant interactions have been seen with low-hyperforin SJW extract. In theory, SJW may inhibit the absorption of iron due to the presence of tannins. Caution is advised when taking red yeast rice or any dietary supplement that is P-glycoprotein regulated.

IMPLICATIONS FOR USE IN PATIENTS WITH CHRONIC KIDNEY DISEASE

Hypericin (SJW's active ingredient) is primarily excreted via the kidneys; thus, as kidney function declines, patients with CKD may not be able to appropriately clear this active ingredient.[96] Given the number of medications taken by patients with CKD, especially those on dialysis, and the potential for interaction with SJW, it is important that patients check with their provider before taking SJW. SJW should not be used in transplant recipients who are taking immunosuppressant medications because of possible organ rejection.[26,96]

Retinol (Vitamin A)

BACKGROUND

Vitamin A, also known as retinol or retinoic acid, is important for vision, growth, cell division, reproduction, and immunity. Vitamin A also has antioxidant properties that might protect cells against the effects of free radicals which are implicated in heart disease, cancer, and other diseases.

The richest sources of vitamin A are spinach, dairy products, and liver. Other sources are foods rich in β-carotene which include green leafy vegetables, carrots, and cantaloupe. The body can convert β-carotene into vitamin A.

Taken orally, vitamin A benefits people who have a poor or limited diet and those with conditions such as pancreatic disease, eye disease, or measles that can increase the need for vitamin A. It is important to note that when vitamin A is taken for antioxidant properties, the supplement might not offer the same benefits as naturally occurring antioxidants in food.[97]

SCIENTIFIC EVIDENCE

Vitamin A deficiency is rare in the United States. In a large clinical trial, individuals at high risk of advanced AMD reduced by 25% their risk of developing the condition by taking a combination of vitamins which also included β-carotene. Vitamin A supplements are recommended for children with measles who can become deficient in the vitamin. Vitamin A deficiency can also cause anemia and dry eyes.

Vitamin A derivatives are used in topical creams to reduce fine wrinkles, splotches, and roughness and to treat acne.[97] An oral form is used to treat severe types of acne (eg, isotretinoin). It is also taken by mouth by some people for GI ulcers, Crohn's disease, parasite in the intestines, gum disease, DM, Hurler syndrome (mucopolysaccharidosis), sinus infections, hay fever, respiratory infections, osteoarthritis, tuberculosis, and

urinary tract infections. It is also used to reduce symptoms of alcoholic hepatitis, multiple sclerosis, and Parkinson disease. Data published to date are insufficient to conclude epidemiological evidence on the association between blood levels or dietary intakes of vitamin A and the risk of Parkinson disease.[98]

DOSAGE

The recommended daily amount of vitamin A is 900 mcg for adult males and 700 mcg for adult females.*[99]

SAFETY

Allergies

There is not enough information available to determine whether vitamin A can cause any types of allergies.

Adverse Effects and Warning

Too much vitamin A can be harmful, causing nausea, vomiting, vertigo, and blurry vision. Taking high-dose vitamin A supplements (>10,000 mcg/d) over a long-term period can cause bone thinning, liver damage, headache, diarrhea, skin irritation, joint pain, and birth defects.[97]

INTERACTIONS WITH MEDICATIONS AND DIETARY SUPPLEMENTS

Taking vitamin A supplements with anticoagulants might increase the risk of bleeding. Taking vitamin A supplements while using the topical cancer drug Bexarotene can increase the risk of the drug's side effects. High doses of supplemental vitamin A can cause liver damage. The risk of liver disease can be increased by taking high doses of vitamin A with other medications known to be harmful to the liver. The weight loss drug Orlistat can decrease the absorption of vitamin A from food sources; thus, use of a multivitamin with vitamin A and β-carotene may be advised. Retinoids and vitamin A supplements should not be taken at the same time as this can increase the risk of high vitamin A levels.[97]

*Specific recommendations for transgender people were not provided.

IMPLICATIONS FOR USE IN PATIENTS WITH CHRONIC KIDNEY DISEASE

Vitamin A levels were assessed in 38 patients receiving HD. Some patients were taking multivitamin preparations containing vitamin A and others were not. Vitamin A concentrations were significantly higher in patients undergoing HD who took the multivitamin preparation that contained vitamin A. Withdrawal of the vitamin A supplements resulted in a significant fall in serum vitamin A concentrations as well as plasma calcium and alkaline phosphatase concentrations. Vitamin A toxicity can contribute to hypercalcemia in patients undergoing HD. Multivitamin preparations containing vitamin A should, therefore, be prescribed with caution in these patients.[100]

Thiamin (Vitamin B1)

BACKGROUND

Thiamin, also known as vitamin B1, is a vitamin found in food and also manufactured as a dietary supplement and medication. Thiamin can be found in whole grains, legumes, and some meats and fish. When processed, the thiamin found in grains can be removed in significant quantities; thus, many countries enrich their cereals and flours with thiamin.[101] Supplements and medications are available to treat and prevent thiamin deficiency and resulting disorders, such as beriberi and Wernicke encephalopathy. Thiamin supplementation is also used to treat maple syrup urine disease and Leigh syndrome. Thiamin supplements are typically taken by mouth, but they may also be given by intravenous or IM injection routes.

SCIENTIFIC EVIDENCE

Research on thiamin use for maple syrup urine disease shows that oral thiamin helps temporarily correct the condition.[102]

Thiamin is known to be reduced in the body in response to various conditions such as DM, drugs, and alcoholism.[95]

DOSAGE

The recommended daily amount of thiamin is 1.2 mg for adult males and 1.1 mg for adult females.* To treat mild deficiency, the WHO recommends daily oral doses of 10 mg thiamin for 1 week, followed by 3 to 5 mg/d for at least 6 weeks.[103] There are other common manifestations for thiamin deficiency. Consultation with the health care provider is needed for the proper recommended thiamin dosage treatment.

SAFETY

Allergies

A very serious allergic reaction to this vitamin is rare.

Adverse Effects and Warnings

Adverse effects are generally few. Allergic reactions including anaphylaxis may occur.

INTERACTIONS WITH MEDICATIONS AND DIETARY SUPPLEMENTS

Although thiamin is not known to interact with any medications, certain medications can have an adverse effect on thiamin levels. It is important to address thiamin status in individuals taking these and other medications on a regular basis. Furosemide (Lasix) is a loop diuretic used to treat patients with HTN and edema via increased urinary output. The use of furosemide has been linked to decreases in thiamin concentrations, possibly to deficient levels, as a result of urinary losses of thiamin. It is not known whether thiamin supplements are effective in preventing thiamin deficiency in patients taking loop diuretics. Further clinical trials are needed to determine this. Fluorouracil (Adrucil) is a chemotherapy agent that is commonly used to treat colorectal and other solid tumor cancers. Several cases

---

*Specific recommendations for transgender people were not provided.

of beriberi or Wernicke encephalopathy resulting from treatment with this medication have been reported. The likely etiology is that the drug might increase thiamin metabolism and block the formation of thiamin pyrophosphate, which is the active form of thiamin. Thiamin supplements may reverse some of these effects.[101]

IMPLICATIONS FOR USE IN PATIENTS WITH CHRONIC KIDNEY DISEASE

Acute thiamin deficiency has been reported with dextrose administration; use caution when the patient's thiamin status is uncertain. Parenteral products may contain aluminum; use caution in patients with impaired kidney function. Furosemide use is common in the later stages of CKD; thus, an increased awareness of possible deficiency is needed in this patient population.

Summary

Evidence regarding the effectiveness, appropriate dosage, risks and benefits, or duration of use of dietary supplements in individuals with CKD is extremely variable. The information presented in this chapter should be used as a general guide for the renal health care provider who needs to counsel patients about the use of dietary supplements and the potential adverse effects and interactions associated with these products. More research is needed on the use of these and other dietary supplements in the population with CKD so that renal care providers can base their recommendations on evidence, rather than extrapolation of data from studies on the general population.

Patients and health care providers are urged to contact MedWatch, the FDA's Medical Products Reporting Program, in the event of any adverse events associated with dietary supplements. The following is the contact information for MedWatch:

- Hotline: 1-888-463-6332
- Website: www.fda.gov/safety/medwatch-fda-safety-information-and-adverse-event-reporting-program

Additional Resources

American Botanical Council: www.herbalgram.org

Consumer Lab: www.consumerlab.com*

Healthline: www.healthline.com

Herb Research Foundation: www.herbs.org

National Institutes of Health, National Center for Complementary and Integrative Health: www.nccih.nih.gov

National Institutes of Health, Office of Dietary Supplements: www.ods.od.nih.gov

Natural Medicines: www.naturalstandard.com*

WedMD: www.webmd.com

World Health Organization: www.who.int

*Paid subscription required.

References

1. Dietary Supplements. US Food and Drug Administration website. August 12, 2020. Accessed August 31, 2020. www.fda.gov/food/dietary-supplements

2. Burrowes JD, Van Houten G. Use of alternative medicine by patients with stage 5 chronic kidney disease. *Adv Chronic Kidney Dis.* 2005;12(3):312-325. doi:10.1016/j.ackd.2005.04.001

3. Nowack R, Balle C, Birnkammer F, et al. Complementary and alternative medications consumed by renal patients in Southern Germany. *J Ren Nutr.* 2009;19(3):211-219. doi:10.1053/j.jrn.2008.08.008

4. Herbal Supplements and Kidney Disease. National Kidney Foundation website. April 17, 2019. Accessed October 27, 2020. www.kidney.org/atoz/content/herbalsupp

5. Luyckx VA. Nephrotoxicity of alternative medicine practice. *Adv Chronic Kidney Dis.* 2012;19(3):129-141. doi:10.1053/j.ackd.2012.04.005

6. Charen E, Harbord N. Toxicity of herbs, vitamins, and supplements. *Adv Chronic Kidney Dis.* 2020;27(1):67-71. doi:10.1053/j.ackd.2019.08.003

7. Nauffal M, Gabardi S. Nephrotoxicity of natural products. *Blood Purif.* 2016;41:123-129. doi:10.1159/000441268

8. Levin A, Stevens PE, Bilous RW, et al. KDIGO 2010 Clinical practice guideline for the evaluation and management of chronic kidney disease. *Kidney Int Suppl.* 2013;3(1):101-102. doi:10.1038/kisup .2012.73

9. Ulbricht CE. *Natural Standard Herb and Supplement Guide: An Evidence-Based Reference.* Mosby Elsevier; 2010:xvii.

10. Vitamin C. Mayo Clinic website. October 2017. Accessed September 8, 2020. www.mayoclinic.org /drugs-supplements-vitamin-c/art-20363932

11. Institute of Medicine Food and Nutrition Board. *Dietary Reference Intakes for Vitamin C, Vitamin E, Selenium, and Carotenoids.* National Academy Press; 2000.

12. Blair D. Vitamin C Supplementation and CKD. Renal & Urology News website. June 2009. Accessed September 8, 2020. www.renalandurologynews .com/home/departments/nutrition/vitamin-c -supplementation-and-ckd

13. Handelman GJ. New insight on vitamin C in patients with chronic kidney disease. *J Ren Nutr.* 2011;21(1):110-112. doi:10.1053/j.jrn.2010.11.003

14. Aloe. RxList website. September 17, 2019. Accessed September 10, 2020. www.rxlist.com/aloe /supplements.htm

15. Aloe. WebMD website. Accessed October 25, 2020. www.webmd.com/vitamins/ai /ingredientmono-607/aloe

16. Breuer L. Food Facts Friday: Aloe Vera. Davita website. June 8, 2018. Accessed October 25, 2020. https://blogs.davita.com/kidney-diet-tips/food-facts -friday-aloe-vera

17. Tabarki B, Al-Hashem A, Alfadhel M. Biotin-thiamine-responsive basal ganglia disease. GeneReviews website. August 20, 2020. Accessed October 25, 2020. www.ncbi.nlm.nih.gov/books/NBK169615/

18. Biotin. MedlinePlus website. Accessed September 11, 2020. https://medlineplus.gov/druginfo/natural /313.html

19. Biotin Side Effects. FastMed website. Accessed September 11, 2020. www.fastmed.com/health -resources/biotin-side-effects

20. Rosner I, Rogers E, Maddrey A, Goldberg DM. Clinically significant lab errors due to vitamin B7 (biotin) supplementation: a case report following a recent FDA warning. *Cureus.* 2019;11(8):e5470. doi:10.7759/cureus.5470

21. Newton KM, Reed SD, LaCroix AZ, et al. Treatment of vasomotor symptoms of menopause with black cohosh, multibotanicals, soy, hormone therapy, or placebo: a randomized trial. *Ann Intern Med.* 2006;145(12):869-879. doi:10.7326/0003-4819 -145-12-200612190-00003

22. Ulbricht CE. Black cohosh. In: *Natural Standard Herb and Supplement Guide: An Evidence-Based Reference.* Mosby Elsevier; 2010:129-131.

23. Chamomile. WebMD website. November 9, 2018. Accessed September 13, 2020. https://webmd.com /diet/supplement-guide-chamomile#1

24. Srivastava JK, Shankar E, Gupta S. Chamomile: a herbal medicine of the past with a bright future. *Mol Med Report.* 2010;3(6):895-901. doi:10.3892/mmr .2010.377

25. Gubili J, ed. Chamomile. The ASCO Post website. August 25, 2016. www.ascopost.com/issues/august -25-2016/chamomile

26. Moore L. Food, food components, and botanicals affecting drug metabolism in transplantation. *J Ren Nutr.* 2013;23(3):e71-e73. doi:10.1053/j.jrn.2013.02 .002

27. Cinnamon. WebMD website. September 2020. Accessed January 18, 2021. www.webmd.com/diet /supplement-guide-cinnamon#2

28. Sahib AS. Anti-diabetic and antioxidant effect of cinnamon in poorly controlled type-2 diabetic Iraqi patients: a randomized-controlled clinical trial. *J Intercult Ethnopharmacol.* 2016;5(2):108-113. doi:10.5455/jice.20160217044511

29. Vitamin B12. NIH website. March 2020. Accessed October 7, 2020. www.ods.od.nih.gov/factsheets /VitmainB12-HealthProfessional

30. Tucker KL, Rich S, Rosenberg I, et al. Plasma vitamin B12 concentrations relate to intake source in the Framingham Offspring Study. *Am J Clin Nutr.* 2000;71(2):514-522. doi:10.1093/ajcn/71.2.514

31. In brief: B vitamins and homocysteine. Harvard Medical School website. March 2014. Accessed January 18, 2020. www.health.harvard.edu/staying -healthy/in_brief_b_vitamins_and_homocysteine

32. Institute of Medicine (US) Standing Committee on the Scientific Evaluation of Dietary Reference Intakes and its Panel on Folate, Other B Vitamins, and Choline. *Dietary Reference Intakes for Thiamin, Riboflavin, Niacin, Vitamin B6, Folate, Vitamin B12, Pantothenic Acid, Biotin, and Choline.* National Academies Press, 1998.

33. Nutrient prescription. In: McCann L, ed. *Pocket Guide for Nutrition Assessment of the Patient With Kidney Disease*. 5th ed. National Kidney Foundation; 2015:4.4–4.5.

34. Ikizler TA, Burrowes JD, Byham-Gray LD, et al; KDOQI Nutrition in CKD Guideline Work Group. KDOQI clinical practice guideline for nutrition in CKD: 2020 update. *Am J Kidney Dis*. 2020;76(3) (suppl 1):S1-S107. doi:10.1053/j.ajkd.2020.05.006

35. Capelli I, Cianciolo G, Gasperoni L, et al. Folic acid and vitamin B12 administration in CKD, why not? *Nutrients*. 2019;11:383. doi:10.3390/nu11020383

36. Amini M, Khosravi M, Baradaran HR, Atlasi R. Vitamin B12 supplementation in end stage renal diseases: a systematic review. *Med J Islam Repub Iran*. 2015;29:167.

37. Arenas-Jal M, Sune-Negre JM, Garcia-Montoya E. Coenzyme Q10 supplementation: efficacy, safety, and formulation changes. *Compr Rev Food Sci Food Saf*. 2020;19:574-594. doi:10.1111/1541 -4337.12539

38. Gupta K. Amazing benefits of coenzyme Q10. QuPro website. June 2018. Accessed October 9, 2020. www.qupro.in/blog/amazing-benefits-of -coenzyme-q10

39. Coenzyme Q10. In: Ulbricht C. *Natural Standard Herb and Supplement Guide: An Evidence-Based Reference*. Mosby Elsevier; 2010:245-248.

40. Coenzyme Q10: CoQ10. WebMD website. April 2019. Accessed January 18, 2021. www.webmd .com/diet/supplement-guide-coenzymeq10 -coq10#1

41. Coenzyme Q10. Mayo Clinic website. November 2020. Accessed January 18, 2021. www.mayoclinic .org/drugs-supplements-coenzyme-q10/art -20362602?p=1

42. Yen C, Chu Y, Lee B, Lin Y, Lin P. Effect of liquid ubiquinal supplementation on glucose, lipids and antioxidant capacity in type 2 diabetes patients: a double-blind, randomized, placebo-controlled trial. *Br J Nutr*. 2018;120(1):57-63. doi:10.1017 /S0007114518001241

43. Herbal supplements market size, share & trends analysis report by product, by formulation, by consumer, and segment forecasts, 2018–2025. Grandview Research website. November 2018. Accessed October 9, 2020. www .grandviewresearch.com/industry-analysis/herbal -supplements-market#

44. Goel V, Lovlin R, Barton R, et al. Efficacy of a standardized echinacea preparation (Echinilin) for the treatment of the common cold: a randomized, double-blind, placebo-controlled trial. *J Clin Pharm Ther*. 2004;29(1):75-83. doi:10.1111/j.1365-2710 .2003.00542.x

45. Barrett B, Brown R, Rakel D, et al. Echinacea for treating the common cold: a randomized controlled trial. *Ann Intern Med*. 2010;153(12):769-777. doi:10 .7326/0003-4819-153-12-201012210-00003

46. Yale SH, Liu K. Echinacea purpurea therapy for the treatment of the common cold: a randomized, double-blind, placebo-controlled trial. *Arch Intern Med*. 2004;164(11):1237-1241. doi:10.1001 /archinte.164.11.1237

47. McCaleb R, Leigh E, Morien K. *The Encyclopedia of Popular Herbs: Your Complete Guide to the Leading Medicinal Plants*. Prima Health; 2000.

48. Kemp DE, Franco KN. Possible leukopenia associated with long-term use of echinacea. *J Am Board Fam Pract*. 2002;15(5):417-419.

49. Omega-3 fatty acids. NIH Office of Dietary Supplements website. October 2020. Accessed January 18, 2021. https://ods.od.nih.gov/factsheets /Omega3FattyAcids-HealthProfessional

50. Omega 3 fatty acids, fish oil, alpha-linolenic acid. In: Ulbricht C. *Natural Standard Herb & Supplement Guide An Evidence-Based Reference*. Mosby Elsevier; 2010:536-540.

51. Hjalmarsdottir F. How much omega-3 should you take per day? Healthline website. December 15, 2019. Accessed March 17, 2021. www.healthline .come/nutrition/how-much-omega-3#

52. Mercury Levels in Commercial Fish and Shellfish (1990–2012). FDA website. October 2014. Accessed October 10, 2020. www.fda.gov/food /metals-and-your-food/mercury-levels-commercial -fish-and-shellfish-1990-2012

53. Pananki Y, Dashti-Khavidaki S, Farnood F, et al. Therapeutic effects of omega-3 fatty acids on chronic kidney disease-associated pruritus: a literature review. *Adv Pharm Bull*. 2016;6(4):509- 514. doi:10.15171/apb.2016.064

54. Hu J, Liu Z, Zhang H. Omega-3 fatty acid supplement as an adjunctive therapy in the treatment of chronic kidney disease: a meta- analysis. *Clinics (Sao Paulo)*. 2017;72(1):58-64. doi:10.6061/clinics/2017(01)10

55. Cortinovis M, Gotti E, Remuzzi G, et al. Omega-3 polyunsaturated fatty acids affect sirolimus exposure in kidney transplant recipients on calcineurin inhibitor-free regimen. *Transplantation*. 2010;89(1):126-127. doi:10.1097/TP.0b013e3181c280df

56. Flax: What You Need to Know. GI Society/Canadian Society of Intestinal Research website. October 2005. Accessed January 18, 2021. https://badgut.org/information-centre/a-z-digestive-topics/flax-what-you-need-to-know

57. Flaxseed and Flaxseed Oil. Mayo Clinic website. October 2017. Accessed October 10, 2020. www.mayoclinic.org/drugs-supplements-flaxseed-and-flaxseed-oil/art-2-366457

58. Flaxseed Oil. WebMD website. Accessed January 18, 2021. www.webmd.com/vitamins/ai/ingredientmono-990/flaxseed-oil

59. Gardner CD, Lawson LD, Block E, et al. Effect of raw garlic vs. commercial garlic supplements on plasma lipid concentrations in adults with moderate hypercholesterolemia: a randomized clinical trial. *Arch Intern Med*. 2007;167(4):346-353. doi:10.1001/archinte.167.4.346

60. Health Benefits of Garlic. Pharmaqz website. March 2014. Accessed October 10, 2020. www.pharmaqz.com/health-benefits-of-garlic

61. El-Saber Batiha G, Beshbishy AM, Wasef LG, et al. Chemical constituents and pharmacological activities of garlic (allium sativum L.): a review. *Nutrients*. 2020;12(3):872. doi:10.3390/nu12030872

62. Borrelli F, Capasso R, Izzo AA. Garlic (allium sativum L.): adverse effects and drug interactions in humans. *Mol Nutr Food Res*. 2007;51(11):1386-1397. doi:10.1002/mnfr.200700072

63. DeKosky ST, Williamson JD, Fitzpatrick AL, et al. Ginkgo biloba for prevention of dementia: a randomized controlled trial. *JAMA*. 2008;300(19):2253-2262. doi:10.1001/jama.2008.683

64. Dodge HH, Zitzelberger T, Oken BS, Howleson D, Kaye J. A randomized placebo-controlled trial of ginkgo biloba for the prevention of cognitive decline. *Neurology*. 2008;70(19 Pt 2):1809-1817. doi:10.1212/01.wnl.0000303814.13509.db

65. Ginko. In: Ulbricht C. *Natural Standard Herb and Supplement Guide: An Evidence-Based Reference*. Mosby Elsevier; 2010:358-361.

66. Ginko. WebMD website. Accessed October 10, 2020. www.webmd.com/vitamins/ai/ingredientsmono-333/ginkgo

67. Davydov L, Stirling AL. Stevens-Johnson syndrome with ginkgo biloba. J *Herb Pharmacother*. 2001;1(3):65-69. doi:10.1080/j157v01n03_06

68. Ginkgo. NIH website. August 2020. Accessed October 10, 2020. www.nccih.nih.gov/health/ginkgo

69. Ginseng. In: Ulbricht C. *Natural Standard Herb and Supplement Guide: An Evidence-Based Reference*. Mosby Elsevier; 2010:362-367.

70. Panax Ginseng. WebMD website. Accessed January 18, 2021. www.webmd.com/vitamins/ai/ingredientmono-1000/panax-ginseng

71. Sawitzke AD, Shi H, Finco MF, et al. The effect of glucosamine and/or chondroitin sulfate on the progression of knee osteoarthritis: a report from the glucosamine/chondroitin arthritis intervention trial. *Arthritis Rheum*. 2008;58(10):3183-3191. doi:10.1002/art.23973

72. Clegg DO, Reda DJ, Harris CL, et al. Glucosamine, chondroitin sulfate, and the two in combination for painful knee osteoarthritis. *N Engl J Med*. 2006;354(8):795-808. doi:10.1056/NEJMoa052771

73. Reichenbach S, Sterchi R, Scherer M, et al. Meta-analysis: chondroitin for osteoarthritis of the knee or hip. *Ann Intern Med*. 2007;146(8):580-590. doi:10.7326/0003-4819-146-8-200704170-00009

74. Glucosamine sulfate. RxList website. September 2019. Accessed January 18, 2021. www.rxlist.com/glucosamine_sulfate/supplements.htm

75. Talbott S. Green tea (Camellia sinensis). In: *Cortisol Control and the Beauty Connection*. Hunter House Publishers; 2007:90-91.

76. Green Tea. NIH website. October 2020. Accessed October 21, 2020. www.nccih.nih.gov/health/green-tea

77. Delimont NM, Haub MD, Lindshield BL. The impact of tannin consumption on iron bioavailability and status: a narrative review. *Curr Dev Nutr*. 2017;1(2):1012. doi:10.3945/cdn.116.000042

78. Green Tea. In: Ulbricht C. *Natural Standard Herb and Supplement Guide: An Evidence-Based Reference*. Mosby Elsevier; 2010:387-389.

79. Milk Thistle. NIH website. August 2020. Accessed October 21, 2020. www.nccih.nih.gov/health/milk-thistle

80. Fallahzadeh MK, Dormanesh B, Sagheb MM, et al. Effect of addition of silymarin to renin-angiotensin system inhibitors on proteinuria in type 2 diabetic patients with overt nephropathy: a randomized, double-bind, placebo-controlled trial. *Am J Kid Dis*. 2012;60(6):896-903. doi:10.1053/j.ajkd.2012.06.005

81. Shane-McWhorter. Milk Thistle. Merck Manual website. July 2020. Accessed October 21, 2020. www.merckmanuals.com/professional/special-subjects/dietary-supplements/milk-thistle

82. Milk Thistle. Mayo Clinic website. October 14, 2017. Accessed October 21. www.mayoclinic.org/drugs-supplements-milk-thistle/art-20362885

83. Noni. In: Ulbricht C. *Natural Standard Herb and Supplement Guide: An Evidence-Based Reference.* Mosby Elsevier; 2010:525-526.

84. West BJ, Deng S, Isami F, Uwaya A, Jensen CJ. The potential health benefits of noni juice: a review of human intervention studies. *Foods.* 2018;7(4):58. doi:10.3390/foods7040058

85. Noni. WebMD website. Accessed October 25, 2020. www.webmd.com/vitamins/ai/ingredientmono-758/noni

86. Bussmann RW, Hennig L, Giannis A, et al. Anthraquinone content in noni (morinda citrifolia L.). *Evid Based Complement Alternat Med.* 2013:208378. doi:10.1155/2013/208378

87. Mueller BA, Scott MK, Sowinski KM, Prag KA. Noni juice (Morinda citrifolia): hidden potential for hyperkalemia? *Am J Kidney Dis.* 2000;35(2):310-312.

88. Gordon AE, Shaughnessy AF. Saw palmetto for prostate disorders. *Am Fam Physician.* 2003;67(6):1281-1283.

89. Bent S, Kane C, Shinohara K, et al. Saw palmetto for benign prostatic hyperplasia. *N Engl J Med.* 2006;354(6):557-566. doi:10.1056/NEJMoa053085

90. Tacklind J, MacDonald R, Rutks I, Stanke JU, Wilt TJ. Serenoa repens for benign prostatic hyperplasia. *Cochrane Database Syst Rev.* 2012;12(CD001423). doi:10.1002/14651858.CD001423.pub3

91. Morgia G, Vespasiani G, Pareo RM, et al. Serenoa repens + selenium + lycopene vs tadalafil 5 mg for the treatment of lower urinary tract symptoms secondary to benign prostatic obstruction: a Phase IV, non-inferiority, open-label, clinical study (SPRITE study). *BJU Int.* 2018;122(2):317-325. doi:10.1111/bju.14209

92. Saw Palmetto. In: Ulbricht C. *Natural Standard Herb and Supplement Guide: An Evidence-Based Reference.* Mosby Elsevier; 2010:641-642

93. Soucy M. The impact of alternative medicine therapies on the nutrition and well-being of the chronic kidney disease (CKD) stage 5 patient. *Renal Nutrition Forum.* 2008;27(2):1-7.

94. Hypericum Depression Trial Study Group. Effect of *Hypericum perforatum* (St John's wort) in major depressive disorder: a randomized controlled trial. *JAMA.* 2002;287(14):1807-1814. doi:10.1001/jama.287.14.1807

95. St. John's Wort. NIH website. October 2020. Accessed October 22, 2020. www.nccih.nih.gov/health/st-johns-wort

96. Mai I, Stormer E, Bauer S, et al. Impact of St John's wort treatment on the pharmacokinetics of tacrolimus and mycophenolic acid in renal transplant patients. *Nephrol Dial Transplant.* 2003;18(4):819-822. doi:10.1093/ndt/gfg002

97. Vitamin A. Mayo Clinic website. October 27, 2017. Accessed October 24, 2020. www.mayoclinic.org/drugs-supplements-vitamin-a/art-20365945

98. Takeda A, Nyssen OP, Syed A, et al. Vitamin A and carotenoids and the risk of Parkinson's disease: a systematic review and meta-analysis. *Neuroepidemiology.* 2014;42(1):25-38. doi:10.1159/000355849

99. Institute of Medicine (US) Panel on Micronutrients. *Dietary Reference Intakes for Vitamin A, Vitamin K, Arsenic, Boron, Chromium, Copper, Iodine, Iron, Manganese, Molydenum, Nickel, Silicon, Vanadium, and Zinc.* National Academies Press; 2001.

100. Farrington K, Miller P, Varghese Z, Baillod RA, Moorhead JF. Vitamin A toxicity and hypercalcaemia in chronic renal failure. *Br Med J (Clin Res Ed).* 1981;282(6281):1999-2002. doi:10.1136/bmj.282.6281.1999

101. Thiamin. NIH website. June 3, 2020. Accessed October 24, 2020. www.ods.od.nih.gov/factsheets/Thiamin-Health Professional

102. Thiamin. Mayo Clinic website. October 25, 2017. Accessed October 24, 2020. www.mayoclinic.org/drugs-supplements-thiamin/art-20366430?p=1

103. Dosage of thiamine supplementation for preventing and treating thiamine deficiency. In: *Thiamine Deficiency and Its Prevention and Control in Major Emergencies.* World Health Organization; 1999:24.

SECTION VI
Special Considerations in Kidney Disease Nutrition Care

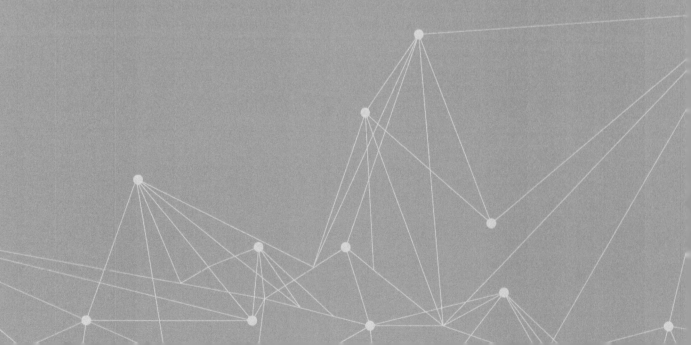

CHAPTER 20

Guidelines for Patients Following Vegetarian, Vegan, or Plant-Based Diets in Kidney Disease

Joan Brookhyser Hogan, RD, CD

Introduction

Plant-based diets are for more than vegans or vegetarians; this pattern of eating can be applied to the meal planning of those patients who have lost a preference for animal-based products as a way to provide needed protein and nutrient intake. These diet preferences are not only safe but can provide notable health benefits compared to kidney diets containing more animal-based products.[1,2]

Plant-based whole grains, legumes, fruits, vegetables, and nuts exert beneficial effects related to cardiometabolic risk factors, such as blood pressure, hyperlipidemia, insulin hemostasis, oxidative stress, inflammatory markers, and endothelial function, all of which are associated with kidney disease and kidney disease progression. Plant-based foods are also high in nutrients, such as magnesium, potassium, vitamin C, and calcium, which contribute to a lower dietary acid load compared to animal products. This alkaline effect has been thought to decrease proteinuria, glomerular hyperfiltration, and kidney disease progression.[3-5]

Other aspects considered to play a role in the value of plant-based foods in kidney disease are improvement in gut microbiota, decreasing inflammation and improving blood sugar and control of uremia. High glycation load from cooked meats might also be a factor in the deleterious impact of animal proteins on kidney disease. In addition, peer reviewed journals are identifying phosphorus absorption from plant-based foods when compared to animal-based protein as a benefit early on in kidney disease prevention and progression.[6,7] As kidney disease progresses, a large phosphorus load leading to elevated parathyroid hormone (PTH) and Fibroblast Growth Factor 23 (FGF-23) levels can further contribute to heart and kidney disease. Studies have shown even 1 week on a vegetarian diet can decrease phosphorus and FGF-23 levels.[8] These same studies are not found with animal protein.[9]

Key areas of focus in planning these diets are requirements for protein while balancing potassium and phosphorus goals and meeting calorie needs to achieve and maintain a weight within a healthy body mass index range.

Protein

Protein options for your patients can differ, depending on their preferences. A patient's definition of a vegan or vegetarian diet can also vary. Defining their preferences early in the nutrition instruction is important as this can impact options for meeting their protein needs.

Types of plant-based diets include the following:

- Pesco-vegetarian: no animal flesh but will eat seafood, fish, eggs, and dairy
- Lacto-ovo vegetarian: no animal flesh, seafood, or fish but will eat eggs and dairy
- Vegan: no animal products, including eggs, dairy, butter, and possibly no honey

- Flexitarian: a style of eating that encourages mostly plant-based foods while allowing meat and other animal products in moderation
- Mediterranean: high in fruits, vegetables, nuts, seeds, legumes, fish, and olive oil, with minimal or rare intake of dairy and red meat

This chapter will focus on the vegan and lacto-ovo vegetarian diets. Protein needs can be met for these patients through a variety of plant-based foods and some dairy products or plant proteins. The most concentrated sources of plant-based protein include dried beans, seit-

an, tofu, tempeh, and nuts, but sources can also include intact grain products (eg, barley, wheat berries, oatmeal, brown and wild rice, spelt, kamut, and millet) or pseudo-cereal grains (eg, quinoa, amaranth, and buckwheat). See Table 20.1 for plant and lacto-ovo protein options. These are general guidelines as nutrient content varies from product to product. Due to the differing amino acid content of plant-based proteins, a variety of sources should be encouraged to meet amino acid and nutrient needs.[10] When limiting dairy intake is necessary, there are many nondairy substitutes that can be incorporated

TABLE 20.1 | Vegan and Lacto-Ovo Vegetarian Foods That Provide Approximately 7 g of Protein per Serving[a]

Protein source		Serving size	Phosphorus (mg)	Potassium (mg)
Dried beans/ peas, cooked	Chickpeas, black beans, pinto beans, navy beans, lentils	½ cup	100-120	200-300
	Edamame	⅓ cup	87	225
Intact grains and pseudo-cereal grains (amaranth, quinoa, millet, oatmeal-non instant, barley, brown or wild rice, wheat berries, spelt, kamut, buckwheat)		1 cup	85-300	150-275
Nut butters (peanut, almond, cashew, sunflower, sesame)		2 tablespoons	100-170	240
Nuts and seeds (chia, almonds, sesame, hemp, cashew, brazil, sunflower, flaxseed)		¼ cup	120-270	50-250
Seitan	Non-high gluten flour	2 oz	130	20
	High gluten flour	½ oz	35	14
Tempeh		¼ cup (40 g)	70-110	130-170
Tofu, firm		⅛ of package or ⅓ cup (90 g)	100-150	160-190
Protein powders— plain	Pea	1 tablespoon	19	25
	Whey	1 tablespoon	65	55
	Rice	1 tablespoon	45	5
Cheese: cheddar, mozzarella, swiss		1 oz	20	130
Egg		1 medium	60	90
Milk[b]	Cow's	1 cup	250	400
	Soy, plain, nonfat	10 oz	260	320
Yogurt	Plain	1 cup	230-355	380-575
	Greek, plain	½ cup	160	160

[a] Information retrieved from:
- https://fdc.nal.usda.gov/about-us.html. Accessed April 2020.
- https://www.livestrong.com/article/294810-the-nutritional-value-of-seitan. Accessed April 2020.
- https://www.healthline.com/nutrition/seitan#seitan. Accessed April 2020.
- https://nutritiondata.self.com. Accessed April 2020.
- https://nkdnutrition.com/products/grass-fed-whey. Accessed April 2020.
- https://nkdnutrition.com/products/organic-brown-rice-protein-powder. Accessed April 2020.

[b] There are several nondairy milks on the market, but most are very marginal in protein (see Table 20.2).

into the diet. See Table 20.2 for the nutritional content of various milk substitutes. Although not a key source of protein, it is good to remember that vegetables can also contribute protein. The amount of protein in vegetables will vary, but it is usually 2 g to 3 g per ½ cup serving. Protein powders from pea, rice, or whey can also be considered for patients when protein needs are not being met by food alone.

TABLE 20.2 | Milk vs Nondairy Milk Comparison[a]

Product (8 oz)	Protein (g)	Phosphorus (mg)	Potassium (mg)
Cow's milk—2%	8	252	390
Almond milk, plain	0-1	40-190	35-255
Rice milk, plain	1	188	25-75
Soy milk, plain/vanilla	7-11	100-250	240-440
Hemp milk	4	400	60-80
Coconut milk	<1	17-199	32-300
Oat milk	2-4	120-270	130-133

[a] Information retrieved from:
- https://nutritiondata.self.com
- https://fdc.nal.usda.gov
- https://healthyeater.com/rice-milk
- https://blogs.davita.com/kidney-diet-tips/soy-milk-or-cows-milk-the-best-choice-for-kidney-diets
- www.jrnjournal.org/action/showPdf?pii=S1051-2276%2808%2900484-6
- www.kidneyhealth.ca/milk-substitutes

Potassium and Phosphorus

Potassium is often seen as the primary concern with plant-based diets and plant-based proteins. If your patient is new to these types of foods in their diet, it would be best to start with those protein foods that are lowest in potassium and phosphorus, such as seitan, tofu, and tempeh. Cooked dried beans and nuts are higher in potassium and phosphorus and, thus, should be added gradually to safely incorporate them into the diet. Prior to developing kidney disease, 90% of a patient's potassium is excreted through their urine. As chronic kidney disease (CKD) progresses, gastrointestinal tract adaptation can occur to the point that over 90% of potassium can be excreted through the stool. Monitoring bowel function, blood sugars, weight loss, and urine output as well as serum bicarbonate and potassium

levels will help determine potassium load tolerance.[11] Constipation is a common problem in the population with CKD, especially those who are on dialysis. Given the higher fiber content of plant-based foods, a gradual switch to a plant-based diet may help with management of constipation. In turn, this may improve potassium management by increasing the amount of potassium eliminated via the gut in these patients.

However, for patients on hemodialysis who maintain higher serum potassium levels with a plant-based diet, adjustments in the dialysate potassium concentration may be needed. The use of potassium-lowering medications, such as sodium polystyrene sulfonate (Kayexalate), sodium zirconium cyclosilicate (Lokelma), or patiromer sorbitex calcium (Veltassa), may also need to be considered for patients on dialysis as well as patients with earlier-stage CKD.[12,13]

Another mineral of concern when promoting a plant-based diet is phosphorus. Diets consist of organic and inorganic phosphorus. Although animal proteins are lower in organic phosphorus when compared to plant-based proteins, the phosphate in plant proteins is estimated to be only 50% bioavailable compared with animal proteins (including milk and cheese) where bioavailability is much higher. This occurs because many plant-based proteins are higher in phytates. This component of fiber binds phosphorus and prevents absorption. Since the 1990s, a surge of phosphate additives, known as inorganic phosphates, have nearly doubled in the typical American diet. This type of phosphate, also known as disodium phosphate, monosodium phosphate, or potassium tripolyphosphate, can be found in many ready-to-eat vegetarian and nonvegetarian products. This includes sweetened beverages, dark sodas, cereals, desserts, and nondairy creamers and toppings. This type of phosphate is estimated to be highly absorbable and should be discouraged. See Table 20.3 on page 434 for a comparison of the phosphorus absorption from foods.

Even with a fractional rate of intestinal absorption with such foods as beans and intact grains, the intake of phosphorus may still lead to higher serum phosphorus levels and, thus, some patients may require phosphate binders.

TABLE 20.3 | Absorbed Phosphorus From Selected Food Groups[a]

Food groups	Estimated percent of absorbed phosphorus
Grains (this does not include leavened breads which may contain yeast-based phytase) Dried beans (cooked) and nuts	20-40
Meat, fish, poultry, and dairy	40-60
Processed food and drinks containing phosphate additives	90-100

[a] Information retrieved from www.ncbi.nlm.nih.gov/pubmed/20093346. Accessed April 2020.

Sodium

Not all vegetarian food items are considered to be a healthy choice. These include meat analogs, packaged vegetarian entrees, tofu hotdogs, commercial veggie burgers, canned soy products, ready-made snacks, pickled vegetables, and vegan cheese. These foods tend to be quite high in sodium, not to mention high in phosphate additives, especially if they contain cheese.

If, on occasion, a patient does use these food products, it is typically not a problem. However, it is best to provide instruction on label reading and suggest the following guidelines:

- Limit packaged entrees containing greater than 500 mg of sodium to one serving per week.
- Limit snack items containing greater than 150 mg of sodium to one serving per week (eg, chips, crackers, packaged nuts, packaged cookies, or pastries).
- Avoid entrees and snacks with phosphate additives listed in the ingredients.

Whether your patient is vegan, vegetarian, or prefers plant-based proteins, it is always best to encourage use of herbs and spices in food preparation. These additions can provide a host of flavor and anti-inflammatory protection. Choices include, but are not limited to, garlic, rosemary, sage, turmeric, cumin, dill, and vinegars.

Calories

Maximizing a patient's energy intake can further help with reduced protein breakdown for energy, weight loss,

risk of related hyperkalemia, and maintenance of visceral and somatic protein stores.[11,14] Additional calories can be added with monounsaturated fats (eg, olive oil, avocado oil, canola oil, or peanut oil) and some polyunsaturated fats (eg, corn oil, soybean oil, sunflower oil, or safflower oil). Low potassium vegetables, herbs, and spices can be blended with these oils to create flavorful sauces that, when added to foods, provide health benefits and extra calories.

Supplements

When eliminating animal-based products from the diet, certain nutrients primarily found in animal-based foods need to be closely monitored. These include vitamin B12, omega-3 fatty acids, and vitamin D. This is especially important for patients who are vegan. Although most patients with CKD should be on a vitamin B complex supplement, which includes vitamin B12, monitoring serum levels of vitamin B12 is important. Certain individuals may not absorb vitamin B12 effectively and will require intramuscular B12 injections to maintain adequate serum vitamin B12 levels.

Omega-3 fatty acids are also important and may be deficient in vegetarian and vegan diets. Of the three main types of omega-3 fatty acids, plant foods typically only contain α-linolenic acid (ALA). ALA is not as active in the body and must be converted to two other forms of omega-3 fatty acid—eicosapentaenoic acid (EPA) and docosahexaenoic acid (DHA)—to bestow the same health benefits. Unfortunately, the body's ability to convert ALA is limited. Only about 5% of ALA is converted to EPA, while less than 0.5% is converted to DHA.[15] Thus, if patients do not supplement with fish oil or get EPA or DHA from their diet, it is important that they eat a good amount of ALA-rich foods to meet their omega-3 fatty acid needs. The recommended minimum omega-3 fatty acid intake per day is 1 g, but it may be higher for some individuals.[16] See Table 20.4 for a list of these foods.

Similar to patients who consume animal products, it can be difficult to meet vitamin D needs with food alone on a plant-based diet. Checking vitamin D levels and supplementing accordingly is recommended.

TABLE 20.4 | Omega-3 Fatty Acid Content of Plant-Based Foods[a]

Food	ALA g/per serving
Flaxseed, whole—1 tablespoon	2.35
Flaxseed oil—1 tablespoon	7.26
Soybean oil—1 tablespoon	0.92
Chia seeds—1 oz	5.06
Canola oil—1 tablespoon	1.28
Algae supplements	Varies

ALA = alpha-linolenic acid
[a]https://ods.od.nih.gov/factsheets/Omega3FattyAcids-HealthProfessional. Accessed April 2020.

Summary

Planning a vegetarian diet for a patient can be challenging to even the most experienced registered dietitian nutritionist. It may require learning about foods that are unfamiliar. It may require exploring new recipes and products to help patients achieve their nutritional goals. Included are three meal plans providing three different amounts of protein (see Box 20.1). These can serve as an example of how patients' diets can be planned. The meal plans limit sodium to less than 1,800 mg. Potassium requirements will vary with each patient, but these

BOX 20.1 | Meal Plans

40 G PROTEIN	60 G PROTEIN	90 G PROTEIN
Breakfast		
1, 8-inch tortilla with	1, 8-inch tortilla with	1, 8-inch tortilla with
• 1 scrambled egg[a] with onion or leeks and ¼ cup mushrooms **or**	• 1 scrambled egg[a] with onion or leeks and ¼ cup mushrooms **or**	• 2 scrambled eggs[a] with onion or leeks and ¼ cup mushrooms **or**
• ⅓ cup scrambled tofu[b] with onions or leeks, and ¼ cup mushrooms **or**	• ⅓ cup scrambled tofu[b] with onions or leeks, and ¼ cup mushrooms **or**	• ⅔ cup scrambled tofu[b] with onions or leeks, and ¼ cup mushrooms **or**
• ½ oz high gluten flour seitan[b] stir fried with onions or leeks, and ¼ cup mushrooms	• ½ oz high gluten flour seitan[b] stir fried with onions or leeks, and ¼ cup mushrooms	• 1 oz high gluten flour seitan[b] stir fried with onions or leeks, and ¼ cup mushrooms
1 cup blueberries	1 cup blueberries	1 cup blueberries
Lunch		
Grain bowl—1 cup cooked whole grain (eg, quinoa, barley, couscous, brown rice) topped with 1 cup fresh vegetables and 1 protein:	Grain bowl—1 cup cooked whole grain (eg, quinoa, barley, couscous, brown rice) topped with 1 cup fresh vegetables and 2 proteins:	Grain bowl—1 cup cooked whole grain (eg, quinoa, barley, couscous, brown rice) topped with 1 cup fresh vegetables and 3 proteins:
• 1 hard-boiled egg **or**	• 2 hard-boiled eggs **or**	• 3 hard-boiled eggs **or**
• ½ oz high gluten flour seitan[b] **or**	• 1 oz high gluten flour seitan[b] **or**	• 1½ oz high gluten flour seitan[b] **or**
• ⅓ cup firm tofu[a,b] **or**	• ⅔ cup firm tofu[a,b] **or**	• 1 cup firm tofu[a,b] **or**
• ¼ cup raw nuts[b]	• ⅓ cup firm tofu and ¼ cup raw nuts[b]	• ⅔ cup firm tofu and ¼ cup raw nuts[b]
Add spices, oil, fresh lemon or lime, balsamic vinegar	Add spices, oil, fresh lemon or lime, balsamic vinegar	Add spices, oil, fresh lemon or lime, balsamic vinegar
Dinner		
½ cup whole wheat pasta and 2 cups fresh vegetables stir fried with 1 protein:	¾ cup cooked chickpea or lentil pasta (15 g protein per cup) and 1 cup fresh vegetables stir fried with 1 protein:	1½ cups cooked chickpea or lentil pasta (15 g protein per cup) and 1 cup fresh vegetables stir fried with 6 proteins:
• ⅓ cup grilled firm tofu[b] **or**	• ⅓ cup grilled firm tofu[b] **or**	• 2 cups grilled tofu[b] **or**
• ½ oz high gluten flour seitan[b] **or**	• ½ oz high gluten flour seitan[b] **or**	• 3 oz high-gluten seitan[a,b] **or**
• ½ cup cooked beans (garbanzo)[a,b]	• ½ cup cooked beans (garbanzo)[a,b]	• ½ cup cooked dried beans with 1⅔ cups tofu[b]
Add oil and spices or lemon juice	Add oil and spices or lemon juice	Add oil and spices or lemon juice
Snacks		
Apple cooked with cinnamon and sweetener of choice, topped with a drizzle of nut milk	Apple cooked with cinnamon and sweetener of choice, topped with ¼ cup plain Greek yogurt or blended tofu[b]	Apple cooked with cinnamon and sweetener of choice, topped with ¼ cup plain Greek yogurt or blended tofu[b]

[a] Protein used in nutrient analysis.
[b] Vegan choices.

examples provide 3,000 mg or less. The phosphorus content is 1,200 mg. Keeping in mind that this phosphorus comes primarily from plant-based food sources, the amount absorbed will be much less than the amount of phosphorus from animal products. This may, in turn, provide more liberalization in the kidney diet.

Further Reading and Meal Preparation Ideas for Vegetarians and Vegans

Palmer S. *The Plant-Powered Diet.* The Experiment; 2012.

Davis B, Melina V. *Becoming Vegan: The Complete Reference to Plant-Based Nutrition.* Book Publishing Co; 2014.

Bittman M. *How to Cook Everything Vegetarian.* Houghton Mifflin Harcourt; 2017.

Bey R. *Cookbook: Vegan's Way—Kidney Health Recipes: Anti-Inflammatory—50 Halal Recipes.* 2017.

Brooksyser Hogan J. *The Vegetarian Diet for Kidney Disease: Preserving Kidney Function With Plant-Based Eating.* 2nd ed. Basic Health Publications, Inc; 2009.

Davis B. Other [Recipes]. Brenda Davis RD website. Accessed April 26, 2021. www.brendadavisrd.com/#recipes

Dr. McDougall website. Accessed April 26, 2021. www.drmcdougall.com/recipes

Vegan. Vegetarian Times website. Accessed April 26, 2021. www.vegetariantimes.com/vegan-vegetarian-recipes/vegan-recipes

References

1. Sparks B. Nutritional considerations for dialysis vegetarian patients, Part one. *J Ren Nutr.* 2018;28(2):e11-e14. doi:10.1053/j.jrn.2017.12.002
2. Gluba-Brzozka A, Franczyk B, Rysz J. Vegetarian diet in chronic kidney disease—a friend or foe. *Nutrients.* 2017;9(4):374. doi:10.3390/nu9040374
3. Hyunju K, Caulfield LE, Garcia-Larsen V, et al. Plant-based diets and incident CKD and kidney function. *Clin J Am Soc Nephrol.* 2019;14(5):682-691. doi:10.2215/CJN.12391018
4. Mirmiran P, Yuzbashin E, Aghayan M, et al. A prospective study of dietary meat intake and risk of incident chronic kidney disease. *J Ren Nutr.* 2020;30(2):111-118. doi:10.1053/j.jrn.2019.06.008
5. Joshi S, Hashmi S, Shah S, et al. Plant-based diets for prevention and management of chronic kidney disease. *Curr Opin Nephrol Hypertens.* 2020;29(1):16-21. doi:10.1097/MNH.0000000000000574
6. Cases A, Cigarran-Guldris S, Mas S, et al. Vegetable-based diets for chronic kidney disease? It is time to reconsider. *Nutrients.* 2019;11(6):1263. doi:10.3390/nu11061263
7. Hepp Z, Dodick DW, Varon SF, et al. Persistence and switching patterns of oral migraine prophylactic medications among patients with chronic migraine: a retrospective claims analysis. *Cephalalgia.* 2017;37(5):470-485. doi:10.1177/0333102416678382
8. Guitierrez OM, Mannstadt M, Isakova T, Rauh-Hain JA, Tamez H, Shah A. Fibroblast growth factor 23 and mortality among patients undergoing hemodialysis. *N Engl J Med.* 2008;359(6):584-592. doi:10.1056/NEJMoa0706130
9. Moe SM, Zidehsarai MP, Chambers MA, et al. Vegetarian compared with meat dietary protein source and phosphorus homeostasis in chronic kidney disease. *Clin J Am Soc Nephrol.* 2011;6(2):257-264. doi:10.2215/CJN.05040610
10. Joshi S, Shah S, Kalantar-Zadeh K. Adequacy of plant-based proteins in chronic kidney disease. *J Ren Nutr.* 2019;29(2):112-117. doi:10.1053/j.jrn.2018.06.006
11. St-Jules DE, Goldfarb DS, Sevick MA. Nutrient non-equivalence: does restricting high-potassium plant foods help to prevent hyperkalemia in hemodialysis? *J Ren Nutr.* 2016;26(5):282-287. doi:10.1053/j.jrn.2016.02.005
12. Choi HY, Ha SK. Potassium balances in maintenance hemodialysis. *Electrolyte Blood Press.* 2013;11(1):9-16. doi:10.5049/EBP.2013.11.1.9
13. Cases A, Gorriz JL. Sodium zirconium cyclosilicate: a new potassium binder for the treatment of hyperkalemia. *Drugs Today (Barc).* 2018;54(10):601-613. doi:10.1358/dot.2018.54.10.2872504
14. Capizzi I, Teta L, Vigotti FN, et al. Weight loss in advanced chronic kidney disease: should we consider individualised, qualitative, ad libitum diets? A narrative review and case study. *Nutrients.* 2017;9(10):1109.
15. Plourde M, Cunnane SC. Extremely limited synthesis of long chain polyunsaturates in adults: implications for their dietary essentiality and use as supplements. *Appl Physiol Nutr Metab.* 2007;32(4):619-634. doi:10.1139/H07-034
16. Trumbo P, Schlicker S, Yates AA, Poos M, Food and Nutrition Board of the Institutes of Medicine, The National Academy. Dietary reference intakes for energy, carbohydrate, fiber, fat, fatty acids, cholesterol, protein and amino acids. *J Am Diet Assoc.* 2002;102(11):1621-1630. doi:10.1016/s0002-8223(02)90346-9

CHAPTER 21

Emergency Meal Planning for Patients on Dialysis

Adapted by Karen Wiesen, MS, RDN, LDN, FNKF

Emergency meal planning is important for all patients on dialysis, especially for those living in areas where power outages are more common. The sample meal plans presented in this chapter have been adapted from materials developed by the Council on Renal Nutrition of the National Kidney Foundation, and combine the recommendations for diabetes and nondiabetes into one document. The meal plan is for use in case of an emergency or a natural disaster when an individual may not be able to attend in-center dialysis or do home dialysis. It is very important for patients to follow a limited diet if dialysis has to be missed. A sample grocery list and a 3-day meal plan for an emergency are presented in Figure 21.1 (page 438) and Figure 21.2 (page 440), and these can be accessed as downloadable handouts. Patients should be aware that the meals plans are much stricter than the usual diet to control the buildup of minerals such as potassium and phosphorus, urea, and fluids that can be life threatening if several dialysis treatments are missed due to the emergency.

What to Expect During an Emergency Situation

During an emergency, services such as water and electricity may be cut off, which may limit preparing meals in the usual way. Depending on the time without electricity, only cold or shelf-stable foods may be available until the crisis is over. Food in the refrigerator will keep for 4 hours if the refrigerator is unopened. A full freezer will hold its temperature up to 48 hours if unopened.[1] It is best to eat the foods from the refrigerator and freezer first before using shelf-stable foods. Distilled or bottled water, disposable plates, and plastic utensils should be kept on hand. Some protein bars may be acceptable to use.

Preparing for an Emergency

Since natural disasters may happen without warning, it is ideal to have foods with a long shelf life available at all times. These foods should be stored in a cool dry place, with attention to checking dates for freshness. Expired foods should be replaced regularly.

The following items are important and useful to have on hand in case of an emergency:

- a 2-week supply of all medicines and vitamins
- the groceries listed in Figure 21.1
- the sample meal plans from Figure 21.2
- emergency phone list with names and phone numbers of doctor, dialysis unit, and the local hospital
- radio with extra batteries
- flashlight with extra batteries
- extra batteries for any other devices (eg, hearing aids)
- candles and matches
- measuring cups and spoons
- plastic forks, spoons, and knives

FIGURE 21.1 | Three-day grocery list for emergencies

FOOD	AMOUNT
Bread/cereal (use 6 to 8 servings per day)	
White bread	1 loaf
Dry cereal: unsalted, sweetened *or* unsweetened puffed wheat *or* rice, shredded wheat	6 single-serving containers *or* 1 box
Vanilla wafers *or* graham crackers *or* unsalted crackers	1 box
Fruits/juices (limit to 2 to 4 servings per day)	
Canned or sealed plastic containers of applesauce, pears, peaches, pineapple, mandarin oranges *or* fruit cocktail	12 single-serving containers
100% cranberry, cran-apple *or* apple juice	12 (4 oz) single-serving pouches or juice boxes
Dairy (limit to ½ cup per day)—buy only one dairy option	
Evaporated milk	3 to 4 cans (8 oz each)
Dry milk powder	2 packages
Fish/meat (limit to 3 oz per day), low sodium or no salt added, canned	
Tuna, salmon, meat, turkey *or* chicken	6 small cans total
Peanut butter, unsalted	1 jar
Sweets (use as desired to increase calories; people with diabetes should use foods marked with ** to treat low blood glucose)	
Marshmallows**	1 large bag
Jelly beans,** sour balls,** hard candies** *or* butter mints**	5 bags total
Honey**	1 jar
White sugar** *or* sugar substitute	1 small bag *or* 1 box of individual packets
Jelly** *or* low-sugar *or* sugar-free jelly	1 jar
Fats (use 6 or more servings per day)	
Vegetable oil	1 bottle
Mayonnaise (perishable after opening)	12 individual packets *or* 3 small jars
Other	
Pouches of premixed fruit punch *or* lemonade without phosphate additives (for people with diabetes use sugar-free fruit punch/lemonade *or* mini sugar-free clear soda)	12 (4 to 6 oz) single serving pouches *or* 12 (7.5 oz mini) sugar-free clear soda
Distilled *or* bottled water	5 one gallon jugs
Gum, sugar-free	1 multipack

- disposable plates, bowls, and cups
- napkins or paper towels
- hand-operated can opener
- 5 gallons distilled or bottled water
- refrigerator thermometer
- enough insulin and supplies on hand, including extra batteries for the glucometer, for people with diabetes

Other Important Considerations

There are several other considerations to make patients aware of when preparing for an emergency:

- Following the diet according to the meal plan given is *very important*.
- Care should be taken to avoid food poisoning when eating perishable foods. If a jar or can is opened, it should not be kept longer than 4 hours unless refrigerated.
- A refrigerator thermometer is necessary to ensure that food is stored at a safe temperature (under 40 °F or 5 °C). Keeping refrigerator and freezer doors closed as much as possible is critical. After 4 hours without electricity, refrigerated food should be transferred to a cooler and filled with ice. If ice is not available, the food must be thrown away. A full freezer will keep food safe for about 48 hours if the door is not opened.[1,2]
- Disposable plates and utensils can be used and thrown away after use.
- Distilled or bottled water can be used for mixing with dry milk or juice, and mixing only 4 oz at a time.
- Fluids should be limited to 2 cups or 16 oz per day. Chewing gum can help reduce thirst.
- Natural salt or salt substitutes should not be used; instead, salt-free foods should be used when possible.
- High-potassium foods should be avoided, limiting the kinds and portion size of fruits eaten to those listed in the handouts.

- For people with diabetes, glucose tablets, sugar, hard candy, low-potassium fruit juices, or sugared soda pop should be kept on hand to treat low blood glucose. High-potassium fruit juices like orange juice should be avoided.
- Sports drinks and vitamin or energy drinks with added sodium, potassium, or phosphate additives are not recommended.
- Foods in nonwaterproof containers that come in contact with flood or dirty water should be discarded. This includes foods with screw-caps, snap lids, pull tops, and crimped tops.[1]

Three-Day Meal Plan for Emergencies

The sample meal plans (Figure 21.2) provide about 40 to 50 g protein, 1,500 mg sodium, 1,500 mg potassium, less than 2 cups or 16 oz fluid for each day, and approximately 1,800 kcal. The meal plans are stricter than a normal kidney diet to keep waste products from building up in the blood during the emergency situation. Fluid is limited to less than 2 cups or 16 oz each day to prevent swelling or shortness of breath. If the disaster should continue for more than 3 days, the meal plan can be repeated, beginning with day 1.

FIGURE 21.2 | Sample meal plans

DAY 1

Breakfast	½ cup milk prepared from 3 tablespoons dry milk powder and ½ cup distilled or bottled water, *or* ¼ cup evaporated milk mixed with ¼ cup distilled or bottled water
	1 single serving of cereal (½ to ¾ cup)
	1 tablespoon sugar (for people with diabetes, use sugar substitute)
	½ cup pineapple (single serving), drained
Morning snack	5 vanilla wafers
	Honey *or* jelly, as desired, on vanilla wafers
	10 sour balls
	Diabetic snack: 5 vanilla wafers
Lunch	2 slices white bread
	¼ cup low-sodium canned tuna (open new can daily)
	1 tablespoon mayonnaise (individual packet or open new jar daily)
	½ cup pears (single serving), drained
	1 pouch of premixed fruit punch *or* lemonade without phosphate additives (for people with diabetes, use 6 oz sugar-free fruit punch/lemonade *or* sugar-free clear soda)
Afternoon snack	6 unsalted crackers
	Honey *or* jelly, as desired, on crackers
	10 jelly beans
	Diabetic snack: 6 unsalted crackers with 1 tablespoon low-sugar *or* sugar-free jelly
Dinner	2 slices white bread
	½ cup (2 oz) canned low-sodium chicken (open new can daily)
	2 tablespoons mayonnaise (individual packet or open new jar daily)
	½ cup peaches (single serving), drained
	½ cup cranberry juice (for people with diabetes, use 6 oz sugar-free fruit punch/lemonade *or* sugar-free clear soda)
Evening snack	3 graham cracker squares
	Honey *or* jelly, as desired, on crackers
	10 butter mints
	Diabetic snack: 3 graham cracker squares

DAY 2

Breakfast	½ cup milk prepared from 3 tablespoons dry milk powder and ½ cup distilled or bottled water, *or* ¼ cup evaporated milk mixed with ¼ cup distilled or bottled water
	1 single serving of cereal (½ to ¾ cup)
	1 tablespoon sugar (for people with diabetes, use sugar substitute)
	½ cup mandarin oranges (single serving), drained
Morning snack	3 graham cracker squares
	Honey *or* jelly, as desired, on graham crackers
	10 hard candies
	Diabetic snack: 3 graham cracker squares

Lunch	2 slices white bread
	¼ cup (1 oz) canned low-sodium turkey (open new can daily)
	1 tablespoon mayonnaise (individual packet or open new jar daily)
	½ cup fruit cocktail (single serving), drained
	1 pouch of premixed fruit punch *or* lemonade without phosphate additives (for people with diabetes, use 6 oz sugar-free fruit punch/lemonade *or* sugar-free clear soda)
Afternoon snack	6 unsalted crackers
	Honey *or* jelly, as desired, on crackers
	10 large marshmallows
	Diabetic snack: 6 unsalted crackers with 1 tablespoon low-sugar *or* sugar-free jelly
Dinner	2 slices white bread
	½ cup (2 oz) canned low-sodium chicken (open new can daily)
	2 tablespoons mayonnaise (individual packets or open new jar daily)
	½ cup pineapple (single serving), drained
	½ cup cranberry juice (for people with diabetes, use 6 oz sugar-free fruit punch/lemonade *or* sugar-free clear soda)
Evening snack	5 vanilla wafers
	Honey *or* jelly as desired (use on wafers)
	10 sour balls
	Diabetic snack: 5 vanilla wafers

DAY 3	
Breakfast	½ cup milk prepared from 3 tablespoons dry milk powder and ½ cup distilled or bottled water, *or* ¼ cup evaporated milk mixed with ¼ cup distilled or bottled water
	1 single serving of cereal (½ to ¾ cup)
	1 tablespoon sugar (for people with diabetes, use sugar substitute)
	½ cup pears (single serving), drained
Morning snack	6 unsalted crackers
	Honey *or* jelly, as desired, on crackers
	10 large marshmallows
	Diabetic snack: 6 unsalted crackers with 1 tablespoon low-sugar *or* sugar-free jelly
Lunch	2 slices white bread
	2 tablespoons unsalted peanut butter
	½ cup peaches (single serving), drained
	1 pouch of premixed fruit punch *or* lemonade without phosphate additives (for people with diabetes, use 6 oz sugar-free fruit punch/lemonade *or* sugar-free clear soda)
Afternoon snack	3 graham cracker squares
	Honey *or* jelly, as desired, on crackers
	10 butter mints
	Diabetic snack: 3 graham cracker squares

Dinner	2 slices white bread
	½ cup (2 oz) canned low-sodium chicken (open new can daily)
	2 tablespoons mayonnaise (individual packets or open new jar daily)
	½ cup mandarin oranges (single serving), drained
	½ cup cranberry juice (for people with diabetes, use 6 oz sugar-free fruit punch/lemonade *or* sugar-free clear soda)
Evening snack	5 vanilla wafers
	Honey *or* jelly, as desired (use on wafers)
	10 sour balls
	Diabetic snack: 5 vanilla wafers

Note for People With Diabetes

You may use 1 tablespoon peanut butter if protein is needed for the evening snack.

You need to continue to monitor your blood glucose on a regular basis.

You need to follow your individual guidelines for insulin reactions and be sure to keep enough supplies on hand.

Best choices for treating low blood glucose levels are fluid-free items such as sugar, hard candy, glucose tablets or gel, or corn syrup. Sugar-sweetened soda and low-potassium juices may also be used but must be counted as part of your 2 cup or 16 oz daily fluid limit.

Adapted with permission from the NKF-CRN Emergency Meal Planning. Accessed May 2019. www.kidney.org

References

1. A Consumer's Guide to Food Safety: Severe Storms and Hurricanes Fact Sheet. USDA Food Safety and Inspection Service website. February 2020. Accessed February 7, 2021. www.fsis.usda.gov/wps/portal/fsis/topics/food-safety-education/get-answers/food-safety-fact-sheets/emergency-preparedness/a-consumers-guide-to-food-safety-severe-storms-and-hurricanes

2. Keep Food Safe After a Disaster or Emergency. Centers for Disease Control and Prevention website. September 2020. Accessed February 7, 2021. www.cdc.gov/foodsafety/keep-food-safe-after-emergency.html

CHAPTER 22

Kidney–Gut Axis: The Connection Between Kidney Disease and the Gut

Lindsey Zirker, MS, RD, CSR

Introduction

The gut microbiota has a wide range of influence on an individual's health. While there is much that is not understood, it is clear that gut microbiota plays a role in chronic disease, including chronic kidney disease (CKD). By better understanding the connection with the gut microbiome, CKD, and the diet, registered dietitian nutritionists (RDNs) are uniquely poised to help improve the quality of life and outcomes for those with CKD.

What Is the Gut Microbiome?

The gut microbiome is a significant ecosystem within the human body consisting of trillions of bacterial cells. In healthy individuals, this ecosystem is symbiotic, providing a cascade of benefits to the host. The colonization of the gut is impacted by a number of factors, including environment (exposure to bacteria in utero; mode of infant delivery; location of residence—region, urban, or rural; and chemical exposure), antibiotics or other medication use, diet, stress, exercise, alcohol use, and intestinal disease.[1,2] Healthy adults have a rich diversity of bacteria—consisting primarily (90%) of two phyla: *Firmicutes* and *Bacteroidetes*. Different bacteria colonize different areas of the gut, with the majority residing in the anaerobic environment of the colon.[1,3] Bacteria in the gut can be separated into two general types of species: saccharolytic and proteolytic. The different types of bacteria present are strongly driven by the type of fuel available and transit time.[4,5]

Saccharolytic bacteria are generally considered beneficial to the host (such as *Bifidobacterium* and *Lactobacillus* species). These bacteria ferment resistant starches and produce short chain fatty acids (SCFA) which support the health and growth of intestinal cells. Saccharolytic bacteria also synthesize vitamins and amino acids, maintain an intact intestinal barrier, compete with pathogenic bacteria for space, produce hormones, and regulate immune function.[1,4,6-8]

Proteolytic bacteria primarily break down or putrefy undigested protein (such as *Clostridium* and *Bacteroides*). This is necessary and important; however, this process produces ammonia, amines, thiols, phenols, and indoles. High amounts of these endotoxins can cause significant inflammation. Phenols and indoles are converted to proinflammatory toxins, such as P-cresyl sulfate (PCS) and indoxyl sulfate (IS). These toxins are known to cause damage to the kidneys and vascular tissue. Normally, these inflammatory factors are generally filtered out by the kidney but are not well filtered with dialysis.[1,4,5,7,9]

INTESTINAL BARRIER AND NORMAL PERMEABILITY

Since the digestive system is on the *outside* of the body, it is important for the intestinal barrier to control what comes *inside* the body. It consists of an epithelial layer along the intestinal lumen which contains mucus bilayers (inner and outer), gut-associated lymphoid tissue, antimicrobial proteins, antibacterial lectins, and defensins.[10,11] This barrier prevents an immune response from the body acting on the microbiota, bacteria translocation (bacteria moving from one part of the intestine to another or into the bloodstream), prevents absorption of toxins and pathogens into the bloodstream, plays a role in immune regulation and function, provides a residence for the bacteria, and allows for selective absorption of nutrients. Tight junctions, gates between the intestinal cells, are a critical part in the selective absorption process, allowing for normal permeability from the intestine to the bloodstream (see Figure 22.1).[11]

What Happens to the Gut Microbiota in Chronic Kidney Disease?

Human and experimental studies show that there are significant differences in the gut microbiota in those patients with CKD. Fecal samples of patients undergoing hemodialysis (HD) showed lower levels of *Bifidobacteria* and higher levels of *Clostridium perfringens*.[4] Patients with uremia were found to have significantly increased amounts of aerobic and anaerobic bacteria not usually present in the small intestine.[3] In those with kidney failure, the most abundant bacteria present in the gut produce IS and PCS.[1] Significant changes to the intestinal barrier have also been found in those with CKD, including decreased tight junctions, decreased villous height, and increased presence of inflammatory cells.[3] These changes all add up to what is generally known as dysbiosis and increased intestinal permeability. Dysbiosis is defined as an imbalance of bacteria in the gut that leads to a disease state.[12] Increased intestinal permeability is a higher permeability in the intestinal barrier due to damage to the mucosal layer and loss of tight junctions.[2] There are several factors that contribute to dysbiosis and intestinal permeability in those with CKD. The flow chart in Figure 22.2 shows the various contributory factors for dysbiosis and increased intestinal permeability.[1]

FIGURE 22.1 | Tight junctions with healthy intestinal barrier vs impaired intestinal barrier[2]

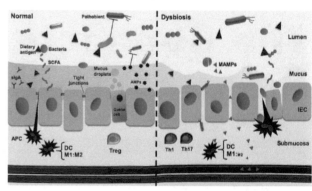

Reproduced with permission from Chan YK, Estaki M, Gibson DL. Clinical consequences of diet-induced dysbiosis. *Ann Nutr Metab.* 2013;63(suppl 2):28-40. doi:10.1159/000354902.[2]

Dysbiosis in Chronic Kidney Disease

CKD contributes to dysbiosis in a number of different ways. As kidney function declines, concentrations of uremic solutes—such as oxalates, uric acid, and urea—increase in the intestine as an adaptive response. Increased urea accumulation increases fuel for proteolytic bacteria and creates an increase of ammonia, which alters pH. Increased uremic solutes cause inflammation and damage the mucosal lining, as well as the vascular and kidney tissues. It is important to note that while dialysis removes some uremic solutes, IS and PCS are protein bound and poorly removed through dialysis.[5,7,8]

Digestive issues are common in those with CKD. Constipation has been found to be as high as 63% in patients on HD (compared to 10%–20% in healthy individuals). Constipation increases the production of toxic byproducts and promotes bacterial overgrowth or bacterial translocation, as more of the small intestine and colon becomes lower in oxygen.[4] Multiple studies show that those with CKD have impaired protein assimilation. The undigested protein provides ample fuel for proteolytic bacteria, creating an increase in the growth of proteolytic bacteria and promoting the increased production of uremic toxins such as IS and PCS. Impaired protein breakdown and assimilation may also contribute to the protein malnutrition and constipation that is often found in this population.[4,5,13]

FIGURE 22.2 | Dysbiosis and influential factors on intestinal permeability

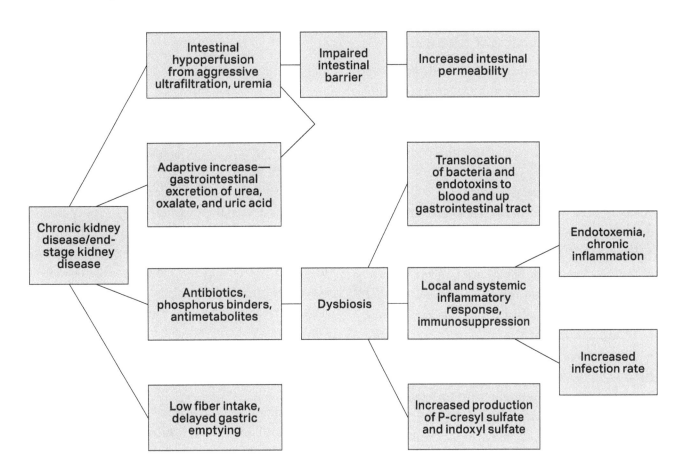

Adapted with permission from Sabatino A, Regolisti G, Brusasco I, Cabassi A, Morabito S, Fiaccadori E. Alteration of intestinal barrier and microbiota in chronic kidney disease. *Nephrol Dial Transplant.* 2015;30(6):924-933. doi:10.1093/ndt/gfu287

Medications also change the intestinal landscape. Antibiotics are the most common medication to impact the gut microbiome. Since they are used prophylactically as well as for treating dialysis access or other infections, many patients on dialysis are frequently exposed to radical shifts in gut microbiota. Phosphorus binders, oral iron, and antireflux medications influence the gut microbiota by binding vitamins in foods, contributing to decreased transit time, and reducing stomach acid. As dysbiosis is better understood and recognized, additional medications will likely be found to contribute to altered gut microbiota.[1,8]

The traditional kidney diet restricts intake of whole grains, fruits, and vegetables, and promotes high intake of protein, especially animal protein for those on dial-

ysis. This dietary pattern further promotes the growth of proteolytic bacteria and the production of IS and PCS and limits the growth of saccharolytic bacteria. This not only makes patients more vulnerable to the damage caused by the increased production of uremic toxins but leaves them without all the other benefits and protection from byproducts of the saccharolytic bacteria. Increased fiber and prebiotic intake promote the growth of saccharolytic bacteria and SCFA, which seems to be protective against dysbiosis, increased removal of potassium via the intestinal tract, decreased transit time, and the production of uremic toxins, slowed progression of CKD, improved gastrointestinal complaints, and decreased complications of obesity, diabetes, and dyslipidemia.[14,15]

Decreased Intestinal Barrier and Increased Permeability in Chronic Kidney Disease

Decreased intestinal barrier and increased intestinal permeability are often associated with a number of chronic conditions—not just kidney disease. However, there are unique features in CKD that contribute to a decreased intestinal barrier and increased intestinal permeability.

It is well established that malnutrition is prevalent in those with CKD and generally has an inflammatory component. In individuals with malnutrition, there are decreased nutrients available for intestinal cell turnover, so intestinal cells are not able to maintain the integrity of the tight junctions. The decreased fuel for bacteria also causes a breakdown of the mucosal layer that is used in the absence of adequate nutrients, leaving a weakened intestinal barrier.[16,17]

Inflammation from the dysbiosis process erodes the tight junctions, which causes gaps rather than controlled gates between the intestinal cells and the release of inflammatory factors.[1,8,13] This increases the passage of pathogens, uremic toxins, partially digested food, antigens, and other inflammatory factors into the bloodstream.[1]

A unique contributor to intestinal permeability in CKD is hypervolemia and aggressive ultrafiltration. Increased volume or edema contributes to edema of the intestinal wall, increasing the release of endotoxin and cytokines, which contributes additional inflammatory damage to tight junctions. Excess ultrafiltration can leave the intestine ischemic due to hypotension. This further compromises the health of the intestinal barrier, increasing inflammation and decreasing the ability to maintain tight junctions.[1,7,10]

IMPACT OF DYSBIOSIS AND IMPAIRED INTESTINAL PERMEABILITY

It is generally accepted that inflammation contributes to the progression of CKD and that those with end-stage kidney disease have high levels of inflammation, heart disease, vascular issues, gastrointestinal issues,

and suppressed or dysfunctional immunity. Research supports that the changes that occur in the gut along with the progression of CKD significantly contribute to these issues.[1,2,8,18] This is not to say that dysbiosis and intestinal permeability are the only factors; as with any chronic disease, there are multiple contributors. In those with CKD who also have dysbiosis, one can expect to find increased production of uremic solutes (especially IS and PCS), a translocation of bacteria, and increased production of endotoxins because the environment of the gut is changed and supports more proteolytic bacterial growth or the growth of saccharolytic bacteria further up the intestine.[5,7,19] This can contribute to other potential issues such as uremic enterocolitis (necrotizing ulcers in the intestinal lymphoid tissue), reflux, small intestine bacterial overgrowth, malabsorption of nutrients and nutrient deficiencies, food allergies, obesity, and other digestive problems.[3,20] Endotoxins are known to contribute to depression and other mental health issues, indicating that dysbiosis may play a key role in mental health issues that also seem to accompany CKD.[15]

Several human and experimental studies have shown that increased production of IS and PCS contributes to nephrotoxicity, inflammation, free radical production, and therefore the progression of CKD.[3,9,12,21] Studies have shown that decreasing serum levels of IS and PCS have the potential to slow CKD progression and improve cardiovascular outcomes.[3,4,19,21] This is one of the mechanisms by which the low protein diet (LPD) and very-low protein diet (VLPD) are thought to be beneficial for those in the earlier stages of CKD. Increased levels of IS have been linked to vascular damage, arterial stiffness, aortic calcification in those with CKD and atherosclerosis, vascular cell dysfunction (hypertrophy of myocardial tissue), and atrial fibrillation in patients on HD. IS and PCS are both associated with increased cardiovascular disease (CVD) risk. IS also increases osteoblast resistance to parathyroid hormone, which encourages the development of adynamic bone disease.[4,19]

Since the increased intestinal permeability not only impacts the protective function of the intestinal lining but also the transport system and uremic toxin levels, it is suspected that the increased level of uremic toxins may downregulate or directly inhibit drug transporters.[11] This may contribute to decreased effectiveness of medications or increase their potential toxicity as they remain longer in the gut.

CKD is one of the many conditions where systemic inflammation and suppressed immunity are both present. While the process is not fully understood, experts believe that the increased intestinal permeability exposes the immune system to so many triggers (bacterial translocation, uremic toxins, partially digested food, antigens, and pathogens) that there is a simultaneous activation of the systemic inflammatory response; however, subsequent safety measures suppress innate and adaptive immunity. This creates a contradictory state where patients with CKD are immunosuppressed but have systemic inflammation.[1,10,11]

Potential Interventions

The understanding of the gut microbiota, dysbiosis, and increased intestinal permeability are in their infant stages. These conditions within the scope of CKD are even less understood. Diagnosing these conditions is challenging and costly, and many health care providers lack training and understanding to interpret these tests. This makes it unlikely that the majority of RDNs and patients will have access to these tests. Because of this and the availability of well-developed resources, the diagnostic tests and methods will not be covered here, but resources for more information and training on dysbiosis and increased intestinal permeability are provided in Box 22.1.

In reviewing the research on interventions for dysbiosis and increased intestinal permeability, many of the studies conducted to investigate potential therapeutic interventions are small, have significant limitations, and include many experimental studies. Some may conclude that "more research or evidence is needed" before implementing any sort of intervention. While research is certainly evidence, that is only one of the many types of evidence. In a climate of an evolving understanding of CKD and gut health where robust studies are not always available, it is important to remember that an evidence-based approach allows for and encourages clinical experience and judgment.[22] Evidence-based medicine is based on clinical judgment, with research and *all* its varying levels of evidence, patient and clinician values, and resources as *supportive* factors.[22] Without the "gold standard" levels of evidence, it can be expected that there will be more variability in results. However, as clinicians implement interventions with this clarified perspective in mind, clinical judgment improves and higher-quality research can be performed. There are many potential helpful and evidence-based interventions that RDNs and other health care providers can implement (see Box 22.2 and Box 22.3 on page 448).

BOX 22.1 | Resources for Dysbiosis and Increased Intestinal Permeability

---

Dietitians in Integrative and Functional Medicine Practice Group, www.integrativerd.org

Advancing Medicine with Food and Nutrients by Ingrid Kohlstadt

Laboratory Evaluations for Integrative and Functional Medicine by Richard S. Lord and J. Alexander Bralley

CKD—Supplements, Gut Health, and Functional/Integrative Nutrition Principles, https://kidneyrd.com/ckd-functional-integrative-nutrition-principles

Institute for Functional Medicine, www.ifm.org/learning-center

Genova Diagnostics, www.gdx.net/clinicians/medical-education

Digestive Health with REAL Food by Aglaee Jacob

Diagnostic Solutions Laboratory, www.diagnosticsolutionslab.com/resource-library

---

BOX 22.2 | List of Potential Immune System Triggers to Remove[1,20]

Possible dietary triggers	gluten, dairy, eggs, yeast, corn, soy, nightshades, nuts, processed foods (possibly due to food additives)
Possible medication triggers	proton pump inhibitors, histamine H2-receptor antagonists (H2 blockers), steroids, aspirin, nonsteroidal anti-inflammatory drugs, sustained release potassium tablets, antibiotics, phosphorus binders, and bisphosphonates
Possible pathogen triggers	small bowel intestinal overgrowth, yeast overgrowth, *Helicobacter pylori*, infection, or parasites
Possible toxin triggers	heavy metals, uremic toxins (from inadequate dialysis or impaired protein digestion)

The 5 R approach is used by many health care providers to help restore balance to the gut microbiota.[20] This approach consists of the following:

- **R**emoving immune or symptom triggers such as foods, toxins, medications, and pathogenic bacteria
- **R**eplacing digestive enzymes, hydrochloric acid, and dietary fiber
- **R**einoculating the gut with friendly bacteria
- **R**epairing the gut lining and mucosa
- **R**educing and managing stress

While practitioners can expect that a patient will get the best results by working through the full protocol, this is not always possible or realistic for many patients with kidney disease. However, better management of gut health may alleviate other issues. For example, while interventions to improve gut health have not been correlated with improved albumin levels, it seems possible that addressing a major source of inflammation would be advantageous. As RDNs come to better understand the impact of the gut microbiota on overall health and potential interventions, more realistic and evidence-based recommendations can be provided to improve gut health. In the following sections, several interventions are reviewed which require no additional training and are likely realistic interventions for patients with CKD.

BOX 22.3 | Guidance on Replacing Digestive Enzymes[20]

For those with low stomach acid, use digestive enzymes with betaine hydrogen chloride.

Broad-spectrum digestive enzymes with this general formulation (prescription may be required) from animal sources include the following:

- Protease 100,000 USP units
- Lipase 20,000 USP units
- Amylase 100,000 USP units

Plant enzymes, such as from papaya, can also be used, but they are less potent.

Digestive bitters, such as Swedish or herbal bitters, can also help with digestion.

These supplements may be available at local health food stores or online from a specific supplement company or supplement dispensaries.

DIET

The diet is one of the most powerful influences on the gut microbiota, which can be beneficial or harmful. For those with CKD and those on dialysis, emerging research supports focusing on dietary patterns of a liberalized diet with an emphasis on eating whole, fresh foods, and getting the right amount and type of protein individualized to the patient's laboratory values, needs, and goals to achieve optimal outcomes.[5,23-26] Specific diet changes to treat dysbiosis and increased intestinal permeability are further discussed in detail.

Increased Fiber Intake

Types of resistant starches or fiber that promote the growth of saccharolytic bacteria are often referred to as prebiotics. All prebiotics are fiber, but not all fiber is considered a prebiotic. Prebiotics increase the production of SCFA, promote a healthy mucosal layer, decrease transit time, and decrease the production of IS and PCS.[1] Dietary fiber (not just prebiotics) can have a positive impact on the gut. Not only does dietary fiber help to decrease transit time, but the dietary fiber to protein intake ratio has been found to be directly related to PCS and IS levels in the blood.[19] Improved cholesterol and blood sugar levels, decreased CVD risk, and improved kidney function are also associated with higher fiber diets—either from food or supplements.[27] Experimental and human studies show that diets higher in fiber have decreased levels of pathogenic bacteria and increased levels of *Bifidobacteria*.[28] See Box 22.4.

BOX 22.4 | Fiber Dosage and Type Used in Human Studies[28-30]

---

15 g high amylose cornstarch (40% digestible starch and 60% resistant starch) daily for 6 weeks significantly reduced indoxyl sulfate and P-cresyl sulfate[28]

14.6 g fiber per day (observation comparing those with higher vs lower fiber intake) had decreased inflammation and all-cause mortality[29]

27 g fiber per day (meta-analysis showed this as the average amount of fiber supplement used in the studies) for various gut health benefits as well as decreased uremic solutes and cardiovascular health[27]

Prebiotics and Probiotics

Prebiotics and probiotics have been shown to improve dysbiosis and increase intestinal permeability.[3,6,18,30] There are no established protocols at this time for species or amount of prebiotics or probiotics. This is not only due to dysbiosis and increased intestinal permeability being only recently recognized issues, but there is limited testing as well as significant variability in the gut microbiota. Reestablishing balance is likely very different for every individual. However, there have been many studies conducted in non-CKD populations that show benefits in using prebiotics and probiotics to address various gastrointestinal issues (eg, irritable bowel syndrome, inflammatory bowel disease, constipation, *Clostridium difficile*, and antibiotic-associated diarrhea). The Yale University Workshop recommendations for probiotic use as well as the Clinical Guide to Probiotics are helpful evidence-based resources in identifying dosages and strain-specific probiotic recommendations.[31,32] While these interventions are not always specifically designed

to resolve dysbiosis or increased intestinal permeability, these gastrointestinal issues are contributing to an unhealthy gut microbiota environment. Helping to resolve them can only benefit patients and their quality of life.

The research on using prebiotics and probiotics to reduce the production of uremic toxins is somewhat limited and has few human studies. A recent systematic review concluded that there is limited evidence to support the use of prebiotics and probiotics in patients with CKD.[33] This is not a surprising conclusion when one considers that diet is rarely considered or controlled for in the studies. Additionally, it is well known that diet can have a significant impact on the gut microbiota as well as on the production of uremic toxins. Without adjusting for diet, it seems unlikely that any significant benefit will be seen from probiotic supplementation. Practitioners hope that as factors contributing to the production of uremic toxins as well as changes to the gut microbiota are better controlled, more high-quality research will be produced to provide clearer guidelines for routine clinical recommendations. In the meantime, prebiotics and probiotics are considered a low-risk intervention.[34,35] So, as with any supplement, making clinical judgments on an *individual basis*, RDNs may recommend prebiotics or probiotics as an evidence-based intervention. Because the availability of probiotic products changes so frequently and is quite extensive, no list is provided in this text. However, referring to The Clinical Guide to Probiotics or Probiotic Advisor (membership required) can give you some guidance on quality products available and their indication.

Prebiotics are found in many probiotic supplements or as individual supplements. However, there are many foods where prebiotics occur naturally. See Box 22.5 on page 450.[36,37]

Appropriate Type and Amount of Protein

For those with CKD stages 3 and 4, the amount and type of protein are critical in slowing CKD progression. The LPD and VLPD with keto analogs have been shown to decrease IS and PCS in those with CKD, thereby resulting in improved dysbiosis and intestinal permeability and showing promising potential interventions for helping to slow the progression of CKD.[38,39]

BOX 22.5 | Prebiotics Naturally Found in Food[36,37]

Vegetables	Jerusalem artichokes,[a] chicory, garlic, onion, leeks, shallots, spring onions, asparagus, beetroot,[a] fennel bulb,[a] green peas, snow peas, sweet corn, savoy cabbage, tomatoes[a]
Legumes	Chickpeas, lentils,[a] kidney beans,[a] baked beans,[a] soy beans
Fruit	Custard apples, nectarines,[a] white peaches,[a] persimmon, tamarillo,[a] watermelon, rambutan, grapefruit,[a] pomegranate, dried fruit[a] (such as figs or dates), bananas[a]
Grains/ starches	Barley, rye, pasta, gnocchi, couscous, wheat bran (whole wheat products),[a] oats, potato starch
Nuts and seeds	Cashews, pistachios[a]

[a] Denotes foods higher in potassium when eaten in generally recommended serving sizes.

BOX 22.6 | Protein Recommendations Used in Studies[38,39]

For patients with chronic kidney disease NOT on dialysis

Low protein diet (0.6 g/kg/d): decreased P-cresyl sulfate (PCS) and other inflammatory factors[38]

Very-low protein diet with keto analogs (0.3 g/kg/d): beneficial changes to gut microbiota, decreased indoxyl sulfate (IS) and PCS, restored intestinal permeability[39]

Vegetarian diet: decreased IS, PCS, urea, and phosphorus[38]

Mediterranean diet (0.8 g/kg/d): beneficial changes to gut microbiota, decreased IS and PCS, restored intestinal permeability[39]

RDNs working with patients undergoing dialysis are used to recommending increased protein intake and supplements to these patients based primarily on low albumin levels. However, the recent Kidney Disease Outcomes Quality Initiative (KDOQI) guidelines encourage multiple factors to be considered when assessing nutritional status and recommending increased protein, such as subjective global assessment, normalized protein catabolic rate, and the malnutrition–inflammation score.[40] This approach seems more likely to ensure that recommendations help patients get adequate protein, rather than excessive amounts—limiting the fuel for proteolytic bacteria. See Box 22.6.

Amount and Type of Fat

Human studies have demonstrated that diets high in saturated fat decrease growth of beneficial bacteria and increase growth of pathogenic bacteria. Conversely, diets higher in unsaturated fats have been found to have the opposite effect and increase beneficial bac-

teria growth and are protective against the growth of pathogenic bacteria.[23,24,41] Some studies suggest fish oil supplementation or Mediterranean diets for those with CKD to increase healthy fat intake and improve gut health.[23,38] Using a more liberal kidney diet would also allow patients undergoing dialysis to follow a Mediterranean style diet, which could have a myriad of potential benefits for the patient.[23] No specific amount per day has been identified at this time; however, an assessment of diet patterns can help to identify whether adjustments to fat intake could be beneficial.

Artificial Sweeteners

Multiple experimental studies have shown that artificial sweeteners can have a negative impact on the gut microbiome and contribute to dysbiosis as well as slow gastric motility.[23,24,42] There are limited high-quality human studies at this time; therefore, eliminating artificial sweeteners for all of those patients with suspected dysbiosis is not currently recommended. However, for those with irritable bowel or who seem to be sensitive to artificial sweeteners, this may be a helpful consideration.[42]

OTHER POTENTIAL INTERVENTIONS

Based on known factors that contribute to dysbiosis and increased intestinal permeability, the following are other possible interventions to consider:

- Use digestive enzymes to improve protein digestion.[20]
- Evaluate use of medications that may have a negative impact on gut health.[20]
- Encourage healthy stress management.[20]
- Correct nutrient deficiencies (utilize physical assessment, food journals, and medication/nutrient interactions if laboratory assessment is not available).[20]
- Improve fluid management—moderating fluid and sodium intake, less aggressive ultrafiltration.[7]

Summary

The gut microbiota provides many benefits when in a healthy state. CKD changes the environment of the gut microbiota and contributes to dysbiosis and increased intestinal permeability. Dysbiosis and increased intestinal permeability can lead to the progression of CKD, as well as other conditions associated with CKD. Dysbiosis and increased intestinal permeability can be corrected by making changes to the diet and using prebiotics and probiotics.

Improving gut health places RDNs in a central role for helping to slow the progression of and improving outcomes in patients with CKD.

References

1. Sabatino A, Regolisti G, Brusasco I, Cabassi A, Morabito S, Fiaccadori E. Alteration of intestinal barrier and microbiota in chronic kidney disease. *Nephrol Dial Transplant*. 2015;30(6):924-933. doi:10.1093/ndt/gfu287

2. Chan YK, Estaki M, Gibson DL. Clinical consequences of diet-induced dysbiosis. *Ann Nutri Metab*. 2013;63(suppl 2):28-40. doi:10.1159/000354902

3. Ramezani A, Raj R. The gut microbiome, kidney disease, and targeted interventions. *J Am Soc Nephrol*. 2014;25(4):657-670. doi:10.1681/ASN.2013080905

4. Evenepoel P, Meijers BK, Bammens BR, Verbeke K. Uremic toxins originating from colonic microbial metabolism. *Kidney Int Suppl*. 2009;(114):S12-S19. doi:10.1038/ki.2009.402

5. Poesen R, Meijers B, Evenepoel P. The colon: an overlooked site for therapeutics in dialysis patients. *Semin Dial*. 2013;26(3):323-332. doi:10.1111/sdi.12082

6. Rossi M, Johnson D, Campbell K. The kidney-gut axis: implications for nutrition care. *J Ren Nutr*. 2015;25(5):399-403. doi:10.1053/j.jrn.2015.01.017

7. Vaziri ND, Zhao Y, Pahl M. Altered intestinal microbial flora and impaired epithelial barrier structure and function in CKD: the nature, mechanisms, consequences and potential treatment. *Nephrol Dial Transplant*. 2016;31:737-746. doi:10.1093/ndt/gfv095

8. Vaziri ND, Wong J, Pahl M, et al. Chronic kidney disease alters intestinal microbial flora. *Kidney Int*. 2013;83(2):308-315. doi:10.1038/ki.2012.345

9. Liabeuf S, Drueke T, Massy Z. Protein-bound uremic toxins: new insight from clinical studies. *Toxins*. 2011;3(7):911-919. doi:10.3390/toxins3070911

10. Anders HJ, Andersen K, Stecher B. The intestinal microbiota, a leaky gut, and abnormal immunity in kidney disease. *Kidney Int*. 2013;83(6):1010-1016. doi:10.1038/ki.2012.440

11. Meijers B, Farre R, Dejongh S, Vicario M, Evenpoel P. Intestinal barrier function in chronic kidney disease. *Toxins*. 2018;10(7):298. doi:10.3390/toxins10070298

12. Ellis R, Small D, Vesey D, et al. Indoxyl sulphate and kidney disease: causes, consequences and interventions. *Nephrology*. 2016;21(3):170-177. doi:10.1111/nep.12580

13. Bammens B, Verbeke K, Vanrenterghem Y, Evenpoel P. Evidence for impaired assimilation of protein in chronic renal failure. *Kidney Int*. 2003;64(6):2196-2203. doi:10.1046/j.1523-1755.2003.00314.x

14. Camerotto C, Cupisti A, D'Alessandro C, Muzio F, Gallieni M. Dietary fiber and gut microbiota in renal diets. *Nutrients*. 2019;11(9):2149. doi:10.3390/nu11092149

15. DeGruttola AK, Low D, Mizoguchi A, Mizoguchi E. Current understanding of dysbiosis in disease in human and animal models. *Inflamm Bowel Dis*. 2016;22(5):1137-1150. doi:10.1097/MIB.0000000000000750

16. Kotanko P, Carter M, Levin NW. Intestinal bacterial microflora—a potential source of chronic inflammation in patients with chronic kidney disease. *Nephrol Dial Transplant*. 2006;21(8):2057-2060. doi:10.1093/ndt/gfl281

17. Schroeder B. Fight them or feed them: how the intestinal mucus layer manages the gut microbiota. *Gastroenterol Rep*. 2019;7(1):3-12. doi:10.1093/gastro/goy052

18. Nallu A, Sharma S, Ramezani A, Muralidharan J, Raj D. Gut microbiome in chronic kidney disease: challenges and opportunities. *Transl Res*. 2017;179:24-37. doi:10.1016/j.trsl.2016.04.007

19. Guldris S, Parra E, Amenos A. Gut microbiota in chronic kidney disease. *Nefrologia*. 2017;37(31):9-19. doi:10.1016/j.nefroe.2017.01.017

20. Kohlstadt I. *Advancing Medicine with Food and Nutrients*. 2nd ed. CRC Press; 2013.

21. Rossi M, Klein K, Johnson DW, Campbell KL. Pre-, pro-, and synbiotics: do they have a role in reducing uremic toxins? A systematic review and meta-analysis. *Int J Nephrol*. 2012;2012:673631. doi:10.1155/2012/673631

22. Lang E. The why and the how of evidence-based medicine. *Mcgill J Med*. 2004;8:90-94.

23. Mafra D, Borges N, Alvarenga L, et al. Dietary components that may influence the disturbed gut microbiota in chronic kidney disease. *Nutrients*. 2019;11(3):496. doi:10.3390/nu11030496

24. Signh R, Chang H, Yan D, et al. Influence of diet on the gut microbiome and implications for human health. *J Trans Med*. 2017;15:73. doi:10.1186/s12967-017-1175-y

25. Welte A, Barnes J. Evaluating the evidence and assessing professional perceptions of the complex renal dietary restriction in hemodialysis. *Renal Nutrition Forum*. 2017;36(4):1-5.

26. Biruete A, Jeong J, Barnes J, Wilund K. Modified nutritional recommendations to improve dietary patterns and outcomes in hemodialysis patients. *J Ren Nutr*. 2017;27(1):62-70. doi:10.1053/j.jrn.2016.06.001

27. Chiavaroli L, Mirrahimi A, Sievenpiper J, Jenkins D, Darling P. Dietary fiber effects in chronic kidney disease: a systematic review and meta-analysis of controlled feeding trials. *Eur J Clin Nutr*. 2015;69(7):761-768. doi:10.1038/ejcn.2014.237

28. Sirich TL, Plummer NS, Gardner CD, Hostetter TH, Meyer TW. Effect of increasing dietary fiber on plasma levels of colon-derived solutes in hemodialysis patients. *Clin J Am Soc Nephrol*. 2014;9(9):1603-1610. doi:10.2215/CJN.00490114

29. Krishnamurthy VM, Wei G, Baird BC, et al. High dietary fiber intake is associated with decreased inflammation and all-cause mortality in patients with chronic kidney disease. *Kidney Int*. 2012;81(3):300-306. doi:10.1038/ki.2011.355

30. Cosola C, Rocchetti M, Sabatino A, Fiaccadori E, Di Iorio B, Gesualso L. Microbiota issue in CKD: how promising are gut-targeted approaches? *J Nephrol*. 2019;32(1):27-37. doi:10.1007/s40620-018-0516-0

31. Floch M, Walker W, Sanders M, et al. Recommendations for probiotic use—2015 update: proceedings and consensus opinion. *J Clin Gastroenterol*. 2015;49(suppl 1):S69-S73. doi:10.1097/MCG.0000000000000420

32. Skokovic-Sunjic D. Clinical guide to probiotic products available in USA. AEProbio website. May 2020. Accessed August 1, 2020. https://usprobioticguide.com

33. McFarlane C, Ramos C, Johnson D, Campbell K. Prebiotic, probiotic and synbiotic supplementation in chronic kidney disease: a systematic review and meta-analysis. *J Ren Nutr*. 2019;29(3):209-220. doi:10.1053/j.jrn.2018.08.008

34. Boyle R, Robins-Browne R, Tang M. Probiotic use in clinical practice: what are the risks? *Am J Clin Nutr*. 2006;83(6):1256-1264. doi:10.1093/ajcn/83.6.1256

35. Vitetta L, Gobe G. Uremia and chronic kidney disease: the role of the gut microflora and therapies with pro- and prebiotics. *Mol Nutr Food Res*. 2013;57(5):824-832. doi:10.1002/mnfr.201200714

36. Zirker L. Benefit and use of prebiotics in patients with chronic kidney disease. *J Ren Nutr*. 2014;25(2):e9-e10. doi:10.1053/j.jrn.2014.12.007

37. Monash University. Prebiotic diet—FAQs. Monash University website. February 2020. Accessed June 26, 2020. www.monash.edu/medicine/ccs/gastroenterology/prebiotic/faq#6

38. Jiang Z, Tang Y, Yang L, Mi X, Qin W. Effect of restricted protein diet supplemented with keto analogues in end-stage renal disease: a systematic review and meta-analysis. *Int Urol Nephrol*. 2018;50(4):687-694. doi:10.1007/s11255-017-1713-9

39. Di Iorio BR, Rocchetti MT, De Angelis M, et al. Nutritional therapy modulates intestinal microbiota and reduces serum levels of total and free indoxyl sulfate and P-cresyl sulfate in chronic kidney disease (Medika Study). *J Clin Med.* 2019;8(9):1424. doi:10.3390/jcm8091424

40. Clinical practice guideline for nutrition in chronic kidney disease: 2019 update. National Kidney Foundation website. December 2019. Accessed December 27, 2019. www.kidney.org/sites/default /files/Nutrition_GL%2BSubmission_101719_Public _Review_Copy.pdf

41. Bibbo S, Ianiro G, Giorgio V, et al. The role of diet on gut microbiota composition. *Eur Rev Med Pharmacol Sci.* 2016;20(22):4742-4749.

42. Spencer M, Gupta A, Dam LV, Shannon C, Menees S, Chey WD. Artificial sweeteners: a systematic review and primer for gastroenterologists. *J Neurogastroenterol Motil.* 2016;22(2):168-180. doi:10.5056/jnm15206

SECTION VII

Practice Recommendations for Nutrition Care in Kidney Disease

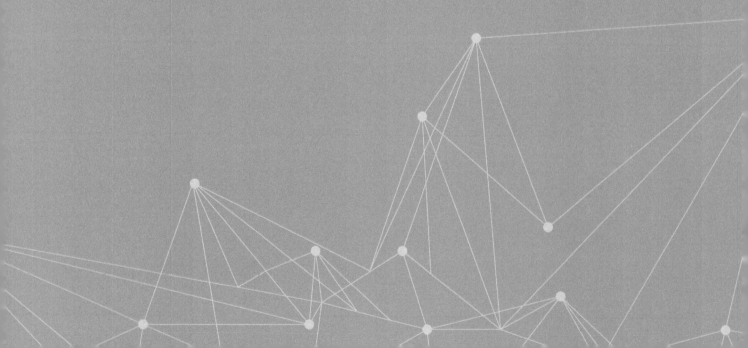

CHAPTER 23

Practice Guidelines, Reimbursement, Scope of Practice, and Continuous Quality Improvement in Kidney Disease

Jessie M. Pavlinac, MS, RDN-AP, CSR, LD, FNKF, FAND

Introduction

Quality patient care comes from following evidence-based practice guidelines, continually improving care, and as federal, state, and facility rules/regulation allows, practicing at the top of your individual scope of practice. This chapter will provide some information and tools to assist renal nutrition practitioners to practice "at the top of their license or certification."

Definition of Medical Nutrition Therapy

The Academy of Nutrition and Dietetics defines medical nutrition therapy (MNT) as follows:

> Medical nutrition therapy is an evidence-based application of the Nutrition Care Process. The provision of MNT (to a patient/client) may include one or more of the following: nutrition assessment/reassessment, nutrition diagnosis, nutrition intervention and nutrition monitoring and evaluation that typically results in the prevention, delay or management of diseases and/or conditions.

> Typically diet modification and counseling leading to the development of a personal diet plan to achieve nutritional goals and desired health outcomes and specialized nutrition therapies, including supplementation with medical foods for those

> unable to obtain adequate nutrients through food intake only; enteral nutrition delivered via tube feeding into the gastrointestinal tract for those unable to ingest or digest food; and parenteral nutrition delivered via intravenous infusion for those unable to absorb nutrients are included.[1]

Nutrition evaluation and monitoring is another step in the Nutrition Care Process (NCP) for providing MNT. The purpose of this step is to determine the degree to which progress is being made toward achieving goals and the desired outcomes of nutrition care are being met (see Chapter 24).[2]

This definition of MNT is broader than what was established in 2002 when Congress passed the Medicare, Medicaid, and State Children's Health Insurance Program Benefits Improvement and Protection Act (BIPA), which authorized Medicare reimbursement for MNT for nondialysis kidney disease (estimated glomerular filtration rate [eGFR] of 13–50 mL/min/1.73 m²), inclusive of post–kidney transplant for up to 36 months, and diabetes (type 1 diabetes mellitus [T1DM], type 2 diabetes mellitus [T2DM], and gestational diabetes mellitus [GDM]). Section 105 of the law defined MNT as "nutritional diagnostic, therapy, and counseling services for the purpose of disease management which are furnished by a registered dietitian or nutrition professional." Effective January 2022, Medicare has expanded the MNT benefit by increasing the eGFR range to 15 - 59 mL/min/1.73 m².[2,3]

Medical Nutrition Therapy and Evidence-Based Guides to Practice

To standardize the NCP, dietetics practitioners use to provide nutrition services, MNT protocols were first developed and published in 1998 in *Medical Nutrition Therapy Across the Continuum of Care*.[4] This publication represented a partnership between the Academy of Nutrition and Dietetics Quality Management Team, the Academy of Nutrition and Dietetics Dietetic Practice Groups, and Morrison Health Care.[5] This publication included a pre–end-stage renal disease (pre-ESRD) protocol for adult patients aged 18 years and older as well as other disease-specific protocols. The initial protocols or practice guidelines were developed by experts in the fields of nutrition care and quality assurance who reached a consensus about the number of recommended nutrition interventions; length of time for each of these interventions; key clinical, behavioral, and functional outcome assessment factors to be measured; and expected outcomes.

With the advent of MNT provider status by the Centers for Medicare & Medicaid Services (CMS), nutrition guidelines for practice must reflect the best clinical evidence.[6-9] In 2000, the Academy of Nutrition and Dietetics House of Delegates approved an evidence grading system for use in the production of future Academy of Nutrition and Dietetics guidelines for practice. This standardized grading system of the evidence helped practitioners determine the impact a particular nutrition intervention has on patient nutritional goals and outcomes. The Academy of Nutrition and Dietetics Quality Management Committee adopted the Institute for Clinical Systems Improvement methodology to grade research evidence.[4] Several guidelines for practice have been published for kidney and transplant patients.[6,7,10] The *Guidelines for Nutrition Care of Renal Patients*, third edition, incorporated the National Kidney Foundation Kidney Disease Outcomes Quality Initiative (KDOQI) clinical practice guidelines that were developed using an evidence rating system.[8,10] These

practice guidelines included the following patients/ conditions: adult with pre-ESRD, adult on dialysis, enteral/parenteral nutrition support for adult on dialysis, adult hospitalized on dialysis, adult in acute renal failure, adult transplant, and adult pregnant with ESRD. The adult pre-ESRD practice guidelines underwent rigorous evidence grading in 2001 and were published separately as the *American Dietetic Association Medical Nutrition Therapy Evidence-Based Guides for Practice: Chronic Kidney Disease (Non-Dialysis) Medical Nutrition Therapy Protocol*.[6] Revision of these 2001 guidelines for chronic kidney disease (CKD) among adults (not on dialysis, including those receiving a kidney transplant) were updated in July 2010 and were made available free to Academy of Nutrition and Dietetics members at the Evidence Analysis Library (EAL) (www.andeal.org).[8]

In 2008, the National Kidney Foundation (NKF) KDOQI published updated nutrition guidelines for children with CKD.[11] In addition, many organizations, dialysis companies, and state, national, and international professional associations have developed their own protocols/guidelines and scope of practice for nutrition care that outline standards and expectations for appropriate MNT, timeframes for initial and follow-up care, expected outcomes, and documentation criteria.

The 2000 NKF KDOQI guidelines and 2010 Academy of Nutrition and Dietetics EAL guidelines were updated in 2020 and published in the *Journal of the Academy of Nutrition and Dietetics* and the *American Journal of Kidney Disease*. The Academy of Nutrition and Dietetics EAL has the details of the grading of the evidence and recommendations that have been included in these publications.[12] These guidelines have recommendations for the following:

- assessment
- medical nutrition therapy
- dietary protein and energy intake
- nutritional supplementation
- micronutrients
- electrolytes

Scope of Practice for the Renal Nutrition Practitioner

The first Standards of Performance for Clinical Dietitians were published in 1978.[13] Twenty years later, the American Dietetic Association Standards of Professional Practice for Dietetics Professionals were published.[14] The most recent publication of the Standards of Practice and Standards of Professional Performance were published in 2018.[15] Nephrology nutrition–specific standards were published in September 2009 and were revised in 2014 and 2021.[16-18] These standards outline three levels of practice: competent, proficient, and expert. The competent registered dietitian nutritionist (RDN) is "learning principles that underpin this focus area and is developing skills for safe and effective nephrology practice." The proficient practitioner has developed a "deeper understanding of nephrology nutrition" and is able to apply evidence-based guidelines. The expert practitioner "displays a range of highly developed clinical and technical skills, and formulates judgments acquired through a combination of education, experience, and critical thinking." This document is a useful tool for identifying the current practice level of the RDN practicing in nephrology nutrition and identifying areas of growth that will lead to the next level of practice with the ultimate goal of achieving expert status.

Reimbursement for Medical Nutrition Therapy

Payment for MNT by third-party payers—Medicare, health maintenance organizations, standard health insurance companies, and state Medicaid programs—was historically limited by the lack of recognition of RDNs as providers. With the passage of BIPA 2000, RDNs and nutrition professionals have been granted status as Medicare providers of MNT. This act provides reimbursement for MNT to all qualifying Medicare Part B beneficiaries with nondialysis kidney disease (glomerular filtration rate 15–59 mL/min/1.73 m^2), inclusive of post–kidney transplantation for up to 36 months,

and diabetes (T1DM, T2DM, and GDM). In 2001, the Academy of Nutrition and Dietetics proposed the first three MNT procedure codes through the American Medical Association code proposal process. The codes defined initial assessment (97802), follow-up (97803), and group MNT (97804). With a physician's referral, Medicare Part B patients who have these conditions are eligible for 3 hours of MNT the first year and 2 hours each subsequent year. The patient's physician can authorize additional hours of MNT based on medical necessity, such as when there is a change in the patient's medical condition. In 2003, CMS added two additional codes for assessment and reassessment of individuals (G0270) and groups (G0271). These codes are used when additional MNT, based on the physician referral, is needed within the same calendar year. Patients receiving dialysis are excluded from this benefit because they already receive MNT as part of the overall conditions for coverage for dialysis units as established by Congress in 1976 and implemented as part of the ESRD program by Medicare.[7]

Medicare requires any qualified RDN or nutrition professional who wishes to provide MNT to Medicare Part B beneficiaries to become a Medicare provider by doing the following[2]:

- Complete an application to become a Medicare provider (CMS855I), and if you work for an organization, complete the Medicare reassignment of benefit form (CMS855R). If you are a member of a group practice, you will need to fill out form CMS855B. Access the Medicare enrollment forms from CMS's website (www.cms.gov/providers /enrollment/forms), from the Medicare carrier's website, or from the Academy of Nutrition and Dietetics website (www.eatright.org/gov).

- Provide proof of qualifications. RDNs must provide proof of the credential from the Commission on Dietetic Registration; nutrition professionals must provide proof of completion of a bachelor of science degree or higher, completion of the nutrition academic requirements, and completion of at least 900 hours of supervised professional practice. In states with licensure or certification,

RDNs and nutrition professionals must show proof of state licensure or certification.[2,3]

- Apply for and receive a unique national provider identifier number from CMS that will be used for billing (https://nppes.cms.hhs.gov).
- Receive a referral from a physician for MNT.[2,3]
- Use specific billing forms, usually CMS1500. However, hospital outpatient nutrition clinics may use the UB92 form if the CMS1500 is not available in the hospital's billing system.
- Use the correct codes. RDNs must use MNT Current Procedural Terminology Codes 97802, 97803, and 97804 (or, if appropriate, G0270, G0271) when billing for these services.[2] Medicare MNT services cannot be billed incident to a physician's services.
- Provide MNT using nationally recognized protocols for diabetes, CKD, and kidney transplantation, such as the Academy of Nutrition and Dietetics *MNT Evidence-Based Guides for Practice.*[8]
- Maintain documentation in the medical record that supports the necessity for MNT.
- Track outcomes data for each Medicare patient who receives MNT services.

Achieving recognition and coverage for Medicare MNT is just the first step in the reimbursement challenge. RDNs should continue to work with their state Medicaid offices and private insurance carriers to be recognized as providers to expand coverage for MNT services.

In March 2020, as part of the Coronavirus Preparedness and Response Supplemental Appropriations Act, physicians and other health care professionals were allowed to bill for Medicare fee-for-service, including MNT by dietitians, for patient care delivered by telehealth during the public health emergency. This legislation allows telehealth service to Medicare Part B beneficiaries by telephone to their current Medicare patients located in their homes.[19] Other possible codes available for dietitians to use in billing for non–dialysis services accepted by CMS and other third-party payers can be found on the eatrightPRO website (www.eatrightpro.org/payment/coding-and-billing/diagnosis-and-procedure-codes/cpt-and-g-codes-for-rdns).

Continuous Quality Improvement in Chronic Kidney Disease

All of the preceding guidelines for nutrition care incorporate the KDOQI Clinical Practice Guidelines for Nutrition in Chronic Renal Failure or nutrition-related segments in other KDOQI practice guidelines, such as diabetes or the Kidney Disease Improving Global Outcomes (KDIGO) practice guidelines for CKD–mineral and bone disorders, hyperlipidemia, and hypertension.[20] The 27 nutrition care guidelines outlined in the 2020 NKF KDOQI/Academy of Nutrition and Dietetics guidelines provide a framework to establish a continuous quality improvement (CQI) or performance improvement program to ensure quality nutrition care for patients with CKD.[12] KDOQI and KDIGO have disease-/condition-specific guidelines for bone and mineral management, anemia management, and so on that can provide further quality improvement topics to be considered. The links to these documents can be found in the additional references at the end of this chapter.

In April 2008, CMS implemented new *Conditions for Coverage for End-Stage Renal Disease Facilities.* This document provides specific guidelines for quality assessment and performance improvement (QAPI) and states, "The important aspects of the QAPI program are appropriately monitoring data/information; prioritizing areas for improvement; determining potential root causes; and developing, implementing, evaluating, and revising plans that result in improvements in care."[21] ESRD Quality Improvement Program (QIP) was the first CMS Value-Based Purchasing program where payment is linked to performance on established quality care measures. Program year 2022 measures include nutrition-relevant measures, including Kt/V dialysis adequacy, hypercalcemia, standardized readmission ratio and hospitalization ratio, percentage of prevalent patients waitlisted for transplant, and medication reconciliation. Dialysis facilities can measure other quality-of-care indicators, in addition to the CMS mandated ones.[22]

Steps in Developing a Continuous Quality Improvement Program

Evidence-based practice indicates that it is the responsibility of practitioners and organizations to utilize practices with the best available evidence when providing care. The guidelines just referenced will have evidence of specific assessment factors and interventions that are proven to be effective. The way to introduce these best practices is through CQI. For example, using the Plan-Do-Study-Act methodology of CQI, you would complete the following steps when integrating evidence-based recommendations of nationally developed guidelines into practice. Implementing evidence-based practice is a process rather than a static event. This process involves a cycle of continuous improvement of care considering evidence-based recommendations.

PLAN THE IMPROVEMENT

Select an improvement topic. Review the evidence-based guidelines and compare these to what you are currently doing in practice. Collect data on how your process currently operates. The challenge is not just to identify inadequate care but also to change clinical practice to improve patient care. To this end, a plan will focus on the changes that have the greatest potential for improvement based on evidenced-based science, linking process to improved outcomes.

IMPLEMENT THE CHANGE

Changing clinical practice requires a systematic approach and strategic planning. In CQI, tools (eg, data collection, metrics, spreadsheets, reminder systems, and order forms) are aids in initiating process change and ensuring consistent care for all patients. This requires diagnostic analysis, development of dissemination and implementation strategy, and a plan to monitor and evaluate the impact of any changes made. When analyzing the available information, identify the following:

- all groups that are affected by or have an influence on the proposed change,

- potential internal and external barriers to needed change, including whether practitioners are willing to change, and
- enabling factors for change (eg, resources and skills).

MONITOR AND EVALUATE

Collect follow-up data (indicators) to evaluate the effectiveness of the change and the degree of compliance and develop strategies to maintain and reinforce change.

ACT TO HOLD THE GAIN AND STANDARDIZE THE IMPROVEMENT

Act on the modifications by repeating the quality cycle to minimize the chance of the change going back to the preimprovement state. At this step, you should have full implementation of actions taken to integrate the best practice. If new information or practice standards are to be used, indicate what they are and where they are located. This can be accomplished through changes in policy and procedures. Educate, communicate, and follow up with training for any practice or coaching that may be required. Be sure to establish a process for training new employees. A systems approach to CQI is an ongoing process that aids in the continual evaluation and improvement on the delivery of health care to patients.

Examples of Possible Continuous Quality Improvement Topics

Topics for CQI for adult patients include:
- Identification of adult malnutrition[23]
- Adult dialysis: evaluation of protein–energy nutritional status
  - Panels of nutritional measures—percentage of usual body weight, percentage of standard body weight, subjective global assessment, dietary interviews and diaries, normalized protein nitrogen appearance, serum creatinine and the creatinine index, and serum cholesterol

- Management of acid-base status—measurement and treatment of serum bicarbonate
- Management of protein and energy intake—dietary protein intake and daily energy intake
- Nutritional intervention, initial and follow-up—intensive nutrition counseling, indications for nutrition support, protein intake during acute illness, and energy intake during acute illness
- Advanced CKD without dialysis
  - Panels of nutritional measures for patients without dialysis
  - Dietary protein intake for patients without dialysis
  - Dietary energy intake for patients without dialysis
  - Intensive nutritional intervention/counseling for patients with CKD
- CKD, dialysis, and transplantation: examples of areas of needed research found in the 2020 NKF/Academy of Nutrition and Dietetics Guidelines[12]
  - Association between handgrip strength and other markers of physical function
  - Testing of predictive energy equations in patients with CKD that can more accurately or precisely determine the individual's unique energy requirements
  - Validity and reliability of the Geriatric Nutrition Risk Index and Subjective Global Assessment tools in older adults with CKD
  - Best methods for dietary assessment among adults diagnosed with CKD stages 1 through 5D and those receiving a kidney transplant
  - Development and testing of dietary assessment tools to integrate technology and assist individuals with limited literacy, vision, and that are culturally appropriate
  - Impact of MNT care on the progression of kidney disease by analyzing the association with risk factors of comorbid conditions

Topics for CQI for pediatric patients include:
- Identification of pediatric malnutrition[24]
- 2008 KDOQI guidelines[11]
  - Evaluation of protein–energy nutritional status
  - Management of acid-base status
  - Urea kinetic modeling
  - Interval measurements of growth and nutritional parameters
  - Energy intake for children treated with maintenance dialysis
  - Protein intake for children treated with maintenance dialysis
  - Vitamin and mineral requirements
  - Nutrition management
  - Nutritional supplementation for children treated with maintenance dialysis

Summary

Perhaps the greatest benefit that clinical practice guidelines/MNT protocols offer to the health care system is improved outcomes for service users through consistent and effective treatment. Promoting interventions with proven benefit can reduce morbidity and mortality risks and improve the quality of life for patients with some conditions, thereby increasing the cost-effectiveness of the care provided.

Additional Resources

To learn more about the Academy of Nutrition and Dietetics *MNT Evidence-Based Guides for Practice*, reimbursement, or continuous quality improvement, consult the following websites:

Academy of Nutrition and Dietetics:
www.eatrightpro.org

> Keywords: medical nutrition therapy, reimbursement, quality management, coding, reimbursement, telehealth

Centers for Medicare & Medicaid Services:
www.cms.hhs.gov

> Keywords: medical nutrition therapy, end-stage renal disease, telehealth

National Kidney Foundation Kidney Disease Outcomes Quality Initiative (KDOQI): www.kidney.org/professionals/guidelines

Clinical Practice Guidelines and Commentaries including Acute Kidney Injury, Anemia, Bone Metabolism in Chronic Kidney Disease (CKD), Cardiovascular Disease in CKD, Classifying CKD, Diabetes, Glomerulonephritis, Hemodialysis Adequacy, Nutrition in CKD, Peritoneal Dialysis Adequacy, and Transplantation

Kidney Disease Improving Global Outcomes (KDIGO) Guidelines: https://kdigo.org/guidelines

CKD Guidelines including Acute Kidney Injury, Anemia, Blood Pressure, CKD Evaluation and Management, Mineral and Bone Disorder, Diabetes, Glomerulonephritis, and Lipids, Living Kidney Donors, Transplant Candidate, and Transplant Recipient

References

1. Academy of Nutrition and Dietetics Definition of Terms List, September 2019. Accessed April 2020. eatrightPRO website. www.eatrightpro.org/~/media/eatrightpro%20files/practice/scope%20standards%20of%20practice/academy-definition-of-terms-list.ashx

2. Medicare Program; CY 2022 Payment Policies Under the Physician Fee Schedule and Other Changes to Part B Payment Policies; Medicare Shared Savings Program Requirements; Provider Enrollment Regulation Updates; and Provider and Supplier Prepayment and Post-Payment Medical Review Requirements. Final Rule. Federal Register 86;221 (2021) (codified at 42 CFR parts 403, 405, 410, 411, 414, 415, 423, 424 and 425). Accessed August 4, 2022. www.govinfo.gov/content/pkg/FR-2021-11-19/pdf/2021-23972.pdf

3. Williams ME, Chianchiano D. Medicare medical nutrition therapy: legislative process and product. *J Ren Nutr.* 2002;12:1-7. doi:10.1053/jren.2002.31187

4. American Dietetic Association; Morrison Health Care. *Medical Nutrition Therapy Across the Continuum of Care.* American Dietetic Association; 1998.

5. Myers ES, Pritchett E, Johnson EQ. Evidence-based practice guides vs. protocols: what's the difference? *J Am Diet Assoc.* 2001;101:1085-1090. doi:10.1016/S0002-8223(01)00270-X

6. American Dietetic Association. *The American Dietetic Association Medical Nutrition Therapy Evidence-Based Guides for Practice: Chronic Kidney Disease (Non-dialysis) Medical Nutrition Therapy Protocol* CD-ROM. American Dietetic Association; 2002.

7. Wiggins KL. *Guidelines for Nutrition Care of Renal Patients.* 3rd ed. American Dietetic Association; 2001.

8. The Academy of Nutrition and Dietetics Evidence Analysis Library. Academy of Nutrition and Dietetics Evidence Analysis Library website. Accessed February 2020. www.andeal.org

9. Conditions for Coverage of Suppliers of End-Stage Renal Disease (ESRD) Services. Revised 2000. Codified at 42 CFR §405.2102.

10. National Kidney Foundation. Kidney Disease Outcomes Quality Initiative (KDOQI) clinical practice guidelines for nutrition in chronic renal failure. *Am J Kidney Dis.* 2000;35(suppl 2):S1-S140. doi:10.1053/ajkd.2001.20748

11. National Kidney Foundation Kidney Disease Outcomes Quality Initiative 2008 update of nutrition in children with chronic kidney disease. National Kidney Foundation website. Accessed February 2020. http://kidneyfoundation.cachefly.net/professionals/KDOQI/guidelines_ped_ckd/index.htm

12. Ikizler TA, Burrowes JD, Byham-Gray LD, et al. KDOQI Nutrition in CKD Guideline Work Group. KDOQI clinical practice guideline for nutrition in CKD: 2020 update. *Am J Kidney Dis.* 2020;76(3)(suppl 1):S1-S107. doi:10.1053/j.ajkd.2020.05.006

13. Scheel JP, McClusky KW. Standards of performance developed for clinical dietitians. *Hospitals.* 1978;52(6):157-158,160,161.

14. The American Dietetic Association Standards of Professional Practice for dietetics professionals [published correction appears in J Am Diet Assoc 1998 Mar;98(3):264]. *J Am Diet Assoc.* 1998;98(1):83-87. doi:10.1016/S0002-8223(98)00023-6

15. Academy Quality Management Committee. Academy of Nutrition and Dietetics: Revised 2017 Standards of Practice in Nutrition Care and Standards of Professional Performance for Registered Dietitian Nutritionists. *J Acad Nutr Diet.* 2018;118(1):132-140.e15. doi:10.1016/j.jand.2017.10.003

16. Brommage D, Karalis M, Martin C, et al. American Dietetic Association and the National Kidney Foundation standards of practice and standards of professional performance for registered dietitians (generalist, specialty, and advanced) in nephrology care. *J Am Diet Assoc.* 2009;109:1617-1625.e33. doi:10.1053/j.jrn.2009.06.020

17. Kent P, McCarthy M, Burrowes JD, et al. Academy of Nutrition and Dietetics and National Kidney Foundation: revised 2014 standards of practice and standards of professional performance for registered dietitian nutritionists (competent, proficient, and expert) in nephrology nutrition. *J Acad Nutr Diet.* 2014;114(9):1448-1457.e45. doi:10.1016/j.jand.2014.05.006

18. Pace R, Kirk J. Academy of Nutrition and Dietetics and National Kidney Foundation: revised 2020 standards of practice and standards of professional performance for registered dietitian nutritionists (competent, proficient, and expert) in nephrology nutrition. *J Ren Nutr.* 2021;31(2):100-115.e41. doi:10.1053/j.jrn.2020.12.001

19. HR 6074 Coronavirus Preparedness and Response Supplemental Appropriations Act, 2020. Congress. gov website. Accessed April 2020. www.congress .gov/bill/116th-congress/house-bill/6074

20. National Kidney Foundation Kidney Disease Outcomes Quality Initiatives. National Kidney Foundation website. Accessed August 2020. www.kidney.org/professionals/guidelines

21. Centers for Medicare and Medicaid Services Condition for Coverage for End Stage Renal Disease Facilities; Federal Register. Centers for Medicare and Medicaid Services website. April 15, 2008. Accessed April 2020. www.cms.hhs.gov /CFCsAndCoPs/downloads/ESRDfinalrule0415.pdf

22. ESRD Quality Incentive Program. Centers for Medicare and Medicaid Services website. January 29, 2021. Accessed February 2021. www.cms.gov /Medicare/Quality-Initiatives-Patient-Assessment -Instruments/ESRDQIP/06_MeasuringQuality

23. White J, Guenter P, Jensen G, et al. Consensus Statement: Academy of Nutrition and Dietetics and American Society for Parenteral and Enteral Nutrition: Characteristics recommended for the identification and documentation of adult malnutrition (undernutrition). *J Acad Nutr Diet.* 2012;(112)5:730-738. doi:10.1177 /0148607112440285

24. Becker P, Carney L, Corkins M, et al. Consensus statement of the Academy of Nutrition and Dietetics/American Society for Parenteral and Enteral Nutrition: Indicators recommended for the identification and documentation of pediatric malnutrition (undernutrition). *J Acad Nutr Diet.* 2014;114(12):1988-2000. doi:10.1177 /0884533614557642

CHAPTER 24

The Nutrition Care Process Model in Nephrology Nutrition

Donna E. Gjesvold, RDN, LD, CCTD, and Michelle Bump, MS, RD, LD

The Nutrition Care Process (NCP) is a systematic method, framework, or road map used by nutrition and dietetics practitioners to provide high-quality, comprehensive nutrition care.[1,2] The NCP consists of four interconnected, yet distinct steps. The first two steps, Nutrition Assessment and Reassessment and Nutrition Diagnosis, focus on problem identification. The third and fourth steps, Nutrition Intervention and Nutrition Monitoring and Evaluation, focus on problem-solving.[2]

The Nutrition Care Process Model (NCPM) describes the NCP by illustrating the workflow of care delivery in a variety of settings at both the individual and population levels. Multiple benefits of using the NCPM have been identified related to nutrition care and research, critical thinking, care documentation, recognition of the value of nutrition care by other professions, and greater utilization of evidence-based guidelines.[2] Adopted formally by the Academy of Nutrition and Dietetics in 2003 for use in the United States, the NCP and NCPM have roots as far back as the 1970s and foundational work even earlier. The NCP and NCPM are being increasingly implemented by international dietetics associations as they highlight the unique contribution of nutrition and dietetics practitioners to care outcomes and establish a global standard for the provision of care.[3]

To ensure that the NCPM is consistent with current practice, it is updated about every 5 years to coincide with updates in other related Academy of Nutrition and Dietetics resources, such as Evidence-Based Nutri-

tion Practice Guidelines.[2,4,5] The current version of the NCPM was published by the Academy of Nutrition and Dietetics in 2017 and is the result of an update completed by a panel of 24 experts in a global consensus building process (see Figure 24.1 on page 464). Three themes emerged in the update review and are highlighted in the current NCPM: use of concise language in the NCPM, promotion of professionals' responsibility for outcomes management, and support for people-centered care.[2]

Work on terminology to support and describe the NCP began in 2003.[6] A printed manual, *International Dietetics and Nutrition Terminology Reference Manual: Standardized Language for the Nutrition Care Process*, was published in 2007. It was subsequently converted to an electronic database, the Electronic Nutrition Care Process and Terminology (eNCPT), in 2014 as this standardized language outgrew the capacity of a printed manual.[7] Updated annually, the eNCPT is available in multiple languages, and translations in progress are expanding its implementation internationally. Using Nutrition Care Process Terminology (NCPT) generates data that can be collected and used to study nutrition care and the NCP specifically.[2] In 2014, the Academy of Nutrition and Dietetics launched the Academy of Nutrition and Dietetics Health Informatics Infrastructure (ANDHII). ANDHII is an NCPT-based platform that provides tools for tracking outcomes of the NCP. Using ANDHII in practice contributes anonymous data to the national Dietetics Outcomes Registry.[7] As indi-

FIGURE 24.1 | The Nutrition Care Process Model[2]

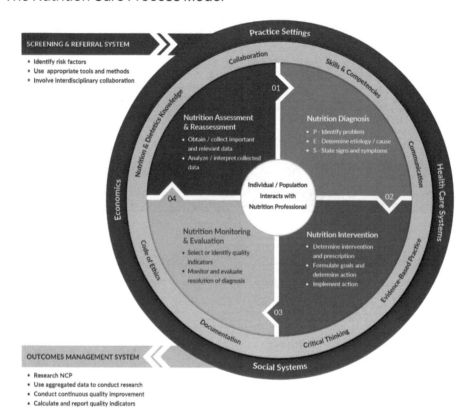

vidual practitioners contribute data, they strengthen the aggregate data that provide evidence of the impact and efficacy of nutrition care.[8] While documentation of care using the NCPM and NCPT is not mandated, the NCP is evolving to become the international standard of care delivery for nutrition and dietetics. As such, it seems reasonable that clinical notes would recognize the steps outlined in the model and use standard language, when possible, to facilitate outcomes research and demonstrate the impact of nutrition intervention.[2]

Applications of the Nutrition Care Process and Model in Nephrology Nutrition

The NCP and NCPM are valuable tools for providing nutrition care in the management of kidney disease as it progresses from early stage chronic kidney disease (CKD) to end-stage kidney disease (ESKD) requiring dialysis or kidney transplant. The NCP in nephrology nutrition ensures

that care is organized to address a specific diagnosis, and it follows certain outcomes over time until the nutrition diagnosis is resolved with the underlying goal of delaying the progression of kidney disease, when possible, and mitigating complications and comorbidities at all stages. The NCPM supports comprehensive, evidence-based care and enables ongoing monitoring to determine which nutrition diagnoses predominate and which interventions produce desired outcomes, thereby promoting effective and efficient nutrition care in the nephrology setting. The use of standardized language in the NCPM streamlines communication between professionals, advancing coordination of care among registered dietitian nutritionists (RDNs) and other health care professionals.

The mandates for ESKD care described in the Conditions for Coverage (CfCs) were published in the Federal Register in April 2008 and align well with the NCP.[9,10] The four steps of the NCP and the NCPT that support it can be coordinated with the categories of documentation required in the CfCs and Interpretive Guidelines

(IGs), as shown in Box 24.1.[11] Organ Transplant Conditions of Participation also mandate that nutrition assessment, intervention, and a patient-specific nutrition plan be documented for all transplant recipients and living donors in all phases of their clinical care.[12]

Use of Nutrition Care Process Terminology

The most current and complete list of NCP terminology exceeds 1,700 terms and is available through the Academy of Nutrition and Dietetics with an online subscription to the eNCPT. There are a variety of practice tools, including NCP snapshots for each step of the NCP, critical thinking suggestions, and comparative standards, in addition to the term lists and their definitions. Worksheets provide suggested etiologies and possible signs and symptoms for each diagnosis, along with references used by the expert committee.[13] These resources will continue to be updated routinely as are other major classification systems in health care.

Getting Started in Clinical Practice

To support the adoption of the NCP, NCPM, and NCPT, the Academy of Nutrition and Dietetics has developed online video modules that use practical case studies to illustrate the NCP and the organization of the eNCPT. The Nutrition Care Process Tutorial Modules, available on eatrightPRO (www.eatrightpro.org), are free for Academy of Nutrition and Dietetics members and can be used for continuing professional education. Dietetic practice group publications are another valuable source of information on application of the NCP, NCPM, and NCPT in specific practice settings.[14]

Case Study: Sample Documentation

The following case study provides an example of implementing the NCP in clinical practice. The patient described is a 46-year-old Black female, a new patient on in-center hemodialysis (ICHD) with ESKD due to hypertension (HTN) (see Figure 24.2 on page 466). At the end of the assessment, the interdisciplinary team (IDT) determined that this patient was stable, in keeping with the definition provided in the IGs that were published to guide surveyors in interpreting the CfCs (see Box 24.2 and 24.3 on page 467).[9] Thus, her first reassessment will be in 3 months in accordance with the IGs and an example is provided in Box 24.4 on page 468.

BOX 24.1 | Comparison of Nutrition Care Process and Conditions for Coverage Mandates

NUTRITION CARE PROCESS (NCP) STEPS[1]	COUNTERPARTS IN CONDITIONS FOR COVERAGE WITH SUPPORTING INTERPRETIVE GUIDELINES (IG) TAGS NOTED[9,10]
Assessment	§494.80 describes requirements for patient assessment. IG Tags V500 to 515 describe information to be included in assessments (509 is specific to nutrition; topics discussed in other tags, such as factors associated with renal bone disease, also relate to nutrition and may be completely or partially addressed by the nephrology dietitian in accordance with accepted practice patterns at the end-stage kidney disease facility).
Diagnosis	Not mandated, but should be included as this is step 2 in the NCP.
Intervention (includes care plan) Monitoring and evaluation	§494.90 states that the interdisciplinary team must develop and implement a comprehensive plan of care that describes services needed (interventions) and outcomes (monitoring and evaluation step of NCP). IG Tag 545 sets expectations for an outcome-oriented plan of care related to nutritional status.

FIGURE 24.2 | Initial documentation: assessment of new patient undergoing in-center hemodialysis

PATIENT OVERVIEW
46-year-old Black female with ESKD due to HTN, initiated ICHD 1 week ago.

FOOD/NUTRITION-RELATED HISTORY
- Patient reports good appetite. States no recent GI issues, such as nausea/vomiting/constipation/diarrhea. No chewing/swallowing problems or food preferences. Takes 2 meals/d with 1 to 2 snacks.

- Patient recalls brief kidney diet education with hospital RDN prior to discharge. Patient states she has been avoiding high potassium foods since she received education. Reports she always limits salt intake.

- Ambulatory; reports that she typically uses cardio machines three times a week at the gym for 30 to 45 minutes but has been too tired to exercise since her recent hospitalization for dialysis initiation.

- Pertinent medications: 3 sevelamer carbonate (Renvela) with meals (reports none with snacks), 1 Dialyvite daily, 2 mcg doxercalciferol injection (Hectorol IV) per treatment.

- Also reports taking daily OTC multivitamins, no herbal supplements.

BIOCHEMICAL DATA, MEDICAL TESTS, AND PROCEDURES

	Results	Dialysis goal
Potassium (K)	5.0 mEq/L	3.5-5.5
Carbon dioxide (CO2)	24.0 mEq/L	22-27
Blood urea nitrogen (BUN)	48 mg/dL	60-80
Creatinine (Cr)	6.8 mg/dL	2-18
Albumin	3.4 g/dL	3.5; optimal 4.0
Normalized protein catabolic rate (nPCR)	1.0 g/kg	1.0-1.4
Glucose, non-fasting	80 mg/dL	80-180
Calcium (Ca)	9.0 mg/dL	8.4-10.2
Corrected calcium	9.5 mg/dL	8.4-10.2
Phosphorus	6.2 mg/dL	3.0-5.5
Intact parathyroid hormone (iPTH)	345 ng/L	150-600
spKt/V*	1.6	>1.2
Urea reduction ratio (URR)	83.3%	>65
Cholesterol, non-fasting	124 mg/dL	<200
Triglycerides (TG)	102 mg/dL	<200
Hemoglobin (Hgb)	10.9 g/dL	10-12; avoid transfusion

*spKt/V = a measure of dialysis adequacy.
Dialysis prescription: 3 times a week, 240 minutes, 2 K+, 2.5 Ca bath

ANTHROPOMETRIC MEASUREMENTS
Height 162.6 cm, target weight 60.2 kg. Weight after last ICHD 59.8 kg (target weight being challenged), body mass index of 23 (using 60.2 kg). Patient reports gaining about 10 lb in the last 2 months prior to initiating ICHD, likely due to fluid. Interdialytic weight gains range from 0.5 to 2 kg over the last week.

NUTRITION FOCUSED PHYSICAL FINDINGS
Patient appears well nourished with no signs of muscle or fat wasting. +1 edema on lower extremities. No wounds present.

PATIENT HISTORY
- Social history: Lives with spouse and two school-aged children.

- Past medical history: ESKD on HD, AV fistula placement, HTN

- Family history: paternal grandmother with CKD, father with HTN

AV = arteriovenous | CKD = chronic kidney disease | ESKD = end-stage kidney disease | GI = gastrointestinal | HD = hemodialysis | HTN = hypertension | ICHD = in-center hemodialysis | OTC = over-the-counter | RDN = registered dietitian nutritionist

BOX 24.2 | 24-Hour Diet Recall of Case Study Patient From Initial Nutrition Assessment

APPROXIMATE TIME	FOOD ITEM	AMOUNT
7:30 AM	Coffee	12 oz
	Milk added	(amount uncertain)

12 PM	Tuna salad sandwich:
	    2 slices whole wheat bread
	    1 can tuna in water
	    1 slice processed cheese
	    1 tablespoon mayonnaise
	    1 tablespoon relish
		1 sandwich

	Apple	1 medium
	Grapes	~15
	Iced tea with sugar substitute	16 oz
6 PM	Chicken breast half	4 oz
	Rotini pasta with cheese sauce	1 cup, cooked
	Salad with romaine lettuce, carrot, tomato, croutons, Italian dressing	2 cups salad ~2 tablespoons dressing
	Iced tea with sugar substitute	16 oz
10 PM	Homemade brownie with nuts	2" square
	Milk, nonfat	8 oz

BOX 24.3 | Initial Documentation: Nutrition Diagnoses and Plan of Care

Nutrition diagnoses (Problem—Etiology—Signs and Symptoms or PES)

Problem (or diagnosis): Excessive phosphorus intake related to Etiology: lack of thorough kidney diet and phosphate binder education as evidenced by Signs and Symptoms: reported consumption of high phosphorus foods and phosphorus of 6.2 mg/dL.

Problem (or diagnosis): Excess vitamin and mineral intake related to Etiology: lack of knowledge of vitamin/mineral needs as evidenced by Signs and Symptoms: consumption of daily multivitamin in addition to renal vitamin.

Nutrition prescription

1,800 to 2,100 kcal/d (30–35 kcal/kg), 60 to 72 g protein (1.0–1.2 g/kg), 2,300 mg sodium, 2,000 mg potassium, 1,000 mg phosphorus, plus daily renal vitamin.

Intervention

Nutrition education: Provided education on recommended kidney diet modifications, including phosphorus restriction and vitamin/mineral needs on dialysis. Discussed limiting high phosphorus foods and discontinuing daily over-the-counter multivitamin.

Coordination of nutrition care: Collaborated with nephrologist on Renvela prescription to clarify dosage for meals and snacks (3 with meals, 1 to 2 with snacks). Communicated dosage information to patient.

Patient goals	• Substitute beverage choice at bedtime with water daily.
	• Discontinue daily multivitamins.
	• Start taking 1 to 2 Renvela with snacks daily.

Monitoring and Evaluation

Nutrition care indicator	Criteria
Serum phosphorus	Phosphorus 3.0–5.5 mg/dL in 1 month
Vitamin and mineral intake	Discontinued use of daily multivitamin per patient report in 1 month

BOX 24.4 | Three-Month Reassessment Documentation

Progress: Three-month reassessment and plan of care outcomes

Patient has successfully met outcome criteria from initial assessment; however, potassium levels have increased and patient reports consuming high-potassium foods most days.

Food/nutrition-related history

Patient continues with good appetite, no gastrointestinal symptoms. Reports consumption of high potassium fruits (bananas, avocado) most days of the week. Discontinued use of over-the-counter multivitamins.

Pertinent medications: 3 sevelamer carbonate (Renvela) with meals and 1 to 2 with snacks, 1 Dialyvite daily, 6 mcg doxercalciferol injection (Hectorol IV) per treatment

Biochemical data, medical tests, and procedures

Last monthly laboratory results included potassium 6.2 mEq/L, albumin 3.8 g/dL, phosphorus 5.2 mg/dL, Kt/V 1.6, urea reduction ratio (URR) 76%.

Dialysis prescription: no change.

Nutrition prescription

1,800 to 2,100 kcal/d (30–35 kcal/kg), 60 to 72 g protein (1.0–1.2 g/kg), 2,300 mg sodium, 2,000 mg potassium, 1,000 mg phosphorus, plus daily renal vitamin.

Nutrition focused physical findings

No edema, no change in muscle/fat status.

Previous nutrition diagnoses

Excessive phosphorus intake related to lack of thorough kidney diet and phosphate binder education as evidenced by reported consumption of high-phosphorus foods and phosphorus of 6.2 mg/dL—resolved.

Excess vitamin and mineral intake related to lack of knowledge of vitamin/mineral needs as evidenced by consumption of daily multivitamin in addition to renal vitamin—resolved.

Nutrition diagnosis

Excess potassium intake related to consumption of high-potassium foods as evidenced by potassium of 6.2 mEq/L.

Intervention

Nutrition education: Provided education on recommended daily potassium intake and high/medium/low potassium foods.

Patient goal: Substitute one high-potassium food choice daily with a low-potassium food choice from education handout provided.

Monitoring and Evaluation

Nutrition care indicator	Criteria
Serum potassium	Potassium 3.5 to 5.5 mEq/L within 1 month

References

1. Lacey K, Pritchett E. Nutrition care process and model: ADA adopts road map to quality care and outcomes management. *J Am Diet Assoc.* 2003;103:1061-1071. doi:10.1016/s0002-8223(03)00971-4

2. Swan WI, Vivanti A, Hakel-Smith NA, et al. Nutrition care process and model update: toward realizing people-centered care and outcomes management. *J Acad Nutr Diet.* 2017;117(12):2003-2014. doi:10.1016/j.jand.2017.07.015

3. Hammond MI, Myers EF, Trostler N. Nutrition care process and model: an academic and practice odyssey. *J Acad Nutr Diet.* 2014;114(12):1879-1894. doi:10.1016/j.jand.2014.07.032

4. Papoutsakis C, Moloney L, Sinley RC, et al. Academy of Nutrition and Dietetics methodology for developing evidence-based nutrition practice guidelines. *J Acad Nutr Diet.* 2017;117(5):794-804. doi:10.1016/j.jand.2016.07.011

5. Writing Group of the Nutrition Care Process/Standardized Language Committee. Nutrition care process and model, part I: the 2008 update. *J Am Diet Assoc.* 2008;108(7):1113-1117. doi:10.1016/j.jada.2008.04.027

6. Writing Group of the Nutrition Care Process/Standardized Language Committee. Nutrition care process and model, part II: using the international dietetics and nutrition terminology to document the nutrition care process. *J Am Diet Assoc.* 2008;108(8):1287-1293. doi:10.1016/j.jada.2008.06.368

7. Murphy WJ, Steiber AL. A new breed of evidence and the tools to generate it: introducing ANDHII. *J Acad Nutr Diet.* 2015;115(1):19-22. doi:10.1016/j.jand.2014.10.025

8. Murphy WJ, Yadrick MM, Steiber AL, Mohan V, Papoutsakis C. Academy of Nutrition and Dietetics Health Informatics Infrastructure (ANDHII): a pilot study on the documentation of the nutrition care process and the usability of ANDHII by registered dietitian nutritionists. *J Acad Nutr Diet.* 2018;118(10):1966-1974. doi:10.1016/j.jand.2018.03.013

9. Medicare and Medicaid Programs: Conditions for coverage for end-stage renal disease facilities. *Fed Regist.* April 2008. 73(73):20370-20484. Accessed April 15, 2020. www.cms.hhs.gov/center/esrd.asp

10. ESRD Surveyor Training Interpretive Guidance, Part 494 Conditions for Coverage for End-Stage Renal Disease Facilities. October 2008. Accessed April 15, 2020. www.cms.gov/Medicare/Provider-Enrollment-and-Certification/GuidanceforLawsAndRegulations/Downloads/esrdpgmguidance.pdf

11. McCarthy M, Asbell D. Nephrology nutrition and the nutrition care process (NCP): where does nutrition diagnosis fit in the new conditions for coverage? *Renal Nutrition Forum.* 2009;28(2):20-23.

12. Interpretive Guidelines for the Organ Transplant Conditions of Participation (CoPs). May 2016. Centers for Medicare & Medicaid Services website. Accessed April 15, 2020. www.cms.gov/Medicare/Provider-Enrollment-and-Certification/SurveyCertificationGenInfo/Downloads/Survey-and-Cert-Letter-16-10.pdf

13. Academy of Nutrition and Dietetics. *Abridged Nutrition Care Process Terminology (NCPT) Reference Manual: Standardized Terminology for the Nutrition Care Process.* Academy of Nutrition and Dietetics; 2017.

14. Therrien, M. Utilizing the nutrition care process and nutrition-focused physical exam in the care of the medically complex patient on hemodialysis. *Renal Nutrition Forum.* 2013;32(1):1-8.

CHAPTER 25

Counseling and Communication Skills for the Renal Dietitian

Kathleen Hunt, RD, CSR

Chronic Kidney Disease: The Disease and The People

According to the National Institutes of Health, approximately one of seven Americans (over 14%) will experience some form of kidney disease in their lifetime.[1,2] If kidney disease progresses into chronic kidney disease (CKD), management is complex and a major part of the care rests on the individual with the disease. Lifestyle, daily routine, and personal choices are heavily impacted for both the individual and for their support system.

Not everyone with CKD is equipped for a new and unsolicited burden of care. Some individuals can follow recommended change, some need time or help to make the change, and some individuals may never adapt to change. The ability to follow long-term, complicated medication regimes, diet or fluid restrictions, frequent medical appointments, treatment monitoring, and keep physically active varies with each individual. As a result, many people with CKD who do not quickly adapt to the changes are labeled "noncompliant." In one hemodialysis study, nonadherence to recommendations ranged from 8.5% to 86%.[3] Sadly, with nonadherence comes more medical complications, an increase in symptoms, a lower quality of life, and a higher risk of mortality.

See Box 25.1 for more on diet nonadherence and common issues for patients with CKD that may limit their chance for success.[4-6]

All of the intrinsic and extrinsic factors remind professionals that the diet for patients with CKD is up against many roadblocks. The task of the renal registered dietitian nutritionist (RDN) to help individuals make changes is big and sometimes feels like a near-impossible task. Achieving a healthy understanding of people and gaining the skills that promote changing habits will lessen the gap between the kidney diet and kidney diet adherence.

BOX 25.1 | Common Barriers to Changing Eating Behavior[4-6]

INTRINSIC FACTORS	EXTRINSIC FACTORS
Age	Family dysfunction
Time on treatment	Lack of social support
Omission (forgetting)	Cultural food patterns
Motivation level	Poverty
Distorted perception of adherence	Limited access to healthy foods
Limited perception of the benefit	Food marketing and advertising

Skills and Tools for the Renal Registered Dietitian Nutritionist

RIGHT ATTITUDE

Trust is the cornerstone of effective communication. Without trust, there is very little that can be achieved.

It starts with the professional's unspoken attitude and body language that tells people if they are in the presence of someone genuinely caring and confident of their success.

Building respect and trust comes from remembering that people with CKD:

- may not have a clear perception of the disease,
- may be fighting for a sense of control over their own lives,
- may fear or lack confidence in their abilities (self-efficacy) related to the diet,
- may lack social support or role models for making change,
- may struggle in relationships with health care providers, or
- may be confused about how to prioritize kidney diet requirements with dietary requirements for other chronic diseases.

Before interviews, education, or counseling sessions begin, some self-checks and reminders are valuable.

PATIENT-BASED EDUCATION

The foundation of well-rounded nutrition education is content accuracy and evidence-based science behind the content. While quality of information is critical, presentation is also essential so that a patient can perceive the message that is being communicated. To improve patient understanding of the content, include a variety of learning style approaches and include the support system or caregivers who help the patient on a regular basis (see Box 25.2).[7,8]

NUTRITION COUNSELING—HELPING OTHERS MAKE CHANGES

The everyday clinical practice of an RDN goes beyond dispensing well-designed nutrition education. Learning to practice behavior-change counseling skills enables patients to rethink their eating behavior and discover solutions to their dietary issues. Effective use of counseling skills opens the doors to tough conversations while maintaining the patient's dignity and autonomy.

BOX 25.2 | Checklist for Improving Educational Programs, Materials, and Presentations[7,8]

Is the information easy, practical, positive, and interactive?

Is there backup education for those who respond to more detailed information?

Is the desirable eating behavior modeled through photographs, skill demonstrations, or workshops?

Are there opportunities to learn in both one-on-one encounters and in group settings?

Are the families, helpful friends, or caregivers included in the education process?

Are there other members of the health care team who can support the changes?

Can the education include the success of others through testimonies, stories, or connections with peer mentors?

Does information on various materials provided to client/patient possibly cause confusion?

The core of behavior-change skills includes:

- listening more,
- talking less,
- using more open-ended questions in conversations, and
- ending each session asking what helped the most that day or what will be the easiest or hardest to implement.

This approach encourages the patient to think more for themselves. Each skill, theory, or behavior-change listed will overlap, so mastering one method will likely prepare the RDN for learning additional methods.

STAGES OF CHANGE: THE TRANSTHEORETICAL MODEL

The stages of change in the transtheoretical model, developed by Prochaska and DiClemente, uses interview techniques that encompass a broader audience than motivational interviewing (MI). This model creates tools for people not-ready-to-change, for people who are thinking about change, and for people actively making behavior changes. Box 25.3 contains a brief description of the stages and some coinciding interview questions.

MOTIVATIONAL INTERVIEWING

MI provides a deep level of patient engagement to overcome ambivalence and promote behavior change. It is a tool to help the patient move through the stages of change, from precontemplation to action. The RDN guides the conversation with the patient using a technique of OARS: Open-Ended Questions, Affirmation, Reflection, and Summarization. This allows the RDN to show empathy, listen, and set patient-centered goals. Box 25.4 shows some brief examples of how MI progresses in conversation.

COGNITIVE BEHAVIOR THERAPY

Cognitive behavior therapy (CBT) helps an individual work through difficult thoughts, feelings, and behavior so that new thoughts and behaviors can be created. CBT requires advanced training beyond the RDN scope of practice. However, some of the CBT strategies

---

BOX 25.3 | Stages of Change Conversations[9]

Precontemplation: Not doing and not thinking about change	Are you thinking about changing?
	What do you know about…?
	How do you feel about making a change? When you are ready, I can help you.
Contemplation: Not doing, but thinking about change	What are the pros and cons of making the change?
	What would make it easier to change?
	What do you need to be successful?
	What can I do to help?
Preparation: Not doing, but planning on changing in 1 to 6 months	When do you plan on starting?
	How will you do it?
	How will your life improve?
	How can I help you?
Action: Now doing the change	What are you doing differently?
	What helped you make the change?
	What problems are you having?
Maintenance: Doing the change most of the time	How do you handle times when you slip up? What obstacles are you facing?
	What issues have you solved?
	What will help you keep on…?
Relapse: Stopped doing the change	What will help you to get back on track? What worked before?
	Why didn't it work?
	What will you do differently?
	What can I do to help?

BOX 25.4 | Motivational Interview Conversations

GUIDING STATEMENT	QUESTIONS
Open with permission	Is it okay to…?
	Do I have your permission to…?
Open-ended starter	Tell me about…
	Help me understand…
	How do you feel about…?
Further probes	Give me some words that describe…
	What else…?
Universal safe reflections	It sounds like you are…
	So, you are saying that…
	It almost sounds like…
	It's been _____ for you to…
Gentle confrontation (for incongruence)	I'm confused…. How do these fit together?
	What you are telling me now is different than what you said earlier about…
	You say you want _____, but what I see you doing is _____.
Creating solutions	What would it take to…?
	What do you see as the solution?
	Would you like to see more choices?
	What can I do to help you?
End-building self-efficacy	I am confident you will find a plan that's best for you.
	I am confident that your choice to _____ will work for you.

are useful tools when working through renal diet issues with a patient (see Box 25.5).

MINDFUL EATING THERAPY: EATING WITH ATTENTION AND AWARENESS

In the age of multitasking and strong food marketing campaigns, mindless eating has become a social normative. To enhance awareness of personal eating decisions and reduce automatic reactions, the patients learn more about their own eating cues. The what, when, and how much they eat are linked to their feelings and environment.[10]

Studies of early stages of CKD have had positive results using mindful eating to decrease weight and body mass index.[11] Further randomized control trials are needed specifically in the renal population.

BOX 25.5 | Cognitive Behavior Therapy Strategies for the Registered Dietitian Nutritionist

Self-monitoring tools	Common examples: patient-oriented reports for tracking their own results to their actions (recording blood glucose and blood pressure levels, or laboratory findings). The report will often provide ideas or options on how the patient can improve their results.
	Follow-up with the practitioner gives patients an opportunity to speak about what the patients have learned, what they plan to do differently, what they may not understand, and where they would like help or further support.
Goal setting	In place of trying to achieve a big goal, the patient builds short-term, smaller, and attainable goals. These small steps build patient confidence.
	Follow-up with the practitioner gives the patient an opportunity to discuss what worked, what did not work, and what might be the next steps to take to work toward achieving the bigger goal.
Problem-solving	Both patient and practitioner brainstorm solutions for achieving a desired goal. The patient chooses what change or action they will attempt. The practitioner closes the conversations with a statement of confidence and affirmation.

Pause and Reflect: the Registered Dietitian Nutritionist and Behavior Counseling Skills

Patience, empathy, and nonjudgmental care of individuals with a chronic disease can be a challenge for the professional when patients do not quickly make the recommended changes in food choices. Often, it helps to remember the following:

- No single counselor, educator, technique, or skill will reach everyone.
- Behavior strategies are useful tools, but they do not guarantee success; they simply provide a positive environment for change.[12]
- Most people can only succeed in making one small change before they tackle the next.
- All individuals struggle at one time or another when faced with challenges—even the professional!

With time, the reward of watching more patients succeed in a few more choices in their diet will build the confidence of both the RDN and the population they serve. It will also solidify the knowledge that the counseling skills and tools listed are integral to improving the lives of individuals with CKD.

Additional Resources

General information on behavior-change theories and skills is available through many reliable internet searches. While not a complete list, the following are books on counseling geared toward the RDN:

Saunter C, Constance A. *Inspiring & Supporting Behavior Change: A Food, Nutrition & Health Professional's Counseling Guide.* 2nd ed. Academy of Nutrition and Dietetics; 2017.

Holli BB, Beto JA. *Nutrition Counseling and Education Skills: A Guide for Professionals.* 7th ed. Wolters Kluwer Health; 2018.

A program for dietetic interns and RDNs to improve counseling techniques. www.mollykellogg.com

Training opportunities in motivational interviewing. www.trainingwithdrellen.com

References

1. Centers for Disease Control and Prevention. Chronic Kidney Disease Surveillance System website. March 2020. Accessed January 22, 2020. https://nccd.cdc.gov/CKD

2. US Renal Data System 2019 Annual Data Report: epidemiology of kidney disease in the United States. *Am J Kidney Dis.* 2020;75(1 suppl 1):A6-A7. doi:10.1053/j.ajkd.2019.09.003

3. Matteson ML, Russell C. Interventions to improve hemodialysis adherence: a systematic review of randomized-controlled trials. *Hemodial Int.* 2010;14(4):370-382. doi:10.1111/j.1542-4758.2010.00462.x

4. Oquendo LG, Asencio JMM, de las Nieves CB. Contributing factors for therapeutic diet adherence in patients receiving hemodialysis treatment: an integrative review. *J Clin Nurs.* 2017;26(23-24):3893-3905. doi:10.1111/jocn.13804

5. Stevenson J, Tong A, Campbell KL, Craig JC. Perspectives of healthcare providers on the nutritional management of patients on haemodialysis in Australia: an interview study. *BMJ Open.* 2018:8(3):e020023. doi:10.1136/bmjopen-2017-020023

6. Stevenson J, Tong A, Gutman T, et al. Experiences and perspectives of dietary management among patients on hemodialysis: an interview study. *J Ren Nutr.* 2018;28(6):411-421. doi:10.1053/j.jrn.2018.02.005

7. Lopez-Vargas PA, Tong A, Howell M, Craig JC. Educational interventions for patients with CKD: a systematic review. *Am J Kidney Dis.* 2016;68(3):353-370. doi:10.1053/j.ajkd.2016.01.022

8. Anderson CAM, Nguyen HA. Nutrition education in the care of patients with chronic kidney disease and end-stage renal disease. *Semin Dial.* 2018;31(2):115-121. doi:10.1111/sdi.12681

9. Holli BB, Beto JA. *Communication and Education Skills for Dietetics Professionals.* 7th ed. Wolters Kluwer Health; 2018.

10. Winkens L, van Strien T, Barrada J, Brouwer I, Penninx B, Visser M. The mindful eating behavior scale: development and psychometric properties in a sample of Dutch adults aged 55 years and older. *J Acad Nutr Diet.* 2018;118(7):1277-1290. doi:10.1016/j.jand.2018.01.015

11. Timmerman G, Tahir M, Lewis R, Samoson D, Temple H, Forman M. Self-management of dietary intake using mindful eating to improve dietary intake for individuals with early stage chronic kidney disease. *J Behav Med.* 2017;40(5):702-711. doi:10.1007/s10865-017-9835-1

12. Raynor H, Champagne C. Position of the Academy of Nutrition and Dietetics: intervention for the treatment of overweight and obesity in adults. *J Acad Nutr Diet.* 2016;116(1):129-147. doi:10.1016/j.jand.2015.10.031

Appendix: Resources for Kidney Disease

Sara Colman Carlson, RDN, CDCES, and Melissa Prest, DCN, MS, RDN, CSR, LDN

This appendix provides professional resources of value to specialists in renal nutrition. It focuses on web-based resources for the renal nutrition professional, beginning with two well-known websites. Of course, the challenge is to be general enough so as not to be quickly outdated and yet detailed enough to be of use to specialists. These sites have been deemed highly accurate. The sites reviewed were active in August 2022. The following professional organizations for renal registered dietitian nutritionists are well known to most of us.

Renal Dietitians Dietetic Practice Group of the Academy of Nutrition and Dietetics

Membership information is available on the Academy of Nutrition and Dietetics website (www.eatrightPRO .org, search Renal Dietetic Practice Group). The Renal Dietitians Dietetic Practice Group (RPG) also has its own page for members (www.renalnutrition.org). This page includes archives of the Renal Nutrition Forum (from the summer of 2003 to the present), member resources, information about RPG awards and stipends, and patient education tools. The Academy of Nutrition and Dietetics membership also includes access to the Evidence Analysis Library, which provides practice guidelines and recommendations in chronic kidney disease management.

Council on Renal Nutrition of the National Kidney Foundation

Extensive information about the Council on Renal Nutrition (CRN) of the National Kidney Foundation (NKF), including the how-to of membership and programs for local and national meetings, is available (www.kidney.org/professionals/CRN). CRN is a contributor to NKF's *RenaLink*, a joint newsletter of the Council of Nephrology Nurses and Technicians, the Council of Nephrology Social Work, and CRN. You will find links to the Kidney Disease Outcomes Quality Initiative (KDOQI) and the global nonprofit foundation, Kidney Disease: Improving Global Outcomes (KDIGO) practice guidelines on the NKF website. On this page, the menu item for patients offers many resources, including the full list of NKF patient education handouts, which may be downloaded as PDF files.

Box A.1 and Box A.2 identify additional organizations and materials of interest to health professionals, patients, and families.

BOX A.1 | Resources for Kidney Disease

SITE NAME / URL	AUDIENCE	SOURCE	CONTENTS
eatrightPRO www.eatrightpro.org	Professionals	Academy of Nutrition and Dietetics	Scope of Practice, Evidence Analysis Library, Advocacy, Position and Practice Papers, Code of Ethics, Continuing Education (paid membership required to access content).
eatRIGHT www.eatright.org	Professionals, patients, family	Academy of Nutrition and Dietetics	Source for science-based food and nutrition information. Find an expert, recipes, videos, and articles.
American Association of Kidney Patients (AAKP) https://aakp.org	Patients, family	AAKP	Information on chronic kidney disease, dialysis, transplant, advocacy.
American Kidney Fund (AKF) www.kidneyfund.org	Patients, family	AKF	Educational resources, recipes, financial assistance, and advocacy for patients with kidney disease (English and Spanish).
American Society of Nephrology (ASN) www.asn-online.org	Professionals	ASN	Abstracts for Kidney Week and other resources (paid membership required to access content).
Centers for Medicare & Medicaid Services (CMS) www.cms.hhs.gov/CFCsAndCoPs/13_ESRD.asp	Professionals	Department of Health and Human Services/CMS	End-stage renal disease Conditions for Coverage.
Diabetes Advanced Network Access (DANA) https://danatech.org	Professionals, patients, family	Association of Diabetes Care and Education Specialists (ADCES)	Search, compare, and evaluate diabetes devices, platforms, mobile apps, and more. Evaluates and rates apps on performance, data management, privacy and security. Free content but requires account to log in.
DaVita Kidney Care www.davita.com	Professionals, patients, family	DaVita Kidney Care	Information about kidney disease, treatment options, education articles, recipes, Food Analyzer, diet and nutrition tools and resources, dialysis center locator, Kidney Smart classes (English and Spanish).
Dialysis and Transplantation (D&T) https://onlinelibrary.wiley.com/loi/19326920	Professionals	Wiley Online Library	Index and PDF files of D&T articles.
Dialysis Patient Citizens (DPC) www.dialysispatients.org	Patients, family	DPC	Patient education, advocacy, resources.

Continued on next page

Continued from previous page

SITE NAME / URL	AUDIENCE	SOURCE	CONTENTS
Epocrates https://online.epocrates.com	Professionals	Athena Health Service	Free access to review prescription and over-the-counter medication information.
Explore Transplant https://exploretransplant.org	Professionals, patients, family	National consortium of experts in transplant and health literacy	Transplant education and decision-making tools for patients and donors.
Fresenius Kidney Care www.freseniuskidneycare.com	Professionals, patients, family	Fresenius Medical Care–North America (FMCNA)	Information about kidney disease, treatment options, education articles, recipes, dialysis center locator (in English and Spanish).
Hypertension, Dialysis and Clinical Nephrology www.hdcn.com	Professionals	Education program of ASN and Renal Physicians Association (RPA)	Current news headlines, meeting highlights, calculators, practice guidelines; some material subscription only.
Journal of Renal Nutrition (JRN) www.jrnjournal.org	Professionals	WB Saunders Company/ Elsevier/ NKF	JRN issues, subscriptions. Each journal includes patient education material (paid subscription required to access content).
Kidney School www.kidneyschool.org	Professionals, patients, family	Medical Education Institute, Inc (Sponsored by: FMCNA, Baxter Healthcare, Rockwell Medicine)	16 kidney education modules. Topics range from kidney function to treatment options and nutrition (in English and Spanish). Available to download or as an audio book.
Library of Congress www.congress.gov	Professionals, patients, family	Library of Congress	Contacts for US senators and representatives, congressional records, committee lists.
Medical Education Institute (MEI) http://meiresearch.org	Professionals, patients, family	MEI (A nonprofit 501(c)(3) dedicated to helping people with chronic diseases learn to manage and improve their health)	Resource library, continuing education credits, patient testimonies, and education. Other sites associated: Life Options; Kidney School; Home Dialysis Central; KDQOL (Kidney Disease Quality of Life) Complete; My Dialysis Choice.
Medline Plus https://medlineplus.gov /healthtopics.html	Professionals, patients, family	US National Library of Medicine and National Institutes of Health (NIH)	Many nutrition and kidney and urinary health topics (in English and Spanish).
National Institute of Diabetes and Digestive and Kidney Diseases (NIDDK) www.niddk.nih.gov	Professionals, patients, family	NIDDK and NIH	Many diabetes and kidney disease education tools. Some materials in Spanish.

Continued on next page

Continued from previous page

SITE NAME / URL	AUDIENCE	SOURCE	CONTENTS
National Kidney Foundation (NKF) www.kidney.org	Professionals, patients, family	NKF	Kidney disease resources. Peer mentoring, education materials, Kidney Disease Outcomes Quality Initiative (KDOQI)/Kidney Disease Improving Global Outcomes (KDIGO) practice guidelines, glomerular filtration rate calculator (in English and Spanish).
The Nephcure Foundation https://nephcure.org	Professionals, patients, family	Nephcure Kidney International	Kidney disease education, patient support, and research with focus on protein-spilling kidney diseases.
The Nephron Information Center http://nephron.com	Professionals, patients, family	Steven Z. Fadem, MD, FACP	Top news stories. Comprehensive resources/links. Legislative stories/links.
Polycystic Kidney Disease (PKD) Foundation https://pkdcure.org	Professionals, patients, family	PKD Foundation	PKD education and resources.
Pub Med https://pubmed.ncbi.nlm.nih.gov	Professionals, patients, family	US National Library of Medicine	Free access to MEDLINE search capabilities.
RenalRD Listserv www.mailman.srv.ualberta.ca/mailman/listinfo/renalrd	Professionals	NKF cyber Nephrology	Discussion forum for renal dietitians.
Renal Support Network (RSN) www.rsnhope.org	Professionals, patients, family	RSN (nonprofit patient organization)	Patient education, advocacy, resources, social networking, forums.
UKidney Internet School of Nephrology https://ukidney.com	Professionals	TalkTMA (thrombotic micro-angiopathy), St. Michael's Hospital Nephrology, The CPD (continuing professional development) Network Endorsed by ASN, Canadian Society of Nephrology, International Society of Nephrology	Internet school of nephrology. Resource content.
US Department of Agriculture (USDA) Food and Nutrition Information Center (FNIC) www.nal.usda.gov/fnic	Professionals, patients, family	USDA and FNIC	Links to various food composition databases. International bibliographies. Information on dietary supplements. Food safety. MyPlate and Historical Food Pyramid.

Continued on next page

Continued from previous page

SITE NAME / URL	AUDIENCE	SOURCE	CONTENTS
United States Renal Data System (USRDS) www.usrds.org	Professionals	USRDS Coordinating Center, funded by the NIDDK	Extensive data reports and reference tables. Slides taken from data reports. Researchers' guide. Related links.

BOX A.2 | Resources Related to Complementary, Alternative, and Integrative Therapies

SITE NAME / URL	AUDIENCE	SOURCE	CONTENTS
ConsumerLab.com www.consumerlab.com	Professionals, patients, family	ConsumerLab.com, LLC	Some content by subscription only. Laboratory test results for many supplements.
National Center for Complementary and Integrative Health (NCCIH) www.nccih.nih.gov	Professionals, patients, family	NIH	Government agency dedicated to exploring complementary and integrative health practices; consumer information.
National Institutes of Health (NIH) Office of Dietary Supplements (ODS) https://ods.od.nih.gov	Professionals, patients, family	NIH	Links to dietary supplement fact sheets; dietary supplement use and safety; nutrient recommendations (in English and Spanish).
Natural Medicines Therapeutic Research Center https://naturalmedicines .therapeuticresearch.com	Professionals	Natural Medicines is impartial; not supported by any interest group, professional organization, or product manufacturer.	Seeks to answer questions about natural medicines by systematically identifying, evaluating, and applying scientific information. Provides safety, effectiveness, and interaction ratings. Based on strict evidence-based criteria and "strength of recommendation" rating.

Continuing Professional Education

This third edition of *Clinical Guide to Nutrition Care in Kidney Disease* offers readers 10 hours of Continuing Professional Education (CPE) credit. Readers may earn credit by completing the interactive quiz at:

https://publications.webauthor.com/clinicalguide_kidneydisease_3e

Index

Page numbers followed by *b*, *f* and *t* refer to boxes, figures and tables, respectively.

calcium oxalate stones, 289
    acid-ash and alkaline-ash foods, 303*b*
    acid-forming foods and protein, 302–303
    medical management, 299–300
    nutritional management, 300–302
calcium-phosphorus- PTH balance, 103–104
calcium polycarbophil (Equalactin, Fiber Tabs), 371*b*
calcium-sensing receptors (CaSRs), 185, 227
calcium stones
    calcium oxalate stones, 289, 299–303
    calcium phosphate stones, 303
    crystal formation, 191
    crystals, 189
calorie load, 94
canagliflozin (Invokana), 368*b*
cancer, 52*b*, 130
    bladder, 51
    long-term posttransplant period, 130
candesartan (Atacand), 364*b*
CAPD. *See* continuous ambulatory peritoneal dialysis (CAPD)
capsaicin, 165
captopril (Capoten), 364*b*
carbamylation of hemoglobin, 154
carbohydrate, 338
    absorption, determinant of, 160*f*
    adult renal transplant patient, 118–119
    consistency, 161
    counting (carb counting), 160–161
    management, dietary strategies for, 159–161
    sparing dialysate solutions, 151
carbonated beverages, 167
carbonyl stress, 67
cardiac diastolic dysfunction, 149
cardiac dysfunction, 40
cardiac mortality, 190
cardiac muscle pathology, 225
cardiac overload and acceleration, 150
cardiac pathology, 224–225
cardiovascular autonomic neuropathy, 166
cardiovascular death, 71
cardiovascular disease (CVD), 14, 39–41
    abnormal mineral metabolism, 226–228
    anticoagulation, 230
    cardiac pathology, 224–225
    congestive heart failure (CHF), 223
    diabetes-related complications, comorbidities and concerns, 168
    dyslipidemia, 225–226
    homocysteinemia, 228–229

    hypertension, 228
    inflammation, 229
    kidney transplant and cardiovascular disease, 229–230
    prevalence, 224
    registered dietitian nutritionist's role in, 230–233
    risk factors, 223, 224*b*
cardiovascular disease (CVD) and chronic kidney disease, medication
    α-adrenergic agonists, 365*b*
    angiotensin-converting enzyme (ACE) inhibitors, 364*b*
    angiotensin II receptor blockers (ARBs), 364*b*
    antiadrenergics, 363*b*
    antiarrhythmics, 362*b*
    antithrombotic agents, 361*b*
    calcium channel blockers, 364*b*
    cardiac glycosides (inotropic agents), 364*b*
    combination medication used for heart failure, 365*b*
    diuretics, 362*b*
    dyslipidemia, 365*b*
    vasodilators, 363*b*
    vasopressin V2-receptor antagonist, 365*b*
cardiovascular mortality, 232
Cardiovascular risk Reduction by Early Anemia Treatment with Epoetin Beta (CREATE) trial, 231
carotid and aortic stiffness, 225
carteolol hydrochloride (Cartrol), 363*b*
carvedilol (Coreg), 363*b*
catabolic hormones, 67
catch-up growth, 259
catheter-related infections, 66
CCPD. *See* continuous cyclical peritoneal dialysis (CCPD)
Centers for Disease Control and Prevention, 14
Centers for Medicare & Medicaid Services (CMS), 82, 456
CfCs. *See* Conditions for Coverage (CfCs)
CGM. *See* continuous glucose monitoring (CGM)
chamomile (*Matricaria recutita*), 402–403
change conversations, stages, 472*b*
chemical-induced diabetes mellitus, 140
chemotherapy, 61
child's midparental, 248
chlorothiazide (Diuril), 362*b*
chlorpropamide (Diabinese), 367*b*
chlorthalidone (Thalitone), 362*b*
cholecalciferol, 6, 187
cholestasis, 334
cholesterol, 22
    and low-density lipoprotein, 83
    and triglycerides, adult peritoneal dialysis patient, 100–101
cholestyramine (Questran, Prevalite), 168, 366*b*, 378

peripheral parenteral nutrition (PPN), 327, 337

peripheral vascular disease (PVD), 148

peritoneal dialysate, 54

peritoneal dialysis (PD), 11, 53, 87, 150–152, 155, 192, 237

    adequacy of dialysis, 91

    adequacy targets, 92*b*–93*b*

    diabetes, 103

    equilibration rates, 91

    fluid management and adequacy of dialysis, 102

    gastrointestinal concerns, 103–104

    history, 88

    KDOQI adequacy guidelines, 93*b*

    malnutrition, 104–105

    nutrient recommendations, 94–102, 101*b*–102*b*

    nutrition assessment, 94

    obesity, 102–103

    peritoneal membrane, 90–91, 91*b*

    peritonitis, 105–106

    process, 89–90, 89*f*

    rates, 80

    side effects and and potential interventions, 106*b*

    solutes and fluid, removal, 91

    types, 88*b*

peritoneal equilibration test (PET), 91, 151

peritoneal membrane

    classifications, 91*b*

    peritoneal dialysis, adult patient on, 90–91

peritoneal protein losses, 94

peritonitis, 61, 105–106

personal eating awareness, renal dietitian, 473

pesco vegetarian, 431

PET. *See* peritoneal equilibration test (PET)

PEW. *See* protein energy wasting (PEW)

phenols, 443

phosphate

    buffers intracellular fluid, 3

    in medications and supplements, 202

    phosphate transporter-1, 206

    phosphate transporter-2, 206

    sodium phosphate-2b, 206

    tenapanor, 206–207

    transport inhibitors, 206–207

phosphate binders, 21, 191, 203*t*, 337

    calcium-based, 189

    calcium-containing, 168

    chronic kidney disease (CKD), 375*b*

    mineral and bone disorders and kidney disease, 202–206

    non-calcium-based, 204

phosphorus

    in acute kidney injury, 57

    adult peritoneal dialysis patient, 100

    calcium and vitamin D, 270–274, 273*t*

    CKD-MBD, 21

    control, mineral and bone disorders and kidney disease, 209

    mineral and bone disorders and kidney disease, 198–202, 214

    mineral and hormonal abnormalities, 188

    natural *vs.* added, 200–202

    removal, 208

    removal during dialysis, 208

    restriction and mortality, 199

physical activity, long-term posttransplant period, 129–130

physical conditioning and exercise, 172

pindolol (Visken), 363*b*

pioglitazone (Actos), 368*b*

pituitary dysfunction, 19

Plan-Do-Study-Act methodology of CQI, 459

plant-based protein, 162

polycystic kidney disease, 15

polyethylene glycol (Miralax), 372*b*

polysaccharide iron complex (Niferex, Nu-Iron), 360*b*

polythiazide (Renese), 362*b*

polyuria, 339

post-dialysis BUN, 66

post hoc subgroup analysis, 54

postprandial glucose monitoring, 155

postrenal AKI, 51

posttransplant, 8. *See also* long-term posttransplant period

    mineral bone disorders (MBD), 213

    monitoring, 152

    nutrition concerns, 121–127

    quality of life, 245

posttransplantation diabetes (PTDM), 152

posttreatment fatigue, 150

potassium, 56

    in acute kidney injury, 56–57

    adult peritoneal dialysis patient, 99

    adult kidney transplant patient, 120

    -binding medications, 72

    considerations, 163

    diffuse, 89

    excretion, 39

    -free lactated Ringer's solution, 90

    in pediatric patient, 276–277

    and phosphorus, 433–434

    restriction, 82

    salt form, 56–57

    -sparing diuretics, 72